[

Memory in neurodegenerative disease

Cognitive impairment in late life is a growing clinical and public health problem, with Alzheimer's disease the most prevalent of the progressive dementias. Memory disorders are the commonest and most disabling feature of neurodegenerative disease, and this book is the first to review in depth the neurobiological and clinical characteristics of memory and its disorders in this group of patients. In addition to Alzheimer's disease it presents current information about memory disorders in Huntington's and Parkinson's diseases and in other neurological conditions such as progressive supranuclear palsy, Creutzfeldt – Jakob disease and HIV-associated dementia.

The contributors are among the most distinguished working in this field. They present the neuroanatomical and neurochemical basis of memory disorders in neurodegenerative disease, and review the contribution of neuroradiology and neuropathology to the understanding of memory and amnesia. Different types of memory are differently affected in these conditions, and the clinical and neuropsychological implications are thoroughly explored. Diagnosis, assessment and treatment issues are discussed, as are ethical and legal considerations and topics of emerging interest such as the early detection of dementia, preserved cognitive functions and neurosurgical interventions. The book is in three parts, each with an integrative summary from a leading authority.

Bringing together biological, cognitive and clinical information, this book will be an essential reference for neuropsychologists, neurologists and psychiatrists, experimental psychologists and other neuroscientists. As memory disorders are so fundamental to neurodegenerative disease, it also serves as an authoritative and up-to-date overview of the dementias and the prospects for treating them.

ALEXANDER I. TRÖSTER is Associate Professor of Neurology and Director, Center for Neuropsychology and Cognitive Neuroscience at the University of Kansas Medical Center.

Memory in Neurodegenerative Disease

Biological, Cognitive, and Clinical Perspectives

Edited by

ALEXANDER I. TRÖSTER

Department of Neurology,
University of Kansas Medical Center

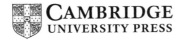
CAMBRIDGE
UNIVERSITY PRESS

PUBLISHED BY THE PRESS SYNDICATE OF THE UNIVERSITY OF CAMBRIDGE
The Pitt Building, Trumpington Street, Cambridge CB2 1RP, United Kingdom

CAMBRIDGE UNIVERSITY PRESS
The Edinburgh Building, Cambridge CB2 2RU, UK http://www.cup.cam.ac.uk
40 West 20th Street, New York, NY 10011-4211, USA http://www.cup.org
10 Stamford Road, Oakleigh, Melbourne 3166, Australia

First published 1998

Printed in the United Kingdom at the University Press, Cambridge

Typeset in Ehrhardt 9/12pt, in QuarkXpress™ [SE]

A catalogue record for this book is available from the British Library

Library of Congress cataloguing in publication data

Memory in neurodegenerative disease : biological, cognitive, and
   clinical perspectives / edited by Alexander I. Tröster.
        p.   cm.
     Includes index.
     ISBN 0 521 57192 8 (hbk.)
      1. Memory disorders.   2. Nervous system – Degeneration.
   I. Tröster, Alexander I.
   RC394.M46M52   1998
   616.8′3–dc21   97-46776 CIP

ISBN 0 521 57192 8 hardback

Every effort has been made in preparing this book to provide accurate and up-to-date
information which is in accord with accepted standards and practice at the time of publication.
Nevertheless, the authors, editors and publisher can make no warranties that the information
contained herein is totally free from error, not least because clinical standards are constantly
changing through research and regulation. The authors, editors and publisher therefore
disclaim all liability for direct or consequential damages resulting from the use of material
contained in this book. Readers are strongly advised to pay careful attention to information
provided by the manufacturer of any drugs or equipment that they plan to use.

Contents

Contributors

Tai-Kyoung Baik

Department of Anatomy, College of Medicine, Hangyang University, Seoul, Korea

Fiona Bardenhagen

Department of Psychology, University of Melbourne, Neurosciences Care Centre, St Vincent's Hospital, 41 Victoria Parade, Fitzroy, Victoria 3065, Australia

William W. Beatty

Department of Psychiatry and Behavioral Sciences, University of Oklahoma Health Sciences Center, Center for Alcohol and Drug Related Studies, Suite 410, Rogers Building, Oklahoma City, OK 73109-4602, USA

Thomas Benke

Klinik für Neurologie, University of Innsbruck, Anichstrasse 35, A-6020 Innsbruck, Austria

Stanley Berent

Neuropsychology Division (0840), University of Michigan Hospitals, Ann Arbor, MI 48109-0840, USA

Mark W. Bondi

Department of Psychology, California State University San Marcos, San Marcos, CA 92096-0001, USA

David C. Bowlby

Department of Psychiatry and Behavioral Sciences, University of Oklahoma Health Sciences Center, Center for Alcohol and Drug Related Studies, Suite 410, Rogers Building, Oklahoma City, OK 73190-4602, USA

Roger A. Brumback

Department of Pathology, BMSB 451, University of Oklahoma Health Sciences Center, 940 Stanton L. Young Blvd, Oklahoma City, OK 73104, USA

Deborah A. Cahn

Butler Hospital, Brown University, 345 Blackstone Blvd, Providence, RI 02906, USA

Thomas C. Cannon

Department of Pathology, BMSB 451, University of Oklahoma Health Sciences Center, 940 Stanton L. Young Blvd, Oklahoma City, OK 73104, USA

Rosemary Fama

Department of Psychiatry and Behavioral Sciences, Stanford University School of Medicine, Stanford, CA 94305-5548, USA

Julie A. Fields

Department of Neurology, University of Kansas Medical Center, 3901 Rainbow Blvd, Kansas City, KS 66160-7314, USA

J. Vincent Filoteo

Department of Psychology, University of Utah, Salt Lake City, UT 84112, USA

Joseph W. Fink
Neuropsychology Program, Department of Psychiatry, University of Chicago, 5841 South Maryland Avenue, MC-3077, Chicago, IL 60637, USA

Bruno Giordani
Neuropsychology Division (0840), University of Michigan Hospitals, Ann Arbor, MI 48109-0840, USA

Louis T. Giron Jr
Neurology Service, Department of Veterans Affairs Medical Center, 4801 East Linwood Blvd, Kansas City, MO 64128-2295, USA

Joni R. Graber
Department of Psychiatry and Behavioral Sciences, University of Oklahoma Health Sciences Center, Center for Alcohol and Drug Related Studies, Suite 410, Rogers Building, Oklahoma City, OK 73190-4602, USA

Michael J. Harnish
Department of Psychiatry and Behavioral Sciences, University of Oklahoma Health Sciences Center, Center for Alcohol and Drug Related Studies, Suite 410, Rogers Building, Oklahoma City, OK 73190-4602, USA

William C. Heindel
Department of Psychology, Brown University, Providence, RI 02912, USA

Diane M. Jacobs
Department of Neurology and Gertrude H. Sergievsky Center, Columbia University College of Physicians and Surgeons, 630 West 168th Street, New York, NY 10032-3702, USA

Raymond P. Kesner
Department of Psychology, University of Utah, Salt Lake City, UT 84112-0251, USA

Robert G. Knight
Department of Psychology, University of Otago, PO Box 56, Dunedin, New Zealand

William C. Koller
Department of Neurology, University of Kansas Medical Center, 3901 Rainbow Blvd, Kansas City, KS 66160-7314, USA

Richard W. Leech
Department of Pathology, BMSB 451, University of Oklahoma Health Sciences Center, 940 Stanton L. Young Blvd, Oklahoma City, OK 73104, USA

Tara T. Lineweaver
Department of Psychology, San Diego State University, San Diego, CA 92093-0948, USA

Hans J. Markowitsch
Department of Physiological Psychology, University of Bielefeld, PO Box 10 01 31, 33501 Bielefeld, Germany

Andrew R. Mayes
Department of Clinical Neurology, University of Sheffield, Royal Hallamshire Hospital, Glossop Road, Sheffield S10 2JF, UK

Edison Miyawaki
Department of Neurology, Brigham and Women's Hospital, Harvard University Medical School *and* Department of Neurology, University of Kansas Medical Center, 3901 Rainbow Blvd, Kansas City, KS 66160-7314, USA

Andreas U. Monsch
>   Memory Clinic, Kantonsspital, University of Basel, Hebelstrasse 10, 4031
>   Basel, Switzerland

Suzanne Norman
>   Department of Psychology, Xavier University, Dana Avenue, Cincinnati, OH
>   45207-6511, USA

Paula K. Ogrocki
>   Bryan Alzheimer's Disease Research Center, Department of Psychiatry and
>   Human Behavior, Duke University Medical Center, 2200 West Main Street,
>   Suite A-230, Durham, NC 27713, USA

Marlene Oscar-Berman
>   Department of Neurology, Boston University Medical Center, M-902, 80 E
>   Concord Street, Boston, MA 02118, USA

Adrian M. Owen
>   MRC Applied Psychology Unit, 15 Chaucer Road, Cambridge CB2 2EF, UK

Anthony M. Paolo
>   University of Kansas Medical Center, 3901 Rainbow Blvd, Kansas City, KS
>   66160-7831, USA

Robert H. Paul
>   Department of Psychiatry and Behavioral Sciences, University of Oklahoma
>   Health Sciences Center *and*
>   Center for Alcohol and Drug Related Studies, Suite 410, Rogers Building,
>   Oklahoma City, OK 73190-4602, USA

Christopher Randolph
>   Department of Neurology, Loyola University Medical Center, 2160 South
>   First Avenue, Maywood, IL 60153, USA

Trevor W. Robbins
>   Department of Experimental Psychology, University of Cambridge, Downing
>   Site, Cambridge CB2 3EB, UK

Barbara J. Sahakian
>   Department of Psychiatry, University of Cambridge, Box 189, Addenbrooke's
>   Hospital, Cambridge CB2 2QQ, UK

David P. Salmon
>   Department of Neurosciences (0948), University of California, San Diego,
>   9500 Gilman Drive, La Jolla, CA 92093-0948, USA

Peter Schofield
>   Department of Neurology and Gertrude H. Sergievsky Center, Columbia
>   University College of Physicians and Surgeons, 630 West 168th Street, New
>   York, NY 10032-3702, USA

Paula K. Shear
>   Department of Psychology, University of Cincinnati, PO Box 210376,
>   Cincinnati, OH 45221, USA

Kristy A. Straits-Tröster
>   Primary Care, Department of Veterans Affairs Medical Center, 4801 East
>   Linwood Blvd, Kansas City, MO 64128-22965, USA

Edith V. Sullivan
>   Department of Psychiatry and Behavioral Sciences, Stanford University
>   School of Medicine, Stanford, CA 94305-5717, USA

Kirsten I. Taylor
Department of Psychology, University of Zürich, 8091 Zürich, Switzerland

Julie A. Testa
Department of Psychiatry and Behavioral Sciences, University of Oklahoma Health Sciences Center, 940 Stanton L. Young Blvd, Oklahoma City, OK 73104–4602, USA

Alexander I. Tröster
Department of Neurology, University of Kansas Medical Center, 3901 Rainbow Blvd, Kansas City, KS 66160-7314, USA

Kathleen A. Welsh-Bohmer
Bryan Alzheimer's Disease Research Center, Department of Psychiatry and Human Behaviour, Duke University Medical Center, 2200 West Main Street, Suite A-230, Durham, NC 27713, USA

Steven B. Wilkinson
Division of Neurosurgery, University of Kansas Medical Center, 3901 Rainbow Blvd, Kansas City, KS 66160-7383, USA

Martin D. Zehr
Research Medical Center, 2316 E Mayer Blvd, Kansas City, MO 64132, USA

Preface

Many volumes are dedicated to studies of memory, which might be considered the essence of the rich tapestry of life. Some volumes describe normal memory, others disordered memory. This book is designed to fill a gap by focusing specifically on memory in neurodegenerative conditions. The explosion of neuroscience research dealing with this topic has left many seeking a single source which might familiarize them with the basics of research outside their own area of expertise. Although no book can be everything to everyone, and cover every relevant topic, this book attempts to bring together biological, cognitive and clinical perspectives, so that neuropsychologists, neurologists, psychiatrists and neuroscientists can familiarize themselves with allied research outside their immediate area of expertise. An effort is made to present research of recent and emerging interest, for example, preclinical detection of dementia, the description of prospective memory and the renaissance of surgery for movement disorders due to neurodegenerative processes. Often neglected topics, such as ethical and legal issues, are also addressed.

I thank my wife, Kristy Straits-Tröster, for her immense patience and understanding while bearing countless solitary hours during the completion of this project. My parents, Guy and Christine Tröster, continue to understand that work load sometimes necessitates putting up with an 'alien' son, and their understanding and inspiration is, as always, greatly appreciated.

The invaluable assistance of Julie Fields in the completion of this volume is most gratefully acknowledged, as is the encouragement and support of Dr Richard Barling, Director of Medical Publishing at Cambridge University Press, who demonstrated great faith in taking on this project. Tremendous gratitude also goes to the editorial and production staff at Cambridge University Press, and especially to Mr Joe Mottershead, without whose professionalism and arduous effort this volume might still be in press several years from now. I also extend my thanks and deep appreciation to the authors contributing to this book. Not only did they all deliver superb chapters in a short time frame, but they patiently endured my editorial whims and rewrites. A final word of gratitude goes to William Bartholome, MD, and Mr Don Lambert, who familiarized me with 'Grandma' Layton's inspiring art.

To my family

For their love, support, patience, and above all, encouragement

To the many thousand individuals participating in the research that is the subject of this book

For giving selflessly of themselves in the hope of helping others

PART I

Biological perspectives

1

Nonhuman primate models of memory dysfunction in neurodegenerative disease: contributions from comparative neuropsychology

MARLENE OSCAR-BERMAN
AND FIONA BARDENHAGEN

INTRODUCTION

Results of nonhuman animal research can provide new information that human experimentation does not allow, usually for ethical considerations or because of limited control over complex environmental influences. The new knowledge can then be used to help understand human disorders. In the present chapter, we review the application of behavioral methods – developed in nonhuman animal laboratories and modified for human use – toward clarifying memory dysfunction in human neurodegenerative disease. Implicit in nonhuman research models of human brain functioning is the assumption of homologous structural-functional relationships among the species (Riley and Langley 1993; Wasserman 1993). Research on brain mechanisms underlying behaviors across species, contributes to the discovery of common and divergent principles of brain-behavior relationships, ultimately to understand how the brain functions. With understanding comes the potential for assessment and treatment of human neurobehavioral disorders.

One approach to understanding interspecies brain functions, comparative neuropsychology, involves the direct evaluation of human clinical populations by employing experimental paradigms originally developed for nonhuman animals (Weiskrantz 1978; Oscar-Berman 1984, 1994; Roberts and Sahakian 1993). Over many decades of animal research, the paradigms were perfected to study the effects of well-defined brain lesions on specific behaviors and many of the paradigms still are used widely

to link specific deficits with localized areas of neuropathology (for reviews, see Medin 1977; Deutsch 1983; Arnold 1984; Stuss and Benson 1986; Meador et al. 1987; Mitchell and Erwin 1987; Fuster 1989; Sahgal 1993). The comparative neuropsychological approach employs simple tasks that can be mastered without relying upon language skills. Precisely because these simple paradigms do not require linguistic strategies for solution, they are especially useful for working with patients whose language skills are compromised, or whose cognitive skills may be minimal (Oscar-Berman 1991, 1994; Oscar-Berman et al. 1991). Comparative neuropsychology contrasts with the traditional approach of using tasks that rely upon linguistic skills, and that were designed to study human cognition (Walsh 1987; Vallar and Shallice 1990; Lezak 1995). As important ambiguities about its heuristic value had not been addressed empirically, only recently has comparative neuropsychology become popular for implementation with brain-damaged patients (for reviews see Oscar-Berman 1994; Squire 1992; Roberts and Sahakian 1993; Seidman et al. 1995). Within the past decade it has had prevalent use as a framework for comparing and contrasting the performances of disparate neurobehavioral populations on similar tasks.

An historical context provides the necessary forum for presenting current-day examples of the usefulness of the approach; therefore, we provide a brief history of comparative neuropsychology, beginning with the early experiments of E.L. Thorndike (1911) in the context of the Darwinian thinking of the time. Next, we review evidence showing that human and nonhuman primates do solve many so called animal tasks in similar ways. Moreover, results of numerous research studies already have clearly demonstrated that the tasks – despite their apparent simplicity – are sensitive to specific cognitive impairments after brain damage in humans and nonhumans alike. Performances of patients with various forms of neurodegenerative disease on comparative neuropsychological tasks are reviewed, and the implications of these findings are discussed in terms of comparative neuropsychological models of working memory and declarative memory.

HISTORICAL CONTEXT

During the first half of this century, neuropsychology was not a separate subdiscipline as we know it today; rather, neuropsychology was subsumed under physiological psychology, the study of the relationship between the brain and behavior. Research in physiological psychology relied mainly on animal subjects. Until the 1950s, only a handful of behavioral laboratories were conducting research with human neurological patients. The research was led by the following investigators, to mention a few: Wechsler (1944), Hebb (1949), Teuber (1955), Penfield (1958), Pribram (1958), Reitan (1962) and Milner (1964) in North America; Russell (1959) and Whitty and Zangwill (1966) in the United Kingdom; and Luria (1966) in Russia. Around that same time, Frank Beach was the editor of the *Journal of Comparative and Physiological Psychology*, a journal devoted to research on the biological underpinnings of behavior. Beach was intrigued by the observation that most studies appearing in the journal relied upon data collected on one laboratory species, the rat. Consequently, he reviewed all of the articles published in the *Journal of Comparative and Physiological Psychology* since its inception in the 1930s (Beach 1960) and discovered that approximately 60% of the papers used laboratory rats, 10% used submammalian vertebrates or invertebrates and 30% employed other mammals (mostly nonhuman primates). In other words, until at least the 1950s, inferences about brain–behavior relationships in people were based principally upon studies of nonhuman species, especially the rat. To understand how the emphasis on rat research occurred, it is important to go back further in time (for additional historical informa-

tion see also Bitterman 1960, 1975; Masterton et al. 1976).

Darwinian influence and Thorndikian connectionism

In 1871, Darwin published *The Descent of Man and Selection in Relation to Sex*. In addition to morphological continuity along the phylogenetic scale, Darwin also considered behavioral continuity. For Darwin, continuity was not compatible with novelty. Darwin tried to demonstrate that seemingly unique characteristics of animals were not really unique at all; rather, . . . 'some hint or promise of it always could be discovered at an earlier point in the series' (Bitterman 1960, p. 704). According to Darwin, then, phylogenetic differences were more quantitative than qualitative.

Psychologists at the end of the nineteenth century were reluctant to accept Darwin's ideas, not because they questioned his conclusions, but because they had little faith in his data. Darwin relied mainly on anecdotal reports from naturalists and zookeepers instead of controlled laboratory experimentation. In the 1890s, one of these skeptics was a doctoral student, E.L. Thorndike, who wanted to explore the derivation of human intelligence. Thorndike was critical of the anecdotal approach, and to collect data for his doctoral dissertation, he built experimental equipment in which to quantify animal behavior. The equipment included puzzle boxes or problem boxes. The animals could see food outside the boxes, and they could escape to retrieve the food by performing simple actions such as pulling a loop, pressing a lever or stepping on a treadle. Thorndike recorded the time it took animals to escape and retrieve the food on each of a series of trials, and he observed that time decreased over trials. In addition, there was transfer, or facilitation, from one experimental situation to another. The terms *learning set* and *learning to learn* (Harlow 1949; Jarrard 1971) later were used to describe gradual improvement over similar problems. Today, terms such as *procedural memory* and *implicit learning* (Tulving 1985; Roediger and Craik 1989; Squire 1992) are applied to the same general phenomenon.

Thorndike's methods had the following advantages over anecdotal reports: objectivity and quantification of the measure (time across trials); reproducibility; flexibility in the experimenter's control over the complexity of the task; and efficiency, because observations could be made on many subjects. Furthermore, using Thorndike's methods, researchers could observe a wide variety of species, with each species relying on its own unique sensory, motor, and motivational characteristics to solve the problems.

In addition to problem boxes, Thorndike used mazes and other experimental devices to study discrimination learning (i.e. the ability to consistently choose one of two or more stimuli presented together over trials). By the early 1900s, numerous investigators interested in measuring animal intelligence, were studying many species of animals in a variety of Thorndikian situations. No matter what the experimental situations, different species behaved similarly: they all gradually increased the speed and number of correct responses, and they all gradually decreased incorrect responding. Figure 1.1 shows a maze designed for measuring animal intelligence, along with learning curves from three different species obtained by three different investigators. The curves show decreases in errors with each run through the maze, expressed as a proportion of the number of errors that were made on the first run. One curve is for a rat (Small 1901); one curve is for a sparrow (Porter 1904); and one curve is for a monkey (Kinnaman 1902). All showed a gradual increase in correct responding, and a gradual decrease in errors.

As more species were tested in a variety of experimental situations, the resultant learning curves suggested that Darwin's ideas about phylogenetic continuity might apply to learning. There were no major differences in the ways different animal species solved the problems, only the rapidity with which task solution was acquired. In 1911, Thorndike published *Animal Intelligence: Experimental Studies*, in which he described the behavior of many different species, and he summarized his theoretical ideas. Thorndike concluded that the principles of learning are the same throughout the phylogenetic scale, and that because of differences in their sensory capacity, motor agility and motivation, animals differ only in the speed of learning, and in the type of learnable material. Thorndike wrote: 'If my analysis is true, the evolution of behavior is a rather simple matter. Formally, the crab, fish, turtle, dog, cat, monkey, and baby have very similar intellects and characters. All are systems of connections subject to change by the laws of exercise and effect' (1911, pp. 280–281). The Law of Exercise states that every response in the presence of a stimulus tends to increase the strength of the tendency for the stimulus to evoke the response; learning is gradual and incremental. The Law of Effect

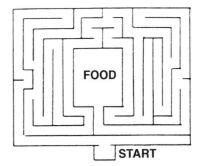

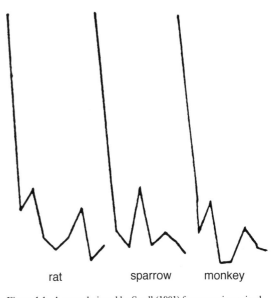

rat   sparrow   monkey

Figure 1.1. A maze designed by Small (1901) for measuring animal intelligence, along with learning curves from three different species trained in the maze. The curves show decreases in errors with each run through the maze, expressed as a proportion of the number of errors that were made on the first run. One curve is for a rat (Small 1901); one curve is for a sparrow (Porter 1904); and one curve is for a monkey (Kinnaman 1902). From Bitterman, M.E. In *Animal Learning*, ed. M.E. Bitterman et al., 1979, pp. 1–23, Plenum Press, with permission.

states that the strength of the stimulus–response bond is increased by pleasant consequences and decreased by unpleasant consequences; in other words, learning depends on reinforcement.

As years went by, Thorndike's Stimulus–Response (or S–R) Reinforcement principle became popular, with men like Clark Hull, Kenneth Spence and B.F. Skinner being among its most vocal supporters (Hilgard and Bower 1975). Others viewed S–R Reinforcement theory with skepticism, and they provided alternative theories (Hilgard and Bower 1975; Oscar-Berman 1991). Although the theorists disagreed on which law of learning might be the universal one, there was overall agreement that the same principles would apply to all species. Consequently, the laboratory rat – an inexpensive and convenient research subject – was commonly used as a representative animal model.

Reversal learning and probability learning: control by systematic variation

From the 1950s to the 1970s, investigators tested the idea that the same laws of learning would apply to all species. One of these investigators was M.E. Bitterman, a comparative psychologist in Pennsylvania. As it was impossible to arrange a set of conditions that made the same sensory, motor and motivational demands for all species, Bitterman (1960) introduced another approach: *Control by systematic variation*. Thus, Bitterman and his colleagues developed a range of standardized testing situations to accommodate the specific sensory and motor capacities of different species of animals, and testing took place under a range of drive states (Bitterman et al. 1979). Standard situations used by Bitterman and his colleagues were *reversal learning* and *probability learning* paradigms. Reversal learning requires subjects first to learn to choose one of two stimuli consistently (e.g. to go *left* when given a choice of responding to two identical stimuli located on the left and the right sides, or to pick *black* when given a choice between a black and a white stimulus). After making the correct choice, the subjects next must learn to switch, or reverse, their choice to the previously unrewarded stimulus (go *right* instead of left, or pick *white* instead of black). The subjects are given a series of such reversals.

Probability learning situations present subjects with choices that differ in amount of payoff. For example, in a 70:30 probability learning condition, 70% of the time the right side (or a black stimulus) will be correct, and 30% of the time the left side (or a white stimulus) will be rewarded. The distribution of reward is reliable but random, such that the subject can not know when a reward will be given for a response to either choice. When one alternative is rewarded more than the other (e.g. 70:30), it is most efficient to maximize the choice of the higher of two payoffs, but many animals, including humans commonly match their responses to the reinforcement distributions in a systematic way.

In reversal tasks and probability learning paradigms, using spatial cues or visual cues, rats could be tested in a T-maze (running response), or in a Skinner box (pressing levers). Similarly, fish could be tested in a water maze, or by swimming against one of two switches. The motivation level or drive state of each species was varied systematically in terms of percentage body weight. Bitterman and his colleagues reasoned that if, under conditions of control by systematic variation, a specific behavioral pattern appeared in one species but not in another, interspecies differences in underlying neural mechanisms of learning would be a tenable explanation; artifacts based on sensory–motor abilities and hunger would be ruled out (Bitterman 1960, 1975; Bitterman et al. 1979).

Using this approach, different species were ordered hierarchically according to learning abilities (see Table 1.1). Bitterman concluded that rats, monkeys and people are subject to the same laws of learning on these tasks. Differences in learning ability by other species begin to appear as neocortical tissue decreases in size.

OTHER BEHAVIORAL PARADIGMS IN COMPARATIVE PSYCHOLOGY

By the 1970s, behaviorists were employing a wide variety of experimental paradigms to assess animal cognition, and monkeys were more commonly being studied than in earlier times. Among the many paradigms popular at the time were learning set tasks, delayed reaction tasks, and delayed conditional discrimination tasks.[1] Each of these classes of tasks will be described in turn.

Learning set paradigms
Harry Harlow (1949, 1951; Harlow et al. 1971) and his colleagues at the University of Wisconsin developed paradigms to compare learning and memory abilities across primate species (Jarrard 1971). Comparisons among primate groups is facilitated by species similarities in sensory systems, as well as the ability to respond with the hands and fingers. Common testing situations used by Harlow

---

[1] For further information about a variety of learning and memory paradigms used in comparative psychology and comparative neuropsychology, see Masterton et al. 1976; Medin 1977; Arnold 1984; Meador et al. 1987; Sahgal 1993.

Table 1.1. *Bitterman's comparative scheme*

Animal	Spatial tasks		Visual tasks	
	Successive reversals	Probability learning	Successive reversals	Probability learning
Human	Yes	M	Yes	M
Monkey	Yes	M	Yes	M
Rat	Yes	M	Yes	M
Pigeon	Yes	M	Yes	Random
Turtle	Yes	M	No	Random
Decorticated Rat	Yes	M	No	Random
Fish	No	Random	No	Random
Cockroach	No	Random	?	?
Earthworm	No	?	?	?

Notes:
'Yes' represents progressive improvement in performance over successive reversals and 'no' represents absence of progressive improvement. 'M' stands for matching of responses to reinforcement distributions in a systematic way, or maximizing the choice of the higher of two payoffs; 'random' refers to matching with no defined strategy. No data were obtained in cases where the '?' appears.
Source: Bitterman 1960, 1975.

and his colleagues were *learning sets*, i.e. series of simple problems where the stimuli or response requirements change from problem to problem, but the principle to be learned remains the same. For example, in visual object learning sets, two distinctly different stimulus items are presented on the left and right sides of a stimulus tray in a Wisconsin General Test Apparatus (Figure 1.2). The objects cover reinforcement wells, only one of which contains a reward, e.g. a piece of food or a coin. To obtain the reward, the subject must learn a *win-stay, lose-shift* strategy, i.e. to choose the object consistently being rewarded, and to avoid the other object. Incorrect strategies include choosing only one side, e.g. the left; alternating sides; alternating objects; choosing randomly; etc. With practice, different species of primates, including children, were observed to show precipitous improvement, as though they had learned to learn the problems (illustrated in Figure 1.3). Investigators ranked species in terms of numbers of problems required to achieve the win-stay, lose-shift strategy, such that only one information trial was needed to solve a problem. The rankings paralleled the

phylogenetic scale, again supporting the idea that similar laws of learning apply to all animals.

Learning-to-learn is the formation of learning sets; the principles to be acquired are not limited to the simple win-stay, lose-shift strategy. In some experiments, the principle to be learned may be *win-shift, lose-stay* (i.e., reversal learning). Other principles are *matching to sample* (MTS) and *nonmatching to sample* (NMTS) (discussed in **Delayed conditional discrimination tasks**); here subjects must choose one of two stimuli that is the same (or different from) a sample stimulus in an array of three stimuli. Another principle requires subjects to alternate responding between two stimuli (as in *object alternation* or OA), while ignoring the irrelevant left-right spatial positions of the stimuli.

Delayed reaction tasks
Delayed reaction tasks (Figure 1.2), such as *delayed response* (DR) and *delayed alternation* (DA), are spatial tasks (usually relying upon visual input) that measure a subject's ability to bridge a time gap (Goldman-Rakic 1987; Fuster 1989; Oscar-Berman et al. 1991). This ability has been termed working memory, which is a transient form of memory (Goldman-Rakic 1987). Working memory is multimodal in nature, and it serves to keep newly-incoming information available on-line; it acts much like a mental clip-board for use in problem solving, planning, etc. In the classical DR task, the experimenter places a piece of food (or some other reward) into a reinforcement-well under one of two identical stimuli. The subject is able to see the experimenter put a reward there, but can not reach it. After the experimenter covers the food-wells with the stimuli, she/he lowers a screen, obscuring the stimulus tray. After a delay period, usually between 0 and 60 s, the experimenter raises the screen to allow the subject to make a choice. The subject then pushes one of the stimuli away and, with a correct choice, takes the reward; attentional and spatial memory skills are needed to do this.

DA shares important features with DR. Both are spatial tasks, and both have a delay between stimulus-presentation and the opportunity to make a response. In DA, however, subjects must learn to alternate responding from left to right. On each trial, the side not previously chosen is rewarded, and a brief delay (usually 5 s) is interposed between trials. Instead of having to notice and remember the location of a reward placed there by the experimenter

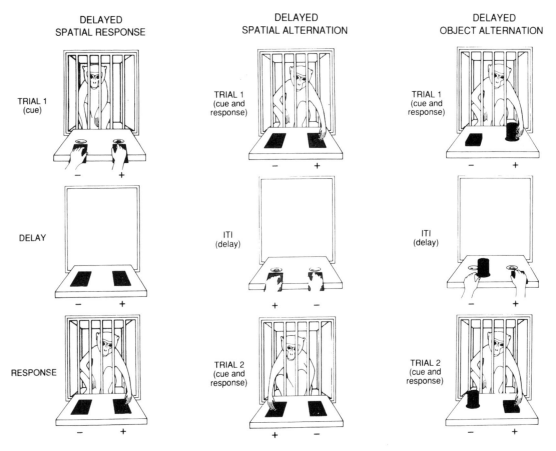

Figure 1.2. Three different tasks presented to Rhesus monkeys in a Wisconsin General Test Apparatus. The tasks illustrated can test working memory skills. The delayed reaction tasks, delayed response (DR) and delayed alternation (DA), rely heavily on spatial memory. The object alternation (OA) task is highly sensitive to perseverative responding. From H.R. Friedman and P.S. Goldman-Rakic, 1988, *Journal of Neuroscience*. 8: 4693–4706, Society for Neuroscience, with permission.

(in DR), subjects must remember the side last chosen, and whether or not a reward had been available. Subjects must also learn to inhibit, on each trial, the previously rewarded response (i.e. they must not perseverate with consecutive responses to one side only). Rankings of the performance levels of a wide range of mammals, including children, on delayed reaction tasks have been reported to parallel the phylogenetic scale (Jarrard 1971; Masterton et al. 1976).

Neuroanatomical systems in delayed reaction task performance.
Delayed reaction tasks have a unique characteristic: they are very sensitive to damage of prefrontal cortical-subcortical brain systems. For over half a century, researchers have observed that monkeys with bilateral lesions of the prefrontal cortex perform poorly on DR and DA, even with very short delays (Warren and Akert 1964; Arnold 1984; Goldman-Rakic 1987; Fuster 1989; Oscar-Berman et al. 1991). In monkeys, two large subdivisions of the prefrontal cortex have been recognized to be important in normal performance on delayed reaction tasks: the dorsolateral surface of the prefrontal cortex (especially area 46 in the principal sulcus), and the ventral prefrontal region including the orbitofrontal surface and inferior convexity. A schematic representation of the two systems is reproduced in Figure 1.4, where it can be seen that, from top to bottom, their connections run through different regions of virtually the same brain structures.

Figure 1.3. Performance by different species of primates, including children, on two-choice object learning-set problems. The curves illustrate precipitous improvement or learning-to-learn the win-stay, lose-shift strategy. From J.L. Fobes and J.E. King, 1982, In *Primate Behavior*, ed. J.L. Fobes and J.E. King pp. 289–326, Academic Press, with permission.

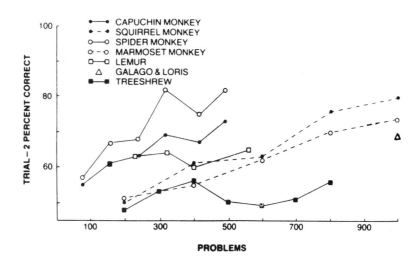

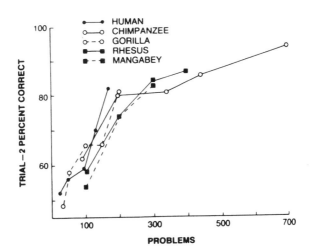

The dorsolateral and ventral subdivisions of prefrontal cortex have correspondingly different cytoarchitectonics, neurochemical sensitivities and connections with the rest of the brain (Warren and Akert 1964; Arnold 1984; Goldman-Rakic 1987; Fuster 1989; Oscar-Berman et al. 1991). The dorsolateral system maintains more intimate connections with other neocortical sites than the ventral system. The dorsolateral system's connections with limbic sites are less striking than the orbitofrontal system's. Visuospatial memory and attentional functions are thought to be compromised with dorsolateral lesions. Although the classical DR and DA paradigms overlap in sensitivity to deficits in spatial working memory, DR is more sensitive than DA to visuospatial attentional deficits

(Oscar-Berman and Hutner 1993). By contrast, functions involved in response inhibition have been linked to orbitofrontal cortex. The ventral frontal system, of which the orbitofrontal cortex is a part, is intimately connected with basal forebrain and limbic structures, but its connections with other neocortical regions are not as extensive as the dorsolateral system's, and, like the dorsolateral system, the ventral system supports successful performance on DA and DR, but it is especially important for DA performance. DA is more sensitive than DR to abnormal perseverative responding (Oscar-Berman and Hutner 1993).

We noted in a previous section that OA, like DA, is an alternation task. OA uses a simple object reversal

Figure 1.4. Schematic representation of two frontal lobe brain systems, illustrating the pathways that run through different regions of many of the same structures. From M. Oscar–Berman et al. 1991, In *Frontal Lobe Function and Injury*, ed. H.S. Levin, H.M. Eisenberg and A.L. Benton, pp. 120–138, Oxford University Press, with permission. Copyight (c) 1991 by H.S. Levin et al.

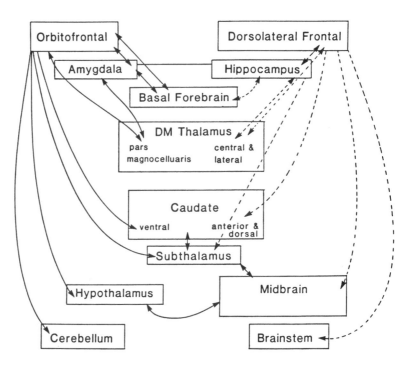

procedure which, like DA, requires memory for the previous response, response inhibition, and rule learning, but in OA, unlike DA, irrelevant spatial cues must be ignored. As it turns out, it has been shown that OA is even more sensitive than DA to perseveration, and OA is highly sensitive to prefrontal brain damage (Oscar-Berman and Hutner 1993; Freedman et al. 1998).

To test the sensitivity of DR, DA and OA tasks to bilateral prefrontal damage in humans, we administered these tasks to patient groups with bilateral frontal lobe lesions (Freedman and Oscar-Berman 1986a; Freedman et al. 1998). We found significant abnormalities in patients with focal prefrontal lesions documented with computed tomography (CT) scans. In addition, we and other investigators tested patients with a variety of disorders affecting frontal brain systems, and many of the patient groups were impaired on DR, DA and/or OA (Pribram et al. 1964; Chorover and Cole 1966; Park and Holzman 1992; Weinberger et al. 1992; Seidman et al. 1995; Gansler et al. 1996; Partiot et al. 1996; Postle et al. 1997). In these studies (which are reviewed later) the resultant profiles of the deficits across the patient populations differed. The different profiles were interpreted to reflect damage to distinct frontal systems (for reviews, see Olton et al. 1985; Overstreet and Russell 1991; Squire

1992; Oscar-Berman and Hutner 1993; Wasserman 1993; Albert and Moss 1996).

Delayed conditional discrimination tasks

Human amnesic patients have been tested on other tasks designed to measure memory in monkeys, and researchers have found that the tasks are sensitive to human memory dysfunction. These tasks include *concurrent discrimination learning* (CL), *delayed matching to sample* (DMTS), and *delayed nonmatching to sample* (DNMTS). In CL, subjects are rewarded for choosing an arbitrarily designated correct item from a set of two stimuli. Several pairs of different stimuli are presented to the subjects, and after the first presentation of the list and a delay interval, the list is presented again. Subjects are rewarded for choosing the previously correct stimulus from each pair. The list is repeated several times to allow subjects to learn to identify the correct stimuli. CL therefore relies on a win-stay, lose-shift strategy, requires memory for stimuli over time, and is reinforced through stimulus–reward associations. Like monkeys with limbic system lesions, amnesic patients perform poorly on this task (Kessler et al. 1986; Aggleton et al. 1988, 1992; Gaffan et al. 1990).

In DMTS, the subject views a stimulus, and then after a delay, must choose that same stimulus from a test pair comprised of the familiar stimulus and a novel one. DNMTS differs from DMTS only in the response required: in DNMTS, subjects must choose the novel stimulus when presented with the test pair. In humans, several studies have shown that performance on DMTS and DNMTS deteriorates when the duration of stimulus exposure is shortened, or when stimulus complexity, or delay-to-test intervals are increased (Mishkin 1982; Oscar-Berman and Bonner 1985, 1989; Squire et al. 1988). These findings show that memory for specific target stimuli over a temporal delay is an important component of DMTS and DNMTS (Oscar-Berman and Bonner 1989).

DMTS, DNMTS and CL are different from delayed reaction tasks in a number of ways. They require memory for specific and multiple stimulus characteristics, often over long delays, and the tasks are sensitive to lesions in the limbic system. The type of memory they involve has been called declarative – or explicit – memory (Tulving 1985; Squire 1992). Declarative memory differs from working memory in that the former is archival in nature; declarative memory can be demonstrated by tasks that require free recall, stimulus recognition or familiarity judgments (Mishkin 1982; Squire et al. 1988; Olton et al. 1992; Squire 1992).

Neuroanatomical systems in delayed conditional discrimination task performance

Nonhuman animal research using DMTS, DNMTS and CL tasks has contributed to our understanding of the structures involved in new learning. It is widely accepted that a limbic brain system, comprised of regions within the temporal lobes, diencephalon and basal forebrain, is necessary for the formation of declarative memories (Mishkin and Appenzeller 1987; Squire 1992; Zola-Morgan and Squire 1993). Mishkin and others have proposed that a combined interruption of two memory-related pathways is necessary for amnesia. One pathway travels the fornix from the hippocampus to the mammillary bodies, then progresses along the mamillothalamic tract to the anterior nucleus of the thalamus, and possibly to the cingulate cortex, before returning to the hippocampus. The other pathway connects the amygdala and medial thalamic nuclei (e.g. the magnocellular portion of the dorsomedial thalamic nucleus), possibly linking with the orbitofrontal cortex, and from there, feeding back to the amygdala (Mayes et al. 1988). Recent evidence shows that the amygdala is not critical in the formation of declarative mem-

ories, but it plays a significant role in forming stimulus–reward and cross-modal associations (for reviews, see Dudai 1989; Zola-Morgan and Squire 1993).

Unlike tests of working memory (or of other prefrontal functions), tests of declarative memory are not reliably sensitive to damage of different subregions of the limbic system. Impaired performance on DMTS, DNMTS and CL, therefore, can indicate disruption anywhere in the two aforementioned limbic-memory pathways, or possibly in connected prefrontal sites as well. The limbic system, however, does seem to be necessary for the consolidation and retrieval of more enduring representations of uni-, poly- and supramodal information (Dudai 1989). Hence the distinction between (1) declarative or archival memories mediated by the limbic system, and (2) the short-term manipulation of memories in prefrontal working memory.

PATIENTS WITH NEURODEGENERATIVE DISEASES OR OTHER NEUROBEHAVIORAL CONDITIONS

The original work on behavioral and neuroanatomical systems involved in comparative neuropsychological tests was based upon nonhuman models. More recently, researchers studying human neurobehavioral disorders have used comparative neuropsychological tests to clarify the functional significance of human prefrontal cortex and limbic system structures. Tasks such as those described earlier have been used with patients because of the sensitivity to prefrontal and limbic system dysfunction in monkeys. Most often, DA, DR and OA have been used in human disorders where frontal system damage is known or suspected. Delayed conditional discrimination learning tasks such as DMTS, DNMTS and CL generally have been used in patient groups with limbic dysfunction and declarative memory impairments. Table 1.2 lists groups tested on behavioral paradigms from comparative neuropsychology.

In humans, evidence regarding functional brain specificity is not as clear as with monkeys. One reason for this relates to the diffuse involvement of several brain systems in many human neurological diseases, in sharp contrast to the precise lesions induced in animal research. Although many of the disorders listed in Table 1.2 involve overlapping pathology of the dorsolateral and the ventral

Table 1.2. *Performance by patient groups*

Tasks							
Prefrontal			Limbic			Neurobehavioral	
DR	DA	OA	DMTS	DNMTS	CL	Disorders	References
++	++	++	++	?	?	Alzheimer's disease	Freedman and Oscar-Berman 1986b; Freedman 1990; Sahgal et al. 1992.
−−	++	?	?	?	++	Huntington's disease	Oscar-Berman and Zola-Morgan 1980; Oscar-Berman et al. 1982.
++	±	++	?	?	?	Parkinson's disease with dementia	Freedman and Oscar-Berman 1986b; Freedman 1990; Partiot et al. 1996.
−−	−−	++	?	?	?	Parkinson's disease without dementia	Freedman and Oscar-Berman 1986b; Canavan et al. 1990; Freedman 1990.
++	++	?	?	?	?	Progressive supranuclear palsy	Partiot et al. 1996.
−−	++	?	?	?	?	Olivopontocerebellar atrophy	El-Awar et al. 1991.
?	?	?	++	?	?	Senile dementia of the Lewy body type	Sahgal et al. 1992.
++	++	++	?	?	?	Bilateral frontal lobe lesions	Pribram et al. 1964; Freedman and Oscar-Berman 1986a; Freedman et al. 1998.
−−	++	++	?	?	?	Closed head injury	Gansler et al. 1996.
−−	±	?	?	?	?	Anterior communicating artery disease	Freedman and Oscar-Berman 1986a.
±	±	?	?	?	±	Nonfrontal lesions, and unilateral frontal lesions	Chorover and Cole 1966; Oscar-Berman et al. 1982; Canavan et al. 1990; Verin et al. 1993.
?	?	?	++	?	++	Encephalitis	Aggleton et al. 1992.
±	++	?	++	++	++	Alcoholic Korsakoff's syndrome	Oscar-Berman and Zola-Morgan 1980; Oscar-Berman et al. 1982, 1992; Oscar-Berman and Bonner 1985, 1989; Freedman and Oscar-Berman 1986a; Kessler et al. 1986; Aggleton et al. 1988; Squire et al. 1988; Gaffan et al. 1990
−−	−−	−−	±	±	±	Alcoholism (without Korsakoff's syndrome)	Oscar-Berman et al. 1982, 1992; Oscar-Berman and Bonner 1985, 1989; Freedman and Oscar-Berman, 1986a; Aggleton et al. 1988, 1992; Bowden et al. 1992; Bardenhagen and Bowden 1995.
±	++	++	?	?	?	Schizophrenia	Park and Holzman 1992; Weinberger et al. 1992; Seidman et al. 1995.
−−	++	−−	?	?	?	Depression	Freedman 1994.
++	−−	++	++	++	?	Post-traumatic stress disorder	Koenen et al. 1997.

Notes:

Delayed Response (DR), Delayed Alternation (DA), Object Alternation (OA), Delayed Matching-to-Sample (DMTS), Delayed Nonmatching-to-Sample (DNMTS), and Concurrent Learning (CL) tasks.

++ = Impairment; −− = No impairment; ± = Impairment in some patients; ? = Not tested.

prefrontal systems, for example, findings from individual studies suggest that some groups are more heavily influenced by dorsolateral than by ventral prefrontal dysfunction (e.g. patients with Parkinson's disease and dementia: Freedman and Oscar-Berman 1986b, 1987; Freedman 1990), while other groups appear to be more heavily influenced by ventral than by dorsolateral dysfunction (e.g. patients with olivopontocerebellar atrophy or late-stage Huntington's disease: El-Awar et al. 1991; Oscar-Berman et al. 1982). Other patients performed poorly on all of the prefrontal tasks (i.e. Alzheimer's disease patients: Freedman and Oscar-Berman 1986b; Freedman 1990); in these patients, there is damage to both systems. It is important to note that the dichotomy is not strict; it is used to emphasize quantitatively different degrees of dysfunction and damage.

Fewer patient groups have been studied using declarative memory tests than working memory tests, but the results shown in Table 1.2 are consistent with predictions based on the neuropathology of these conditions. Amnesic patients with alcoholic Korsakoff's syndrome (involving diencephalic, limbic, basal forebrain and cortical damage: Harper and Kril 1990; Hunt and Nixon 1993) or herpes simplex encephalitis (thought to involve temporal lobe damage: Aggleton et al. 1992) perform poorly on both DMTS and CL. An interesting finding is that of impaired DMTS and CL performance in some groups of non-Korsakoff alcoholics (Aggleton et al. 1988; Bowden et al. 1992). This shows that DMTS and CL are more sensitive to subtle changes in memory functioning than conventional neuropsychological measures, and may signal the presence of undiagnosed neuropathology involving limbic system sites in nonamnesic alcoholics (Bowden 1990; Bowden et al. 1992). We expect that impairments on DMTS, DNMTS and CL tasks would also be apparent in other neurodegenerative conditions where gross or subtle memory impairments are noted.

DMTS deficits also have been recorded in patients with dementia of the Alzheimer type (Sahgal et al. 1992), and senile dementia of the Lewy body type (characterized by senile plaque formation and variable limbic, neocortical and subcortical Lewy body formation; Sahgal et al. 1992). Several of the neurobehavioral disorders represented in Table 1.2 involve overlapping pathology of prefrontal and limbic systems. Findings of deficits on tasks sensitive to both prefrontal and limbic dysfunction can be interpreted as reflecting underlying involvement of both systems in the disorder in question, but possible interactions between prefrontal and limbic regions in memory functioning should also be considered.

Research is needed to determine whether there is a dissociation between impairments on tasks sensitive to prefrontal and limbic damage, respectively, in patients with discrete prefrontal or limbic lesions. Indeed, although the sensitivity of comparative neuropsychological tests to brain lesions is well established, few well-controlled studies have set out to determine the neuroanatomical specificity of these tasks in humans. Important control factors are homogeneity of the lesion site within patient groups (Freedman and Oscar-Berman 1986a); the delay between occurrence of the lesion and testing (Verin et al. 1993); and methodological consistency (Bardenhagen and Bowden 1998). It is possible that a number of comparative neuropsychological tasks will prove to be sensitive, but not specific, to prefrontal or limbic lesions in human subjects. Until the specificity of these tests in humans is demonstrated definitively, it is important to interpret research findings cautiously, in terms of patterns of impairment and damage within functional systems.

COMPARATIVE NEUROPSYCHOLOGY AND MODELS OF MEMORY

Comparative neuropsychological research has provided a framework that is helpful for understanding memory dysfunction in neurodegenerative disorders. In some neurodegenerative diseases (e.g. Parkinson's disease and progressive supranuclear palsy), patients may have working-memory and attentional impairments resulting from prefrontal system damage (Freedman and Oscar-Berman 1986b; Partiot et al. 1996; Postle et al. 1997). In other disorders (e.g. herpes encephalopathy), there may be new learning impairments suggestive of disruptions in declarative memory and limbic system damage (Aggleton et al. 1992). Models of working memory and of declarative memory recognize the complexity of neuroanatomical and neurochemical systems underlying behavior, and they can be used to explain the heterogeneity of neurobehavioral symptoms observed within and between neurodegenerative diseases (Wickelgren 1997).

Goldman-Rakic's (1987) model of prefrontal working memory postulates that prefrontal cortex receives sensory and mnemonic representations of reality as well as symbolic representations (e.g. concepts, plans) which have been elaborated in other cerebral areas. This sensory and mnemonic information is maintained by the prefrontal cortex in representational memory until a decision or operation is required, when it is used to modulate behavior. Responses are initiated as a motor command. Prefrontal working memory is thus thought to regulate behavior through the manipulation of representational knowledge. This model explains why so-called frontal lobe symptoms can be seen in patients with lesions in non-frontal parts of the brain. The sensory and mnemonic information that comprises representational memory is gained from other cortical areas; therefore, disruptions in transmission of information from those areas may lead to a breakdown in the frontal lobe's use of representational memory in modulating complex behaviors.

Goldman-Rakic (1990) has noted that the prefrontal cortex is part of a larger network of cortical areas, and that the heterogeneity of frontal lobe symptoms might be due to disruptions in different parts of the network. In addition, others have argued against viewing the functions of different areas of the prefrontal cortex separately, stating that they should be considered as parts of the integrative functions of the circuits in which they are involved (Groenewegen et al. 1990). These views are echoed by Berman and Weinberger (1990, p. 522), who have stated that 'disruption anywhere along the complex circuitry connecting prefrontal cortex with other brain areas can cause a clinically significant syndrome of abnormal behavior suggestive of prefrontal lobe dysfunction'. Given the extensive anatomical connections of prefrontal and limbic circuits, it has also been suggested that prefrontal lesions may cause impairments on tasks thought to represent limbic system dysfunction (Dudai 1989).

Declarative memory impairments resulting from limbic system damage have been demonstrated in neurobehavioral disorders characterized by amnesia. Although much is known about the neuroanatomy of declarative (or explicit) memory, less is known about the structures subserving procedural (or implicit) memory (Tulving 1985; Saint-Cyr and Taylor 1992; Squire 1992). Procedural memory (described earlier in the discussion of Learning Sets) applies to learning of rules, habits, and skills. Procedural memory is more robust than declarative memory in classical amnesic disorders (Oscar-Berman and Zola-Morgan 1980; Squire 1992); however, it may be impaired in conditions involving the basal ganglia, such as

Parkinson's and Huntington's diseases (for a review, see Saint-Cyr and Taylor 1992). For example, Verin et al. (1993) suggested that the striatum, which is considered to be the substrate of pre-elaborated motor programs, could also be viewed as the anatomic substrate of pre-elaborated routine behavioral programs. Two types of behavioral organizations involving the prefronto–striato–pallido–thalamo–prefrontal loop were proposed. The first requires elaboration of new behavioral schemata by a learning process, permitting adaptation of the subject to new environmental situations. The second is independent of the environment, concerns routine and stereotyped behaviors and is generated by subcortical structures that are normally repressed by prefrontal cortex. Lesions in prefrontal cortex may, therefore, release control of these stereotyped behaviors. This is consistent with the suggestion that basal ganglia (striatal)–frontal lobe circuitry contributes to procedural memory functions (Saint-Cyr and Taylor 1992). The striatum is thought to be a procedural memory buffer, necessary to mobilize new procedures and to select among known procedures; it is designed to function intuitively and nonconsciously. Prefrontal working memory oversees the use of this mechanism, and intervenes when opportunities for solutions are apparent. Breakdowns in the cooperative interaction between striatal procedural memory functions and prefrontal explicit working memory processes may be responsible for intrusive errors of motor sequences seen in Huntington's disease, and also the bradyphrenia and bradykinesia of Parkinson's disease (Saint-Cyr and Taylor 1992).

Comparison of working memory tasks and declarative memory tasks

Differences between declarative and working memory tasks are illustrated by research conducted with human subjects in Australia (alcoholics and nonalcoholic controls; Bardenhagen and Bowden 1995; Bardenhagen and Bowden 1998). In this research, we manipulated knowledge of the response rules in DMTS and OA. The response rule in DMTS is a simple matter of choosing the familiar stimulus. Provision of this rule, prior to and during testing on DMTS, had a small effect on performance of the subjects, but the major determinant of performance was the length of the list to be remembered. All subjects performed very well on lists of one item, but there was a significant decrease in correct responding as list length increased to two and four items, and all subjects performed near chance on lists of eight items. The results indicated that memory for stimuli over time, not rule knowledge, was crucial to task performance (Bardenhagen and Bowden 1995).

In contrast to DMTS where provision of the response rule had only a minor effect on performance, instruction in the response rule had a major effect on OA performance. There are two response rules in OA: the alternation rule (the reward alternates between objects on successive trials) and the correction rule (a trial is not over until the correct object is chosen). Performance is measured in terms of perseverative and nonperseverative errors. By definition, the first error on any trial is nonperseverative; subsequent errors on that trial are perseverative. Results with OA tasks are summarized in Figure 1.5. Subjects who were provided with the alternation rule performed almost without errors, which suggests that knowledge of the alternation rule is a major requirement for task success. Subjects who were provided with the correction rule made no perseverative errors, but made the same number of nonperseverative errors as subjects who were given neither rule. These results indicate that the ability to induce rules was a necessary precondition to success on OA and suggest that a proportion of perseverative errors may be due to a lack of knowledge of the response rules (Bardenhagen and Bowden 1998).

The results of these two studies emphasize the differences in mnemonic requirements of declarative and working memory tests: declarative tests rely heavily on memory for stimuli over temporal intervals in order to recognize or recall the target stimuli, and working memory tasks rely upon manipulation of representational memories to solve problems, or induce rules. Our data also highlight the need for intact working memory skills in DMTS performance, as provision of the response rule was helpful to some subjects. Thus, it is likely that people (and monkeys) induce the response rule in DMTS, DNMTS and CL tasks. The response rule in declarative memory tasks requires a simple stimulus–reward association, hence the lesser effect of knowledge of the DMTS response rule on task performance. At this point it should be noted that most tasks draw on procedural memory processes for access to previously acquired behavioral programs and knowledge of the response rule. For example, in DMTS subjects learn to choose the familiar stimulus and in OA they learn to alternate correctly.

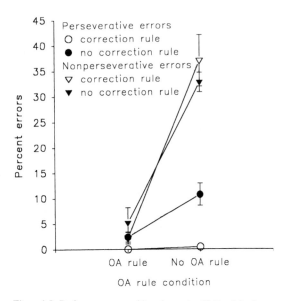

Figure 1.5. Performance on an object alternation (OA) task by four groups (five subjects per group of combined alcohol-dependent and non alcoholic controls). Points represent mean perseverative or nonperseverative errors (mean errors expressed as a percentage of trials completed), and bars depict standard errors of the means. Adapted from Bardenhagen and Bowden 1998.

CONCLUSIONS AND IMPLICATIONS

Comparative neuropsychological tests are much the same today as in earlier versions of the tasks used to investigate learning in the context of Darwin's ideas about phylogenetic continuity. Research with nonhuman animals demonstrated that the same laws of learning apply to rats, monkeys and humans, but the methods of comparative neuropsychology have been applied to human neurobehavioral disorders only recently. Some modifications have been made to the tests to facilitate the transfer to testing human subjects, generally involving changing the reward from food to money. The standard administration of the tasks in humans still involves minimal instructions, thus necessitating a degree of procedural learning in humans, as in nonhuman animals.

Findings from research with human neurobehavioral disorders has supported the models of memory hypothesized from experiments with nonhuman animals. These different forms of memory are tied to different functional systems of the brain. Disruptions to structures or tracts involved in the limbic system, a complex circuit of diencephalic, medial temporal and basal forebrain structures, is known to result in impaired new learning, recall and recognition of information. This form of memory is often called declarative memory. Declarative memory is contrasted with procedural memory, which involves acquisition of habits, skills and other information not available for conscious recall or recognition (and thought to involve circuitry of prefrontal cortex and basal ganglia). Damage to prefrontal brain systems results in impairments on tasks requiring the integration of memories, plans and ideas over short temporal intervals; this form of memory has accordingly been named prefrontal working memory. Disruptions to the neuroanatomical or neurochemical systems in the limbic and frontal networks may result in impairments in declarative, procedural or working memory abilities.

When neurodegenerative conditions have a localized onset, memory impairments related to the area affected will be apparent; therefore, in groups with putative medial-temporal or diencephalic pathology (e.g. herpes encephalitis), declarative memory impairments might be evident. These would manifest as forgetfulness, anterograde or retrograde amnesia, or poor performance on DMTS or CL. In cases with suspected frontal lobe involvement (e.g. closed head injury), impairments in working memory may be seen as deficits in planning or integration of information, and abnormal perseverative responding, for example. Deficits in delayed reaction tasks also are expected. Diseases involving the basal ganglia (e.g. Huntington's disease, Parkinson's disease, progressive supranuclear palsy) might result in problems with routine or stereotyped behaviors, i.e. impairments in a form of procedural memory. As neurodegenerative diseases are often diffuse in their effects, either early or late in the clinical course, impairments in any of these three memory systems may be apparent. This would apply to the later stages of the diseases mentioned above, but also to earlier stages of conditions like vascular dementias, demyelinating conditions, Creutzfeldt–Jakob disease, mitochondrial

disorders and other metabolic conditions, and schizophrenia. Ideally, research with memory disordered populations would employ tasks sensitive to prefrontal and limbic system damage to help identify impairments of the different types of memory in these disorders. This information could, in turn, be used to help devise rehabilitation and treatment strategies for people with memory disorders.

In summary, behavioral paradigms from comparative neuropsychology have provided sensitive tools for assessing declarative and working memory impairments, but further research needs to be conducted to determine the specificity of these tools. Experimental manipulations are a promising way of further understanding the cognitive and theoretical aspects of the tests, and to help further understanding of normal memory processes. Despite the unknown specificity of the tests in humans, the sensitivity of comparative neuropsychological tests ensures their utility in examining performance in a wide range of neurobehavioral disorders. As we begin to learn about performance profiles of patients with different neurobehavioral disorders on these tasks, about behavioral patterns on different forms of the tests, and about the neuroanatomical systems involved in memory, an integrative approach to understanding human brain functioning emerges. An integrative approach recognizes the interconnectivity of the different functional systems, and it accounts for the heterogeneity of neuropsychological symptoms between and within different neurobehavioral disorders.

ACKNOWLEDGMENTS

The writing of this chapter was supported by funds from the US Department of Health and Human Services, NIAAA (F37-AA07112 and K05-AA00219) to Boston University and by funds from the Medical Research Service of the US Department of Veterans Affairs.

REFERENCES

Aggleton, J.P., Nicol, R.M., Huston, A.E. and Fairbairn, A.F. 1988. The performance of amnesic subjects on tests of experimental amnesia in animals: Delayed matching-to-sample and concurrent learning. *Neuropsychologia*. 26: 265–272.

Aggleton, J.P., Shaw, C. and Gaffan, E.A. 1992. The performance of postencephalitic amnesic subjects on two behavioural tests of memory: Concurrent discrimination learning and delayed matching-to-sample. *Cortex*. 28: 359–372.

Albert, M.S. and Moss, M.B. 1996. Neuropsychology of aging: Findings in humans and monkeys. In *Handbook of the biology of aging*, 4th ed., ed. E.L. Schneider and J.W. Rowe, pp. 217–233. San Diego, CA: Academic Press.

Arnold, M.B. 1984. *Memory and the brain*. London: Lawrence Erlbaum.

Bardenhagen, F.J. and Bowden, S.C. 1995. Does knowledge of the response rule determine human performance on an animal test of amnesia? *Neuropsychology*. 9: 573–579.

Bardenhagen, F.J. and Bowden, S.C. 1998. Cognitive components of perseverative and nonperseverative errors on the object alternation task. *Brain and Cognition*. (In press.)

Beach, F.A. 1960. Experimental investigations of species-specific behavior. *American Psychologist*. 15: 1–18.

Berman, K.F. and Weinberger, D.R. 1990. The prefrontal cortex in schizophrenia and other neuropsychiatric diseases: In vivo physiological correlates of cognitive deficits. *Progress in Brain Research*. 85: 521–537.

Bitterman, M.E. 1960. Toward a comparative psychology of learning. *American Psychologist*. 15: 704–712.

Bitterman, M.E. 1975. The comparative analysis of learning. *Science*. 188: 699–709.

Bitterman, M.E., LoLordo, V.M., Overmier, J.B. and Rashotte, M.E. (ed.) 1979. *Animal learning: Survey and analysis*. New York: Plenum Press.

Bowden, S.C. 1990. Separating cognitive impairment in neurologically asymptomatic alcoholism from Wernicke–Korsakoff syndrome: Is the neuropsychological distinction justified? *Psychological Bulletin*. 107: 355–366.

Bowden, S.C., Benedikt, R. and Ritter, A. 1992. Delayed matching to sample and concurrent learning in nonamnesic humans with alcohol dependence. *Neuropsychologia*. 30: 427–435.

Canavan, A.G.M., Passingham, R.E., Marsden, C.D., Quinn, N., Wyke, M. and Polkey, C.E. 1990. Prism adaptation and other tasks involving spatial abilities in patients with Parkinson's disease, patients with frontal lobe lesions and patients with unilateral temporal lobectomies. *Neuropsychologia*. 28: 969–984.

Chorover, S.L. and Cole, M. 1966. Delayed alternation performance in patients with cerebral lesions. *Neuropsychologia*. 4: 1–7.

Darwin, C. 1871. *The descent of man and selection in relation to sex*, vol. 1. New York: Appleton.

Deutsch, J.A. (ed.) 1983. *The physiological basis of memory*. New York: Academic Press.

Dudai, Y. 1989. *The neurobiology of memory: Concepts, findings, trends*. Oxford: Oxford University Press.

El-Awar, M., Kish, S., Oscar-Berman, M., Robitaille, Y., Schut, L. and Freedman, M. 1991. Selective delayed alternation deficits in dominantly inherited olivopontocerebellar atrophy. *Brain and Cognition*. 16: 121–129.

Fobes, J.L. and King, J.E. 1982. Measuring primate learning abilities. In *Primate behavior*, ed. J.L. Fobes and J.E. King, pp. 289–326. New York: Academic Press.

Freedman, M. 1990. Object alternation and orbitofrontal system dysfunction in Alzheimer's and Parkinson's disease. *Brain and Cognition*. 14: 134–143.

Freedman, M. 1994. Frontal and parietal lobe dysfunction in depression: Delayed alternation and tactile learning deficits. *Neuropsychologia*. 32: 1015–1025.

Freedman, M., Black, S., Ebert, P. and Binns, M. 1998. Orbitofrontal function, object alternation, and perseveration. *Cerebral Cortex*. 8: 18–27.

Freedman, M. and Oscar-Berman, M. 1986a. Bilateral frontal lobe disease and selective delayed-response deficits in humans. *Behavioral Neuroscience*. 100: 337–342.

Freedman, M. and Oscar-Berman, M. 1986b. Selective delayed response deficits in Parkinson's and Alzheimer's disease. *Archives of Neurology*. 43: 886–890.

Freedman, M. and Oscar-Berman, M. 1987. Tactile discrimination learning deficits in Alzheimer's and Parkinson's diseases. *Archives of Neurology*. 44: 394–398.

Friedman, H.R. and Goldman-Rakic, P.S. 1988. Activation of the hippocampus and dentate gyrus by working-memory: A 2-deoxyglucose study of behaving Rhesus monkeys. *Journal of Neuroscience*. 8: 4693–4706.

Fuster, J.M. 1989. *The prefrontal cortex.* New York: Raven Press.

Gaffan, E.A., Aggleton, J.P., Gaffan, D. and Shaw, C. 1990. Concurrent and sequential pattern discrimination learning by patients with Korsakoff amnesia. *Cortex.* 26: 381–397.

Gansler, D.A., Covall, S.B, McGrath, N. and Oscar-Berman, M. 1996. Measures of prefrontal dysfunction after closed head injury. *Brain and Cognition.* 30: 194–204.

Goldman-Rakic, P.S. 1987. Circuitry of primate prefrontal cortex and regulation of behavior by representational memory. In *Handbook of physiology, section I: The nervous system,* vol. V. *Higher functions of the brain,* part 1, ed. V.B. Mountcastle, F. Plum, and S.R. Geiger, pp. 373–417. Bethesda: American Physiological Society.

Goldman-Rakic, P.S. 1990. Cellular and circuit basis of working memory in prefrontal cortex of nonhuman primates. *Progress in Brain Research.* 85: 325–336.

Groenewegen, H.J., Berendse, H.W., Wolters, J.G. and Lohman, A.H.M. 1990. The anatomical relationship of the prefrontal cortex with the striato-pallidal system, the thalamus and the amygdala: Evidence for a parallel organization. *Progress in Brain Research.* 85: 95–118.

Harlow, H.F. 1949. The formation of learning sets. *Psychological Review.* 56: 51–65.

Harlow, H.F. 1951. Primate learning. In *Comparative psychology,* 3rd ed., ed. C.P. Stone, pp. 183–238. Englewood Cliffs, New Jersey: Prentice-Hall.

Harlow, H.F., Harlow, M.K., Schlitz, K.A. and Mohr, D.J. 1971. The effect of early adverse and enriched environments on the learning ability of Rhesus monkeys. In *Cognitive processes of nonhuman primates,* ed. L.E. Jarrard, pp. 121–148. New York: Academic Press.

Harper, C.G. and Kril, J. 1990. Neuropathology of alcoholism. *Alcohol and Alcoholism.* 25: 207–216.

Hebb, D.O. 1949. *The organization of behavior: A neuropsychological theory.* New York: Wiley.

Hilgard, E.R. and Bower, G.H. 1975. *Theories of learning.* Englewood, New Jersey: Prentice-Hall.

Hunt, W.A. and Nixon, S.J. (ed.) 1993. *Alcohol-induced brain damage, NIAAA research monograph No. 22.* Rockville, Maryland: USDHHS, NIH Publications.

Jarrard, L.E. (ed). 1971. *Cognitive processes of nonhuman primates.* New York: Academic Press.

Kessler, J., Irle, E. and Markowitsch, H.J. 1986. Korsakoff and alcoholic subjects are severely impaired in animal tasks of associative memory. *Neuropsychologia.* 24: 671–680.

Kinnaman, A.J. 1902. Mental life of two Macacus rhesus monkeys in captivity. II. *American Journal of Psychology.* 13: 173–218.

Koenen, K.C., Driver, K.L., Schlesinger, L.K., Roper, S.J., Oscar-Berman, M. and Wolfe, J. 1997. Measures of prefrontal functioning in post-traumatic stress disorder (PTSD). *Proceedings of the American Psychological Society Convention.* pp. 98–99.

Lezak, M. 1995. *Neuropsychological assessment,* 3rd ed. New York: Oxford University Press.

Luria, A.R. 1966. *Higher cortical functions in man.* New York: Basic Books.

Masterton, R.B., Bitterman, M.E., Campbell, C.B.G. and Hotton, N. (ed.) 1976. *Evolution of brain and behavior.* New York: Wiley.

Mayes, A.R., Meudell, P., Mann, D. and Pickering, A. 1988. Location of lesions in Korsakoff's syndrome: Neuropsychological and neuropathological data on two patients. *Cortex.* 24: 367–388.

Meador, D.M., Rumbaugh, D.M., Pate J.L. and Bard, K.A. 1987. Learning, problem solving, cognition, and intelligence. In *Comparative primate biology,* vol. 2, part B: *Behavior, cognition, and motivation,* ed. G. Mitchell and J. Erwin, pp. 17–83. New York: Alan R. Liss.

Medin, D.L. 1977. Information processing and discrimination learning set. In *Behavioral primatology,* vol. 1, ed. A.M. Schrier, pp. 33–69. Hillsdale, New Jersey: Lawrence Erlbaum.

Milner, B. 1964. Some effects of frontal lobectomy in man. In *The frontal granular cortex and behavior,* ed. J.M. Warren and K. Akert, pp. 313–334. New York: McGraw-Hill.

Mishkin, M. 1982. A memory system in the monkey. *Philosophical Transactions of the Royal Society, London (Biology).* 298: 85–95.

Mishkin, M. and Appenzeller, T. 1987. The anatomy of memory. *Scientific American.* 256: 62–71.

Mitchell, G. and Erwin, J. (ed.) 1987. *Comparative primate biology,* vol 2, part B, *Behavior, cognition, and motivation.* New York: Alan R. Liss.

Olton, D.S., Gamzu, E. and Corkin, S. (ed.) 1985. Memory dysfunctions: An integration of animal and human research from preclinical and clinical perspectives. *Annals of the New York Academy of Sciences.* 444: 1–449.

Olton, D.S., Markowska, A.L. and Voytko, M.L. 1992. Working memory: Animals. In *Encyclopedia of learning and memory,* ed. L.R. Squire, pp. 635–638. New York: Macmillan.

Oscar-Berman, M. 1984. Comparative neuropsychology and alcoholic Korsakoff's disease. In *Neuropsychology of memory,* ed. L. Squire and N. Butters, pp. 194–202. New York: Guilford Press.

Oscar-Berman, M. 1991. Clinical and experimental approaches to varieties of memory. *International Journal of Neuroscience*. 58: 135–150.

Oscar-Berman, M. 1994. Comparative neuropsychology: Brain function in nonhuman primates and human neurobehavioral disorders. In *Neuropsychological explorations of memory and cognition: A tribute to Nelson Butters*, ed. L. Cermak, pp. 9–30. New York: Plenum Press.

Oscar-Berman, M. and Bonner, R.T. 1985. Matching- and delayed-matching-to-sample performance as measures of visual processing, selective attention, and memory in aging and alcoholic individuals. *Neuropsychologia*. 23: 639–651.

Oscar-Berman, M. and Bonner, R.T. 1989. Nonmatching- (oddity) and delayed nonmatching-to-sample performance in aging, alcoholic, and alcoholic Korsakoff individuals. *Psychobiology*. 17: 424–430.

Oscar-Berman, M. and Hutner, N. 1993. Frontal lobe changes after chronic alcohol ingestion. In *Alcohol-induced brain damage, NIAAA Research Monograph No. 22*, ed. W.A. Hunt and S.J. Nixon, pp. 121–156. Rockville, Maryland: USDHHS, NIH Publications.

Oscar-Berman, M. and Zola-Morgan, S.M. 1980. Comparative neuro-psychology and Korsakoff's syndrome. II: Two-choice visual discrimination learning. *Neuropsychologia*. 18: 513–526.

Oscar-Berman, M. Hutner, N. and Bonner, R.T. 1992. Visual and auditory spatial and nonspatial delayed-response performance by Korsakoff and non-Korsakoff alcoholic and aging individuals. *Behavioral Neuroscience*. 106: 613–622.

Oscar-Berman, M., McNamara, P. and Freedman, M. 1991. Delayed response tasks: Parallels between experimental ablation studies and findings in patients with frontal lesions. In *Frontal lobe function and injury*, ed. H.S. Levin, H.M. Eisenberg, and A.L. Benton, pp. 120–138. New York: Oxford University Press.

Oscar-Berman, M., Zola-Morgan, S.M., Oberg, R.G.E. and Bonner, R.T. 1982. Comparative neuropsychology and Korsakoff's syndrome. III: Delayed response, delayed alternation, and DRL performance. *Neuropsychologia*. 20: 187–202.

Overstreet, D.H. and Russell, R.W. 1991. Animal models of memory disorders. In *Neuromethods*, vol. 19: *Animal models in psychiatry II*, ed. A. Boulton, G. Baker, and M. Martin-Iverson. Totowa, New Jersey: The Humana Press.

Park, S. and Holzman, P.S. 1992. Schizophrenics show spatial working memory deficits. *Archives of General Psychiatry*. 49: 975–982.

Partiot, A., Verin, M., Pillon, B, Teixeira-Ferreira, C., Agid, Y. and Dubois, B. 1996. Delayed response tasks in basal ganglia lesions in man: Further evidence for a striato-frontal cooperation in behavioural adaptation. *Neuropsychologia*. 34: 709–721.

Penfield, W. 1958. *The excitable cortex in conscious man*. Springfield, Illinois: Charles C. Thomas.

Porter, J.P. 1904. A preliminary study of the psychology of the English sparrow. *American Journal of Psychology*. 15: 313–346.

Postle, B.R., Jonides, J., Smith, E.E., Corkin, S. and Growdon, J.H. 1997. Spatial, but not object, delayed response is impaired in early Parkinson's disease. *Neuropsychology*. 11: 171–179.

Pribram, K.H. 1958. *Comparative neurology and evolution of behavior: Behavior and evolution*. New Haven: Yale University Press.

Pribram, K.H., Ahumada, A., Hartog, J. and Roos, L. 1964. A progress report on the neurological processes disturbed by frontal lesions in primates. In *The frontal granular cortex and behavior*, ed. J.M. Warren and K. Akert, pp. 28–55. New York: McGraw-Hill.

Reitan, R.M. 1962. Psychological deficit. *Annual Review of Psychology*. 13: 415–444.

Riley, D.A., and Langley, C.M. 1993. The logic of species comparisons. *Psychological Science*. 4: 185–189.

Roberts, A.C. and Sahakian, B.J. 1993. Comparable tests of cognitive function in monkey and man. In *Behavioral neuroscience: A practical approach*, vol. 1, ed. A. Sahgal, pp. 165–184. New York: Oxford University Press.

Roediger, H.L. and Craik, F.I.M. (ed.) 1989. *Varieties of memory and consciousness: Essays in honor of Endel Tulving*. Hillsdale, New Jersey: Erlbaum.

Russell, W.R. 1959. *Brain: Memory: Learning*. Oxford: Clarendon Press.

Sahgal, A. (ed.) 1993. *Behavioral neuroscience. A practical approach*, vol. 1. New York: Oxford University Press.

Sahgal, A., Galloway, P.H., McKeith, I.G., Lloyd, S., Cook, J.H., Ferrier, N. and Edwardson, J.A. 1992. Matching-to-sample deficits in patients with senile dementias of the Alzheimer and Lewy body types. *Archives of Neurology*. 49: 1043–1046.

Saint-Cyr, J.A. and Taylor, A.E. 1992. The mobilization of procedural learning: The 'key signature' of the basal ganglia. In *Neuropsychology of memory*, 2nd ed., ed. L. R. Squire and N. Butters, pp. 188–202. New York: Guilford Press.

Seidman, L.J., Oscar-Berman, M., Kalinowski, A.G., Ajilor, O., Kremen, W.S., Faraone, S.V. and Tsuang, M.T. 1995. Experimental and clinical neuropsychological measures of prefrontal dysfunction in schizophrenia. *Neuropsychology*. 9: 481–490.

Small, W.S. 1901. Experimental study of the mental processes of the rat. *American Journal of Psychology*. 12: 206–239.

Squire, L.R. 1992. Memory and the hippocampus: A synthesis from findings with rats, monkeys, and humans. *Psychological Review*. 99: 195–231.

Squire, L.R., Zola-Morgan, S. and Chen, K.S. 1988. Human amnesia and animal models of amnesia: Performance of amnesic patients on tests designed for the monkey. *Behavioral Neuroscience*. 102: 210–221.

Stuss, D.T. and Benson, D.F. (ed.) 1986. *The frontal lobes*. New York: Raven Press.

Teuber, H.-L. 1955. Physiological psychology. *Annual Review of Psychology*. 6: 267–296.

Thorndike, E.L. 1911. *Animal intelligence: Experimental studies*. New York: Macmillan.

Tulving, E. 1985. How many memory systems are there? *American Psychologist*. 40: 385–398.

Vallar, G. and Shallice, T. (ed.) 1990. *Neuropsychological impairments of short-term memory*. Cambridge: Cambridge University Press.

Verin, M., Partiot, A., Pillon, B., Malapani, C., Agid, Y. and Dubois, B. 1993. Delayed response tasks and prefrontal lesions in man: Evidence for self-generated patterns of behaviour with poor environmental modulation. *Neuropsychologia*. 31: 1379–1396.

Walsh, K.W. 1987. *Neuropsychology: A clinical approach*, 2nd ed. New York: Churchill Livingstone.

Warren, J.M. and Akert, K. (ed.) 1964. *The frontal granular cortex and behavior*. New York: McGraw-Hill.

Wasserman, E.A. 1993. Comparative cognition: Beginning the second century of the study of animal intelligence. *Psychological Bulletin*. 113: 211–228.

Wechsler, D.A. 1944. *The measurement of adult intelligence*, 3rd ed. Baltimore: Williams and Wilkins.

Weinberger, D.R., Berman, K.F., Suddath, R. and Torrey, E.F. 1992. Evidence of dysfunction of a prefrontal-limbic network in schizophrenia. *American Journal of Psychiatry*. 149: 890–897.

Weiskrantz, L.A. 1978. A comparison of hippocampal pathology in man and other animals. In *Functions of the septo-hippocampal system: Ciba Foundation Symposium 58*, ed. K. Elliott and J. Whelan, pp. 373–406. New York: Elsevier Science.

Whitty, C.W.M. and Zangwill, O.L. 1966. *Amnesia*. London: Butterworths.

Wickelgren, I. 1997. Getting a grasp on working memory. *Science*. 275: 1580–1582.

Zola-Morgan, S. and Squire, L.R. 1993. Neuroanatomy of memory. *Annual Review of Neuroscience*. 16: 547–563.

2

Nonprimate animal models of motor and cognitive dysfunction associated with Huntington's disease

RAYMOND P. KESNER
AND J. VINCENT FILOTEO

INTRODUCTION

The purpose of this chapter is to present the neuropathological, neurochemical and neuroanatomical substrates of Huntington's disease (HD) followed by a discussion of the extant animal models aimed at mimicking the neuropathological, neurochemical and neuroanatomical characteristics of this disease. Then, the neurological, behavioral and cognitive dysfunctions of HD are reviewed, and this review is followed by a discussion of possible parallel functions associated with models of caudate dysfunction aimed at mimicking the neurological, behavioral and cognitive characteristics of HD. Unfortunately, there is a paucity of studies that have examined cognitive dysfunction in the best models of HD. Thus, in order to determine whether the caudate in animals, especially the rat, mediates motor and cognitive functions that parallel similar caudate mediated functions in humans, the patterns of motor and cognitive deficits in animals with caudate dysfunction induced by multiple means will be described. To the extent that there are caudate mediated parallels in motor and cognitive functions between animals and humans, there would be a greater impetus to study in more detail the cognitive dysfunctions of animal models of HD.

NEUROPATHOLOGICAL FEATURES OF HUNTINGTON'S DISEASE

At a macroscopic level, the primary area of pathology in HD is the head of the caudate nucleus and, to a lesser extent, the putamen (see also Chapter 3). In a large scale postmortem study, Vonsattel et al. (1985) found that the dorsomedial aspects of the caudate appear to be the locus of greatest cell loss in this structure with the ventrolateral aspects of this nucleus becoming more affected as the disease progresses. Other brain regions also appear to be affected in HD but, again, the brunt of the pathology occurs in the striatum. De La Monte et al. (1988) examined standardized coronal slices of 30 HD patients and found a volumetric reduction of over one-half in the caudate nucleus and putamen, whereas the cerebral cortex, white matter and thalamus only experienced a reduction of approximately one-fourth their normal volumes. In vivo examination of HD patients' brains using computed tomography (CT) and magnetic resonance imaging (MRI) often reveals normal volumetric indices in the early course of the disease and the hallmark caudate atrophy in the later courses of the disease (Cala et al. 1990). Positron emission tomography (PET) studies, however, have identified striatal hypometabolism in HD even in the absence of structural changes (Kuhl et al. 1982; Chapter 6), which suggests that abnormal metabolic activity may be a precursor to the later morphological changes. From a gross anatomical perspective, the brains of HD patients can often exhibit cortical atrophy (i.e. sulcal widening and gyral atrophy), particularly in the frontal regions (Forno and Jose 1973; Cummings and Benson 1992).

Several other neuropathological hallmarks of HD can be observed at the microscopic level. Although there appear to be at least six types of cells within the striatum, HD tends to have a predilection for the smaller neurons. In particular, the medium-sized spiny neurons tend to be most affected in this disease, whereas aspiny and larger neurons are not as affected (Graveland et al. 1985; Ferrante et al. 1987; Kowall et al. 1987). Once the medium-sized spiny neurons have deteriorated in the striatum, they appear to be replaced by astrocytes (Vonsattel et al. 1985). The medium-sized spiny neurons contain gamma-aminobutyric acid (GABA) and the death of these cells leads to a substantial depletion (approximately 80%) of this neurotransmitter in the basal ganglia of patients with HD (Bird et al. 1973; McGeer et al. 1973; Stahl and Swanson 1974; Perry and Hansen 1990), although other neurochemicals also appear to be decreased in this disease, including choline acetyl transferase, enkephalin, dynorphin and substance P (Stahl and Swanson 1974; Wu et al. 1979; Beal et al. 1988a,b). Increases in some neurochemicals, such as somatostatin and neuropeptide Y, have also been reported (Beal et al. 1988b).

Given the fact that HD results in characteristic changes at both the macro- and microscopic level, Vonsattel et al. (1985) have developed a pathological severity scale for HD which takes into account changes at both the morphological and neuronal levels. An examination of this scale is instructive because it provides a description of the neuropathological progression of the disease. The scale uses a rating system with five grades (0–4). Grade 0 reflects no macro- or microscopic abnormalities despite the clear presence of HD symptomatology in vivo. Grade 1 brains demonstrate normal striatums at the macroscopic level, whereas at a microscopic level, astrocytosis is readily apparent in the medial aspects of the caudate. Grade 2 reflects macroscopic atrophy of the head of the caudate with microscopic neuronal loss and astrocytosis in the head, body and tail of the caudate. Grade 3 is indicative of severe striatal atrophy at the macroscopic level with early involvement of the nucleus accumbens and globus pallidus, and the microscopic changes include astrocytosis in all aspects of the caudate, mild astrocytosis in the dorsal putamen and relative sparing of the nucleus accumbens. The final grade, Grade 4, reflects almost complete obliteration of the caudate at both macroscopic and microscopic levels, and with the nucleus accumbens demonstrating moderate astrocytosis.

There are several important issues related to the neuropathology of HD which should be taken into consideration when attempting to develop an animal model of this disease. First, the neuropathology associated with HD varies as a function of the stage of the disease. For example, it appears that the head of the caudate nucleus is the brain region most affected in this disease, despite the fact that other parts of the caudate may be affected earlier in the course of the disorder. Thus, researchers attempting to

develop an animal model of HD must take into consideration which stage of the disease they are attempting to mimic. The use of the rating system developed by Vonsattel et al. (1985) could help in gauging the degree of pathology which is attempted to be mimicked by any given animal model. Second, there are both macro- and microscopic pathological features that are hallmarks of this disease, and therefore the level at which the model is being developed must be taken into consideration. It is not enough to simply reproduce the neuropathology at a macroscopic level (e.g. introducing lesions into the head of the caudate); a good model of this disease must also mimic the disorder at a micro-anatomical level. Third, not all patients with HD demonstrate the same behavioral manifestations of the disease, which suggests that there may be patient-to-patient variation in the neuropathological features of this disease. This latter point argues for the notion that a single model of HD may not be viable and several models may need to be developed, each specific to the particular subtypes of this disease.

DEVELOPMENT OF ANIMAL MODELS OF HUNTINGTON'S DISEASE

In order to generate an animal model of HD, it is very important to mimic the pattern of cell loss and subsequent changes in neurotransmitter function observed in the caudate-putamen. The earliest and still most important animal models of HD are based on the assumption that overproduction of glutamate in cortical connections to the caudate results in excitotoxic damage to caudate neurons. The first rat model was based on intracranial injections of kainic acid into the caudate of rats resulting in the destruction of intrinsic striatal neurons and spared axons of afferent origin (Coyle and Schwarcz 1976; McGeer and McGeer 1976). There are, however, a few serious problems with the kainic acid model, in that kainate, probably due to its convulsive properties, produces severe extrastriatal damage which includes the limbic system. Furthermore, damage includes the small, aspiny interneurons containing somatostatin and neuropeptide Y as well the enzyme dihydronicotinamide adenine dinucleotide phosphate diaphorase (NADPH). These neurons do not degenerate in HD (Beal 1994). Finally, the slow progressive disorder of HD cannot be triggered by a single injection of kainic acid.

The second, and currently the best animal (rat) model of HD, results from an intracranial injection of quinolinic acid (QUIN; 2,3-pyridine decarboxylic acid), an NMDA antagonist, into the caudate of rats resulting in intra-striatal neuronal loss and sparing of afferent axons (Schwarcz et al. 1983). In this model QUIN first produces swelling of dendrites and, later, degeneration of postsyn-aptic processes followed by gliosis. The area of neuronal degeneration is spherical and remains confined to the area of injection. Thus, in contrast to kainic acid injections, the lesions induced by QUIN do not extend beyond the caudate nucleus. QUIN produces neurochemical changes that are similar to those observed in the caudate of HD patients. For example, there is depletion of neurochemical markers of spiny neurons including GABA and substance P, an increase in neurochemical markers of aspiny neurons including somatostatin and neuropeptide Y, but no change in the enzyme NADPH (Beal et al. 1986). It should be noted that Davies and Roberts (1987) did not find selective sparing of somatostatin and NADPH con-taining striatal neurons following QUIN injections. There are increases in serotonin levels and neurotensin immuno-reactivity, decreases in choline acetyltransferase activity levels, but no changes in dopamine levels (Beal 1994). QUIN induced lesions result in marked depletion of NMDA receptors similar to that observed in HD patients (Greenamyre and Young 1989). It is important to note that QUIN, which is an endogenous tryptophan metabo-lite, is present in rats and human brains (Wolfensberger et al. 1983) and 3HAO, the enzyme responsible for the bio-synthesis of QUIN, is enhanced in the caudate–putamen complex of the brain of HD patients (Schwarcz et al. 1987). Finally, the observation that a single injection of QUIN into the caudate leads to a slow progressive reduc-tion in the size of the caudate nucleus proceeding outward from the lesion zone (Beal et al. 1986), coupled with the observation that QUIN is not very toxic in the develop-ing rat striatum (Foster et al. 1983), suggests that QUIN induced lesions might mimic the pathology of late onset HD. Other animal models emphasize an impairment in energy metabolism within the caudate–putamen complex which is characteristic of HD patients (Beal 1994). More work is needed to determine whether the anatomical and biochemical changes in this model match the pattern observed in HD patients.

COGNITIVE AND BEHAVIORAL CHANGES IN HUNTINGTON'S DISEASE AND ITS ANIMAL MODELS

Over the past 20 years our understanding of the nature and pattern of neuropsychological deficits in HD has become increasingly clear. From a global standpoint, the overall pattern of cognitive deficits observed in this disease appears to be very different from that observed in patients with primarily cortical dementias, such as Alzheimer's disease (AD) (Chapters 8, 10, 11, 12 and 18). In general, patients with AD display a marked anomia, a rapid rate of forgetting and constructional apraxia. In contrast, patients with HD do not demonstrate an anomia, and their memory impairment is characterized by deficient retrieval processes. Patients with HD dementia exhibit deficits in problem solving, abstract reasoning, information pro-cessing speed and certain components of attention (McHugh and Folstein 1975; Mendez 1994; Morris 1995).

Although HD typically results in global cognitive deterioration (i.e. dementia), only some cognitive func-tions are affected early in the course of the disease. An understanding of which specific areas of cognition are affected in patients with HD is important, because the goal of any animal model of this disease should be to recreate very similar behavioral abnormalities. The following sec-tions provide brief reviews of the specific cognitive deficits observed in patients with HD, and of behavioral deficits in rats with damage to the caudate.

Motor functioning

Choreiform movements, which are involuntary jerking movements, are the unmistakable hallmark of HD. Initially evident in the hands and face, they progress to eventually involve the rest of the body. Huntington's disease also affects voluntary movements. For example, HD patients often demonstrate akinesia (an impairment in initiating voluntary movement) and bradykinesia (slowness in vol-untary movement once initiated). Several studies have examined the specific nature of the voluntary movement abnormalities observed in HD. For example, Bradshaw et al. (1992) found that HD patients were impaired in the initiation of sequential movements, and that this deficit was even more pronounced in the absence of preparatory cues. These investigators also found that the time HD patients take to carry out a motor sequence (i.e. movement time) was not aided by the use of preparatory cues, whereas normal controls were able to utilize this information to reduce their movement time. Interestingly, HD patients' deficits in movement initiation and speed were associated with the degree of their functional incapacity, a finding which suggests that impairments in voluntary movements may be a good predictor of everyday functioning (Girotti et al. 1988).

A similar pattern of voluntary movement abnormalities has been observed in rats with caudate lesions. For example, ibotenic or QUIN lesions of the lateral caudate result in significant impairments in movement initiation and reaching movements of the tongue and forelimbs, in the use and accuracy of forelimb movement, in swimming speed, in changes in the frequency and duration of a variety of motor movements, and in reversal of limb preference (Whishaw et al. 1986; Pisa 1988; Sanberg et al. 1989; Pisa and Cyr 1990; Block et al. 1993). These changes in movement initiation, programming, frequency, duration and amplitude parallel the motor problems observed in HD patients.

There is also evidence of important regional specificity in the behavioral changes produced by caudate lesions. Ibotenic or QUIN lesions of the medial caudate, in contrast to the lateral caudate, do not produce any, or only mild, changes in motor activity (Pisa 1988; Pisa and Cyr 1990; Furtado and Mazurek 1996).

Declarative learning and memory in Huntington's disease

The ability to consciously recollect information is among the most widely studied phenomena in HD. Several studies have demonstrated that HD patients are impaired on standardized measures of memory, and that their profile of memory deficits differs from that in other memory impaired patients. For example, in contrast to patients with damage primarily to the medial temporal lobes (e.g. AD patients) or dorsomedial nucleus of the thalamus (e.g. Korsakoff's patients), patients with HD tend to commit a higher number of perseverative errors, recall more words from the recency portion of a word list, demonstrate relatively better recognition than free recall and have a relatively normal rate of forgetting (Butters et al. 1988; Massman et al. 1990; Delis et al. 1991; Tröster et al. 1993). HD patients have also been shown to be impaired on tasks that require learning of associations among stimuli (Sprengelmeyer et al. 1995a). Together, these results suggest that HD is associated with mildly deficient encod-

ing, intact storage but markedly deficient initiation of systematic retrieval strategies (Butters et al. 1985, 1986).

In addition to their deficits in learning new information (i.e. anterograde amnesia), HD patients have difficulty with tasks that require recall of information learned in the past (i.e. retrograde amnesia). For example, HD patients are deficient in recalling famous faces and historical information (Albert et al. 1981; Beatty et al. 1988); however, the pattern of their retrograde memory impairment is qualitatively different than that observed in patients with AD or Korsakoff's disease. Patients with HD are equally impaired in recalling information from all past decades, whereas AD and Korsakoff's patients are differentially impaired in recalling more recent memories (Albert et al. 1981; Beatty et al. 1988).

Nondeclarative memory and learning in Huntington's disease

There is accumulating evidence that patients with HD also are impaired on a broad range of tasks that require the acquisition and retention of novel skills or procedures, but do not require the conscious recollection of previously encountered information. For example, Martone et al. (1984) found that HD patients were deficient in improving their performance across multiple trials of a mirror-reading task. Similarly, Paulsen et al. (1993) observed that HD patients neither adapted to viewing a spatial target through prisms that shifted central fixation 20 degrees to the right or left, nor demonstrated the normal after effects of prism adaptation after removing the viewing apparatus. Patients with HD are also impaired in learning the pursuit-rotor test, a task which requires subjects to maintain continuous contact between a rod and a point on a moving turntable (Heindel et al. 1989). Using a serial reaction time task, Knopman and Nissen (1991) demonstrated that, compared to normal controls, patients with HD were deficient in decreasing their reaction times over multiple trials when pressing four buttons in a set sequence. HD patients also demonstrate a deficit in developing a sensory–motor bias. Specifically, Heindel et al. (1991) administered a weight-biasing task to a group of HD patients in which subjects were asked to rate the perceived weight of a set of test weights after having been previously exposed (i.e. biased) to a heavier or lighter set of weights. The normal controls in this study rated the set of test weights as being heavier if they had been biased with the lighter weights, but as lighter if they had been biased with heavier weights. In contrast, moderately demented HD patients did not demonstrate this biasing effect, which suggests that they were unable to adapt to the sensory–motor feedback provided by the biasing weight set.

The deficits of HD patients on these various tasks of skill or procedural learning are in marked contrast to their relatively intact performances on other tasks that do not require the learning of a novel skill or procedure (i.e. tasks that have limited motor requirements), but nevertheless also require the unconscious recollection of previously experienced material. For example, HD patients have been shown to be relatively unimpaired on priming tasks that require lexical processes, semantic processes or visuoperceptual processes (Shimamura et al. 1987; Salmon et al. 1988; Heindel et al. 1989, 1990), and there is some evidence to suggest that these types of memories in HD patients are relatively stable over extended periods of time (Bylsma et al. 1991). Thus, it appears that HD patients' deficits on tasks that do not require the conscious recollection of information are somewhat specific to the motor domain. This has lead Heindel et al. (1993) to argue for the notion that dysfunction of the striatum in HD patients leads to a deficit in the establishment of motor programs, a view which is consistent with that of other investigators (e.g. Saint-Cyr and Taylor 1992).

At first glance it might appear that HD patients' deficits in motor-based learning and memory are due to the motor impairments observed in this disease; however, several studies have indicated that the patients' poor performances on these tasks are not associated with the degree of their motor symptoms, but rather with their overall level of cognitive status (Heindel et al. 1991; Paulsen et al. 1993). This suggests that the motor impairment of HD cannot completely account for the deficient motor-based learning and memory in this disease.

Learning and memory in animals with caudate lesions

Based on research with animals it has been assumed that the basal ganglia, including the caudate nucleus, mediate procedural learning as exemplified by the learning of stimulus–response associations or habits (Mishkin and Petri, 1984; Phillips and Carr 1987). Support for this idea comes from the findings that visual pattern discrimination and concurrent visual object discrimination are disrupted in monkeys with lesions of either the putamen or the tail of the caudate, but not in monkeys with lesions of the hip-

pocampus (Mishkin 1982; Wang et al. 1990). It should be noted, however, that monkeys with lesions in the tail of the caudate have difficulty only in remembering new visual object discriminations, not previously acquired ones.

It has been suggested that in rats the caudate mediates the sensory–motor integration involved in learning of stimulus–response associations as required by tasks in which a particular motor response is reinforced in the presence of a single cue, or by tasks that require a consistent choice of direction, or a consistent choice to initiate or withhold responding (Phillips and Carr 1987; McDonald and White 1993). Support for this idea comes from a large number of studies indicating that damage to the dorsal caudate impairs brightness discrimination (Schwartzbaum and Donovick 1968), tactile discrimination (Colombo et al. 1989), conditional visual discrimination (Reading et al. 1991), right/left maze discrimination (Cook and Kesner 1988), runway learning (Kirkby et al. 1981), eight-arm maze learning (Colombo et al. 1989; Packard and White 1990), cued radial arm or Morris water maze learning (Whishaw et al. 1987; Packard and White 1990). In this latter task, only an approach response to the correct visual cue location is required. Furthermore, lesions of the caudate have resulted in inappropriate selection of fixed-interval schedules (Hansing et al. 1967). It should be noted that rats with hippocampal lesions are not impaired on the above mentioned tasks (McDonald and White 1993). As lesions of the caudate in rabbits impair classical conditioning of an eye-blink response, but not heart rate conditioning (Powell et al. 1978), it is likely that the caudate is involved only in stimulus-somatic motor response associations.

There is some evidence for regional specificity in caudate lesions' effects on behavior. In a conditional visual discrimination (fast versus slow frequency of light flashes) task requiring a choice bar press response, only ibotenic acid lesions of the lateral, but not the medial caudate, result in task acquisition impairments. A similar impairment in learning a stimulus–response association (entering an arm of an eight-arm maze if cued by a light) following lateral caudate lesions was also reported by McDonald and White (1993). These findings suggest that the lateral caudate is necessary for the acquisition of response rules to perform accurately on conditional visual discrimination tasks (Reading et al. 1991).

The major problem in interpreting the exact involvement of the caudate in stimulus–response association learning derives from the difficulty in determining whether the impairment is due to a failure in detecting the sensory stimulus, a deficiency in learning stimulus–reward associations or a defect in shifting attentional set. With respect to visual information, it can be shown that caudate lesioned rats are not impaired in recognizing visual stimuli, learning stimulus–reward associations or in shifting attention (Kesner et al. 1993; McDonald and White 1993; Ward and Brown 1996). Furthermore, it is possible to demonstrate that increased firing of single cells within the caudate, associated with a learned head movement in response to an auditory cue, is context dependent. In other words, caudate cells respond only when the auditory cue elicits a head movement (Gardiner and Kitai 1992). In general, there is overwhelming support that the caudate, and more specifically the lateral caudate, mediates procedural learning, as exemplified by stimulus–response learning, in nonprimates. Even though there are no data on stimulus-response learning in rats following QUIN lesions of the caudate, the above mentioned animal studies suggest a parallel between HD patients' and caudate lesioned rats' procedural memory impairments.

Executive and attentional functions

Patients with HD also demonstrate deficits outside the memory domain. 'Executive function' deficits have long been reported in this disease (Caine et al. 1978; Fedio et al. 1979). In particular, patients with HD consistently perform poorly on tasks that emphasize novel problem solving, planning and concept formation (Brandt and Butters 1986; Lange et al. 1995), e.g. the Wisconsin Card Sorting Test. This test requires subjects to sort cards so that the cards match one of four stimulus cards on one of three predetermined dimensions (the dimension is not explicitly revealed to the subject). The subject must thus deduce from the examiner's feedback about the correctness of each response, the dimension along which cards are to be matched. After a predetermined number of correct sorts, the sorting rule is changed (without explicit instruction to the subject). The subject must shift response strategy based on the examiner's verbal feedback about the correctness of the previous response. On this test, HD patients are often impaired in switching to a new rule once they have established a sorting principle (i.e. they perseverate; Josiassen et al. 1983). Other studies have also demonstrated that HD patients are impaired on tests that

place a heavy emphasis on switching between cognitive sets (Starkstein et al. 1988).

Different components of attention also appear to be affected in patients with HD. For example, these patients often demonstrate impairments on tasks that require mental tracking and manipulation of information, such as serial sevens, mental arithmetic and backward digit span (Folstein et al. 1990; Pillon et al. 1991). HD patients also demonstrate impairments on tasks requiring them to maintain vigilance over extended periods of time, or to divide their attention between different stimuli (Sprengelmeyer et al. 1995b). Certain attentional inhibitory mechanisms are also impaired in this disease (Sprengelmeyer et al. 1995b; Swerdlow et al. 1995). For example, using a task that has been employed extensively in animals, Swerdlow et al. (1995) demonstrated that patients with HD do not show the normal pattern of decreased acoustic or tactile startle response following a prepulse, suggesting that these patients are impaired in sensory–motor gating. Patients with HD do not appear to be impaired in their ability to shift attention between spatial locations, such as on the Posner task (Tsai et al. 1995) or between different levels of visual hierarchical stimuli (Filoteo et al. 1995).

HD patients also show impairments on working-memory tasks (Chapter 8) which require subjects to recall motor-based responses. In a preliminary study, Duncan-Davis et al. (1996) administered tests of spatial and motor working-memory to a small group of HD patients. During the study phase of the spatial memory task, subjects were shown a subset of six stimulus locations (X's) randomly selected from a set of 16 and presented in a sequential manner. In the test phase immediately following the study phase, two stimulus locations (X's) were presented simultaneously. The subject was asked to indicate which location they had seen during the study phase. During the study phase of the motor working-memory task, subjects were shown sequential presentations of six hand positions randomly selected from a set of 16, and they were asked to imitate the hand position. During the test phase, subjects were shown two pictures of different hand positions and were asked to determine which one they had seen in the study phase. The preliminary results of this study are shown in Figure 2. 1. Relative to normal controls, the HD patients were differentially impaired in the motor memory task. Interestingly, a recent study by Pasquier et al. (1994) demonstrated that HD patients were impaired on a task

Figure 2.1. Mean percentage correct for Huntington's disease (HD) patients and control subjects based on working memory tests for hand positions and spatial locations.

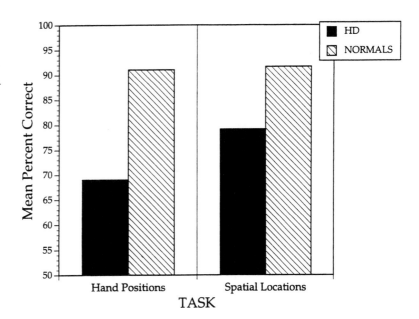

requiring them to recall the spatial displacement of a handle on the apparatus. The results of that study, along with our preliminary findings, suggest that patients with HD are impaired on working-memory tasks, particularly when the task places a heavy demand on motor processes.

Similar patterns of working-memory deficits have also been demonstrated in rats with caudate lesions. For example, electrolytic lesions in the medial caudate impair rats' memory for a specific motor response (right-left turn), but not memory for a visual object or for a spatial location (Kesner et al. 1993). The performances of control and caudate lesioned rats on motor and spatial delayed matching to sample procedures (using short delays (1–4 s) between the study and test phases), are illustrated in Figure 2.2. Caudate lesioned rats were impaired only on the motor delayed matching to sample task. Medial caudate lesions also do not disrupt working memory for eight spatial locations on an eight-arm maze (Cook and Kesner 1988; Colombo et al. 1989). The pattern of greater impairment on motor than spatial working memory tasks in caudate lesioned rats closely parallels that observed by Duncan-Davis et al. (1996) in HD patients.

With respect to the ability to switch strategies, it has been shown that rats with ibotenate lesions of the medial caudate have difficulty in selecting alternative strategies in cue and place water navigation tasks (Whishaw et al. 1987) and in spatial reversal learning (Kolb 1977). These results,

too, are consistent with observed deficits in HD patients (Caine et al. 1978).

To evaluate covert attention in caudate lesioned rats, rats were tested with a Posner paradigm involving the presentation of valid and invalid spatial cues following unilateral, large 6-OHDA lesions of the caudate. The results indicated that these lesions only increased mean reaction times contralateral to the side of the lesion, but the reaction times did not change differentially as a function of the requirements to disengage, maintain or shift attention. Rats following caudate lesions thus appear not to have any deficits in directing attention. Instead, the deficit on the Posner paradigm is probably due to an impairment in motor activity (Ward and Brown 1996). This lack of effect of caudate lesions on rats' covert attention is similar to that reported for HD patients (Filoteo et al. 1995).

In general then, it appears that the medial caudate mediates 'executive' functions as indicated by its involvement in working memory for motor responses and in the selection of alternate strategies. The medial caudate does not, however, mediate covert attentional processes.

Spatial orientation

Patients with HD are also impaired on visual tasks, even when such tasks do not place heavy emphasis on motor responding. For example, patients with HD demonstrate deficits on tests of visual confrontation naming; however,

Figure 2.2. Mean percentage correct performance for caudate lesioned and control rats as a function of 1–4 s delays for memory for a motor response (right/left turn) and memory for a spatial location.

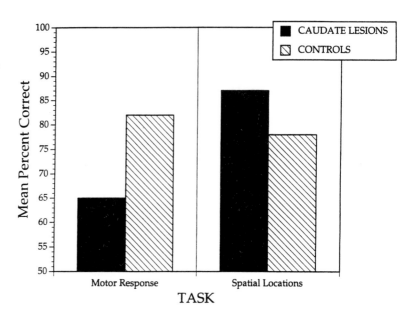

their deficit reflects misperception of the stimuli rather than an impairment in language processes per se (Hodges et al. 1990). Patients with HD are also impaired on tasks requiring the accurate perception of faces (Jacobs et al. 1995) and on numerous other measures which assess visual–spatial information processing (Mohr et al. 1991). Visuoconstructional deficits have also been consistently reported in patients with HD (Rouleau et al. 1992; Phillips et al. 1994), although it is difficult to parse out the differential contributions of visuoperceptual and motor impairments on such tasks.

Several studies have reported an interesting dissociation in HD between performance on egocentric (i.e. how one's own body is oriented in space) and allocentric (i.e. how two objects relate in space) tasks. Specifically, patients with HD tend to be more impaired on tasks that emphasize egocentric as opposed to allocentric orientation. Patients with AD, in contrast, tend to demonstrate the opposite pattern of impairment. For example, Brouwers et al. (1984) found that HD patients were more impaired on a task that required right-left judgments (an egocentric task), than on visuoconstructional tasks (allocentric tasks). Bylsma et al. (1992) found that HD patients were impaired on a right-left judgment task, as well as on a route-walking task.

A comparable pattern of greater egocentric than allocentric task impairments has also been reported in studies of caudate lesioned animals. For example, rats

and monkeys with caudate lesions show deficits on tasks such as delayed response, delayed alternation, and delayed matching to position (Divac et al. 1967; Sanberg et al. 1978; Oberg and Divac 1979; Dunnett 1990). One salient feature of delayed response, delayed alternation and delayed matching to position tasks is the maintenance of spatial orientation to the baited food well relative to the position of the subject's body, i.e. egocentric localization. Similar egocentric spatial orientation problems probably account for the mild deficits observed in caudate lesioned animals on the Morris water maze (Block et al. 1993; Popoli et al. 1994; Furtado and Mazurek 1996).

Rats with caudate lesions are deficient in learning a maze requiring alternate right-left turns, but not a maze not requiring right-left alternations (Borst et al. 1970). Such lesioned animals are also impaired on a radial arm maze task requiring them to find a goal box, the position of which is determined relative to the rat's starting position (Potegal 1982), and on a 'return from passive transport' task. In the latter task rats are tested in a visually homogeneous, octagonal enclosure with a water spout at each corner. The animal is allowed to drink from one spout while confined in an enclosed wagon. The back of the wagon is closed off and the rat is transported away from, and at a right angle to, the goal spout. As the animal must navigate on the basis of vestibular feedback, return within the passive transport task can be considered to be a test of egocentric localization. It should be noted that hippocampal, unlike caudate lesions, do not disrupt performance on this task (Abraham et al. 1983).

In a more explicit test of egocentric localization, Cook and Kesner (1988) placed rats at the end of a randomly selected arm in an eight-arm maze and reinforced them for running to the immediately adjacent right or left arm. No reinforcements were available in the remaining five arms. The animals were allowed only one choice per trial. The same animals were also trained in a different eight-arm maze, using the standard eight-arm maze learning procedure (Olton and Samuelson 1976). After training on both tasks, rats received medial caudate lesions. Two weeks later they were retested for retention of the two tasks. The caudate lesioned rats had no retention of the previously learned 'adjacent arm' egocentric task, i.e. they performed at chance levels. These same animals showed no deficits on the standard eight-arm radial maze task. Similar results have been reported by others (e.g. Colombo et al. 1989).

Wiener (1993) has reported that cells in the caudate increase their firing rates based on a rat's location, heading direction and timing of the initiation and execution of displacement movements within an egocentric space. These data show that the caudate mediates egocentric spatial orientation, which is consistent with the views of Potegal (1982), Kesner and DiMattia (1987) and Robbins and Brown (1990).

There is only a limited set of studies of egocentric spatial orientation in rats with QUIN lesions, but the pattern of results is consistent with that of other animal studies suggesting a role of the caudate in egocentric orientation.

NEUROANATOMICAL CORRELATES OF COGNITIVE DEFICITS

One important consideration in the development of an animal model of HD is the exact neuropathological underpinnings of the cognitive impairment observed in these patients. Given the neuropathological characteristics of HD, many investigators have concluded that the underlying neuropathological correlate of cognitive impairment in this disease is atrophy of the caudate; however, the caudate nucleus has reciprocal connections with frontal lobe structures (Alexander et al. 1986), and many investigators have argued that the cognitive impairment in HD is associated with frontal lobe dysfunction secondary to

caudate atrophy. Although it is difficult to parse out the exact contributions of frontal lobe and caudate pathology to cognitive impairment in this disease, several studies have indicated that caudate abnormalities tend to be more strongly associated with cognitive deficits in these patients than are frontal lobe abnormalities (Starkstein et al. 1988; Weinberger et al. 1988; Bamford et al. 1989). In contrast, the motor deficits in HD tend to be more strongly associated with putaminal abnormalities. These studies indicate that pathology in the caudate nucleus per se may be the most important neuropathological corollary of HD patients' cognitive deficits. As such, these studies provide preliminary support for the utility of animal models that focus on lesioning the caudate nucleus in order to better understand the cognitive deficits seen in patients with HD.

Within the caudate nucleus of the rat there also appears to be some regional specificity with respect to caudate mediated behavioral and cognitive functions. The lateral, but not medial, caudate nucleus receives its major inputs from somatosensory and motor cortex (Wise and Jones 1977; Ebrahami et al. 1992). It is not surprising, then, that the lateral caudate appears to mediate primarily the initiation and programming of motor movements, changes in frequency, duration and amplitude of motor movements, as well as procedural (stimulus–response) learning. The lateral caudate would thus be functionally more related to the putamen in monkeys and humans. In contrast, the medial caudate nucleus receives its major inputs from the medial prefrontal cortex (anterior cingulate, prelimbic and infralimbic cortex). It appears to mediate executive functions including working memory and strategy selection (Groenewegen et al. 1990). The medial caudate would thus be functionally related to dorsolateral prefrontal cortex in monkeys and humans. It is possible, then, that heterogeneity in the locus of caudate pathology, and consequently the behavioral functions affected, is responsible for the variability seen in the symptomatology of individual HD patients.

CONCLUSIONS

Even though cognitive functions in rats are not identical to those in humans, it is remarkable that there are a number of close parallels in caudate mediated cognitive functions as indicated by parallel patterns of dysfunction observed in caudate lesioned rats and in humans with HD. Some of these parallels include similar alterations in motor function, impairments in procedural learning, impairments in executive functions based on working memory and strategy selection, and deficiencies in the use of egocentric space. At the same time there are similarities in residual (preserved) cognitive functions, including working memory for allocentric spatial information and covert attention. The QUIN lesion of the caudate appears to be the best current model to mimic the *pathology* and *biochemistry* of caudate dysfunction in HD. Few studies have evaluated the *behavioral* effects of QUIN caudate lesions in rats. Consequently, there remains a need to examine the behavioral effects of QUIN injections into the lateral and medial caudate in rats in order to model the richness of cognitive deficits seen in HD patients.

REFERENCES

Abraham, L., Potegal, M. and Miller, S. 1983. Evidence for caudate nucleus involvement in an egocentric spatial task: Return from passive transport. *Physiological Psychology*. 11: 11–17.

Albert, M.S., Butters, N. and Brandt, J. 1981. Patterns of remote memory in amnesic and demented patients. *Archives of Neurology*. 38: 495–500.

Alexander, E., DeLong, M.R. and Strick, P.L. 1986. Parallel organization of functionally segregated circuits linking basal ganglia and cortex. *Annual Review of Neuroscience*. 9: 357–381.

Bamford, K.A., Caine, E.D., Kido, D.K., Plassche, W.M. and Shoulson, I. 1989. Clinical-pathologic correlation in Huntington's disease: A neuropsychological and computed tomography study. *Neurology*. 39: 796–801.

Beal, M.F. 1994. Huntington's disease. In *Neurodegenerative diseases*, ed. G. Jolles and J. M. Stutzmann, pp. 169–181. New York: Academic Press.

Beal, M.F., Ellison, D.W., Mazurek, M.I., Swartz, K.J., Malloy, J.R., Bird, E.D. and Martin, J.B. 1988a. A detailed examination of substance P in pathologically graded cases of Huntington's disease. *Journal of Neurological Science*. 84: 51–61.

Beal, M.F., Kowall, N.W., Ellison, D.W., Mazurek, M.F., Swartz, K.J. and Martin, J.B. 1986. Replication of the neurochemical characteristics of Huntington's disease by quinolinic acid. *Nature*. 321: 168–171.

Beal, M.F., Mazurek, M.F., Ellison, D.W. Swartz, K.J., McGarvey, U., Bird, E.D. and Martin, J.B. 1988b. Somatostatin and neuropeptide Y concentrations in pathologically graded cases of Huntington's disease. *Annals of Neurology*. 20: 489–495.

Beatty, W.W., Salmon, D.P., Butters, N., Heindel, W.C. and Granholm, E.L. 1988. Retrograde amnesia in patients with Alzheimer's or Huntington's disease. *Neurobiology of Aging*. 9: 181–186.

Bird, E.D., Mackay, A.V.P., Rayner, C.N. and Iversen, L.L. 1973. Reduced glutamic-acid-decarboxylase activity of post-mortem brain in Huntington's chorea. *Lancet*. 1: 1090–1092.

Block, F., Kunkel, M. and Schwarz, M. 1993. Quinolinic acid lesion of the striatum induces impairment in spatial learning and motor performance in rats. *Neuroscience Letters*. 149: 126–128.

Borst, A., Delacour, J. and Libauban, S. 1970. Effets chez le rat de lesions du noyau caude sur le conditionnement de reponse alternee. *Neuropsychologia*. 8: 89–102.

Bradshaw, J.L., Phillips, J.G., Dennis, C., Mattingley, J.S., Andrewes, D., Chiu, E., Pierson, J. M. and Bradshaw, J.A. 1992. Initiation and execution of movement sequences in those suffering from and at-risk of developing Huntington's disease. *Journal of Clinical and Experimental Neuropsychology*. 14: 179–192.

Brandt, J. and Butters, N. 1986. The neuropsychology of Huntington's disease. *Trends in Neurosciences*. 9: 118–120.

Brouwers, P., Cox, C., Martin, A., Chase, T. and Fedio, P. 1984. Differential perceptual-spatial impairment in Huntington's and Alzheimer's dementias. *Archives of Neurology* 41: 1073–1076.

Butters, N. Salmon, D.P., Cullum, C.M., Cairns, P., Tröster, A.I., Jacobs, D., Moss, M. and Cermak, L.S. 1988. Differentiation of amnesic and demented patients with the Wechsler Memory Scale - Revised. *The Clinical Neuropsychologist*. 2: 133–148.

Butters, N., Wolfe, J., Granholm, E. and Martone, M. 1986. An assessment of verbal recall, recognition and fluency abilities in patients with Huntington's disease. *Cortex*. 22: 11–22.

Butters, N., Wolfe, J., Martone, M., Granholm, E. and Cermak, L.S. 1985. Memory disorders associated with Huntington's disease: Verbal recall, verbal recognition, and procedural memory. *Neuropsychologia*. 23: 729–743.

Bylsma, F.W., Brandt, J. and Strauss, M.E. 1992. Personal and extrapersonal orientation in Huntington's disease and those at risk. *Cortex*. 28: 113–122.

Bylsma, F.W., Rebok, G.W. and Brandt, J. 1991. Long-term retention of implicit learning in Huntington's disease. *Neuropsychologia*. 29: 1213–1221.

Caine, E.D., Hunt, R.D., Weingartner, H. and Ebert, M.H. 1978. Huntington's dementia: Clinical and neuropsychological features. *Archives of General Psychiatry*. 35: 377–384.

Cala, L.A., Black, J.L., Collins, D.W., Ellison, R.M. and Zubrick, S.A. 1990. Thirteen years longitudinal study of computed tomography, visual electrophysiology and neuropsychological changes in Huntington's chorea patients and 50% at-risk asymptomatic subjects. *Clinical and Experimental Neurology*. 27: 43–63.

Colombo, P.J., Davis, H.P. and Volpe, B.T. 1989. Allocentric spatial and tactile memory impairments in rats with dorsal caudate lesions are affected by preoperative behavioral training. *Behavioral Neuroscience*. 103: 1242–1250.

Cook, D. and Kesner, R.P. 1988. Caudate nucleus and memory for egocentric localization. *Behavioral and Neural Biology*. 49: 332–343.

Coyle, J. T. and Schwarcz, R. 1976. Lesion of striatal neurones with kainic acid provides a model for Huntington's chorea. *Nature*. 263: 244–246.

Cummings, J.L. and Benson, D.F. 1992. *Dementia: A clinical approach*. Stoneham, MA: Butterworth-Heinemann.

Davies, S.W. and Roberts, P.J. 1987. No evidence for preservation of somatostatin-containing neurons after intrastriatal injections of quinolinic acid. *Nature*. 327: 326.

Delis, D.C., Massman, P.J., Butters, N., Salmon, D.P., Cermak, L.S. and Kramer, J.H. 1991. Profiles of demented and amnesic patients on the California Verbal Learning Test: Implications for the assessment of memory disorders. *Psychological Assessment*. 3: 19–26.

De La Monte, S.M., Vonsattel, J.P. and Richardson, E.P. 1988. Morphometric demonstration of atrophic changes in the cerebral cortex, white matter and neostriatum in Huntington's disease. *Journal of Neuropathology and Experimental Neurology*. 47: 516–525.

Divac, I., Rosvold, H.E. and Szwarcbart, M.K. 1967. Behavioral effects of selective ablation of the caudate nucleus. *Journal of Comparative and Physiological Psychology*. 63: 184–190.

Duncan-Davis, J., Filoteo, V. and Kesner, R. 1996. *Memory impairment for spatial location and motor movements in patients with Huntington's disease*. Paper presented at the annual meeting of the Cognitive Neuroscience Society, San Francisco, March 31–April 2, 1996.

Dunnett, S.B. 1990. Role of prefrontal cortex and striatal output systems in short-term memory deficits associated with ageing, basal forebrain lesions, and cholinergic-rich grafts. *Canadian Journal of Psychology*. 44: 210–232.

Ebrahimi, A., Pochet, R. and Roger, M. 1992. Topographical organization of the projections from physiologically identified areas of the motor cortex to the striatum in the rat. *Neuroscience Research*. 14: 39–60.

Fedio, P., Cox, C.S., Neophytides, A., Canal-Frederick, G. and Chase, T.N. 1979. Neuropsychological profile of Huntington's disease: Patients and those at risk. In *Advances in neurology*, vol. 23, ed. T. N. Chase, N. S. Wexler, and A. Barbeau, pp. 239–271. New York: Raven Press.

Ferrante, R.J., Kowall, N.W., Beal, M.F., Martin, J.B., Bird E.D. and Richardson, E.P. 1987. Morphologic and histochemical characteristics of a spared subset of striatal neurons in Huntington's disease. *Journal of Neuropathology and Experimental Neurology*. 46: 12–27.

Filoteo, J.V., Delis, D.C., Roman, M.J., Demadura, T., Ford, E., Butters, N., Salmon, D.P., Paulsen, J., Shults, C.W., Swenson, M. and Swerdlow, N. 1995. Visual attention and perception in patients with Huntington's disease: Comparisons with other subcortical and cortical dementias. *Journal of Clinical and Experimental Neuropsychology*. 17: 654–667.

Folstein, S.E., Brandt, J. and Folstein, M.F. 1990. Huntington's disease. In *Subcortical dementia*, ed. J. L. Cummings, pp. 87–107. New York: Oxford University Press.

Forno, L.S. and Jose, C. 1973. Huntington's chorea: A pathological study. In *Advances in neurology*, vol. 1, ed. A. Barbeau, T. N. Chase and G. W. Paulson, pp. 453–470. New York: Raven Press.

Foster, A.C., Collins, J.F. and Schwarcz, R. 1983. On the excitotoxic properties of quinolinic acid, 2,3-piperidine dicarboxylic acids and structurally related compounds. *Neuropharmacology*. 22: 1331–1342.

Furtado, J.C.S. and Mazurek, M.F. 1996. Behavioral characterization of quinolinate-induced lesions of the medial striatum: Relevance for Huntington's disease. *Experimental Neurology*. 138: 158–168.

Gardiner, T.W. and Kitai, S.T. 1992. Single-unit activity in the globus pallidus and neostriatum of the rat during performance of a trained head movement. *Experimental Brain Research*. 88: 517–530.

Girotti, F., Marano, R., Soliveri, P., Geminiani, G. and Scigliano, G. 1988. Relationship between motor and cognitive deficits in Huntington's disease. *Journal of Neurology*. 235: 454–457.

Graveland, G.A., Williams, R.S. and DiFiglia, M. 1985. Evidence for degenerative and regenerative changes in neostriatal spiny neurons in Huntington's disease. *Science*. 227: 770–773.

Greenamyre, J.T. and Young, A.B. 1989. Synaptic localization of striatal NMDA, quisqualate and kainate receptors. *Neuroscience Letters*. 101: 133–137.

Groenewegen, H.J., Berendse, H.W., Wolters, J.G. and Lohman, A.H.M. 1990. The anatomical relationship of the prefrontal cortex with the striatopallidal system, the thalamus and the amygdala: Evidence for a parallel organization. *Progress in Brain Research*. 85: 95–118.

Hansing, R.A., Schwartzbaum, J.S. and Thompson, J.B. 1967. Operant behavior following unilateral and bilateral caudate lesions in the rat. *Journal of Comparative and Physiological Psychology*. 66: 378–388.

Heindel, W.C., Salmon, D.P. and Butters, N. 1990. Pictorial priming and cued recall in Alzheimer's and Huntington's disease. *Brain and Cognition*. 13: 282–295.

Heindel, W.C., Salmon, D.P. and Butters, N. 1991. The biasing of weight judgment in Alzheimer's and Huntington's disease: A priming or programming phenomenon? *Journal of Clinical and Experimental Neuropsychology*. 13: 189–203.

Heindel, W.C., Salmon, D.P. and Butters, N. 1993. Cognitive approaches to the memory disorders of demented patients. In *Comprehensive Handbook of Psychopathology*, 2nd ed., ed. P. B. Sutker and H. E. Adams, pp. 735–761. New York: Plenum Press.

Heindel, W.C., Salmon, D.P., Shults, C.W., Walicke, P.A. and Butters, N. 1989. Neuropsychological evidence for multiple implicit memory systems: A comparison of Alzheimer's, Huntington's and Parkinson's disease patients. *Journal of Neuroscience*. 9: 582–587.

Hodges, J.R., Salmon, D.P. and Butters, N. 1990. The nature of the naming deficit in patients with Alzheimer's and Huntington's disease. *Brain*. 114: 1547–1558.

Jacobs, D., Shuyren, J. and Heilman, K.M. 1995. Impaired perception of facial identity and facial affect in Huntington's disease. *Neurology*. 45: 1217–1218.

Josiassen, R.C., Curry, L.M. and Mancall, E.L. 1983. Development of neuropsychological deficits in Huntington's disease. *Archives of Neurology*. 40: 791–796.

Kesner, R., Bolland, B.L. and Dakis, M. 1993. Memory for spatial locations, motor responses, and objects: Triple dissociation among the hippocampus, caudate nucleus, and extrastriate visual cortex. *Experimental Brain Research*. 93: 462–470.

Kesner, R.P. and DiMattia, B.V. 1987. Neurobiology of an attribute model of memory. *Progress in Psychobiology and Physiological Psychology*. 12: 207–277.

Kirkby, R.J., Polgar, S. and Coyle, I.R. 1981. Caudate nucleus lesions impair the ability of rats to learn a simple straight-alley task. *Perception and Motor Skills*. 52: 499–502.

Knopman, D. and Nissen, M.J. 1991. Procedural learning is impaired in Huntington's disease: Evidence from the serial reaction time task. *Neuropsychologia*. 29: 245–254.

Kolb, B. 1977. Studies of the caudate-putamen and dorsomedial thalamic nucleus of the rat: Implications for mammalian frontal-functions. *Physiology and Behavior*. 18: 237–244.

Kowall, N.W., Ferrante, R.J. and Martin, J.B. 1987. Neuropathology of Huntington's disease – reply. *Trends in Neurosciences*. 10: 404–406.

Kuhl, D.E., Phelps, M.E., Markham, C.H., Metter, E.J., Riege, W.H. and Winter, J. 1982. Cerebral metabolism and atrophy in Huntington's disease determined by 18FDG and computed tomographic scan. *Annals of Neurology*. 12: 425–434.

Lange, K.W., Sahakian, B.J., Quinn, N.P., Marsden, C.D. and Robbins, T.W. 1995. Comparison of executive and visuospatial memory function in Huntington's disease and dementia of the Alzheimer type matched for degree of dementia. *Journal of Neurology, Neurosurgery and Psychiatry*. 58: 598–606.

Martone, M., Butters, N., Payne, M., Becker, J. and Sax, D.S. 1984. Dissociations between skill learning and verbal recognition in amnesia and dementia. *Archives of Neurology*. 41: 965–970.

Massman, P.J., Delis, D.C., Butters, N., Levin, B.E. and Salmon, D.P. 1990. Are all subcortical dementias alike? Verbal learning and memory in Parkinson's and Huntington's disease patients. *Journal of Clinical and Experimental Neuropsychology*. 12: 729–744.

McDonald, R.J. and White, N.M. 1993. A triple dissociation of memory systems: Hippocampus, amygdala and dorsal striatum. *Behavioral Neuroscience*. 107: 3–22.

McGeer, E.G. and McGeer, P.L. 1976. Duplication of biochemical glutamic and kainic acids. *Nature*. 263: 517–519

McGeer, P.L., McGeer, E. and Fibiger, H.C. 1973. Choline acetylase and glutamic acid decarboxylase in Huntington's chorea. *Neurology*. 23: 912–917.

McHugh, P.R. and Folstein, M.F. 1975. Psychiatric syndromes of Huntington's chorea. In *Psychiatric aspects of neurological disease*, ed. D.F. Benson and D. Blumer, pp. 267–286. New York: Grune & Stratton.

Mendez, M.F. 1994. Huntington's disease: Update and review of neuropsychiatric characteristics. *International Journal of Psychiatry and Medicine*. 24: 189–208.

Mishkin, M. 1982. A memory system in the monkey. *Philosophical Transactions of the Royal Society, London B*. 298: 85–95.

Mishkin, M. and Petri, H.L. 1984. Memories and habits: Some implications for the analysis of learning and retention. In *Neuropsychology of memory*, ed. L.R. Squire and N. Butters, pp. 287–296. New York: Guilford Press.

Mohr, E., Brouwers, P., Claus, J.J., Mann, U.M., Fedio, P. and Chase, T.N. 1991. Visuospatial cognition in Huntington's disease. *Movement Disorders*. 6: 127–132.

Morris, M. 1995. Dementia and cognitive changes in Huntington's disease. In *Advances in neurology*, vol. 65, ed. W.J. Weiner and A.E. Lang, pp. 187–199. New York: Raven Press.

Oberg, R.G.E. and Divac, I. 1979. 'Cognitive' functions of the neostriatum. In *The neostriatum*, ed. I. Divac and R.G E. Oberg, pp. 291–313. Oxford: Pergamon.

Olton, D.S. and Samuelson, R.J. 1976. Remembrance of places passed: Spatial memory in rats. *Journal of Experimental Psychology*. 2: 97–116.

Packard, M.G. and White, N.M. 1990. Lesions of the caudate nucleus selectively impair 'Reference Memory' acquisition in the radial maze. *Behavioral and Neural Biology*. 53: 39–50.

Pasquier, F., Van Der Linden, M., Lefebvre, V., Lefebvre, C., Bruyer, R. and Petit, H. 1994. Motor memory and the preselection effect in Huntington's and Parkinson's disease. *Neuropsychologia*. 32: 951–968.

Paulsen, J.S., Butters, N., Salmon, D.P., Heindel, W.C. and Swenson, M.R. 1993. Prism adaptation in Alzheimer's and Huntington's disease. *Neuropsychology*. 7: 73–81.

Perry, T.L. and Hansen, S. 1990. What excitotoxin kills striatal neurons in Huntington's disease: Clues from neurochemical studies. *Neurology*. 40: 20–27.

Phillips, A.G. and Carr, G.D. 1987. Cognition and the basal ganglia: A possible substrate for procedural knowledge. *Canadian Journal of Neurological Science*. 14: 381–385.

Phillips, J.G., Bradshaw, J.L., Chiu, E. and Bradshaw, J. A. 1994. Characteristics of handwriting of patients with Huntington's disease. *Movement Disorders*. 5: 521–530.

Pillon, B., Dubois, B., Ploska, A. and Agid, Y. 1991. Severity and specificity of cognitive impairment in Alzheimer's, Huntington's and Parkinson's diseases and progressive supranuclear palsy. *Neurology*. 41: 634–642.

Pisa, M. 1988. Motor functions of the striatum in the rat: Critical role of the lateral region in tongue and forelimb reaching. *Neuroscience*. 24: 453–463.

Pisa, M. and Cyr, J. 1990. Regionally selective roles of the rat's striatum in modality-specific discrimination learning and forelimb reaching. *Behavioral Brain Research*. 37: 281–292.

Popoli, P., Pezzola, A., Domenici, M.R., Sagratella, S., Diana, G., Caporali, M.G., Bronzetti, E., Vega, J. and De Carolis, A.S. 1994. Behavioral and electrophysiological correlates of the quinolinic acid rat model of Huntington's disease in rats. *Brain Research Bulletin*. 35: 329–335.

Potegal, M. 1982. Vestibular and neostriatal contributions to spatial orientation. In *Spatial abilities: Development and physiological foundations*, ed. M. Potegal, pp. 361–387. New York: Academic Press.

Powell, D.A., Mankowski, D. and Buchanan, S.L. 1978. Concomitant heart rate and corneoretinal potential conditioning in the rabbit (Oryctolagus cuniculus): Effects of caudate lesions. *Physiology and Behavior*. 20: 143–150.

Reading, P.J., Dunnett, S.B. and Robbins, T.W. 1991. Dissociable roles of the ventral, medial and lateral striatum on the acquisition and performance of a complex visual stimulus-response habit. *Behavioral Brain Research*. 45: 147–161.

Robbins, T.W. and Brown, V.J. 1990. The role of the striatum in the mental chronometry of action: A theoretical review. *Reviews of Neuroscience*. 2: 81–213.

Rouleau, I., Salmon, D.P., Butters, N., Kennedy, C. and McGuire K. 1992. Quantitative and qualitative analyses of clock drawings in Alzheimer's and Huntington's disease. *Brain and Cognition*. 18: 70–87.

Saint-Cyr, J.A. and Taylor, A.E. 1992. The mobilization of procedural learning: The 'key signature' of the basal ganglia. In *Neuropsychology of memory*, 2nd ed., ed. L. R. Squire and N. Butters, pp. 188–210. New York: Guilford Press.

Salmon, D.P., Shimamura, A.P., Butters, N. and Smith, S. 1988. Lexical and semantic priming deficits in patients with Alzheimer's disease. *Journal of Clinical and Experimental Neuropsychology*. 10: 477–494.

Sanberg, P.R., Calderon, S.F., Giordano, M., Twe, J.M. and Norman, A.B. 1989. The quinolinic acid model of Huntington's disease: Locomotor abnormalities. *Experimental Neurology*. 105: 45–53.

Sanberg, P. R., Lehmann, J. and Fibiger, H. C. 1978. Impaired learning and memory after kainic acid lesions of the striatum: A behavioral model of Huntington's disease. *Brain Research*. 149: 546–551.

Schwarcz, R., Okuno, E., Speciale, C. Kohler, C. and Whetsell, W.O., Jr. 1987. Neuronal degeneration in animals and man: The quinolinic acid connection. In *Neurotoxins and their pharmacological implications*, ed. P.G. Jenner, pp. 19–33. New York: Raven Press.

Schwarcz, R., Whetsell, W.O., Jr. and Mangano, R.M. 1983. Quinolinic acid: An endogenous metabolite that produces axon-sparing lesions in rat brain. *Science*. 219: 316.

Schwartzbaum, J.S. and Donovick, P.J. 1968. Discrimination reversal and spatial alternation associated with septal and caudate dysfunction in rats. *Journal of Comparative and Physiological Psychology*. 65: 83–92.

Shimamura, A.P., Salmon, D.P., Squire, L.R. and Butters, N. 1987. Memory dysfunction and word priming in dementia and amnesia. *Behavioral Neuroscience*. 101: 347–351.

Sprengelmeyer, R., Canavan, A.G.M., Lange, H.W. and Homberg, V. 1995a. Associative learning in degenerative neostriatal disorders: Contrasts in explicit and implicit remembering between Parkinson's and Huntington's diseases. *Movement Disorders*. 10: 51–65.

Sprengelmeyer, R., Lange, H. and Homberg, V. 1995b. The pattern of attentional deficits in Huntington's disease. *Brain*. 118: 145–152.

Stahl, W.L. and Swanson, P.D. 1974. Biochemical abnormalities in Huntington's chorea brains. *Neurology*. 24: 813–819.

Starkstein, S.E., Brandt, J., Folstein, S., Strauss, M., Berthier, M.L., Pearlson, G.D., Wong, D., McDonnell, A. and Folstein, M. 1988. Neuropsychological and neuroradiological correlates of Huntington's disease. *Journal of Neurology, Neurosurgery and Psychiatry*. 51: 1259–1263.

Swerdlow, N.R., Paulsen, J., Braff, D.L., Butters, N., Geyer, M.A. and Swenson, M.R. 1995. Impaired prepulse inhibition of acoustic and tactile startle response in patients with Huntington's disease. *Journal of Neurology, Neurosurgery and Psychiatry*. 58: 192–200.

Tröster, A.I., Butters, N., Salmon, D.P., Cullum, C.M., Jacobs, D., Brandt, J. and White, R.F. 1993. The diagnostic utility of savings scores: Differentiating Alzheimer's and Huntington's diseases with the Logical Memory and Visual Reproduction Tests. *Journal of Clinical and Experimental Neuropsychology*. 15: 773–788.

Tsai, T.T., Lasker, A. and Zee, D.S. 1995. Visual attention in Huntington's disease: The effect of cueing on saccade latencies and manual reaction times. *Neuropsychologia*. 33: 1617–1626.

Vonsattel, J.P., Myers, R.H., Stevens, T.J., Ferrante, R.J., Bird, E.D. and Richardson, E.P. 1985. Neuropathological classification of Huntington's disease. *Journal of Neuropathology and Experimental Neurology*. 44: 559–577.

Wang, J., Aigner T. and Mishkin M. 1990. Effects of neostriatal lesions on visual habit formation in rhesus monkeys. *Society of Neuroscience Abstracts*. 16: 617.

Ward, N.M. and Brown, V.J. 1996. Covert orienting of attention in the rat and the role of striatal dopamine. *Journal of Neuroscience*. 16: 3082–3088.

Weinberger, D., Berman, K.F., Iadorola, M., Driesen, A. and Zec, R.F. 1988. Prefrontal cortical blood flow and cognitive function in Huntington's disease. *Journal of Neurology, Neurosurgery and Psychiatry*. 51: 94–104.

Whishaw, I.Q., Mittleman, G., Bunch, S.T. and Dunnett, S.B. 1987. Impairments in the acquisition, retention and selection of spatial navigation strategies after medial caudate-putamen lesions in rats. *Behavioral Brain Research*. 24: 125–138.

Whishaw, I.Q., O'Connor, W.T. and Dunnett, S.B. 1986. The contributions of motor cortex, nigrostriatal dopamine and caudate-putamen to skilled forelimb use in the rat. *Brain*. 109: 805–843.

Wiener, S.I. 1993. Spatial and behavioral correlates of striatal neurons in rats performing a self-initiated navigation task. *Journal of Neuroscience*. 13: 3802–3817.

Wise, S.P. and Jones, E.G. 1977. Cells of origin and terminal distribution of descending projections of the rat somatic sensory cortex. *Journal of Comparative Neurology*. 175: 129–158.

Wolfensberger, M., Amsler, U., Cuenod, M., Foster, A.C., Whetsell, W.O., Jr. and Schwarcz, R. 1983. Identification of quinolinic acid in rat and human brain tissue. *Neuroscience Letters*. 41: 247–252.

Wu, J.Y., Bird, E.D., Chen, M.S. and Huang, W. M. 1979. Studies of neurotransmitter enzymes in Huntington's chorea. In *Advances in neurology*, vol. 23, ed. T.N. Chase, N.S. Wexler and A. Barbeau, pp. 527–536. New York: Raven Press.

3 Neuropathology and memory dysfunction in neurodegenerative disease

JULIE A. TESTA, ROGER A. BRUMBACK, TAI-KYOUNG BAIK, RICHARD W. LEECH AND THOMAS C. CANNON

INTRODUCTION TO DEMENTIA

Research in the field of dementia has increased exponentially over the last 30 years, leading to a wealth of information on the epidemiology, psychology, neuropathology, biochemistry and genetics of Alzheimer's, Parkinson's and other neurodegenerative diseases. Interdisciplinary approaches have begun to combine the information gathered from the various fields of study into theories regarding the etiology, prevention and treatment of these disorders. This chapter will focus on the neuropathology of several neurodegenerative diseases, including Alzheimer's disease, Parkinson's disease and progressive supranuclear palsy, diffuse Lewy body disease, Huntington's disease, corticobasal degeneration, Pick's disease and prion disease. Vascular dementia is beyond the scope of this chapter and will not be discussed. The currently known neuropathological changes will be discussed in relation to the cognitive impairments of each neurodegenerative disease. Clinical and neuropathological criteria for the various neurodegenerative diseases are presented in Tables 3.1 and 3.2.

Due to the considerable overlap of clinical and neuropathological symptoms among neurodegenerative diseases, guidelines have been published to aid in the collection of information important for an accurate diagnosis. The American Academy of Neurology has recommended the following diagnostic tests be performed on patients with dementia to rule-out potentially treatable disorders: complete blood cell count, serum electrolytes, serum glucose, blood urea nitrogen, serum creatinine, liver function tests, syphilis serology and serum vitamin B_{12} level (Lanska 1996). Although in most clinical settings, detailed medical and neuropsychological information is often not gathered on each patient, collection of such data in research programs is important for providing clues to the causes and progression of various types of dementia.

ALZHEIMER'S DISEASE

Alzheimer's disease (AD) is the leading cause of dementia, comprising more than 50% of all cases (Tomlinson et al. 1970), and will continue to be a major health care problem in the twenty-first century due to the increased number of individuals living beyond 65 years of age. The prevalence of dementia increases exponentially with age, doubling in frequency every 5 years for individuals between the ages of 65 and 85 years (Katzman and Kawas 1994). Approximately 10% of individuals over the age of 65 years are diagnosed with AD, with an age-related prevalence ranging from 3% among individuals 65–74 years, to 19% among individuals 75–84 years and 47% among individuals older than 85 years (Bachman et al. 1993) (Figure 3.1). Hereditary factors play a role in the predisposition to this disease. Genes on four different chromosomes have been identified but the exact interrelationship between the genetic predisposition and nongenetic factors is not yet clear (Levy-Lahad and Bird 1996).

The recent literature has focused on cognitive impairments associated with AD and the underlying patho-

Table 3.1. *Neuropathological criteria for neurodegenerative diseases*

Alzheimer's disease (Khachaturian, 1985; Mirra et al. 1991, 1993)

A. Age-related plaque score derived from frequency of neuritic plaques in sections of frontal, temporal, or parietal cortex and patient's age at time of death. Neurofibrillary tangles are not required for diagnosis.

| Age of Patient at time of death | Age-related plaque score | | | |
	None	Sparse	Moderate	Frequent
<50 years	0	C	C	C
50–75 years	0	B	C	C
>75 years	0	A	B	C

B. Neuropathological criteria for diagnosis of Alzheimer's disease:

Definite='C' age-related plaque score *and* clinical history of dementia *and* presence or absence of other neuropathological lesions likely to cause dementia;

Probable='B' age-related plaque score *and* clinical history of dementia *and* presence or absence of other neuropathological lesions likely to cause dementia;

Possible='A' age-related plaque score *and* clinical history of dementia *and* presence or absence of other neuropathological lesions likely to cause dementia; or, 'B' or 'C' age-related plaque score and absence of clinical manifestations of dementia

Parkinson's disease (Gibb, 1992)

A. Nerve cell loss in the substantia nigra pars compacta with associated Lewy bodies

B. Additional nerve cell loss in locus ceruleus, ventral tegmental area, nucleus basalis of Meynert, raphe nucleus and thalamus

Huntington's disease (Vonsattel et al. 1985)

Degree of neuropathological involvement of striatum is graded on a five-point scale:

Grade 0: No discernible gross or microscopic abnormalities characteristic of Huntington's disease

Grade 1: No macroscopic abnormalities; microscopic mild neuronal cell loss and astrocytic gliosis in paraventricular region of caudate nucleus and dorsal region of putamen

Grade 2: Macroscopic evidence of caudate atrophy; microscopic mild neuronal loss and reactive astrocytosis

Grade 3: Macroscopic appearance of the ventricular outline of the head of the caudate nucleus is a straight line; microscopic evidence of moderate, diffuse cell loss and gliosis throughout caudate nucleus

Grade 4: Caudate nucleus appears severely shrunken, and the putamen and internal capsule are also atrophic; microscopic evidence shows nerve cell depletion and fibrillary astrocytosis throughout the caudate nucleus and putamen

Diffuse Lewy body disease (McKeith et al. 1996)

Essential for diagnosis: Cortical and brainstem Lewy bodies (substantia nigra or locus ceruleus)

Associated but not essential for diagnosis: Lewy body-related neurites, plaques, neurofibrillary tangles, regional neuronal loss (mainly brain stem and nucleus basalis of Meynert), microvacuolation and synapse loss, and neurochemical abnormalities and neurotransmitter deficits

Pick's disease (Litvan et al. 1996b)

Lobar atrophy of the frontal and anterior temporal lobes, with Pick argyrophilic inclusions (Pick bodies), and occasionally atrophy of the caudate nucleus, pallidum, basal ganglia or substantia nigra

Other lesions include balloon cells (Pick cells), massive neuronal loss, astrogliosis and spongiosis

Clinical history compatible with Pick's disease

Corticobasal degeneration (Litvan et al. 1996b)

A. Circumscribed or lobar atrophy in parietal or frontoparietal areas

B. Tau-positive neurons in the cerebral cortex; swollen and achromatic neurons, basophilic inclusions, numerous neuropil threads, and severe neuronal loss in the substantia nigra, basal ganglia or dentatorubrothalamic tract

C. Astrogliosis and spongiosis in subcortical white matter

Progressive supranuclear palsy (Hauw et al. 1994)

Numerous neurofibrillary tangles and/or neuropil threads in the basal ganglia and brainstem:

1) Two or more neurons with neurofibrillary tangles or neuropil threads must be found in the same field in at least three of the following brain areas: pallidum, subthalamic nucleus, substantia nigra, and pons; and

2) One or more neurons with neurofibrillary tangles or neuropil threads must be found in the same field in at least three of the following brain areas: striatum, oculomotor complex, medulla and dentate nucleus

Human prion diseases (Budka et al. 1995)

Creutzfeldt – Jakob disease (sporadic, iatrogenic, or familial):

1) Spongiform encephalopathy in cerebral and/or cerebellar cortex and/or subcortical gray matter; and/or

2) Encephalopathy with PrP^{Sc} immunoreactivity (plaques and/or diffuse synaptic and/or patchy/perivacuolar types)

Gerstmann–Sträussler–Scheinker disease (in family with dominantly inherited progressive ataxia and/or dementia): Encephalo(myelo)pathy with multicentric PrP^{Sc} plaques

Familial fatal insomnia (in family with PRNP^{178} mutation): thalamic degeneration, with focal cerebral spongiform change

Kuru (in the Fore population)

Table 3.2. *Criteria for clinical diagnosis of Alzheimer's disease*

American Psychiatric Association (DSM-IV)	NINCDS-ADRDA
I. The development of multiple cognitive deficits manifested by both: 1) memory impairment (impaired ability to learn new information or recall previously learned information) 2) one (or more) of the following cognitive disturbances: • aphasia (language disturbance) • apraxia (impaired ability to carry out motor activities despite intact motor function) • agnosia (failure to recognize or identify objects despite intact sensory function) • disturbance in executive functioning (i.e. planning, organizing, sequencing, abstracting)	I. The criteria for the clinical diagnosis of PROBABLE Alzheimer's disease include: • dementia established by clinical examination and documentation by the Mini-Mental State Exam, Blessed Dementia Scale, or some similar examination, and confirmed by neuropsychological tests; • deficits in two or more areas of cognition; • progressive worsening of memory and other cognitive functions; • no disturbance of consciousness; • onset between ages 40 and 90, most often age 65 years; and • absence of systemic disorders or other brain diseases that in and of themselves could account for the progressive deficits in memory and cognition
II. The cognitive deficits in Criteria I.1 and I.2 cause significant impairment in social or occupational functioning and represent a significant decline from a previous level of functioning	
III. The course is characterized by gradual onset and continuing cognitive decline	II. Clinical diagnosis of POSSIBLE Alzheimer's disease: • may be made on the basis of the dementia syndrome, in the absence of other neurological, psychiatric, or systemic disorders sufficient to cause dementia, and in the presence of variations in the onset, in the presentation, or clinical course; • may be made in the presence of a second systemic or brain disorder sufficient to produce dementia, which is not considered to be the cause of the dementia; and • should be used in research studies when a single, gradually progressive severe cognitive deficit is identified in the absence of other identifiable causes
IV. The cognitive deficits in Criteria I.1 and I.2 are not due to any of the following: • other central nervous system conditions that cause progressive deficits in memory and cognition • systemic conditions that are known to cause dementia • substance-induced conditions	
V. The deficits do not occur exclusively during the course of a delirium	III. Criteria for diagnosis of DEFINITE Alzheimer's disease include: • the clinical criteria for probable Alzheimer's disease and • histopathological evidence obtained from a biopsy or autopsy
VI. The disturbance is not better accounted for by another Axis I disorder	

Source: Adapted from American Psychiatric Association 1994.

physiological changes. It is first necessary to understand the pathological changes which occur in AD and other dementias prior to making assumptions regarding the correlation of pathology with cognitive impairment. Furthermore, because most dementias afflict individuals after the age of 60 years, the changes which occur with normal aging are additive to changes attributable to any neurodegenerative disorder (Terry et al. 1994). Changes in both verbal and nonverbal memory occur in healthy elderly people. Age-related losses are greater in magnitude if memory is tested with recall procedures than on recognition tests. Verbal memory changes with normal aging pos-

sibly correlate with the observed age-related reduction in size of the hippocampus and surrounding medial temporal lobe (Golomb et al. 1993). The pattern of memory loss in AD patients is similar to that of normal aging, but the severity of loss is much greater in AD and the deficits are almost as severe with recognition as with recall tests (Janowsky et al. 1996).

Brain imaging and autopsy studies of normal elderly individuals have demonstrated only minimal cerebral atrophy; however, by the time an individual reaches the age of 60 years, up to 30% of central nervous system neurons can be lost as a normal process of aging (Terry et al. 1987).

Figure 3.1. Estimated prevalence of Alzheimer's disease by decades for the century and a half from 1900 to 2050, calculated from United States census data and epidemiological studies of Alzheimer's disease. Adapted from R.A. Brumback and R.W. Leech, 1994, with permission.

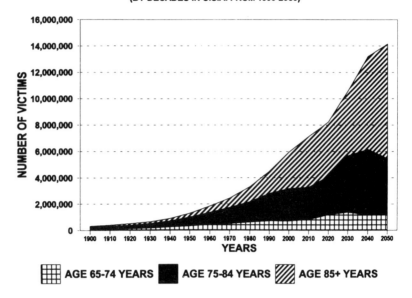

PREVALENCE OF ALZHEIMER'S DISEASE
(BY DECADES IN U.S.A. FROM 1900-2050)

Marked neurological or neuropsychological deficits usually do not become apparent until a large percentage of neurons in a particular area are destroyed (more than the safety margin for neuronal function), thus the normal age-related loss is not clinically apparent (Brumback and Leech 1994).

Neuropathology of Alzheimer's disease

Thus far, histopathological confirmation is the only method of definitively establishing the diagnosis of AD. In AD, neuronal death is accelerated in association with the appearance of amyloid plaques and neurofibrillary changes (Terry et al. 1991) (Figure 3.2).

Pathological criteria for the diagnosis of AD have been published by Khachaturian (1985) and Mirra et al. (1993). These diagnostic criteria only take into account the neuritic plaques, ignoring the neurofibrillary tangles which can also be found in other neurodegenerative diseases. The pathological criteria for AD contain an age factor, i.e. more plaques are necessary to make the diagnosis in older individuals. Thus, these criteria adhere to the concept that plaque formation is a normal aging phenomenon that is just accelerated by the process of AD. The idea that AD represents only early aging comes from the nineteenth century German neuropsychiatrists who studied the pathological substrate of 'senile' dementia (dementia occurring after the age of 65 years). Dementia after age 65 years was considered a normal part of aging and the presence of neurofibrillary tangles and neuritic plaques in senile dementia was considered to be the pathological explanation of this aging process. Alois Alzheimer in 1907, described dementia in a 51-year-old woman with the pathological changes of neuritic plaques and neurofibrillary tangles (Alzheimer 1987). It was suggested that age of onset could be used to differentiate presenile dementia (subsequently named Alzheimer's disease) from senile dementia (Kraepelin 1987, original paper 1910). The presence of plaques and tangles in an individual with dementia under age 65 years (presenile dementia) was considered to be evidence of 'precocious senility' (Amaducci et al. 1986; Schwartz and Stark 1992). The notion of senile dementia as a normal aging phenomenon was not generally abandoned until the early 1990s, although some still cling to this concept. Currently, most investigators believe that AD is a disorder that can begin at almost any age during adulthood and its presence is indicated by the finding of Alzheimer plaques and neurofibrillary tangles (Amaducci et al. 1986).

Alzheimer's disease is associated with loss of pyramidal cells in cortical layers III and V, and with lesser neuronal loss in layers II and VI (Arnold et al. 1994). Neurofibrillary tangles and Alzheimer plaques represent the destructive

Figure 3.2. Graph depicting cerebral neuronal loss over the lifetime of an individual. In most people, up to 30% of neurons can be lost due to the wear and tear of normal life, but this loss is far less than the approximately 80% reduction necessary to produce clinical symptomatology (the safety margin for clinical symptoms). In Alzheimer's disease, there is progressive destruction of neurons over a 30+ year period such that the number of remaining neurons is less than the number necessary for normal clinical function. When too few neurons remain, the patient presents with clinical symptoms. Adapted from Brumback and Leech, 1994, with permission.

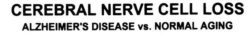
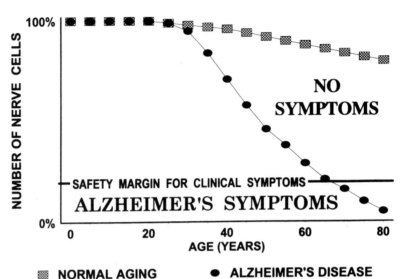

change in the nervous system (Brumback and Leech 1994), with the plaques being found throughout all layers of the cerebral cortex, as well as to a lesser extent in the hypothalamus, claustrum, tegmentum of the midbrain and rostral pons, and cerebellar cortex (Figure 3.3). The highest density of plaques and tangles is observed in the hippocampus and adjacent neocortex, areas important for memory and cognition (Terry et al. 1994).

A variety of Alzheimer plaques occur, differing in appearance and composition (Figures 3.4, 3.5, 3.6). *Diffuse amyloid plaques* have a loose accumulation of β/A4–amyloid without surrounding abnormal neurites. Diffuse amyloid plaques are considered to be precursors to neuritic plaques (Gooch and Stennett 1996). The typical *mature neuritic plaque* consists of a dense central core of β/A4–amyloid and is surrounded by a halo and a ring of abnormal neurites (dystrophic neurites) associated with wisps of β/A4–amyloid. *Primitive (immature) plaques* contain a loose accumulation of β/A4–amyloid surrounded by abnormal neurites. *Hypermature (burnt-out) plaques* have a dense core of β/A4–amyloid surrounded by reactive astrocytes but without abnormal neurites (Roberts et al. 1995). Diffuse amyloid plaques do not appear to be correlated to cognitive changes in AD possibly because they are most numerous in the brains of patients with early stage disease (Nagy et al. 1995).

The β/A4–amyloid of Alzheimer plaques derives from an amyloid precursor protein (APP) produced by a gene on chromosome 21 (Ashall and Goate 1994). Amyloid precursor protein is a transmembrane protein found mainly at nerve terminals. Abnormal degradation of this protein can produce peptide fragments which aggregate into the insoluble β/A4–amyloid, which is thought to be toxic to neurons and interfere with synaptic transmission (Yankner et al. 1989). Mutations of the amyloid precursor protein gene have been associated with early-onset AD (usually in the 40s and 50s), hereditary cerebral hemorrhage with amyloidosis-Dutch type (HCHWA-D), or with congophilic angiopathy (Bornebroek et al. 1996) (Figure 3.7).

Plaques containing β/A4–amyloid found at autopsy in the brains of apparently nondemented individuals probably represent a preclinical stage of AD (Mirra et al. 1993), although nondemented elderly individuals with densities of plaques insufficient to meet the criteria for the pathological diagnosis for AD are often given the equivocal diagnosis of 'Alzheimer's changes' (Terry et al. 1994).

Neurofibrillary tangles result from the abnormal hyperphosphorylation of tau (τ) proteins which are a normal component of the axonal microtubules. The hyperphosphorylated tau protein polymerizes into insoluble paired helical filaments. When observed in the neuronal cell body,

Figure 3.3. Examples of two types of neurofibrillary tangles found in Alzheimer's disease. (a) Flame-shaped neurofibrillary tangle in hippocampal pyramidal neuron. (b) Globular (globose) neurofibrillary tangle in cholinergic neuron in the nucleus basalis of Meynert. (Bielschowsky stain).

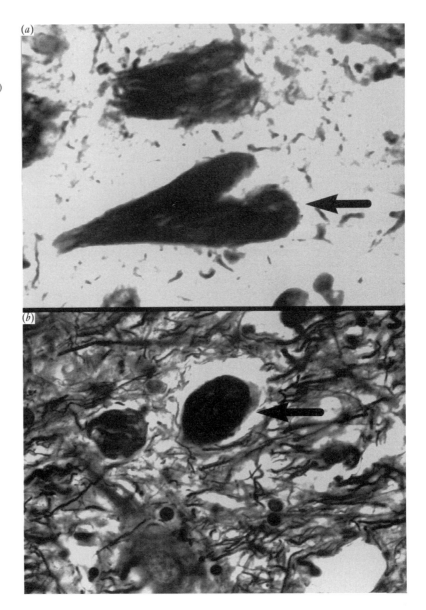

these paired helical filaments are called neurofibrillary tangles, but when visualized in neuronal processes away from the cell body, they are termed dystrophic neurites or neuropil threads (Delaère et al. 1989).

Neurofibrillary tangles (Figure 3.8) are prominent in up to 90% of AD patients, and are located in greatest quantity in the hippocampus, entorhinal cortex and temporal lobe neocortex (Hyman 1997). It has been suggested that the accumulation of the paired helical filaments found in tangles may be injurious to neurons, resulting in cell death;

however, extensive neuronal loss occurs in the neocortex of AD patients with few or no tangles (Terry et al. 1994). Neurofibrillary tangles are heavily concentrated in cortical layers II, III, V and VI in AD (Arnold et al. 1994). The finding of any tangles (but not their density in any particular case) increased with age in a series of unselected autopsies (patients with and without known clinical dementia) from 37% in the 70s to 90% in the 90s (Hubbard et al. 1990). Tangles are not unique to AD but are also found in progressive supranuclear palsy, encephalitis lethargica,

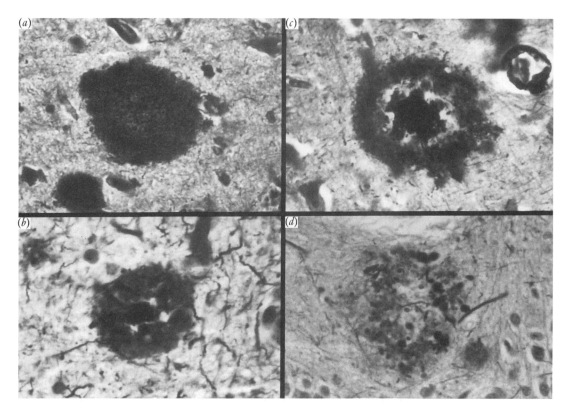

Figure 3.4. Examples of the various types of plaques seen in Alzheimer's disease. Plaques are thought to progress from diffuse amyloid plaque (a), to primitive (immature) neuritic plaque with loose amyloid core and scattered abnormal neurites (b), to mature neuritic plaque with a dense core of amyloid, surrounding halo, and a concentrated ring of abnormal neurites (c), and finally to the hypermature (burnt-out) plaque with its dense core of amyloid surrounded by reactive astrocytes but few if any neurites (d). Bielschowsky stain.

post-encephalitic parkinsonism, cerebral trauma and dementia pugilistica (Tomlinson 1992).

Neuropil threads are scattered, short, sometimes curly, thread-like structures in the neighborhood of plaques and neurofibrillary tangles. Delaère et al. (1989) found that severity of dementia was correlated with the densities of Alzheimer plaques and neurofibrillary tangles and the number and size of tau-positive fibers (neuropil threads) in the plaques.

Other pathological features of AD include the presence of Hirano bodies and granulovacuolar bodies. Hirano bodies are eosinophilic, highly refractive, rod-like structures adjacent to pyramidal neurons in the hippocampal formation (Figure 3.9). Granulovacuolar bodies of Simchowicz are small vacuoles containing a dense central granule found in the cytoplasm of hippocampal pyramidal neurons (Figure 3.10). They are nondiagnostic as they can be found in both AD and Pick's disease, as well as other neurodegenerative disorders.

The number of synaptic contact areas per neuron is significantly reduced in demented individuals compared to age-matched controls in the hippocampal dentate gyrus, molecular layer and cerebellar granular layer (Bertoni-Freddari et al. 1996). Such decreases in synapses have been correlated with cognitive deficits (DeKosky and Scheff 1990) and synapse density in the cerebral cortex has been found to be the best correlate of dementia severity in AD (Dekosky and Scheff 1990; Terry et al. 1991; Samuel et al. 1994). Anderson (1996) suggested that the greatest synaptic loss involves axons with the greatest length. It is likely that the loss of synapses is indicative of a loss of neuron-to-neuron connectivity, which is the basic

Figure 3.5. (a, b) Examples of plaques in the hippocampus in Alzheimer's disease viewed at low power. Note the large number of readily identifiable plaques in each microscopic field. Intense reactive astrocytosis can also be seen in some cases (b). Bielschowsky stain.

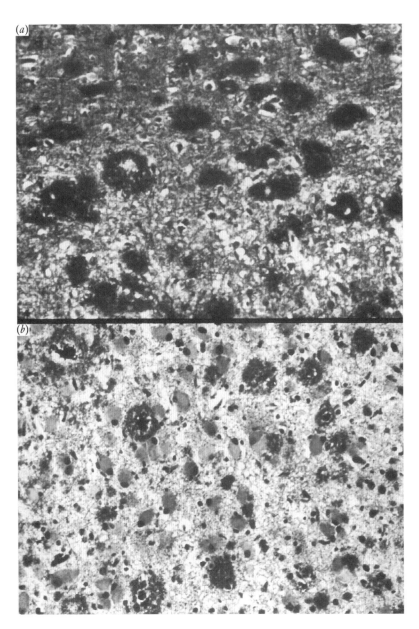

underlying mechanism for the dementia (Terry et al. 1991).

Neurotransmitter changes in Alzheimer's disease
The 'cholinergic hypothesis' has been used to explain much of the memory dysfunction in AD (Chapter 4). Choline acetyltransferase (ChAT) activity in the hippocampal and limbic cortical areas is reduced by as much as 60–90%, and is associated with a decrease of acetylcholine (ACh) synthesis, and reduced acetylcholinesterase activity (AChE) (Davies and Maloney 1976; Perry et al. 1978). Loss of up to 20% of muscarinic cholinergic receptors in the cerebral cortex has been found in one study (Mash et al. 1985), although other studies have reported normal numbers (Perry et al. 1978). Structural changes include a greater than 75% neuronal loss in the nucleus basalis of Meynert

Figure 3.6. Example of single
primitive plaque in hippocampus in
Alzheimer's disease. With the
ordinary hematoxylin and eosin
stain the amyloid core is readily
visible (a). With a fluorescent stain
for amyloid (thioflavin S stain) the
amyloid is brightly visible against
the dark background (b).

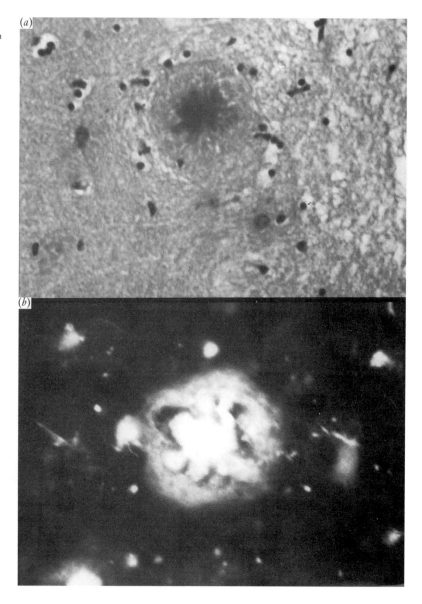

(Whitehouse et al. 1982; Rogers et al. 1985), which is a major site of cholinergic neurons. Alzheimer plaques and neurofibrillary tangles in the cerebral cortex exhibit high levels of AChE activity and ChAT activity (Perry et al. 1978; Whitehouse et al. 1982). Further support for the cholinergic hypothesis comes from the observation that administration of scopolamine (an anticholinergic drug) to research subjects alters cognitive ability (particularly memory) in a manner similar to AD (Drachman and Leavitt 1974), although scopolamine fails to model all memory deficits associated with AD.

In addition to changes in the cholinergic system, AD patients have disruptions in other neurotransmitter systems. Neuronal loss in the dorsal raphe nucleus reduces cerebral cortical concentrations of serotonin and its metabolite 5-hydroxyindole acetic acid (5-HIAA) (Curcio and Kemper 1984). Behavioral changes such as depression have been linked to this serotonin dysregulation.

Figure 3.7. Cerebral amyloid angiopathy accompanies amyloid deposition in plaques in Alzheimer's disease. The amyloid accumulates in the walls of subarachnoid vessels (a, b, e, f) and intraparenchymal vessels (c, d). a, c, e: thioflavin S fluorescent stain; b, d, f: hematoxylin and eosin stain.

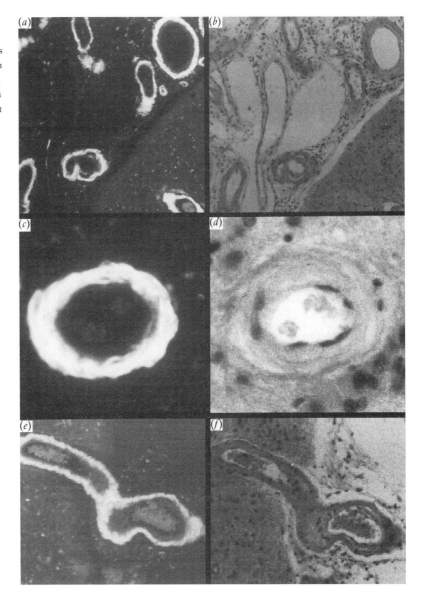

Decreased levels of serotonin in the prosubiculum have been associated with psychotic symptoms in AD patients who have a hastened cognitive decline (Zubenko et al. 1991; Kirby and Lawlor 1995). Loss of neurons in the locus ceruleus is associated with a reduction in levels of norepinephrine in the hippocampus and cerebral cortex (Bondareff et al. 1981).

Clinical and neuroanatomic changes in Alzheimer's disease

Grossly visible changes in the brain are more commonly observed in moderate to severely demented individuals and in patients with earlier onset AD. Brain weight remains within the normal range until approximately the seventh year of clinically evident disease (Figure 3.11). Gross atrophy of the gyri is prominent in the fronto-temporal and parietal areas (Figure 3.12), with lesser

Figure 3.8. Comparison of the pathological changes in the hippocampus in Alzheimer's disease. Neurofibrillary tangles can be identified with the Congo red stain as apple green birefringence under polarized light (a) or with the Bielschowsky silver stain (b, c, d, e). Neurofibrillary tangles are the hyperphosphorylated tau protein accumulated in the neuronal cell body. Similar hyperphosphorylated tau protein in neuronal processes (axons or dendrites) is termed neuropil threads or dystrophic neurites (arrow in c). With the silver stain, neurofibrillary tangles have a denser and fibrillary appearance in comparison to plaques (f).

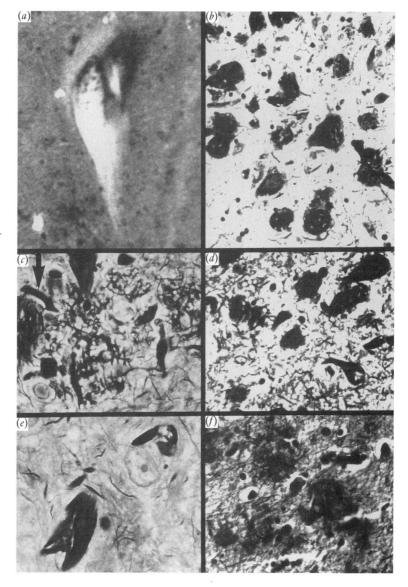

involvement of the occipital lobe. There is striking involvement of the temporal lobe inferiomedially where the parahippocampal gyrus is usually severely atrophic. The olfactory bulb and tract are also often grossly atrophic, while other cranial nerves appear normal. Other findings include thinning of the cerebral cortical ribbon, enlargement of the lateral ventricles, shrinkage of the hippocampus and amygdala, and pallor of the locus ceruleus (but with normal coloration of the substantia nigra) (Terry et al. 1994).

Grundman et al. (1996) found significant magnetic resonance imaging (MRI) identified cerebral cortical atrophy in AD patients, including a mean reduction of 16% in the size of the mesial temporal cortex (defined as the uncus, amygdala, hippocampus and parahippocampal gyrus). The mesial temporal lobe is involved with feeding behaviors and appetite (as well as memory and emotion) and is affected early in the course of AD which may explain why the reduced cerebral cortical thickness correlated with a separate index of decreased body mass. The reduction in

Figure 3.9. Arrows indicate three Hirano bodies adjacent to pyramidal neurons in hippocampal formation in Alzheimer's disease. Hematoxylin and eosin stain.

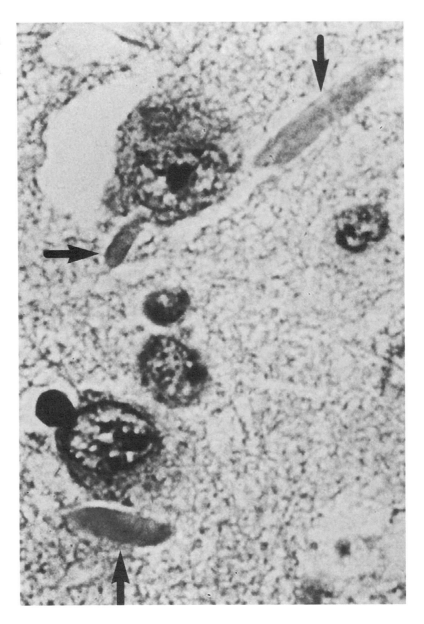

mesial temporal cortex volume also significantly correlated with cognitive function measured with the Dementia Rating Scale, Mini-Mental State Exam and Blessed-Information-Memory-Concentration Test.

Clinical and cognitive symptoms of AD progress in a fairly predictable manner starting with memory impairment, followed by language impairment, personality changes and parietal lobe symptoms, and are explainable by atrophy of the appropriate brain structures (Figure 3.13). Braak and Braak (1991) defined six stages of damage in AD that correlated with neuropsychological deterioration (Figures 3.14 and 3.15). During stages I and II, which are associated with no apparent cognitive changes, neurofibrillary tangles form in the transentorhinal region. In stages III and IV, the entorhinal area fills with neurofibrillary tangles and neuropil threads, and changes appear in the hippocampus and spread through the temporal isocortex. Subtle cognitive changes appear in stages

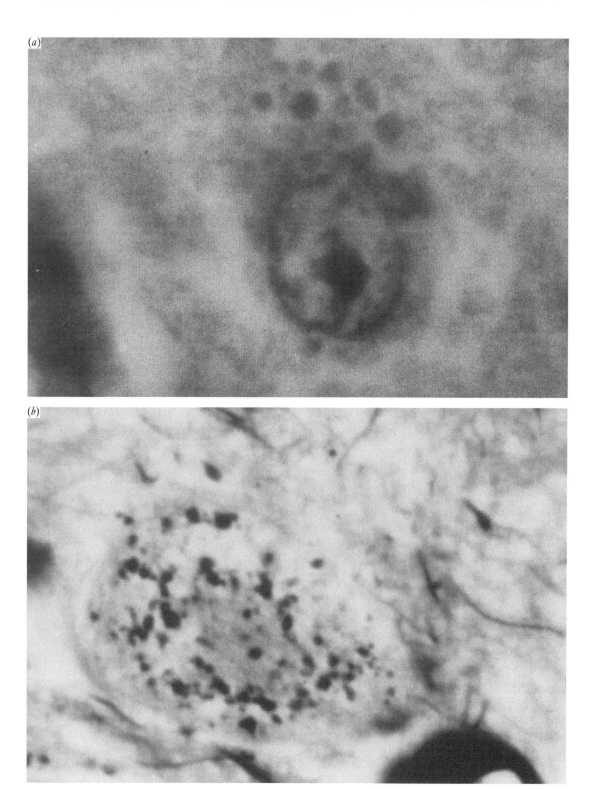

Figure 3.10. Granulovacuolar bodies of Simchowicz in Alzheimer's disease are evident as dense eosinophilic, highly refractile bodies surrounded by a halo in the cytoplasm of hippocampal pyramidal neurons (a). Haematoxylin and eosinstain. The granulovacuolar bodies also are stained by silver stains (b). Bielschowsky stain.

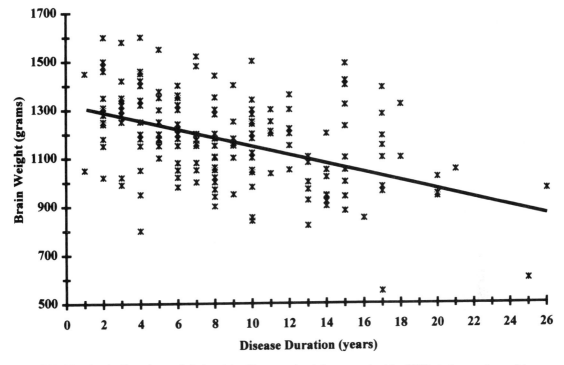

Figure 3.11. There is a significant decrease in brain weight with increased duration of Alzheimer's disease. In a sample of 191 brains confirmed to have Alzheimer's disease, the brain weight tended to drop below a normal weight of 1200 g in the seventh year of the disease.

III and IV. Fully developed AD can be clinically recognized in stages V and VI, at which time the cerebral neocortex has atrophied and many neurofibrillary tangles are noted (Hyman et al. 1990; Braak and Braak 1996). This destruction of afferent neurons of the entorhinal cortex and efferent neurons of the subiculum effectively cuts off the hippocampus from the rest of the cerebral cortex (Hyman et al. 1990).

Terry et al. (1991) correlated the severity of dementia and the neuropathological changes of AD using three very similar tests of overall cognitive function (Dementia Rating Scale, Mini-Mental State Exam and Blessed-Information-Memory-Concentration Test). AD patients were compared to neuropathologically normal matched control patients. Only weak correlations between numbers and distribution of neurofibrillary tangles and neuritic plaques and the various cognitive indexes were found; however, a strong correlation was reported between the density of neocortical synapses and the cognitive measures. It is noteworthy that the normal comparison cases showed virtually no Alzheimer plaques, neurofibrillary tangles or lesions in the hippocampal and entorhinal regions. Similar results have been obtained by DeKosky and Scheff (1990) who investigated synaptic density in the frontal cortex and found a significant correlation between decreased synaptic density and the Mini-Mental State Exam.

Additional research by Samuel et al. (1994) confirmed that the reduced synaptic density in the frontal cortical region strongly correlated with clinical dementia severity. These investigators also found that neurofibrillary tangles in the nucleus basalis of Meynert bore a stronger relationship than synaptic density to overall dementia severity. Further analyses suggested that frontal synaptic destruction contributed to impairments in initiation, conceptualization and attention, while the tangles in the nucleus basalis of Meynert contributed to memory difficulties. Synaptic loss in the neocortex appeared to affect cognition via loss of corticocortical interconnections, while neurofibrillary tangles in the nucleus basalis of Meynert

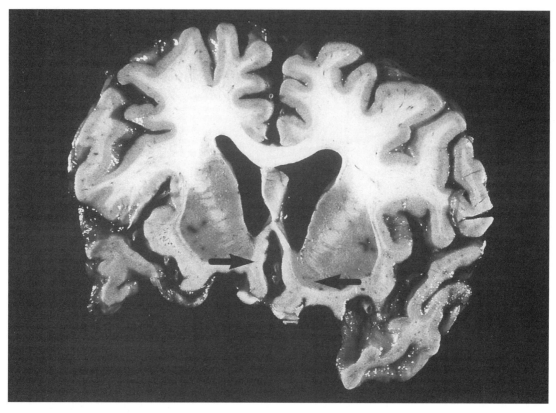

Figure 3.12. Coronal section of a formalin fixed brain with
Alzheimer's disease at the level of the nucleus accumbens septi and
septal nucleus (arrows) displaying marked atrophy.

indicated damage to the cholinergic outflow tracts, known
to be important for learning and memory (Bartus et al.
1985; Davis et al. 1992). Large numbers of neurofibrillary
tangles in the hippocampus and substantia innominata
(which includes the nucleus basalis of Meynert) are indicative of loss of a critical number of neurons (Hubbard et al.
1990). Hubbard and colleagues (1990) suggested that AD
symptoms begin when approximately 30% of neurons
have been lost, and that by the advanced stages of the
disease at least 40% of nerve cells from the hippocampus
and 50% of nerve cells from the substantia innominata
have been lost (Figures 3.16 and 3.17).

Möslä and colleagues (1987) found a strong correlation
between severity of dementia and the occurrence, but not
quantity, of Alzheimer plaques and neurofibrillary tangles
in amygdala, hippocampus and neocortex, although
plaques showed weaker correlations than tangles. In addi-

tion, these investigators found a strong correlation
between severity of dementia and reduced total brain
weight. Lower brain weights correlated with decreased
ability to walk, increased disability, occurrence of dyskinesia in orofacial and truncal areas and presence of primitive
reflexes.

The hypothesis that education relates to a lowered risk
for AD is noteworthy (Chapter 14). Higher education level
can lead to a greater brain reserve (possibly due to
increased neuronal connections) providing better protection from neuronal destruction, thereby lowering the
risk for developing clinical dementia. Doraiswamy et al.
(1995) found convincing evidence that higher educational
levels were significantly related to higher scores on the
Alzheimer's Disease Assessment Scale – Cognitive subscale, even after controlling for age, severity of dementia
(Mini-Mental State Exam score), and gender.

Figure 3.13. Alzheimer's disease results in moderate to severe atrophy of areas of the brain important for memory, language and judgment.

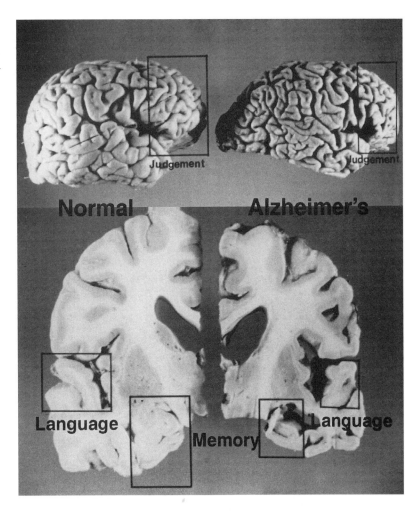

Cognitive changes in Alzheimer's disease

Research on cognitive dysfunction in AD has elucidated patterns of impairment specific for each stage of the disease, similar to the neuropathological stages noted earlier (Braak and Braak 1991). Table 3.3 provides a guide to the common clinical changes which accompany Alzheimer's disease (Corey-Bloom et al. 1994). Although AD also involves declines in cognitive domains other than memory (e.g. language, visuoperceptual skills, praxis and executive functions), we focus here, consistent with the theme of this book, on the hallmark feature of AD, namely memory impairment, as evidenced by the inability to recall previously learned information (i.e. retrograde amnesia) or to learn new information (i.e. anterograde amnesia) (American Psychiatric Association, 1994). Indeed, memory test scores are thought to best discriminate between very

early AD and normal aging (Welsh et al. 1991; Chapters 17 and 18).

Memory impairments in AD can be conceptualized as affecting several independent memory systems which differ in their content and the processes acting upon that content. One distinction is drawn between declarative (or explicit) and nondeclarative (or implicit or procedural) memory. Declarative memory refers to knowledge of facts and events that can be consciously recollected, whereas nondeclarative memory refers to unconscious remembering reflected in the performance of task operations (Butters et al. 1995; Chapter 12). Declarative memory is further divided into episodic and semantic memory. Episodic memory refers to knowledge of events linked to a specific spatial and temporal context. Semantic memory, in contrast, refers to our general knowledge about words,

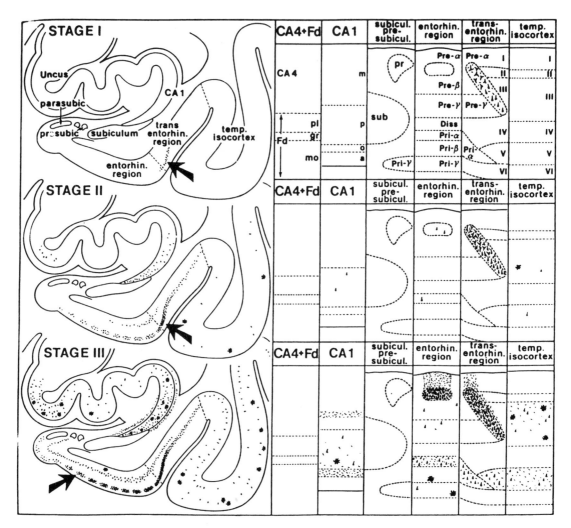

Figures 3.14, 3.15. Summary diagrams of cortical neurofibrillary changes seen in stages I–VI of Alzheimer's disease. Mild and severe destruction of the transentorhinal layer Pre-α characterizes the transentorhinal stages I and II. The two forms of limbic stages (III and IV) are marked by conspicuous involvement of layer Pre-α in both the transentorhinal region and proper entorhinal region. The hallmark of the two forms of isocortical stages (V and VI) is a severe destruction of isocortical association areas. The large arrows point to the leading characteristics, smaller ones indicate additional features. Areas and layers are outlined in stage I. *a*: alveus; CA1: first sector of the Ammon's horn; CA4: fourth sector of the Ammon's horn; Diss: lamina dissecans; entorhin.: entorhinal; Fd: fascia dentata; gr: granule cell layer of the fascia dentata; m: molecular layer of sector CA1; mo: molecular layer of the fascia dentata; o: stratum oriens; *p*: pyramidal cell layers of sector CA1; parasubic: parasubiculum; pl: plexiform layer of the fascia dentata; *pr*: parvocellular layer of the presubiculum; Pre-α, β, γ: lamina principalis externa, layer α, β, γ; Pri-α, β, γ: lamina principalis interna, layer α, β, γ; presubic: presubiculum proper; sub: subiculum; temp.: temporal; transentorhin.: transentorhinal; *I–VI*: isocortical layers. (From H. Braak and E. Braak 1991, with permission, figures 9 and 10). Neuropathological staging of Alzheimer-related changes. *Acta Neuropathologica* (Berl.) 82: 239–259.

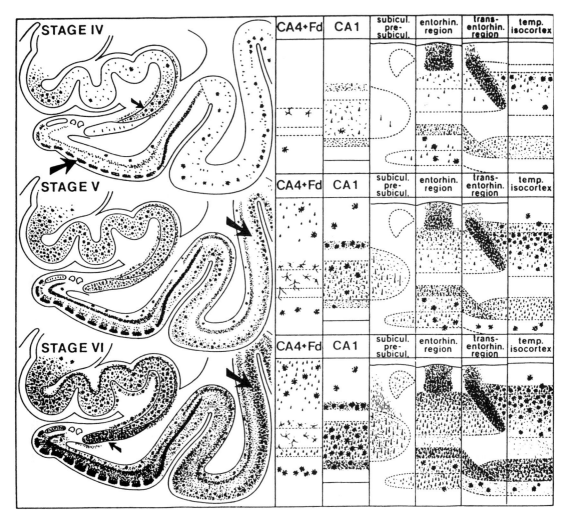

Figures 3.14, 3.15. (*cont.*)

objects, concepts and rules, which is overlearned and relatively resistant to brain damage (Squire et al. 1993).

Alzheimer's disease severely compromises both episodic and semantic memory. With regard to episodic memory, it is well known that AD impairs the ability to learn and retain new information (Martin et al. 1985). This memory impairment is characterized by rapid rates of forgetting and the propensity to commit intrusion errors (i.e., to 'contaminate' recalled information with information extraneous to the task at hand) (Chapter 18). The impairment in learning and retaining new information has been linked to the medial temporal and neocortical pathology of AD. In addition to impairments in learning and retaining

new information, patients with AD experience an impairment in recalling information from the past. Information affected includes personal, autobiographic episodic and semantic memories, spatial information and general knowledge (Kopelman 1989; Beatty and Salmon 1991). This memory loss, at least early in the disease, affects relatively recent memories more than it does memories of events in the distant past, thus giving the impression of a 'temporally graded' retrograde amnesia. This temporal gradient distinguishes the retrograde amnesia of AD from that in 'subcortical dementias', which appears to be similarly severe for all decades of life (Chapter 10). Remote memory loss correlates with tests of frontal lobe function,

Figure 3.16. Comparison of hippocampal CA1 region in normal (a) and Alzheimer's disease (b) brains. Note the hypercellular appearance in Alzheimer's disease due to the marked loss of neurons and replacement by reactive astrocytes. Luxol fast blue–cresyl violet stain.

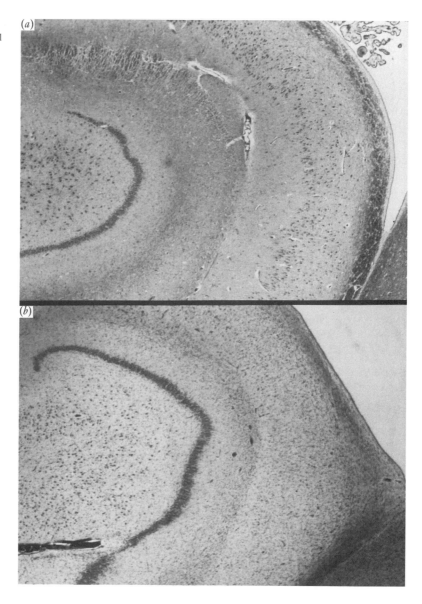

which suggests that pathological changes to the frontal lobes might prevent adequate retrieval of information (Kopelman 1989). As remote memory impairments increase, frontal lobe and limbic-diencephalic pathology likely degrade necessary semantic knowledge in addition to impairing the retrieval of information (Hodges et al. 1992; Beatty et al. 1995).

Alzheimer's disease also leads to a marked compromise of semantic memory, as evidenced by patients' poor performance on verbal fluency and naming tasks (Tröster et al. 1989b; Chertkow and Bub 1990; Hodges et al. 1992). Although the impairment of semantic memory in AD is not disputed, debate continues about the exact cognitive mechanisms underlying the impaired semantic memory task performance, i.e. whereas some authors postulate that conceptual knowledge contained in semantic memory is lost and/or degraded, others hypothesize that semantic memory content is not lost, but rather, is inaccessible (Chapter 11).

The severe impairment in semantic memory seen in

Figure 3.17. Comparison of nucleus basalis of Meynert in normal (a) and Alzheimer's disease (b) brain. Note the marked loss of the large cholinergic neurons in Alzheimer's disease. Luxol fast blue-cresyl violet stain.

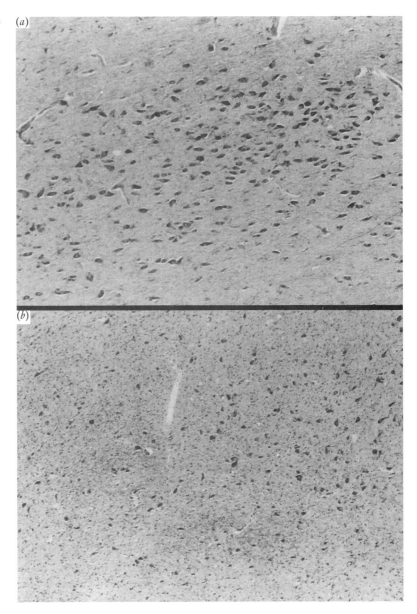

AD patients has been attributed to several neuropathological characteristics of AD, including the loss of neurons in the basal forebrain (nucleus basal of Meynert and septal nuclei), which disrupts cholinergic input to the hippocampus and cerebral cortex. Studies of normal volunteers administered scopolamine (an anticholinergic drug), however, reveal that anticholinergic treatment is *not* associated with transient decrements in verbal intelligence (Drachman and Leavitt 1974) or remote memory (Tröster et al. 1989a). These findings lead one to question the importance of cholinergic dysfunction in AD patients' semantic memory loss. Other possible causes of the decline in semantic memory in AD may be the severe atrophy of the hippocampus and amygdala, structures known to be important for memory (Zola-Morgan et al. 1989) and of the lateral temporal neocortices (Hodges et al. 1992).

Although significantly impaired on declarative (or

Table 3.3. *Clinical features of Alzheimer's disease by stage*

Feature	Early	Intermediate	Late
Cognitive			
Memory	Poor recall of new information; remote memories relatively preserved	Remote memory affected	Untestable
Language	Dysnomia; mild loss of fluency	Nonfluent, poor comprehension, impaired repetition	Near-mutism
Visuospatial	Misplacing objects; difficulty driving	Getting lost; difficulty copying figures	Untestable
Behavioral	Delusions; depression; insomnia	Delusions; depression; agitation; insomnia	Agitation; wandering
Neurological	Abnormal face-hand test; decreased graphesthesia; frontal release signs	Abnormal face-hand test; decreased graphesthesia; frontal release signs; extrapyramidal signs; nonspecific gait disorder	Mutism; incontinence; frontal release signs; rigidity; loss of gait; ± myoclonus

Source: Adapted from Corey-Bloom et al. 1994.

explicit) memory tests, AD patients retain the ability to perform well on certain nondeclarative (or implicit) memory tasks (for a detailed review see Chapter 12). For example, AD and Huntington's disease (HD) patients show a double dissociation on two implicit memory tasks: AD subjects perform well on the pursuit-rotor test, but poorly on verbal priming tasks; HD patients, in contrast, perform well on verbal priming tasks, but do poorly on pursuit-rotor tasks (Eslinger and Damasio 1986; Heindel et al. 1989; Pillon et al. 1993). Heindel et al. (1989) suggested that lexical priming is mediated by the neocortical association areas known to be damaged in AD, while motor skill learning is mediated by the corticostriatal system known to be damaged in HD patients. Similarly, Eslinger and Damasio (1986) suggested that AD subjects can learn a motor skill because the anatomical systems involved (the cerebellum, basal ganglia, thalamus, motor and premotor cortices and related pathways) are unaffected by the disease.

Further evidence of the preservation of procedural or skill learning and performance is evident in the preserved cognitive skills of some AD patients (Chapter 20). Beatty et al. (1994) identified AD patients who retain the ability to perform certain, highly practiced skills despite extensive neuropsychological decline. For example, one patient was able to continue playing the trombone in a Dixieland band, although he could not remember the title of the songs. Another severely demented individual successfully played contract bridge with friends, but could no longer keep the score. Several other patients were able to play dominoes or canasta, or complete jigsaw puzzles. These observations suggest that certain, well-learned information and skills remain intact and accessible in some AD patients.

PARKINSON'S DISEASE

Parkinson's disease (PD) occurs in about 4 per 1000 people (Koller and Megaffin 1994) and presents with characteristic symptoms of: (1) rhythmic resting tremor; (2) bradykinesia (a slowness in the execution of movements with few spontaneous movements); and (3) rigidity. Patients can have a tremor-dominant or akinetic/rigid clinical presentation (Rajput 1994). Environmental factors correlate with the pathogenesis of PD, although genetic and age-related neurobiological processes might also be involved (Shoulson and Kurlan 1993). Changes consistent with PD have been produced following administration of 1-methyl–4-phenyl–1,2,3,6-tetrahydropyridine (MPTP), a toxic contaminant produced during illicit meperidine synthesis (Kopin and Markey 1988). Estimates of the prevalence of dementia in PD patients range from 25 to 50% (Lichter et al. 1988; Hughes et al. 1993) and may reach 65% in patients over age 85 years (Mayeux et al. 1990).

The diagnosis of idiopathic PD is often difficult to make with certainty, as many other disorders mimic symptoms of PD (Table 3.4). The etiology of parkinsonism is

Table 3.4. *Disorders associated with Parkinsonian symptoms*

Idiopathic Parkinson's disease
Postencephalitic parkinsonism
Iatrogenic drug-induced parkinsonism
Arteriosclerotic pseudoparkinsonism
Progressive supranuclear palsy
Multiple-system atrophy
Hypoparathyroidism and basal ganglia calcification
Repeated head injury (dementia pugilistica)
Hydrocephalus
Creutzfeldt-Jakob disease
Gerstmann-Sträussler-Scheinker disease
Alzheimer's disease
Pick's disease
Diffuse Lewy body disease

Source: Adapted from Koller and Megaffin 1994.

diverse and includes infectious, toxic, pharmacological, metabolic, hereditary, and degenerative causes (Koller and Megaffin 1994) and the diagnosis of idiopathic PD can only be made upon the exclusion of other disorders. The considerable overlap between many of these diseases has lead to errors in research focusing on the clinicopathologic correlations in idiopathic PD. In fact, as will be discussed in a later section on diffuse Lewy body disease, investigators cannot agree whether these disorders represent separate pathological entities or subgroups of one disease. Generally, when additional clinical or neuropathological changes accompany symptoms characteristics of PD, the etiology can often be attributed to a different disorder.

Neuropathology of Parkinson's disease

Neuropathological changes in PD include a characteristic loss of neurons in the substantia nigra and locus ceruleus resulting in depigmentation of these structures (Figure 3.18). Consistent with this neuronal loss, there are reduced brain levels of dopamine and norepinephrine (Côté and Crutcher 1991). Collections of melanin containing macrophages and reactive gliosis mark the sites of cell loss, and surviving neurons often contain Lewy bodies or hyaline inclusions (Hansen et al. 1990; Forno 1996) (Figure 3.19). The severity of PD is correlated with neuronal loss in the substantia nigra and is relatively independent of age (Alvord et al. 1974; Rinne et al. 1989). Pathological

changes begin long before clinical symptoms of PD, which emerge only when approximately 80% of neurons from the substantia nigra have been lost (Brumback and Leech 1994).

Additional neuronal loss can be observed in the caudate nucleus and nucleus basalis of Meynert in parkinsonian patients (Braak and Braak 1990). Cortical atrophy has not been typically thought of as a neuropathological change associated with PD. Amyloid accumulation and neurofibrillary changes have been observed in the cerebral cortex of cognitively impaired parkinsonian patients. In one study, amyloid plaques were prevalent in the presubiculum, entorhinal cortex and isocortex, but not in the hippocampal formation (Braak and Braak 1990). Neurofibrillary changes were minimal in the hippocampal formation and isocortical areas but were dense in the entorhinal cortex along with a neuropil thread feltwork. In contrast, AD patients exhibited greater numbers of neurofibrillary tangles in the isocortex and allocortex. This suggested that the cognitive impairments in PD result from bilateral destruction of pathways connecting the isocortex and hippocampal formation.

Neurotransmitter and neuroanatomic changes in Parkinson's disease

Degeneration of the dopaminergic neurons in the substantia nigra pars compacta profoundly reduces concentrations of dopamine, its synthesizing enzymes (tyrosine hydroxylase and dopa-decarboxylase) and its metabolites (homovanillic acid [HVA], 3, 4-dihydroxyphenylacetic acid [DOPAC] and 3-methoxytyramine [MTA]) in structures of the nigrostriatal system (Forno 1992) including the substantia nigra pars compacta (levels reduced up to 90%), putamen, caudate nucleus and globus pallidus. The nigrostriatal dopaminergic neurons which project to the putamen (the motor part of the striatum) suffer heavy losses (85% reduction). The caudate nucleus and nucleus accumbens (the 'cognitive' areas of the striatum) have decreased levels of dopamine and homovanillic acid (75% reduction) (Kopin and Markey 1988) (Figure 3.20).

In PD, neuronal degeneration in the ventral tegmental area reduces concentrations of dopamine and homovanillic acid in areas receiving mesolimbic projections (i.e. nucleus accumbens, medial olfactory area, lateral hypothalamus, amygdaloid nucleus). Mesocortical areas (i.e. paraolfactory, entorhinal, cingulate, hippocampal and frontal cortices) also have reduced dopamine and homovanillic acid

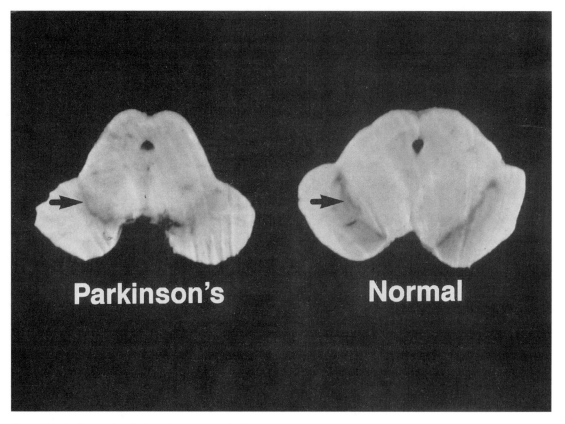

Figure 3.18. Depigmentation of substantia nigra (arrow) in the midbrain in Parkinson's disease.

concentrations from cell loss in both the ventral tegmental area and the substantia nigra. Cortical levels of dopamine and homovanillic acid decrease by more than 50% (Kopin and Markey 1988).

Neuronal loss occurs uniformly throughout the locus ceruleus disrupting noradrenergic pathways to the cerebellum, brainstem, and cerebral cortex (Kish et al. 1984). This is in contrast to AD which causes loss of rostral locus ceruleus neurons disrupting pathways to the cerebral cortex, but preserving caudal locus ceruleus neurons and the projections to the cerebellum and spinal cord (Brumback and Leech 1994) (Figure 3.21).

Additional neurotransmitter systems are affected in PD. Neuronal loss in the dorsal raphe nucleus causes decreased levels of serotonin in frontal and temporal cortical areas (Meara 1996). The loss of cholinergic neurons in the nucleus basalis of Meynert and medial septal area of the basal forebrain has been correlated to subcorticofrontal cognitive impairments (Dubois et al. 1990).

Cognitive changes in Parkinson's disease

PD is characterized by 'subcortical' cognitive changes reflected in poor performance on tests of executive function (including set shifting), verbal fluency, declarative memory, motor function and information processing speed. Cognitive changes are thought to reflect dysfunction of prefrontal and temporal lobe circuitry at the level of the basal ganglia (Cummings and Benson 1984). Significant correlations have been found between motor disability and cognitive dysfunction, which suggests that cognitive deficits of PD are also related to the degeneration of the nigrostriatal dopamine system (Lichter et al. 1988), a proposal supported by the observed lack of improvement in cognitive function with levodopa therapy (Levin et al.

Figure 3.19. Microscopic changes in Parkinson's disease include Lewy bodies in surviving pigmented neurons (arrow in a and inset) and collections of pigment (melanin) laden macrophages (arrowheads in b) indicating the site of cell loss ('tombstones'.) Hematoxylin and eosin stain.

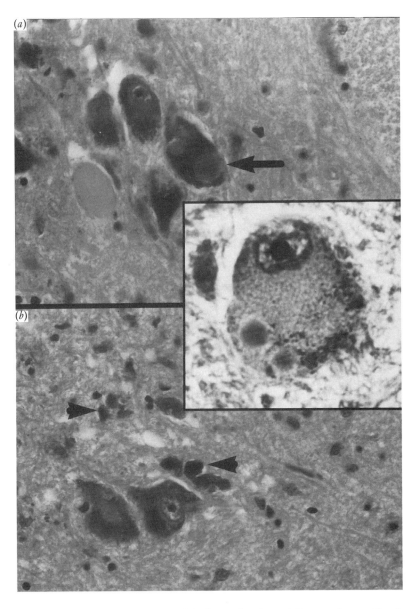

1989). The severity of dementia has also been related to neuronal loss in the nucleus basalis of Meynert (Chui et al. 1986), suggesting that cholinergic dysfunction contributes to cognitive decline.

The bradyphrenia (slowing of thought or information processing) typically observed in patients with PD can be assessed by tests of attention, vigilance or reaction time (Stern et al. 1984). The slowing of cognitive processes is hypothesized to be the result of damage to the locus ceruleus noradrenergic system (Chui 1989). For example,

abnormalities in reaction time, vigilance and general intelligence, along with severity of motor symptoms, are correlated with reduced levels of noradrenergic metabolites (Stern et al. 1984).

Speech deficits, which are more severe in demented than nondemented patients, occur in 70% of PD patients. Speech is characterized by low volume, lack of inflection, slow initiation, reduced articulation, impaired prosody, use of short phrases and a rushed rate of speech (Cummings et al. 1988; Rajput 1994). PD patients have

(a)   (b)

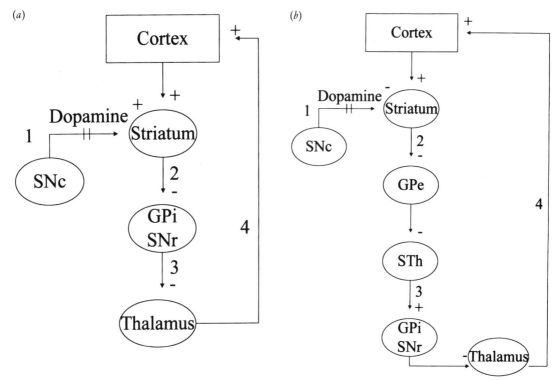

Figure 3.20. Schematic diagram showing how dopamine depletion in Parkinson's disease affects the direct and indirect striatopallidal pathways and movement. In (a) loss of excitatory dopamine input to striatal neurons projecting to GPi and SNr (1), results in relatively reduced inhibition of the GPi and SNr neurons (2). There is then decreased disinhibition of thalamic neurons (3), resulting in slowness and poverty of movement (4). In (b) loss of inhibitory dopamine input to striatal neurons projecting to GPe (1), results in increased inhibition of GPe neurons (2). The disinhibition of STh input to GPi and SNr (3), reinforces the inhibition of unwanted movement (4). GPi: internal segment of globus pallidus; SNr: substantia nigra pars reticulata; Snc: substantia nigra pars compacta; GPe: external segment of globus pallidus; STh: subthalamic nucleus. Adapted from Afifi (1994). Basal ganglia: functional anatomy and physiology. Part 2. *Journal of Child Neurology* 9, 352–361 (figures 10–12), with permission.

relatively preserved linguistic abilities (confrontation naming, word list generation and information content in spontaneous speech) when compared to AD patients with a similar degree of dementia severity (Cummings et al. 1988). Semantic memory in nondemented PD patients is often unimpaired (Tatemichi et al. 1994), although memory for semantic information is disrupted in demented patients (Pillon et al. 1991). Interestingly, Pillon et al. (1991) found a greater impairment of semantic memory in patients with PD and dementia than with AD.

Memory impairments are prominent in PD; however, the deficits are not as severe as those in AD. In PD, declarative memory deficits are evident on measures of both immediate and delayed recall (Levin et al. 1989), and espe-

cially on effort-demanding tasks (Appollonio et al. 1994), but cued recall and recognition are better preserved in PD than AD patients (Koller and Megaffin 1994). This pattern of test performance has been interpreted to mean that the ability to register, store and consolidate information is generally retained, but that retrieval processes (putatively mediated by the fronto-striatal systems) are impaired in early PD (Pillon et al. 1993). Declarative, remote memory impairments in PD are characterized by a flat temporal gradient (i.e. memory loss is similarly severe across all decades of life) (Beatty 1992).

Findings pertaining to nondeclarative memory (motor skill learning) in PD are inconsistent. Some investigators reported no deficit (Beatty 1992), others reported deficits

Figure 3.21. Comparison of neuronal loss in the locus ceruleus in Alzheimer's disease and Parkinson's disease. There is a uniform loss of neurons from the whole rostral-caudal extent of the locus ceruleus in Parkinson's disease due to a metabolic derangement in these catecholaminergic neurons. In contrast, in Alzheimer's disease, the loss involves only those rostral neurons projecting to the cerebral cortex that are normally dependent on neurotrophic factors produced by cerebral cortical neurons, while the caudal neurons projecting to the cerebellum and spinal cord are preserved. Adapted from R.A. Brumback and R.W. Leech (1994), with permission.

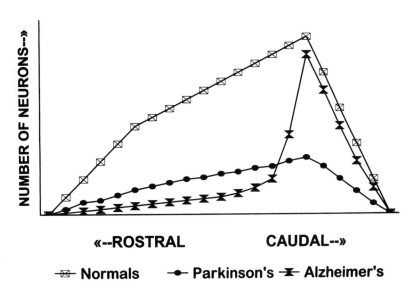

only in demented subjects (Heindel et al. 1989), and yet others reported deficits in all PD patients, demented or not (Harrington et al. 1990).

Chui and colleagues (1986) conducted clinicopathologic examinations in PD patients who had no evidence of concomitant AD. Clinical findings indicated impairments in intellectual functioning, visuospatial ability, orientation and long-term memory and slowed psychomotor ability, but language function was spared. Akinesia and rigidity were correlated to the extent of neuronal loss in the substantia nigra. Based on the strong correlation between cognitive and motor function in PD patients and evidence that the nigrostriatal system is involved in visuospatial integration (Stern et al. 1983) and language formation (Damasio et al. 1982), cognitive deficits were attributed to the same pathological lesions as the motor deficits (Lichter et al. 1988). Disruption of other systems could also explain some of the cognitive disturbances. A second dopaminergic pathway, the mesocorticolimbic system has been implicated in the intellectual and behavioral disturbances in some patients (Agid et al. 1984), and the reduction of norepinephrine levels (important in memory and attention) from loss of locus ceruleus neurons projecting to the cerebral cortex may also explain some of the cognitive deterioration.

DIFFUSE LEWY BODY DISEASE (DEMENTIA WITH LEWY BODIES)

There is confusion in the literature regarding the role Lewy bodies play in dementia, in part due to inconsistencies in nomenclature and pathological criteria for diagnosis (Kosaka et al. 1984; Hansen et al. 1990; Hansen 1994; Hely et al. 1996; McKeith et al. 1996). The presence of Lewy bodies in the neocortex has been alternately proposed to represent a distinct subset of AD (Hansen et al. 1990; Hansen 1994), a component of idiopathic PD (Hely et al. 1996), an asymptomatic form of normal aging or subclinical disease (Forno 1996), or a distinct clinical entity termed diffuse Lewy body disease (Dickson et al. 1991). Another hypothesis proposed a continuum of disorders from asymptomatic cases on one end, diffuse Lewy body disease on the other and idiopathic PD in between (Kosaka et al. 1984). The term 'dementia with Lewy bodies' has been suggested to encompass the range of clinical and pathological variation (McKeith et al. 1996), but diffuse Lewy body disease is the more commonly recognized term. Table 3.5 lists the spectrum of Lewy body disorders (Forno and Langston 1990; McKeith et al. 1996).

Neuropathology of diffuse Lewy body disease
Pathological criteria require the presence of cortical and subcortical Lewy bodies. In addition, the following

Table 3.5. *Diagnostic distinctions of dementias with Lewy bodies*

Lewy body disease
   Group A, diffuse type (diffuse Lewy body disease)
   Group B, transitional type (combined form of A and C)
   Group C, brainstem type (idiopathic Parkinson's disease)
Diffuse cortical Lewy body disease (Lewy body dementia)
Parkinson's disease in Alzheimer's disease
Diffuse Lewy body disease

Alzheimer's disease and Parkinson's disease
Alzheimer's disease with incidental Lewy bodies

Alzheimer's disease with concomitant Lewy body disease
Lewy bodies in Alzheimer's disease
Senile dementia of the Lewy body type
Lewy body variant of Alzheimer's disease

Diffuse Lewy body disease, common form, with plaques and/or tangles
Diffuse Lewy body disease, pure form, with no senile changes

Alzheimer's disease with Lewy bodies

Source: Adapted from Hansen 1994.

Table 3.6. *Clinical criteria for diagnosis of diffuse Lewy body disease*

A. Presence of progressive cognitive decline of sufficient magnitude to interfere with normal social or occupational function. Prominent or persistent memory impairment may not necessarily occur in the early stages but is usually evident with progression. Deficits on tests of attention and of frontal-subcortical skills and visuospatial ability may be especially prominent.

B. Two of the following core features are essential for probable diagnosis, and one is essential for possible diagnosis:
   1) Fluctuating cognition with pronounced variations in attention and alertness
   2) Recurrent visual hallucinations that are typically well formed and detailed
   3) Spontaneous motor features of parkinsonism

C. Features supportive of the diagnosis are: repeated falls, syncope, transient loss of consciousness, neuroleptic sensitivity, systematized delusions, hallucinations in other modalities

Source: Adapted from McKeith et al. 1996.

pathological changes can occur: Lewy body-related neurites in the hippocampus, amygdala, nucleus basalis of Meynert, dorsal vagal nucleus and other brainstem nuclei; diffuse and neuritic plaques; neurofibrillary tangles; neuropil threads; neuronal loss predominantly in the brainstem and nucleus basalis of Meynert; microvacuolation and synaptic loss; and neurotransmitter changes such as a reduction in cortical choline acetyltransferase activity. Clinically, this disease affects patients at a younger age than most other neurodegenerative diseases. Distinct parkinsonian symptoms and accompanying dementia are hallmark features of diffuse Lewy body disease (Hansen 1994).

Lewy bodies are intracytoplasmic eosinophilic neuronal inclusions formed from altered cytoskeletal elements. Lewy bodies have been described as prominent in the neocortical layers V and VI, and in monoaminergic and cholinergic neurons of cerebral cortex, substantia nigra, locus ceruleus and substantia innominata (Hansen 1994). Neocortical Lewy bodies have been found mainly in the temporal lobe, insular cortex and cingulate gyrus (Kosaka et al. 1984). The Lewy bodies appear in elongated forms in nerve cell processes in the nucleus basalis of Meynert, hypothalamus, autonomic ganglia and dorsal motor nucleus of the vagus (Braak and Braak 1990; Hansen 1994; Forno 1996). Some investigators have suggested that Lewy bodies can be found in the neocortex of nearly all patients with parkinsonism (Perry et al. 1991).

Crystal et al. (1990) found progressive dementia, gait impairment, abnormal tone or tremor, abnormal electroencephalograms, agitation, hallucinations, and delusions in a small sample of diffuse Lewy body disease patients. The neurological and neuropsychological symptoms correlated with low choline acetyltransferase activity in cortical areas and amyloid plaques in neocortex. Cholinergic neuronal loss has been reported in the nucleus basalis of Meynert without concomitant AD (Chui et al. 1986; Jellinger 1996) and this neuronal loss has been linked to memory impairment (Drachman and Leavitt 1974; Korczyn et al. 1986). Marked striatal dopamine deficiencies occur in addition to the cholinergic depletion (Galasko et al. 1996), producing a pattern of 'subcortical' neuropsychological deficits (Salmon et al. 1996). Table 3.6 presents clinical criteria for the diagnosis of diffuse Lewy body disease (dementia with Lewy bodies) (McKeith et al. 1996).

Comparison of diffuse Lewy body, Alzheimer's and Parkinson's diseases

In 1974, Alvord and colleagues suggested that two types of parkinsonian degenerative changes occur: (1) Lewy body disease, reflecting idiopathic parkinsonism; and (2) Alzheimer's neurofibrillary tangle disease, in which cortical degeneration is linked to the severity of dementia, and substantia nigra changes are related to the severity of parkinsonism. As more evidence has been collected, the relationship between diffuse Lewy body disease, PD and AD has become less clear, leading to considerable debate (for a review see Forno 1996). One reason for the confusion is the overlap (which increases with advancing age) between the occurrence of AD and PD. To date, studies have found the co-occurrence of AD in up to 33% of PD patients (Hughes et al. 1993) and the occurrence of PD in up to 60% of AD patients (Perry et al. 1991; Hughes et al. 1993).

In addition to the overlap between AD and PD, the existence of diffuse Lewy body disease and Lewy body variant of AD have been proposed. Common pathological changes between certain cases of AD and PD include the existence of neuritic plaques and neurofibrillary tangles in PD cases, and the presence of Lewy bodies in the substantia nigra, locus ceruleus and cerebral cortex along with neuronal loss in the substantia nigra of AD brains (Forno 1992). In addition, the majority of patients with AD and extrapyramidal signs have the pathological changes of PD in the substantia nigra (Ince et al. 1991).

Ince et al. (1991) have attempted to differentiate the changes associated with diffuse Lewy body disease, AD and PD by observing the extent of Alzheimer-type pathology in each group. The presence of Alzheimer-type pathology in the hippocampus (neurofibrillary tangles, granulovacuolar degeneration and Alzheimer plaques) was greatest for patients with AD, followed in density by Lewy body disease cases, PD cases and normal controls. Forno (1992) presented neuropathological evidence suggesting that the occurrence of Lewy bodies in AD patients is substantially higher (one in four) compared to the general autopsy population (one in 15), and that it increases in all cases with advanced age.

Although considerable overlap exists between the features of diffuse Lewy body disease and AD, careful examination can reveal helpful clinical and neuropathological differences between these conditions. Salmon et al. (1996) compared pure diffuse Lewy body disease and AD

patients on neuropsychological measures. Both groups presented with symptoms of slow onset dementia characterized by cognitive decline and memory impairments, but each disease was associated with distinct cognitive profiles. Diffuse Lewy body disease patients exhibited global dementia characterized by impairments in visuospatial abilities, attention, memory, language, executive function and psychomotor performance. The diffuse Lewy body disease patients had only mildly impaired scores on the Mini-Mental State Exam and Dementia Rating Scale, which suggested to these authors a slower progression of diffuse Lewy body disease than AD. The diffuse Lewy body disease subjects had milder memory problems but were more impaired in visuospatial and visuoconstruction tasks. The investigators hypothesized that neuropathological changes in the temporal, frontal, and parietal lobes caused the impairments in memory, language, executive function and visuospatial ability. Damage to the substantia nigra and depleted dopaminergic input to the striatum impaired learning, attention, visuoconstructive abilities and psychomotor performance.

Hansen and colleagues (1990) reported the findings from neuropathological examination of probable AD patients following their demise. One-third of these patients had diffuse neocortical Lewy bodies in addition to the Alzheimer plaques and neurofibrillary tangles, consistent with AD. The cases with Lewy bodies had the Lewy bodies located in the locus ceruleus, substantia nigra or substantia innominata in addition to the neocortex. No purely AD patient had Lewy bodies in the neocortex although some had a few subcortical Lewy bodies present. In comparison to the pure AD brains, those with neocortical Lewy bodies had paleness of the substantia nigra, neuronal hypocellularity in subcortical regions, loss of neurons and Lewy bodies in the substantia nigra, and reduced choline acetyltransferase levels and neurofibrillary tangles in the midfrontal areas.

Patients with neocortical Lewy bodies also had essential tremor and masked faces, and extrapyramidal involvement included bradykinesia, gait abnormality or slowing of rapid alternating movement. Cognitive differences existed between cases of pure AD and those with neocortical Lewy bodies even though the two groups had comparable overall dementia severity and similar memory and language impairments. Patients with neocortical Lewy bodies were significantly more impaired on measures of attention, semantic fluency, letter fluency, visuospatial function and construction ability. The authors noted the association between these cognitive processes affected by 'subcortical forms of dementia' and the associated Lewy bodies and greater neuronal loss in subcortical structures (including the substantia nigra). The greater cognitive dysfunction was related to greater parietal cortex changes, more severe neuronal loss in the substantia innominata, and reduced levels of choline acetyltransferase in frontal and parietal cortex. Hansen et al. (1990) have hypothesized that Lewy body variant of AD represents a combination of cortical and subcortical impairments.

In summary, patients with neocortical Lewy bodies show similar signs to AD with additional mild extrapyramidal signs, hallucinations, more rapid disease course, and more severe deficits in attention, verbal fluency and visuospatial processing (Hansen et al. 1990; Perry et al. 1991; Galasko et al. 1996).

PROGRESSIVE SUPRANUCLEAR PALSY

The concept of subcortical dementia was proposed to describe the neuropsychological changes which accompanied progressive supranuclear palsy (also called Steele–Richardson–Olszewski syndrome; Steele et al. 1964; Albert et al. 1974). This disease was contrasted to cortical dementias for two reasons: (1) the pathological changes involve the basal ganglia, upper brain stem and cerebellar nuclei, and (2) true aphasias, apraxias and agnosias do not occur (Dubois et al. 1996). The characteristic features of the disease include slow information processing, forgetfulness, apathy or depression and an impaired ability to manipulate acquired knowledge. Speech alterations include slurred articulation, hypophonia and eventual mutism. Dementia is present in 25% of patients at disease onset, with the rest developing cognitive deficits later in the disease course (Tomlinson, 1992). Characteristic features include pseudobulbar palsy, truncal rigidity, supranuclear gaze palsy, frequent falls and onset after age 40 years.

Progressive supranuclear palsy occurs in 1.4 per 100 000 people (Golbe and Dickson 1995) making it the most common atypical parkinsonian syndrome (Litvan et al. 1996a), yet, it is still only 1% as common as PD (Golbe and Dickson 1995). The actual prevalence of progressive supranuclear palsy may be considerably higher due to relative late formal diagnosis relative to symptom onset (Golbe and Dickson 1995) or to misdiagnosis (Litvan et al. 1996a). The disease usually lasts between 2 and 11 years, averaging 6 years in duration (Wisniewski 1985). Many disorders resemble progressive supranuclear palsy, especially in the early stages. The more commonly confused diagnoses include PD, AD, diffuse Lewy body disease, Pick's disease, Creutzfeldt–Jakob disease, corticobasal degeneration, rigid forms of Huntington's disease and multisystem atrophy (Hauw et al. 1994). The differences between PD, progressive supranuclear palsy and corticobasal degeneration are described in Table 3.7.

Neuropathology of progressive supranuclear palsy
Neuropathological changes in progressive supranuclear palsy include neurofibrillary tangles, neuropil threads, neuronal loss and reactive astrocytosis in the globus pallidus, subthalamic nucleus, striatum, nucleus basalis of Meynert, brain stem (colliculi, substantia nigra, periaqueductal gray matter, red nucleus, dorsal and median raphe nuclei and inferior olives) and cerebellar dentate nucleus. Rare neuropil threads or neurofibrillary tangles can sometimes be detected in the prefrontal and precentral cortices. Myelin pallor is seen in the brain stem tegmentum, medial longitudinal fasciculus and superior cerebellar peduncles (Hauw et al. 1994; Litvan et al. 1996b). The neurofibrillary tangles contain paired helical filaments and are immunoreactive for hyperphosphorylated tau protein (just as in AD). As these tangles do not occur in the pyramidal-shaped cerebral cortical neurons, but rather in multipolar subcortical neurons, the tangles have a spherical or 'globose' shape (Figure 3.22).

Neurotransmitter changes in progressive supranuclear palsy
Biochemical changes are significant, including up to a 90% decrease of dopamine and homovanillic acid in the substantia nigra and striatum and decreased numbers of striatal dopamine receptors (Ruberg et al. 1985). Slight decreases in choline acetyltransferase in the striatum and cerebral cortex have also been found. Cortical levels of dopamine, norepinephrine and serotonin are relatively preserved. Frontal lobe dysfunction probably results from progressive deafferentation due to reduced input from the basal ganglia and thalamus (Agid et al. 1987; Dubois et al. 1996).

Table 3.7. *Clinical and pathological comparison of progressive supranuclear palsy, corticobasal degeneration, and Parkinson's disease*

Characteristic features	Progressive supranuclear palsy	Corticobasal degeneration	Parkinson's disease
Clinical features			
Motor symptoms	Symmetrical	Asymmetrical	Symmetrical
Rigidity	Axial > limb	Limb > axial	Limb > axial
Postures	Extended	Alien hand	Bowed
Tremor	Uncommon	Uncommon	Common
Ophthalmoplegia	Supranuclear gaze palsy with downward gaze lost first	Supranuclear gaze palsy	Upward and converge lost first
Cognitive changes			
Dementia	20–60%	Rare at onset; more common late in disease	25–50%
Bradyphrenia	Common	Common	Common
Personality changes	Apathy or depression	Apathy or depression	Depression in 50%
Language	Slow and poorly articulated speech	Slow and poorly articulated speech, apraxia, anomia	Slow and poorly articulated speech
Response to levodopa	Little improvement	Little improvement	Substantial improvement
Disease duration	4–8 years	6–10 years	5–15 years
Pathology			
Location	Subthalamic nucleus, red nucleus, substantia nigra, dentate nucleus	Cerebral cortex atrophy, substantia nigra, basal ganglia, thalamus	Substantia nigra, locus ceruleus, ventral tegmental area
Type of change	Globose neurofibrillary tangles, cell loss, granulovacuolar degeneration, gliosis, neuropil threads	Corticobasal inclusion, neurofibrillary tangles, neuropil threads, balloon neurons, status spongiosus	Lewy bodies, cell loss, gliosis

Source: Adapted from Gibb et al. 1989; Gibb 1992, Litvan et al. 1996.

Cognitive changes in progressive supranuclear palsy

Cognitive changes characteristic of progressive supra-nuclear palsy include cognitive slowing, forgetfulness and impaired executive functioning. The cognitive slowing is due to slowed central processing of information and decreased ability to shift mental set, which is evident on tests of executive function (such as the Wisconsin Card Sorting Test). Other impaired executive functions include abstract thinking, concept formation, lexical and design fluency, and problem solving (Dubois et al. 1996).

Declarative memory deficits are thought to be due to changes in the frontal lobes following damage to stri-atofrontal pathways. Patients have deficits in delayed recall but perform much better when cued, suggesting that the temporal lobes are relatively unaffected. Nondeclarative memory deficits are not consistently reported. Impairments have been described in cognitive but not motor procedural learning, and priming appears relatively preserved in progressive supranuclear palsy (Dubois et al. 1996), suggesting an intact association neocortex (Salmon and Heindel 1992).

Comparisons of cognitive function among AD, Huntington's disease (HD), progressive supranuclear palsy and PD groups have demonstrated disease-specific cognitive impairments for each group except PD. In other words, although these diseases have some cognitive impairments in common, certain features of cognitive impairment appear to be unique and differentiate each group from the other. Pillon et al. (1991) found that whereas patients with progressive supranuclear palsy had 'subcorticofrontal' cognitive and behavioral impairments, AD patients had

Figure 3.22. Neurofibrillary tangles in progressive supranuclear palsy have a spherical or 'globose' shape in the multipolar subcortical neurons as shown in the neurons of the pontine nuclei (arrow in a). Neurofibrillary tangles also are found in pigmented neurons of the substantia nigra in progressive supranuclear palsy (b). Bielschowsky stain.

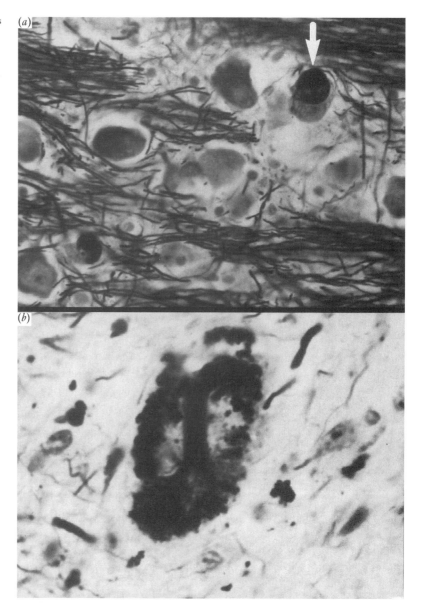

remote memory and orientation impairments, followed later by linguistic disturbances. HD patients exhibited concentration and learning difficulties, but PD patients had no characteristic cognitive deficits distinguishing them from the other patient groups. However, PD patients had impairments on tests of frontal lobe functioning and speech production (Pillon et al. 1991).

PICK'S DISEASE

Pick's disease is a possibly heritable neurodegenerative disorder (Groen and Endtz 1982), appearing 10–20% as often as AD (Tissot et al. 1985). Duration of the disease from diagnosis to death is five to 10 years (Tissot et al. 1985). In Pick's disease patients, brain imaging and autopsy examinations characteristically display progressive frontotemporal lobar atrophy (Figure 3.23); however, only

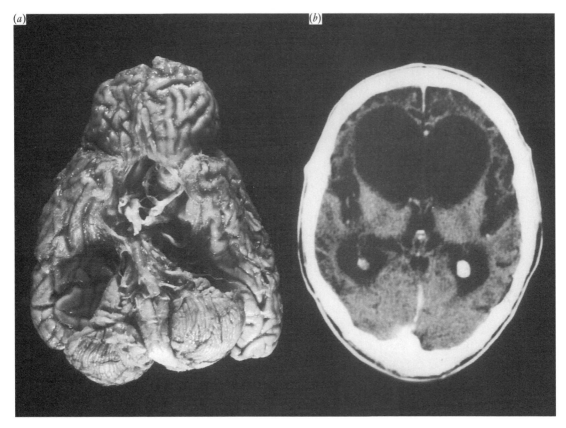

Figure 3.23. Inferior view of the surface of the brain (a) and computerized tomography image in the horizontal plane (b) in Pick's disease showing marked frontal and anterior temporal lobar atrophy with massive enlargement of the frontal horns of the lateral ventricles.

neuropathological diagnostic criteria for Pick's disease have been developed.

Neuropathology of Pick's disease

Neuropathological changes associated with Pick's disease include atrophy of the anterior portion of the frontal lobe and a characteristic atrophy of the anterior portion of the superior temporal gyrus (anterior to the central sulcus) with preservation of the posterior portions of that gyrus. The parietal and occipital lobes are generally spared (Figure 3.24). The atrophy leaves the gyri with a 'knife-edge' appearance. There is also a characteristic, severe loss of the granular neurons that comprise the dentate gyrus of the hippocampal complex. Subcortical structures in which neuronal loss occurs include the basal ganglia, amygdala, nucleus basalis of Meynert, substantia nigra and locus ceruleus (Hansen 1994; Hof et al. 1994).

Neuropathological features of Pick's disease include severe cerebral cortical neuronal loss, Pick bodies and ballooned neurons (Pick cells) (Giannakopoulos et al. 1996) (Figure 3.25). Pick bodies are intracytoplasmic argyrophilic neuronal inclusions which are composed of straight filaments, microtubules and occasional paired helical filaments (similar to those in AD neurofibrillary tangles) (Hof et al. 1994). The lateral ventricles, particularly the frontal horns, are dilated due to the atrophic changes. Although there is some neuronal loss in the nucleus basalis of Meynert, cortical levels of choline acetyltransferase are not reduced in Pick's disease as they are in AD.

Distinct variants of Pick's disease have been reported (Constantinidis et al. 1974): (1) the most common feature of frontal atrophy contributes to the clinical signs of depression, bulimia, gluttony, apraxia and disorientation; (2) some Pick's disease patients with greater frontal lobe

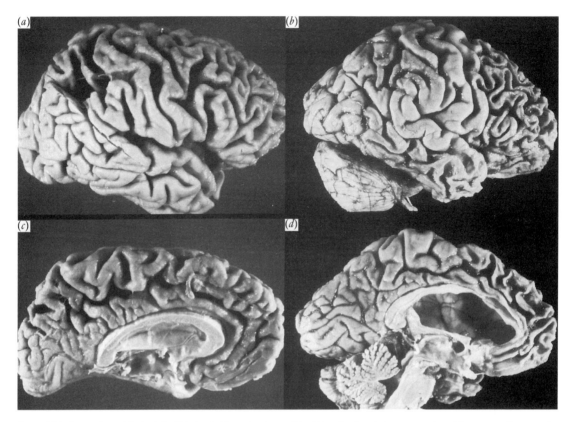

Figure 3.24. Comparison of the brain in Alzheimer's disease (a, c) and Pick's disease (b, d). Note that in Alzheimer's disease there is generalized cortical atrophy involving all lobes of the brain but somewhat less severe occipitally. In contrast, in Pick's disease there is severe atrophy of the frontal lobe and the anterior inferior temporal lobe. Note also the relative preservation of the precentral gyrus and the characteristic atrophy of the anterior portion of superior temporal gyrus (anterior to the central sulcus) with preservation of the posterior portions of that gyrus.

involvement also exhibit palilalia, echolalia and stereotypic behaviors ; (3) when the precentral gyrus is involved, pyramidal and extrapyramidal symptoms and dysarthria can be identified; and (4) atrophy in the hippocampal limbic and frontotemporal areas is associated with wide mood swings and behavioral disinhibition.

Cognitive changes in Pick's disease

There have been only a few large series of Pick's disease cases published, and most references to the disease are based on single case reports. Hodges and Gurd (1994), for example, provided a detailed description of the clinical, neuropsychological, and neuropathological findings of a 67-year-old man with Pick's disease. Slight focal atrophy of the orbitomedial region with ventricular enlargement was shown by computed tomographic (CT) scan. Post-mortem neuropathological examination established the presence of Pick bodies in the hippocampal granular and pyramidal cells; ballooned cells (Pick cells) in the neocortex; mild to moderate atrophy of the orbitomedial frontal lobes, inferior temporal gyrus and parahippocampal gyrus; and ventricular enlargement. The patient displayed significant deficits in memory and frontal lobe function, but had a near-perfect score on the Mini-Mental State Exam. Semantic memory and lexical retrieval abilities deteriorated with disease progression. Anterograde verbal and nonverbal memory were significantly impaired although better performance was observed with recognition versus free recall tasks. Episodic remote memories assessed with the Famous Faces Test were normal when first tested, but fell to a clinically impaired range within 16 months. Similar results were obtained for the Famous

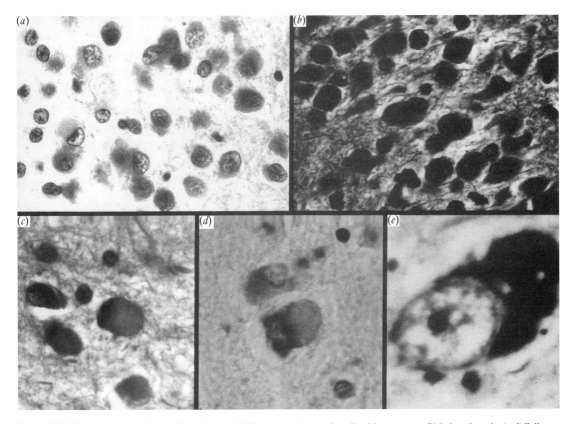

Figure 3.25. Hippocampal pathology in Picks disease: (a) Balloon cells (Pick cells). Luxol fast blue-cresyl violet stain. (b, e) Pick bodies in granular cells of dentate gyrus. Bielschowsky stain. (c, d) Balloon cells (Pick cells). Hematoxylin and eosin stain.

Events test. Short-term working memory (assessed by digit-span forward and backward) was found to be preserved. This pattern of deficits was considered to be typical of the cognitive changes associated with Pick's disease.

Comparison of Pick's and Alzheimer's diseases

Individual clinical presentations of Pick's disease and AD can often be very similar, making diagnosis difficult and necessitating neuropathological confirmation (Arnold et al. 1994). Pick's disease causes extensive atrophy and gliosis throughout the frontal lobe and anterior temporal lobe, most prominent in cortical layer III. Pick bodies are most evident in the insula and inferior temporal cortex. Loss of hippocampal dentate gyrus granular neurons with relatively preserved pyramidal neurons is characteristic of Pick's disease, while in AD there is early loss of hippocampal pyramidal neurons with preservation of the dentate gyrus neurons (Figure 3.26).

Nearly three-quarters of Pick's disease patients display early personality changes and behaviors such as roaming, hyperorality and disinhibition, while less than one-third of AD patients have such symptoms. These behaviors correlate with the greater frontal and anterior temporal lobe damage in Pick's disease. Language changes in Pick's disease are suggestive of 'anterior' (nonfluent) aphasia with reduced speech production, word-finding difficulties and echolalia (Mendez et al. 1993).

In addition to the clinical overlap of Pick's disease with AD, the neuropathological features of Pick's disease overlap with those of frontal lobe dementia, primary progressive aphasia, corticobasal degeneration and multi-system atrophy. Because of the neuropathological similarities, these latter disorders have been grouped together under the heading 'Pick's complex'.

Feany and colleagues (1996) have attempted to differentiate Pick's disease from progressive supranuclear palsy and corticobasal degeneration. All three disorders

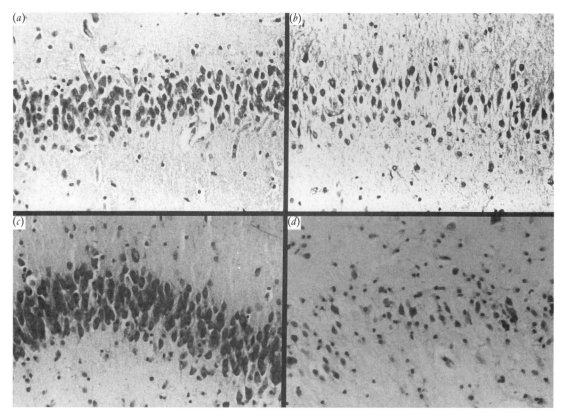

Figure 3.26. Comparison of hippocampal dentate gyrus in Alzheimer's disease (a, c) and Pick's disease (b, d). Note the marked loss of small granular neurons in the dentate gyrus of the hippocampal formation in Pick's disease and preservation in Alzheimer's disease. Luxol fast blue-cresyl violet stain.

involved abnormalities of cortical and subcortical regions; however, Pick's disease showed more cortical involvement, progressive supranuclear palsy more subcortical damage and corticobasal degeneration showed similarly extensive cortical and subcortical pathology. The three disorders all involved significant pathology in the substantia nigra, subthalamic nucleus and locus ceruleus; however, Pick's disease was distinguished by greater numbers of ballooned neurons; corticobasal degeneration was distinguished by numerous neuropil threads in gray and white matter and neurofibrillary tangles in the globus pallidus; progressive supranuclear palsy cases also had numerous tangles in the globus pallidus, but few neuropil threads or ballooned neurons. Thus, although there was significant overlap, neuropathological changes were relatively distinct for each disorder, which suggests separate pathophysiological entities.

CORTICOBASAL DEGENERATION

Corticobasal degeneration is a rare, neurodegenerative disorder which presents with clinical signs of apraxia, asymmetric akinetic-rigid syndrome, supranuclear gaze palsy, alien limb syndrome and dystonia/myoclonus (Gibb et al. 1989). Pathological changes consistent with the disease include neuropil threads, spongiosis and swollen and ballooned neurons present diffusely in the cerebral cortex (predominantly in the parietal or frontoparietal areas) (Gibb et al. 1989; Litvan et al. 1996b). Some patients have neurofibrillary tangles in the brain stem, dentate nucleus, subcortical nuclei, cerebral cortex and spinal cord. Argyrophilic and tau-positive basophilic neuronal inclusions are found in the basal ganglia and substantia nigra (Gibb et al. 1989; Litvan et al. 1996b). Severe neuronal loss and gliosis occur in the putamen, globus pallidus, locus ceruleus, substantia nigra, red nucleus, thalamus and subthalamic nucleus. Neuronal loss in the brain stem monoaminergic nuclei results in decreased levels of dopamine and norepinephrine (Gibb et al. 1989).

Cognitive function is impaired in some patients with corticobasal degeneration. Neuropsychological examinations of patients reveal the following: poor abstraction, word fluency deficits, apraxia, anomia, slowed speech and generalized intellectual loss (Gibb et al. 1989; Beatty et al. 1995). Damage to corticostriatal pathways is hypothesized to cause deficits in verbal fluency and nondeclarative memory (Gibb et al. 1989; Beatty et al. 1995). Declarative memory decline is evident on measures of recall and recognition, but performance on recognition tasks is disproportionately better. Relatively preserved recognition memory is associated with the lack of involvement of the hippocampus and adjacent temporal areas, while deficits in remote memory may be accounted for by degenerative changes in the temporoparietal cortices (Beatty et al. 1995).

HUNTINGTON'S DISEASE

Huntington's disease (HD) is a genetically determined, autosomal dominant disorder with an estimated prevalence of 4–8 per 100 000 (Kokmen et al. 1994). Each child of an affected parent has a 50% chance of inheriting the disease gene. Huntington's disease has a typical onset between ages 35 and 50 years, and leads to death after 15–20 years (Myers et al. 1988). The onset of HD may vary from age 4 to age 70 years, and over 25% of all cases begin after age 50 years while 7% begin before age 20 years.

Clinical features include chorea, dyskinesia, impaired fine motor movements of limbs, visuospatial problems, emotional changes and gaze apraxia (Koroshetz et al. 1993; Tatemichi et al. 1994). Behavioral changes which accompany or precede motor impairments include memory disturbances, depression, irritability and occasionally psychosis. As the disease progresses, cognitive and motor disturbances become increasingly worse, leading to loss of independent function over the course of 10–20 years (Gusella et al. 1993). Juvenile HD patients often manifest features of progressive rigidity (without chorea), dysarthria, mental deterioration, epilepsy, hyperreflexia, oculomotor apraxia, tremor in limbs and bradykinesia (Bruyn and Went 1986; Koroshetz et al. 1993). The duration of juvenile onset HD varies from 2 (Bruyn and Went 1986) to 12 years (Myers et al. 1988).

The genetic mutation underlying HD involves a CAG repeat sequence located on chromosome 4 (4p16) at the G8 locus. Expansion of the repeat sequence to greater than 35 is associated with the disease (Ashizawa et al. 1994; Penney et al. 1997). Normally, the gene codes for a polyglutamine protein called huntingtin, which is essential for normal nervous system development. The mutated form of huntingtin may cause inappropriate apoptotic cell death (programmed cell death), which is enhanced by longer polyglutamine segments of the protein (Nasir et al. 1996). Individuals with longer repeats have symptom onset at an earlier age. Affected children of affected fathers have an earlier onset of symptoms than those with affected mothers due to greater expansion of the trinucleotide repeat sequence (Koroshetz et al. 1993). Through this unusual pattern of inheritance, disease severity can increase and onset occur earlier in successive generations (termed anticipation).

Neuropathology of Huntington's disease

The hallmark pathological change in HD is marked atrophy of the caudate nucleus and putamen, with additional atrophy of thalamus, brain stem and cerebellum (Figure 3.27). Early in the disease process, there is loss of the striatal medium spiny neurons (which compose 80–90% of striatal neurons), first in the caudate and later in the putamen (Koroshetz et al. 1993) (Figure 3.28). Other areas affected include the globus pallidus, subthalamic nucleus, substantia nigra and hypothalamus. Neuronal loss and reactive astrocytosis in cortical layers III, V, and VI lead to a 20–30% overall reduction in thickness of the cerebral cortex (Roos 1986).

The movement disorder (chorea) results from loss of striatal medium spiny neurons (Côté and Crutcher 1991). The medium spiny neurons receive the majority of dopaminergic afferents from the substantia nigra along with glutamatergic afferents from the cortex, and they contain γ-aminobutyric acid (GABA), opiate peptides and substance P (Koroshetz et al. 1993; Gusella et al. 1993). Consistent with the loss of medium spiny neurons in the caudate and putamen are the severely decreased levels of GABA and its synthesizing enzyme, glutamic acid decarboxylase (GAD). Reduction in acetylcholine and the enzyme choline acetyltransferase, enkephalin, substance P and dynorphin also occurs (Tatemichi et al. 1994).

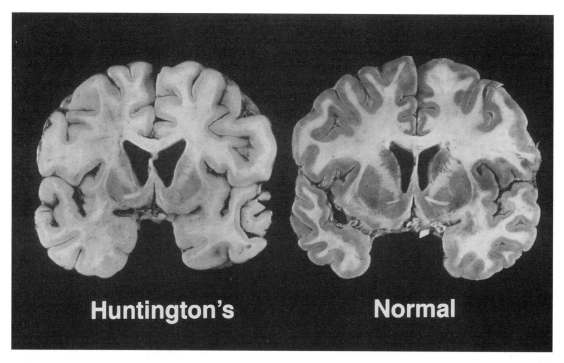

Figure 3.27. Coronal brain section at the level of the anterior commissure in Huntington's disease and normal. Note the marked atrophy of the caudate nucleus, lesser atrophy of the putamen, and dilation of the lateral ventricles in Huntington's disease.

The death of GABA neurons probably relates to glutamate excitotoxicity. This hypothesis is supported by experimental studies injecting excitatory agonists of *N*-methyl-*D*-aspartate (NMDA) receptors (one of the subtypes of glutamate receptors) which produce death of the medium spiny neurons in a pattern similar to that seen in HD (Ellison et al. 1987).

Afifi (1994) reviewed basal ganglia (caudate, putamen, globus pallidus, nucleus accumbens septi and olfactory tubercle) function in HD and PD. There are five anatomical and functional cortico–striato–thalamo–cortical loops: (1) putamen/motor pathway for motor planning and initiation; (2) caudate nucleus/oculomotor pathway important for saccadic eye movements; (3) caudate nucleus/dorsolateral prefrontal pathway important for spatial memory; (4) caudate nucleus/lateral orbitofrontal prefrontal pathway important in set and activity shifting; and (5) ventral striatum/limbic pathway important for emotional and behavioral control. Through these pathways, the basal ganglia are involved in motor preparation and execution, sensory–motor gating, cognition, emotion and behavior. Lesions to the dorsolateral prefrontal circuit result in cognitive and spatial memory disturbances in HD and PD (Afifi 1994).

The five pathways function in similar ways: each cortical area sends excitatory glutamatergic projections to the striatum which produces striatal inhibitory GABAergic effects on thalamic nuclei. Furthermore, there are indirect and direct pathways from the striatum to the output nuclei (internal segment of globus pallidus and substantia nigra pars reticulata) (Figure 3.29). In HD, the loss of striatal GABAergic neurons results in disinhibition of the external segment of globus pallidus, excess inhibition of subthalamic nucleus, decreased excitation of substantia nigra pars reticulata and internal segment of globus pallidus and less inhibition of the thalamus. The result is random unwanted movements (Figure 3.30).

It is of interest to note the opposing symptoms and pathology of HD and PD. Whereas HD causes decreased basal ganglia output with consequent hypotonia and hyperkinesia, PD leads to increased basal ganglia output with resultant hypertonia and hypokinesia (Côté and Crutcher 1991).

Autopsy results from patients with preclinical HD

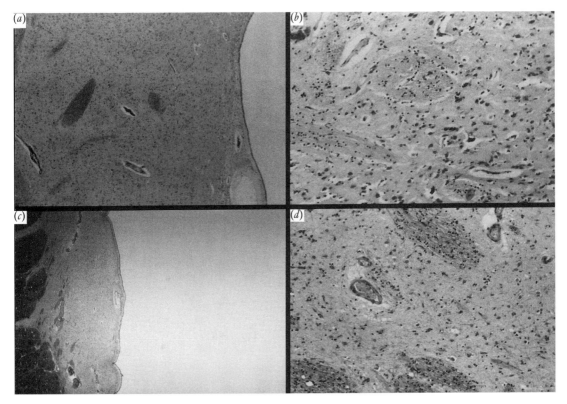

Figure 3.28. Comparison of microscopic appearance of the caudate nucleus in normal brain (a, b) and Huntington's disease (c, d). Note that in Huntington's disease there is severe atrophy of the caudate nucleus (c, low power) and marked neuronal loss (d, high power). Luxol fast blue-periodic acid Schiff-hematoxylin.

indicate that a large percentage of striatal neurons are lost prior to symptom onset (Carrasco and Mukherji 1986). Cognitive changes are numerous and increase in severity as the disease progresses. Motor deficits are linked to changes in the caudate nucleus while emotional and neuropsychological changes are related to cortical atrophy and frontal deafferentation. Dementia in HD is correlated with the degree of caudate atrophy rather than frontal atrophy, although frontal lobe function is significantly affected by the caudate atrophy (Tomlinson 1992).

Cognitive changes in Huntington's disease

Caine and Shoulson (1983) report five categories of neuropsychological changes which occur in HD. Cognitive changes occur in: (1) arousal, attention and concentration; (2) affect and mood; (3) perception; (4) intellectual function; and (5) personality. With regard to memory impairments, Butters et al. (1985) proposed that declarative memory impairments in HD are due to deficits in the initiation and maintenance of memory retrieval strategies. Empirical findings suggest that the retrieval deficit hypothesis is applicable to all declarative memory deficits in HD, regardless of the memory dichotomies invoked (i.e. episodic verus semantic, anterograde versus retrograde). Butters and colleagues discovered that both HD and amnesiac patients demonstrated impaired recall and recognition on an episodic memory test, but that the performance of HD patients improved disproportionately on recognition testing. Similarly, retrieval deficits likely account for HD patients' poor performance on semantic memory (e.g. verbal fluency) tasks (Tröster et al. 1989b). The interpretation that retrieval deficits underlie retrograde amnesia in HD is supported primarily by the observation that the memory impairment is equally severe across all decades of life (i.e. there is a 'flat' temporal gradient) (Beatty et al. 1988). Given the frontosubcortical

(a)

(b)

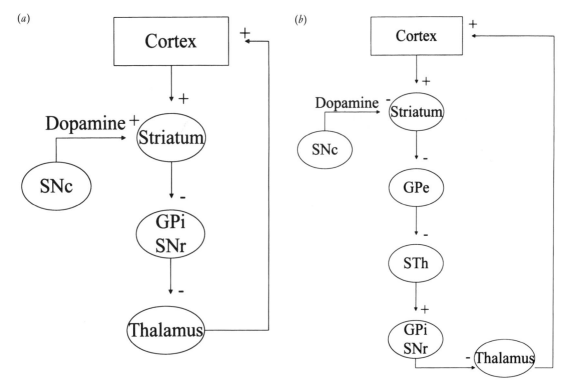

Figure 3.29. Schematic diagram of the direct and indirect striatopallidal pathways in control of normal movement. (a) The direct pathway is excitatory and reinforces wanted behavior. (b) The indirect pathway is inhibitory and suppresses unwanted behavior. GPi: internal segment of globus pallidus; SNr: substantia nigra pars reticulata; SNc: substantia nigra pars compacta; GPe: external segment of globus pallidus; STh: subthalamic nucleus. Adapted from Afifi (1994). Basal ganglia: functional anatomy and physiology. Part 2. *Journal of Child Neurology* 9, 352–361 (figures 10–12), with permission.

pathology of HD, the proposal that retrieval deficits underlie remote memory impairment in HD is also consistent with Kopelman's (1989) contention that frontal dysfunction underlies deficient remote memory retrieval.

Research on nondeclarative memory in HD suggests that the disease involves deficits in motor and cognitive skill learning as assessed with pursuit rotor and Tower of Hanoi tasks (Butters et al. 1985; Heindel et al. 1989). Priming appears to be relatively intact in HD (Heindel et al. 1989). This dissociation between skill learning and priming in HD likely reflects that the former requires an intact corticostriatal system (which is damaged in HD; Pillon et al. 1991), whereas priming is mediated by the relatively unaffected neocortical association areas (Terry and Katzman 1983).

PRION DISEASES

Prion diseases are transmissible neurodegenerative disorders which have been identified in five different human variants: (1) kuru, a disease transmitted through the death rituals in New Guinea; (2) Creutzfeldt–Jakob disease, a world-wide disorder that occurs sporadically; (3) fatal familial insomnia, a heritable disease; (4) atypical prion disease, sporadically occurring or heritable; and (5) Gerstmann–Sträussler–Scheinker syndrome, a heritable disease (Prusiner 1996). Animal variants of prion disease include scrapie in sheep and goats, chronic wasting disease in mule deer and elk, bovine spongiform encephalopathy ('mad cow disease'), exotic ungulate spongiform encephalopathy, feline spongiform encephalopathy and transmissible mink encephalopathy (Prusiner, 1988; Hansen 1994; Gajdusek 1996).

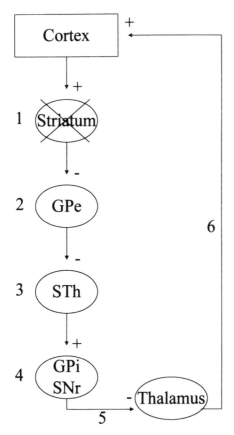

Figure 3.30. Schematic diagram showing how the striatal lesion in Huntington's disease affects the indirect striatopallidal pathway for movement. Loss of matrix neurons projecting to GPe (1), results in disinhibition of GPe (2), which results in excess inhibition of STh (3), which then results in decreased excitation of GPi and SNr (4), resulting in less inhibition of the thalamus (5), producing random unwanted movement (6). GPi : internal segment of globus pallidus; SNr : substantia nigra pars reticulata; GPe : external segment of globus pallidus; STh : subthalamic nucleus. Adapted from Afifi (1994). Basal ganglia: functional anatomy and physiology. Part 2. *Journal of Child Neurology* 9, 352–361 (figures 10–12), with permission.

Table 3.8. *Prion protein gene mutations in prion diseases*

Human prion disease variant	Insertions or codon mutations in PRNP
Familial Creutzfeldt–Jakob disease	178, 200, 210
Fatal familial insomnia	178
Gerstmann–Sträussler–Scheinker syndrome with ataxia, variable spongiform change	102, 117
Mixed Creutzfeldt–Jakob and Gerstmann–Sträussler–Scheinker syndrome with atypically long duration and variable spongiform change	Insertions in octapeptide region; 145 (stop)
Gerstmann–Sträussler–Scheinker syndrome with neurofibrillary tangles	198, 217, 145
Gerstmann–Sträussler–Scheinker syndrome with spastic paralysis	105

Source: Adapted from Richardson and Masters 1995; Ghetti et al. 1996.

Prion diseases (also called subacute spongiform encephalopathies in humans) are both infectious and genetic, but unlike other known infectious agents, prions lack a nucleic acid genome to code for progeny (Prusiner 1996). These diseases are transmissible cerebral amyloidoses which involve the modification of the host precursor protein into insoluble amyloid fibrils (Gajdusek 1996). Prion diseases affect only the central nervous system.

Molecular studies have identified an abnormal isoform of the prion protein, identified as PrP^{Sc}, produced by a conformational change in the normally produced isoform PrP^C (Ghetti et al. 1996). In humans, the prion protein gene (identified as PRNP in the literature) is located on the short arm of chromosome 20 (Prusiner 1988). The normal function of PrP^C is unknown, but mutations of the prion protein gene are associated with several different diseases (DeArmond and Prusiner 1995; Richardson and Masters 1995; Ghetti et al. 1996). Table 3.8 outlines the currently identified genetic mutations associated with prion diseases (Richardson and Masters 1995).

Mechanisms involved in human prion diseases include infection, sporadic occurrence and genetic transmission. The incubation period following infection ranges from several weeks to three decades (Prusiner 1988). Prion diseases have been successfully transmitted in experimental studies to laboratory animals and accidentally to humans from treatment with contaminated growth hormone extract during surgical procedures and from contaminated cadaveric dural grafts (Brown 1994).

It is hypothesized that when a molecule of prion protein PrP^C undergoes a conformational change to PrP^{Sc}, this PrP^{Sc} then serves as a nidus for causing structural alteration of adjacent PrP^C molecules. The conformational change then propagates to all the existing and any newly formed PrP^C molecules. The conformational alteration that produces PrP^{Sc} allows the material to precipitate in β-pleated sheets (amyloid), which are extremely stable and resistant to degradation and are also apparently toxic to central nervous system cells. The PrP^{Sc} is found in enlarging intracellular vacuoles which results in the spongiform microscopic appearance. The original transformation or PrP^C to PrP^{Sc} can occur because of a mutation in the PRNP gene which makes spontaneous structural changes in the molecule possible (thus, the heritable forms of the disease). Entrance of preformed PrP^{Sc} into the nervous system can also serve as the initial nidus (thus, the transmissible nature of the disease). Rare spontaneous aberrant chemical events in the nervous system could alter an otherwise normal PrP^C molecule to the PrP^{Sc} form again resulting in a nidus (thus, the world-wide distribution of the sporadic form of Creutzfeldt–Jakob disease) (Ghetti et al. 1996; Gajdusek 1996).

Creutzfeldt–Jakob disease

Neuropathology of Creutzfeldt–Jakob disease

Neuropathological findings in Creutzfeldt–Jakob disease, the most common of the human prion disorders, include spongiform changes, neuronal loss and profound reactive astrocytosis in the gray matter with no inflammatory response. Kuru plaques, which are round, compact, eosinophilic, extracellular deposits of PrP^{Sc} can sometimes be identified in the cerebellum (Kretzschmar et al. 1996). Early in the course, the spongiform change is a delicate vacuolization of the neuropil of the thalamus, basal ganglia, cerebellar molecular layer, and cerebral neocortex, often leaving the hippocampus unaffected. Status spongiosus occurs in later stages, presumably from coalescence of the delicate vacuoles resulting in large vacuolar spaces accompanied by severe gliosis and profound neuronal loss.

Spongiform changes in the white matter appear in a variant termed panencephalitic Creutzfeldt–Jakob disease. In addition, significant myelin degeneration can be found in brain stem, cerebellum and corticospinal and spinocerebellar tracts. This type of neuropathology has been mainly described in Japanese patients with a longer disease duration (Kretzschmar et al. 1996; Shyu et al. 1996) (Figure 3.31).

Some of the features common to both AD and Creutzfeldt–Jakob disease include similar gender distribution (males and females equally affected), age of onset (67 years in AD, 60 years in Creutzfeldt–Jakob disease), progressive mental deterioration, neuronal loss and gliosis, and amyloid plaques (ß/A4-amyloid in AD and PrP^{Sc} amyloid in Creutzfeldt–Jakob disease) (Hansen 1994). The spongiform changes that are considered pathognomonic of Creutzfeldt–Jakob disease occur in all cortical layers, while loosening of the neuropil secondary to reactive gliosis can produce a spongiform-like change in the upper cortical layers in AD (Kretzschmar et al. 1996) (Figure 3.32).

Initially, there is generalized atrophy of basal ganglia, thalamus and cerebellar folia in Creutzfeldt–Jakob disease. Clinical signs of extrapyramidal movement disorders have been correlated with the changes in the basal ganglia (Shyu et al. 1996). Cortical atrophy becomes severe within 1 year after onset. The appearance of the brain at autopsy is variable, but most brains show some degree of cortical atrophy (thinning) with ventricular enlargement (Hansen 1994). Magnetic resonance images (MRI) of Creutzfeldt–Jakob disease patients have revealed bilateral increased signal intensity in the caudate nucleus and putamen which correlates with the degree of cortical and basal ganglion atrophy. Signal intensity has also been correlated with the degree of astrocytosis and vacuolization of the neuropil (Finkenstaedt et al. 1996).

Cognitive and neurologic changes in Creutzfeldt–Jakob disease

Clinical diagnosis in Creutzfeldt–Jakob disease is based on the appearance of periodic sharp-wave complexes on electroencephalography (EEG) and the presence of two or more of the following features: myoclonus, visual or cerebellar symptoms, akinetic mutism and pyramidal or extrapyramidal signs (Finkenstaedt et al. 1996). MRI often shows increased signal intensity in the thalamus, striatum and cerebral cortex (Gertz et al. 1988).

Neuropsychological and clinical changes are prominent and progress rapidly, with the typical disease course spanning 6 months to 1 year (Matthews 1985; Brown et al. 1986). Due to the rapid progression of Creutzfeldt–Jakob disease, detailed clinical information is often limited (Matthews 1985). Memory disturbances, behavioral abnormalities, dysphasia, dysarthria, agraphia and loss of insight are common with Creutzfeldt–Jakob disease. Neurological symptoms such as myoclonus, spasticity and rigidity, and primitive reflexes are prominent (Matthews 1985; Brown 1994).

Figure 3.31. Pathological changes in prion disease include severe spongiform changes (status spongiosus). The whole cerebral cortical thickness in a gyrus is involved (a). The spongiform appearance is due to numerous intracellular and extracellular vacuoles of varying size; large vacuoles are the result of coalescence of many smaller vacuoles (b; high magnification). Remnant neurons contain large amounts of lipofuscin (c; dark arrow) and large reactive astrocytes with vacuolated cytoplasm are evident (c; white arrow). Hematoxylin and eosin stain.

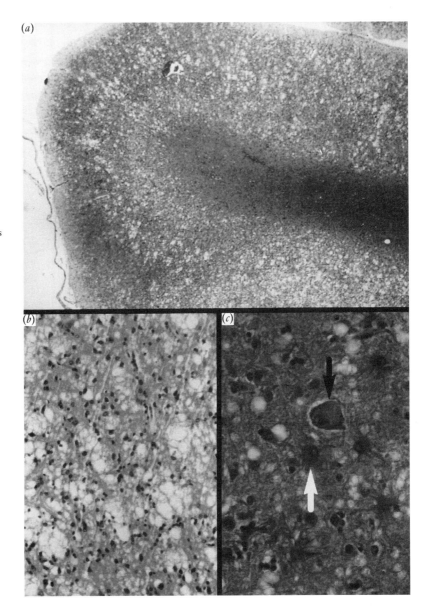

In a series of 230 cases of Creutzfeldt–Jakob disease it was found that the cognitive deterioration apparent at disease onset included memory dysfunction, behavioral abnormalities and higher cortical function deficits (Brown et al. 1986). Neurological changes which began early in the disease were gait disturbance, clumsiness and visual changes. In later stages, all patients became demented and displayed progressively worse cerebellar and extrapyramidal signs. Most patients had myoclonus, gait disturbances or other movement disorders. EEG changes were observed in 80% of the patients. Death occurred within 1 year following symptom onset in 90% of the patients. Although specific cognitive changes were not described, clinical changes correlated with the severity of neuronal loss, spongiform changes and gliosis (Brown et al. 1994).

Gerstmann–Sträussler–Scheinker disease

Gerstmann–Sträussler–Scheinker disease is characterized by progressive ataxia, extrapyramidal signs, spastic paraparesis and dementia. This disease has an autosomal

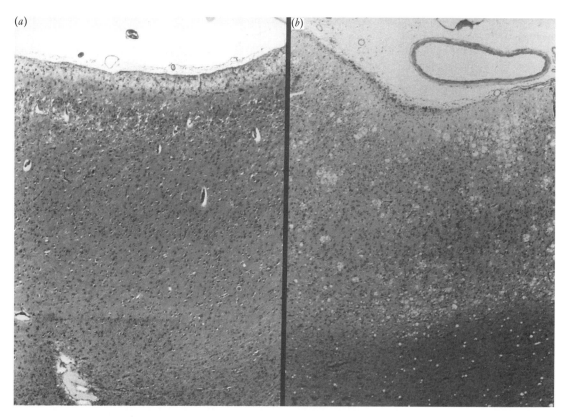

(a)   (b)

Figure 3.32. While loosening of the neuropil in upper cortical layers secondary to reactive gliosis in Alzheimer's disease can simulate spongiform change (a), true spongiform change in prion diseases diffusely involves all cortical layers (b). Hematoxylin and eosin stain.

dominant pattern of inheritance. At least five different mutations to the PRNP gene have been discovered which cause Gerstmann–Sträussler–Scheinker disease, each resulting in a slightly different clinical presentation (Brown 1994; Budka et al. 1995; Ghetti et al. 1996).

Gerstmann–Sträussler–Scheinker disease differs from familial Creutzfeldt–Jakob disease in several ways: (1) higher frequency of cerebellar and pseudobulbar deficits; (2) infrequent presence of myoclonus and abnormal electroencephalographic activity; and (3) longer survival period (4 years for Gerstmann–Sträussler–Scheinker disease versus 1 year for Creutzfeldt–Jakob disease). Neuropathological examination reveals numerous PrP[Sc] amyloid plaques in the central nervous system, particularly in the cerebral cortex and basal ganglia, as well as spongiform changes in all cortical layers (Brown 1994; Budka et al. 1995; Ghetti et al. 1996).

Detailed studies of cognitive changes in Gerstmann–Sträussler–Scheinker disease are rare. In a recent report of three cases, Unverzagt et al. (1997) described a 'global' dementia, characterized by deficits in intelligence, executive function, information processing speed, motor skills and memory, in two cases. In the third case, symptomatic for less than 1 year, deficits in verbal fluency, memory and motor skills were interpreted as suggestive of predominantly subcortical involvement early in the disease.

Kuru

Kuru was characterized by shivering-like tremor, progressive cerebellar ataxia, followed by dysarthria, emotional lability, loss of speech and complete incapacitation. Death typically occurred within 1 year after disease onset. This disease was restricted to the New Guinean highlands where natives practiced an elaborate death ceremony. Following the cessation of this custom, kuru virtually disappeared. Unlike Creutzfeldt–Jakob disease, dementia was rare. Neuropathological changes were characterized by reactive astrocytosis, minimal status spongiosis of cerebral gray matter, neuronal loss and the presence of kuru plaques in 75% of the cases, predominantly in the cerebellum (for reviews see Brown 1994; Gajdusek 1996).

Fatal familial insomnia

Fatal familial insomnia is an autosomal dominant disease which has an onset around age 49 years and a duration of slightly over 1 year. Affected individuals suffer a progressive loss of total sleep time including rapid eye movement (REM) sleep. Electroencephalography shows a nonspecific slowing without the periodic complexes found in Creutzfeldt–Jakob disease. Focal spongiform changes in the anterior ventral and mediodorsal thalamic nuclei underlie the sleep disturbances, as well as autonomic, motor and endocrine dysfunction. Neuropathological changes also include generalized neuronal loss and reactive astrocytosis in the thalamus with lesser changes in the entorhinal cortex and cerebral neocortex. Similar to Gerstmann–Sträussler–Scheinker disease and familial Creutzfeldt–Jakob disease, the etiology can be traced to a mutation of the PRNP gene (Budka et al. 1995).

ACKNOWLEDGMENTS

We thank Tamara R. Sigler for help with many of the figures. The authors also express their appreciation to the Oklahoma Chapter of the Alzheimer's Association for their support. Julie A. Testa was supported by the National Institute of Drug Abuse grant T32-DA07248.

REFERENCES

Afifi, A.K. 1994. Basal ganglia: Functional anatomy and physiology. Part 2. *Journal of Child Neurology*. 9: 352–361.

Agid, Y., Ruberg, M., Dubois, B. and Javoy-Agid, F. 1984. Biochemical substrates of mental disturbances in Parkinson's disease. In *Parkinson-specific motor and mental disorders*, ed. R.G. Hassler and J.F. Christ, pp. 211–218. New York: Raven Press.

Agid, Y., Ruberg, M., Dubois, B. and Pillon, B. 1987. Anatomoclinical and biochemical concepts of subcortical dementia. In *Cognitive neuropharmacology*, ed. S.M. Stahl, S.D. Iverson and E.C. Goodman, pp. 248–271. Oxford: Oxford University Press.

Albert, M.L., Feldman, R.G. and Willis, A.L. 1974. The 'subcortical dementia' of progressive supranuclear palsy. *Journal of Neurology, Neurosurgery and Psychiatry*. 37: 121–130.

Alvord, E.C., Forno, L.S., Kusske, J.A., Kauffman, R.J., Rhodes, J.S. and Goetowski, C.R. 1974. The pathology of parkinsonism: A comparison of degeneration in the cerebral cortex and brainstem. *Advances in Neurology*. 5: 175–193.

Alzheimer, A. 1987. A characteristic disease of the cerebral cortex. In *The early story of Alzheimer's disease*, ed. K. Bick, L. Amaducci and G. Pepeu, pp. 1–4. New York: Raven Press. (Original title: Über eine eigenartige Erkrankung der Hirnrinde. *Allgemeine Zeitschrift für Psychiatrie und Psychisch-Gerichtliche Medizin*. 1907; 64: 146–148.)

Amaducci, L.A., Rocca, W.A. and Schoenberg, B.S. 1986. Origin of the distinction between Alzheimer's disease and senile dementia: how history can clarify nosology. *Neurology*. 36: 1497–1499.

American Psychiatric Association 1994. *Diagnostic and Statistical Manual of Mental Disorders*, 4th ed. Washington, DC: American Psychiatric Association.

Anderson, B. 1996. Axonal length correlates with dementia severity in Alzheimer's disease. *Medical Science Research*. 24: 271–273.

Appollonio, I., Grafman, J., Clark, K., Nichelli, P., Zeffiro, T. and Hallett, M. 1994. Implicit and explicit memory in patients with Parkinson's disease with and without dementia. *Archives of Neurology*. 51: 359–367.

Arnold, S.E., Hyman, B.T. and Van Hoesen, G.W. 1994. Neuropathologic changes of the temporal pole in Alzheimer's disease and Pick's disease. *Archives of Neurology*. 51: 145–150.

Ashall, F. and Goate, A.M. 1994. Role of the ß-amyloid precursor protein in Alzheimer's disease. *Trends in Biochemistry*. 19: 42–45.

Ashizawa, T., Wong, L.-J.C., Richards, C.S., Caskey, C.T. and Jankovic, J. 1994. CAG repeat size and clinical presentation in Huntington's disease. *Neurology*. 44: 1137–1143.

Bachman, D.L., Wolf, P.A., Linn, R.T. et al. 1993. Incidence of dementia and probable Alzheimer's disease in a general population: The Framingham Study. *Neurology*. 43: 515–519.

Bartus, R.T., Dean, R.L., Pontecorvo, M.J. and Flicker, C. 1985. The cholinergic hypothesis: A historical overview, current perspective and future directions. *Annals of the New York Academy of Sciences*. 444: 332–357.

Beatty, W.W. 1992. Memory disturbances in Parkinson's disease. In *Parkinson's disease: Neurobehavioral aspects*, ed. S. Huber and J. Cummings, pp. 49–58. New York: Oxford University Press.

Beatty, W.W. and Salmon, D.P. 1991. Remote memory for visuospatial information in patients with Alzheimer's disease. *Journal of Geriatric Psychiatry and Neurology*. 4: 14–17.

Beatty, W.W., Salmon, D.P., Butters, N., Heindel, W.C. and Granholm, E.L. 1988. Retrograde amnesia in patients with Alzheimer's disease or Huntington's disease. *Neurobiology of Aging*. 9: 181–186.

Beatty, W.W., Scott, J.G., Wilson, D.A., Prince, J.R. and Williamson, D.J. 1995. Memory deficits in a demented patient with probable corticobasal degeneration. *Journal of Geriatric Psychiatry and Neurology*. 8: 132–136.

Beatty, W.W., Winn, P., Adams, R.L., Allen, W., Wilson, D.A., Prince, J.R., Olson K.A., Dean, K. and Littleford, D. 1994. Preserved cognitive skills in dementia of the Alzheimer type. *Archives of Neurology*. 51: 1040–1046.

Bertoni-Freddari, C., Fattoretti, P., Paoloni, R., Caselli, U., Galeazzi, L. and Meier-Ruge, W. 1996. Synaptic structural dynamics and aging. *Gerontology*. 42: 170–180.

Bondareff, W., Mountjoy, C.Q. and Roth, M. 1981. Selective loss of neurons of origin of adrenergic projection to cerebral cortex (nucleus locus coeruleus) in senile dementia. *Lancet*. I: 783–784.

Bornebroek, M., Haan, J., Maat-Schieman, M.L.C., Van Duinen, S.G. and Roos, R.A.C. 1996. Hereditary cerebral hemorrhage with amyloidosis-Dutch type (HCHWA-D): I – A review of clinical, radiologic and genetic aspects. *Brain Pathology*. 6: 111–114.

Braak, H. and Braak, E. 1990. Cognitive impairment in Parkinson's disease: Amyloid plaques, neurofibrillary tangles and neuropil threads in the cerebral cortex. *Journal of Neural Transmission*. 2: 45–57.

Braak, H. and Braak, E. 1991. Neuro-pathological staging of Alzheimer-related changes. *Acta Neuropathologica* (Berlin). 82: 239–259.

Braak, H. and Braak, E. 1996. Evolution of the neuropathology of Alzheimer's disease. *Acta Neurologica Scandinavica*. 165: 3–12.

Brown, P. 1994. Transmissible human spongiform encephalopathy (infectious cerebral amyloidosis): Creutzfeldt–Jakob disease, Gerstmann–Sträussler–Scheinker syndrome and Kuru. In *Neurodegenerative diseases*, ed. D.B. Calne, pp. 839–877. Philadelphia: WB Saunders.

Brown, P., Cathala, F., Castaigne, P. and Gajdusek, D.C. 1986. Creutzfeldt–Jakob disease: Clinical analysis of a consecutive series of 230 neuro-pathologically verified cases. *Annals of Neurology*. 20: 597–602.

Brown, P., Gibbs, C.J., Rodgers-Johnson, P., Asher, D.M., Sulima, M.P., Bacote, A., Goldfarb, L.G. and Gajdusek, D.C. 1994. Human spongiform encephalopathy: The National Institutes of Health series of 300 cases of experimentally transmitted disease. *Annals of Neurology*. 35: 513–529.

Brumback, R.A. and Leech, R.W. 1994. Alzheimer's disease: Pathophysiology and the hope for therapy. *The Journal of the Oklahoma State Medical Association*. 87: 103–111.

Bruyn, G.W. and Went, L.N. 1986. Huntington's chorea. In *Handbook of clinical neurology*, vol. 5 (49), ed. P.J. Vinken, G.W. Bruyn and H.L. Klawans, pp. 267–313. New York: Elsevier.

Budka, H., Aguzzi, A., Brown, P., Brucher, J.M., Bugiani, O., Gullotta, F., Haltia, M., Hauw, J.J., Ironside, J.W., Jellinger, K., Kretzschmar, H.A., Lantos, P.L., Masullo, C., Scholte, W., Tateishi, J. and Weller, R.O. 1995. Neuropathological diagnostic criteria for Creutzfeldt–Jakob disease (CJD) and other human spongiform encephalopathies (prion diseases). *Brain Pathology*. 5: 459–466.

Butters, N., Delis, D.C. and Lucas, J.A. 1995. Clinical assessment of memory disorders in amnesia and dementia. *Annual Review of Psychology*. 46: 493–523.

Butters, N., Wolfe, J., Martone, M., Granholm, E. and Cermak, L.S. 1985. Memory disorders associated with Huntington's disease: Verbal recall, verbal recognition and procedural memory. *Neuropsychologia*. 23: 729–743.

Caine, E.D. and Shoulson, I. 1983. Psychiatric syndromes in Huntington's disease. *American Journal of Psychiatry*. 140: 728–733.

Carrasco, L.H. and Mukherji, C.S. 1986. Atrophy of corpus striatum in normal male at risk of Huntington's chorea. *Lancet.* I: 1388–1389.

Chertkow, H. and Bub, D. 1990. Semantic memory loss in dementia of Alzheimer's type. *Brain.* 113: 397–417.

Chui, H.C. 1989. Dementia: a review emphasizing clinicopathologic correlation and brain-behavior relationships. *Archives of Neurology.* 46: 806–814.

Chui, H.C., Mortimer, J.A., Slager, U., Zarow, C., Bondareff, W. and Webster, D.D. 1986. Pathologic correlates of dementia in Parkinson's disease. *Archives of Neurology.* 43: 991–995.

Constantinidis, J., Richard, J. and Tissot, R. 1974. Pick's disease: Histological and clinical correlations. *European Neurology.* 11: 208–217.

Corey-Bloom, J., Galasko, D. and Thal, L.J. 1994. Clinical features and natural history of Alzheimer's disease. In *Neurodegenerative diseases*, ed. D.B. Calne, pp. 631–645. Philadelphia: Saunders.

Côté, L. and Crutcher, M.D. 1991. The basal ganglia. In *Principles of neural science*, ed. E.R. Kandel, J.H. Schwartz and T.M. Jessell, pp. 647–659. Norwalk: Appleton and Lange.

Crystal, H.A., Dickson, D.W., Lizardi, J.E., Davies, P. and Wolfson, L.I. 1990. Antemortem diagnosis of diffuse Lewy body disease. *Neurology.* 40: 1523–1528.

Cummings, J.L. and Benson, D.F. 1984. Subcortical dementia: Review of an emerging concept. *Archives of Neurology.* 41: 874–879.

Cummings, J.L., Darkins, A., Mendez, M., Hill, M.A. and Benson, D.F. 1988. Alzheimer's disease and Parkinson's disease: Comparison of speech and language alterations. *Neurology.* 38: 680–684.

Curcio, C.A. and Kemper, T. 1984. Nucleus raphe dorsalis in dementia of the Alzheimer type: Neurofibrillary changes and neuronal packing density. *Journal of Neuropathology and Experimental Neurology.* 43: 359–368.

Damasio, A.R., Damasio, H., Rizzo, M., Varney, N. and Gersh, F. 1982. Aphasia with nonhemorrhagic lesions in the basal ganglia and internal capsule. *Archives of Neurology.* 39: 15–20.

Davies, P. and Maloney, A.J.F. 1976. Selective loss of central cholinergic neurons in Alzheimer's disease. *Lancet.* II: 1403.

Davis, K.L., Thal, L.J., Gamzu, E.R., Davis, C.S., Woolson, R.F., Gracon, S.I., Drachman, D.A., Schneider, L.S., Whitehouse, P.J., Hoover, T.M., Morris, J.C., Kawas, C.H., Knopman, D.S., Earl, N.L., Kumar, V., Doody, R.S. and the Tacrine Collaborative Study Group. 1992. A double-blind, placebo-controlled multicenter study of tacrine for Alzheimer's disease. *New England Journal of Medicine.* 327: 1253–1259.

DeArmond, S.J. and Prusiner, S.B. 1995. Prion protein transgenes and the neuropathology in prion diseases. *Brain Pathology.* 5: 77–89.

DeKosky, S.T. and Scheff, S.W. 1990. Synapse loss in frontal cortex biopsied in Alzheimer's disease: Correlation with cognitive severity. *Annals of Neurology.* 27: 457–464.

Delaère, P., Duyckaerts, C., Brion, J.P., Poulain, V. and Hauw, J.J. 1989. Tau, paired helical filaments and amyloid in the neocortex: A morphometric study of 15 cases with graded intellectual status in aging and senile dementia of Alzheimer type. *Acta Neuropathologica* (Berlin). 77: 645–653.

Dickson, D.W., Ruan, D., Crystal, H., Mark, M.H., Davies, P., Kress, Y. and Yen, S.H. 1991. Hippocampal degeneration differentiates diffuse Lewy body disease (DLBD) from Alzheimer's disease: Light and electron microscopic immunocytochemistry of CA2–3 neurites specific to DLBD. *Neurology.* 41: 1402–1409.

Doraiswamy, P.M., Krishen, A., Stallone, F., Martin, W.L., Potts, N.L., Metz, A. and DeVeaugh-Geiss, J. 1995. Cognitive performance on the Alzheimer's Disease Assessment Scale: Effect of education. *Neurology.* 45: 1980–1984.

Drachman, D.A. and Leavitt, J. 1974. Human memory and the cholinergic system. *Archives of Neurology.* 30: 113–121.

Dubois, B., Deweer, B. and Pillon, B. 1996. The cognitive syndrome of progressive supranuclear palsy. *Advances in Neurology.* 69: 399–403.

Dubois, B., Pillon, B., Lhermitte, F. and Agid, Y. 1990. Cholinergic deficiency and frontal dysfunction in Parkinson's disease. *Annals of Neurology.* 28: 117–121.

Ellison, D.W., Beal, M.F., Mazurek, M.F., Malloy, J.R., Bird, E.D. and Martin, J.B. 1987. Amino acid neurotransmitter abnormalities in Huntington's disease and the quinolinic acid animal model of Huntington's disease. *Brain.* 110: 1657–1673.

Eslinger, P.J. and Damasio, A. 1986. Preserved motor learning in Alzheimer's disease: Implications for anatomy and behavior. *Journal of Neuroscience.* 6: 3006–3009.

Feany, M.B., Mattiace, L.A. and Dickson, D.W. 1996. Neuropathologic overlap of progressive supranuclear palsy, Pick's disease and corticobasal degeneration. *Journal of Neuropathology and Experimental Neurology*. 55: 53–67.

Finkenstaedt, M., Szudra, A., Zerr, I., Poser, S., Hise, J.H., Stoebner, J.M. and Weber, T. 1996. MR Imaging of Creutzfeldt–Jakob disease. *Radiology*. 199: 793–798.

Forno, L.S. 1992. Neuropathologic features of Parkinson's, Huntington's and Alzheimer's diseases. *Annals of the New York Academy of Sciences*. 648: 6–16.

Forno, L.S. 1996. Neuropathology of Parkinson's disease. *Journal of Neuropathology and Experimental Neurology*. 55: 259–272.

Forno, L.S. and Langston, J.W. 1990. Lewy bodies and aging. *Journal of Neurology, Neurosurgery and Psychiatry*. 49: 278.

Gajdusek, D.C. 1996. Infectious amyloids: Subacute spongiform encephalopathies as transmissible cerebral amyloidoses. In *Fields' virology*, ed. B.N. Fields, D.M. Knipe and P.M. Howley, pp. 2851–2900. Philadelphia: Lippincott – Raven Publishers.

Galasko, D., Katzman, R., Salmon, D.P. and Hansen, L. 1996. Clinical and neuropathological findings in Lewy body dementias. *Brain and Cognition*. 31: 166–175.

Gertz, H.J., Henkes, H. and Cervos-Navarro, J. 1988. Creutzfeldt–Jakob disease: Correlation of MRI and neuropathologic findings. *Neurology* 38: 1481–1482.

Ghetti, B., Piccardo, P., Frangione, B., Bugiani, O., Giaccone, G., Young, K., Prelli, F., Farlow, M.R., Dlouhy, S.R. and Tagliavini, F. 1996. Prion protein amyloidosis. *Brain Pathology*. 6: 127–145.

Giannakopoulos, P., Hof, P.R., Savioz, A., Guimon, J., Antonarakis, S.E. and Bouras, C. 1996. Early-onset dementia: Clinical, neuropathological and genetic characteristics. *Acta Neuropathologica* (Berlin). 91: 451–465.

Gibb, W.R.G. 1992. Neuropathology of Parkinson's disease and related syndromes. *Neurologic Clinics*. 10: 361–376.

Gibb, W.R.G., Luthert, P.J. and Marsden, C.D. 1989. Corticobasal degeneration. *Brain*. 112: 1171–1192.

Golbe, L.I. and Dickson, D.W. 1995. Familial autopsy-proven progressive supranuclear palsy. *Neurology*. 45(Suppl 4): A255.

Golomb, J., de Leon, M.J., Kluger, A., George, A.E., Tarshish, C. and Ferris, S.H. 1993. Hippocampal atrophy in normal aging. *Archives of Neurology*. 50: 967–973.

Gooch, M.D. and Stennett, D.J. 1996. Molecular basis of Alzheimer's disease. *American Journal of Health-System Pharmacists*. 53: 1545–1557.

Groen, J.J. and Endtz, L.J. 1982. Hereditary Pick's disease. *Brain*. 105: 443–459.

Grundman, M., Corey-Bloom, J., Jernigan, T., Archibald, S. and Thal, L.J. 1996. Low body weight in Alzheimer's disease associated with mesial temporal cortex atrophy. *Neurology*. 46: 1585–1591.

Gusella, J.F., MacDonald, M.E., Ambrose, C.M. and Duyao, M.P. 1993. Molecular genetics of Huntington's disease. *Archives of Neurology*. 50: 1157–1163.

Hansen, L. 1994. Pathology of the other dementia. In *Alzheimer disease*, ed. R.D. Terry, R. Katzman and K.L. Bick, pp. 167–177. New York: Raven Press.

Hansen, L., Salmon, D., Galasko, D., Masliah, E., Katzman, R., DeTeresa, R., Thal, L., Pay, M.M., Hofstetter, R., Klauber, M., Rice, V., Butters, N. and Alford, M. 1990. The Lewy body variant of Alzheimer's disease: A clinical and pathologic entity. *Neurology*. 40: 1–8.

Harrington, D., Haaland, K., Yeo, R. and Marder, E. 1990. Procedural memory in Parkinson's disease: Impaired motor but not visuoperceptual learning. *Journal of Clinical and Experimental Neuropsychology*. 12: 323–329.

Hauw, J.J., Daniel, S.E., Dickson, D., Horoupian, D.S., Jellinger, K., Lantos, P.L., McKee, A., Tabaton, M. and Litvan, I. 1994. Preliminary NINDS neuropathologic criteria for Steele-Richardson-Olszewski syndrome (progressive supranuclear palsy). *Neurology*. 44: 2015–2019.

Heindel, W.C., Salmon, D.P., Shults, C.W., Walicke, P.A. and Butters, N. 1989. Neuropsychological evidence for multiple implicit memory systems: A comparison of Alzheimer's, Huntington's and Parkinson's disease patients. *Journal of Neuroscience*. 9: 582–587.

Hely, M.A., Reid, W.G.J., Halliday, G.M., McRitchie, D.A., Leicester, J., Joffe, R., Brooks, W., Broe, G.A. and Morris, J.G.L. 1996. Diffuse Lewy body disease: Clinical features in nine cases without coexistent Alzheimer's disease. *Journal of Neurology, Neurosurgery and Psychiatry*, 60: 531–538.

Hodges, J.R. and Gurd, J.M. 1994. Remote memory and lexical retrieval in a case of frontal Pick's disease. *Archives of Neurology*. 51: 821–827.

Hodges, J.R., Salmon, D.P. and Butters, N. 1992. Semantic memory impairment in Alzheimer's disease: Failure of access or degraded knowledge? *Neuropsychologia*. 30: 301–314.

Hof, P.R., Bouras, C., Perl, D.P. and Morrison, J.H. 1994. Quantitative neuropathologic analysis of Pick's disease cases: Cortical distribution of Pick bodies and coexistence with Alzheimer's disease. *Acta Neuropathologica*. 87: 115–124.

Hubbard, B.M., Fenton, G.W. and Anderson, J.M. 1990. A quantitative histological study of early clinical and preclinical Alzheimer's disease. *Neuropathology and Applied Neurobiology*. 16: 111–121.

Hughes, A.J., Daniel, S.E., Blankson, S. and Lees, A.J. 1993. A clinicopathologic study of 100 cases of Parkinson's disease. *Archives of Neurology*. 50: 140–148.

Hyman, B.T. 1997. The neuropathological diagnosis of Alzheimer's disease: Clinical-pathological studies. *Neurobiology of Aging*. 18: S27–S32.

Hyman, B.T., Van Hoesen, G.W. and Damasio, A.R. 1990. Memory-related neural systems in Alzheimer's disease: An anatomic study. *Neurology*. 40: 1721–1730.

Ince, P., Irving, D., MacArthur, F. and Perry, R.H. 1991. Quantitative neuropathological study of Alzheimer-type pathology in the hippocampus: Comparison of senile dementia of Alzheimer type, senile dementia of Lewy body type, Parkinson's disease and non-demented elderly control patients. *Journal of Neurological Sciences*. 106: 142–152.

Janowsky, J.S., Carper, R.A. and Kaye, J.A. 1996. Asymmetrical memory decline in normal aging and dementia. *Neuropsychologia*. 34: 527–535.

Jellinger, K.A. 1996. Structural basis of dementia in neurodegenerative disorders. *Journal of Neural Transmission*. 47: 1–29.

Katzman, R. and Kawas, C. 1994. The epidemiology of dementia and Alzheimer disease. In *Alzheimer disease*, ed. R.D. Terry, R. Katzman and K.L. Bick, pp. 105–122. New York: Raven Press.

Khachaturian, Z.S. 1985. Diagnosis of Alzheimer's disease. *Archives of Neurology*. 42: 1097–1105.

Kirby, M. and Lawlor, B.A. 1995. Biologic markers and neurochemical correlates of agitation and psychosis in dementia. *Journal of Geriatric Psychiatry and Neurology*. 8 (Suppl.): S2-S7.

Kish, S.J., Shannak, S., Rajput, A.H., Gilbert, J.J. and Hornykiewicz, O. 1984. Cerebellar norepinephrine in patients with Parkinson's disease and control subjects. *Archives of Neurology*. 41: 612–614.

Kokmen, E., Özekmekçi, F.S., Beard, C.M., O'Brien, P.C. and Kurland, L.T. 1994. Incidence and prevalence of Huntington's disease in Olmsted County, Minnesota (1950 through 1989). *Archives of Neurology*. 51: 696–698.

Koller, W.C. and Megaffin, B.B. 1994. Parkinson's disease and parkinsonism. In *Textbook of geriatric neuropsychiatry*, ed. C.E. Coffey and J.L. Cummings, pp. 434–456. Washington, DC: American Psychiatric Press.

Kopelman, M.D. 1989. Remote and autobiographical memory, temporal context memory and frontal atrophy in Korsakoff and Alzheimer patients. *Neuropsychologia*. 27: 437–460.

Kopin, I.J. and Markey, S.P. 1988. MPTP toxicity: Implications for research in Parkinson's disease. *Annual Review of Neuroscience*. 11: 81–96.

Korczyn, A.D., Inzelberg, R., Treves, T., Neufeld, M., Reider, I. and Rabey, P.M. 1986. Dementia of Parkinson's diseases. *Advances in Neurology*. 45: 399–403.

Koroshetz, W.J., Myers, R.H. and Martin, J.B. 1993. Huntington disease. In *The molecular and genetic basis of neurological disease*, ed. R.N. Rosenberg, S.B. Prusiner, S. DiMauro, R.L. Barchi and L.M. Kunkel, pp. 737–751. Boston: Butterworth-Heinemann.

Kosaka, K., Yoshimura, M., Ikeda, K. and Budka, H. 1984. Diffuse type of Lewy body disease: Progressive dementia with abundant cortical Lewy bodies and senile changes of varying degree: a new disease? *Clinical Neuropathology*. 3: 185–192.

Kraepelin, E. 1987. Senile and pre-senile dementias. In *The early story of Alzheimer's disease*, ed. K.L. Bick, L. Amaducci and G. Pepeu, pp. 32–81. New York: Raven Press. (Original title: Das senile und präsenile Irresein. *Psychiatrie: Ein Lehrbuch für Studierende und Ärzte*, 1910, pp. 533–554; 593–632. Leipzig: Verlag von Johann Ambrosius Barth.)

Kretzschmar, H.A., Ironside, J.W., DeArmond, S.J. and Tateishi, J. 1996. Diagnostic criteria for sporadic Creutzfeldt–Jakob disease. *Archives of Neurology*. 53: 913–920.

Lanska, D.J. 1996. Recommendations of the American Academy of Neurology for evaluation of dementia. *Mayo Clinic Proceedings*. 71: 821.

Levin, B.E., Llabre, M.M. and Weiner, W.J. 1989. Cognitive impairments associated with early Parkinson's disease. *Neurology*. 39: 557–561.

Levy-Lahad, E. and Bird, T.D. 1996. Genetic factors in Alzheimer's disease: A review of recent advances. *Annals of Neurology*. 40: 829–840.

Lichter, D.G., Corbett, A.J., Fitzgibbon, G.M., Davidson, O.R., Hope, J.K.A., Goddard, G.V., Sharpled, K.J. and Pollock, M. 1988. Cognitive and motor dysfunction in Parkinson's disease. *Archives of Neurology*. 45: 854–860.

Litvan, I., Agid, Y., Calne, D., Campbell, G., Dubois, B., Duvoisin, R.C., Goetz, C.G., Golbe, L.I., Grafman, J., Growdon, J.H., Hallett, M., Jankovic, J., Quinn, N.P., Tolosa, E. and Zee, D.S. 1996a. Clinical research criteria for the diagnosis of progressive supranuclear palsy (Steele–Richardson–Olszewski syndrome): Report of the NINDS-PSP International workshop. *Neurology*. 47: 1–9.

Litvan, I., Hauw, J.J., Bartko, J.J., Lantos, P.L., Daniel, S.E., Horoupian, D.S., McKee, A., Dickson, D., Bancher, C., Tabaton, M., Jellinger, K. and Anderson, D.W. 1996b. Validity and reliability of the preliminary NINDS neuropathologic criteria for progressive supranuclear palsy and related disorders. *Journal of Neuropathology and Experimental Neurology*. 55: 97–105.

Martin, A., Cox, C., Brouwers, P. and Fedio, P. 1985. A note on different patterns of impaired and preserved cognitive abilities and their relation to episodic memory deficits in Alzheimer's patients. *Brain and Language*. 26: 181–185.

Mash, D.C., Flynn, D.D. and Potter, L.T. 1985. Loss of M2 muscarine receptors in the cerebral cortex in Alzheimer's disease and experimental cholinergic denervation. *Science*. 228: 1115–1117.

Matthews, W.B. 1985. Creutzfeldt–Jakob disease. In *Handbook of clinical neurology*, vol. 2 (46), ed. J.A.M. Frederiks, pp. 289–299. New York: Elsevier.

Mayeux, R., Chen, J., Mirabello, E., Marder, K., Bell, K., Dooneief, G., Côté, L. and Stern, Y. 1990. An estimate of the incidence of dementia in idiopathic Parkinson's disease. *Neurology*. 40: 1513–1517.

McKeith, I.G., Galasko, D., Kosaka, K., Perry, E.K., Dickson, D.W., Hansen, L.A., Salmon, D.P., Lowe, J., Mirra, S.S., Byrne, E.J., Lennox, G., Quinn, N.P., Edwardson, J.A., Ince, P.G., Bergeron, C., Burns, A., Miller, B.L., Lovestone, S., Collerton, D., Jansen, E.N.H., Ballard, C., de Vos, R.A.I., Wilcock, G.K., Jellinger, K.A. and Perry, R.H. 1996. Consensus guidelines for the clinical and pathologic diagnosis of dementia with Lewy bodies (DLB): Report of the consortium on DLB International Workshop. *Neurology*. 47: 1113–1124.

Meara, J. 1996. Serotonin and the extrapyramidal system: A neurological perspective. *Human Psychopharmacology*. 11: S95-S102.

Mendez, M.F., Selwood, A., Mastri, A.R. and Frey, W.H. 1993. Pick's disease versus Alzheimer's disease: A comparison of clinical characteristics. *Neurology*. 43: 289–292.

Mirra, S.S., Hart, M.N. and Terry, R.D. 1993. Making the diagnosis of Alzheimer's disease. *Archives of Pathology and Laboratory Medicine*. 117: 132–144.

Mirra, S.S., Heyman, A., McKeel, D., Sumi, S.M., Crain, B.J., Brownlee, L.M., Vogel, F.S., Hughes, J.P., van Belle, G. and Berg, L. 1991. The Consortium to Establish a Registry for Alzheimer's Disease (CERAD) II: Standardization of the neuropathological assessment of Alzheimer's disease. *Neurology*. 41: 479–486.

Möslä, P.K., Säkö, E., Paljärvi, L., Rinne, J.O. and Rinne, U.K. 1987. Alzheimer's disease: Neuropathological correlates of cognitive and motor disorders. *Acta Neurologica Scandinavica*. 75: 376–384.

Myers, R.H., Vonsattel, J.P., Stevens, T., Cupples, L.A., Richardson, E.P., Martin, J.B. and Bird, E.D. 1988. Clinical and neuropathologic assessment of severity in Huntington's disease. *Neurology*. 38: 341–347.

Nagy, Z.S., Esiri, M.M., Jobst, K.A., Morris, J.H., King, E.M.F., McDonald, B., Litchfield, S., Smith, A., Barnetson, L. and Smith, A.D. 1995. Relative roles of plaques and tangles in the dementia of Alzheimer's Disease: Correlations using three sets of neuropathological criteria. *Dementia*. 6: 21–31.

Nasir, J., Goldberg, P. and Hayden, M.R. 1996. Huntington disease: New insights into the relationship between CAG expansion and disease. *Human Molecular Genetics*. 5: 1431–1435.

Penney, J.B., Vonsattel, J.P., MacDonald, M.E., Gusella, J.F. and Myers, R.H. 1997. CAG repeat number governs the development rate of pathology in Huntington's disease. *Annals of Neurology*. 41: 689–692.

Perry, E.K., McKeith, I., Thompson, P., Marshall, E., Kerwin, J., Jabeen, S., Edwardson, J.A., Ince, P., Blessed, G., Irving, D. and Perry, R.H. 1991. Topography, extent and clinical relevance of neurochemical deficits in dementia of Lewy body type, Parkinson's disease and Alzheimer's disease. *Annals of the New York Academy of Sciences*. 640: 197–202.

Perry, E.K., Tomlinson, B.E., Blessed, G., Bergman, K., Gibson, P.H. and Perry, R.H. 1978. Correlation of cholinergic abnormalities with senile plaques and mental test scores in senile dementia. *British Medical Journal*. 2: 1457–1459.

Pillon, B., Deweer, B., Agid, Y. and Dubois, B. 1993. Explicit memory in Alzheimer's, Huntington's and Parkinson's diseases. *Archives of Neurology*. 50: 374–379.

Pillon, B., Dubois, B., Ploska, A. and Agid, Y. 1991. Severity and specificity of cognitive impairment in Alzheimer's, Huntington's and Parkinson's disease and progressive supranuclear palsy. *Neurology*. 41: 634–643.

Prusiner, S.B. 1988. Prion diseases and brain dysfunction. In *Aging and the brain*, ed. R.D. Terry, pp. 219–242. New York: Raven Press.

Prusiner, S.B. 1996. Prion biology and disease – Laughing cannibals, mad cows and scientific heresy. *Medicinal Research Reviews*. 16: 487–505.

Rajput, A.H. 1994. Clinical features and natural history of Parkinson's disease (special consideration of aging). In *Neurodegenerative diseases*, ed. D.B. Calne, pp. 555–571. Philadelphia: WB Saunders.

Richardson, E.P. and Masters, C.L. 1995. The nosology of Creutzfeldt–Jakob disease and conditions related to the accumulation of PRP^{CJD} in the nervous system. *Brain Pathology*. 5: 33–41.

Rinne, J.O., Rummukainen, J., Paljärvia, L. and Rinne, U.K. 1989. Dementia in Parkinson's disease is related to neuronal loss in the medial substantia nigra. *Annals of Neurology*. 26: 47–50.

Roberts, G.W., Gentleman, S.M. and McKenzie, J. 1995. Molecular pathogenesis of the cerebral amyloidoses. In *Molecular neuropathology*, ed. G.W. Roberts and J.M. Polak, pp. 109–137. Cambridge: Cambridge University Press.

Rogers, J.D., Brogan, D. and Mirra, S.S. 1985. The nucleus basalis of Meynert in neurological disease: A quantitative morphological study. *Annals of Neurology*. 17: 163–170.

Roos, R.A.C. 1986. Neuropathology of Huntington's chorea. In *Handbook of clinical neurology*, vol. 5 (49), ed. P.J. Vinken, G.W. Bruyn and H.L. Klawans, pp. 315–326. New York: Elsevier.

Ruberg, M., Javoy-Agid, F., Hirsch, E., Scatton, B., Leheureux, R., Hauw, J., Duyckaerts, C., Gray, F., Morelmaroger, A., Rascol, A., Serdaru, M. and Agid, Y. 1985. Dopaminergic and cholinergic lesions in progressive supranuclear palsy. *Annals of Neurology*. 18: 523–529.

Salmon, D.P., Galasko, D., Hansen, L.A., Masliah, E., Butters, N., Thal, L.J. and Katzman, R. 1996. Neuropsychological deficits associated with diffuse Lewy body disease. *Brain and Cognition*. 31: 148–165.

Salmon, D.P. and Heindel, W.C. 1992. Impaired priming in Alzheimer's disease: Neuropsychological implications. In *Neuropsychology of memory*, 2nd ed., ed. L. Squire and N. Butters, pp. 170–187. New York: Guilford Press.

Samuel, W., Terry, R.D., DeTeresa, R., Butters, N. and Masliah, E. 1994. Clinical correlates of cortical and nucleus basalis pathology in Alzheimer dementia. *Archives of Neurology*. 51: 772–778.

Schwartz, M.F. and Stark, J.A. 1992. The distinction between Alzheimer's disease and senile dementia: Historical considerations. *Journal of the History of Neuroscience*. 1: 169–187.

Shoulson, I. and Kurlan, R. 1993. Inherited disorders of the basal ganglia. In *The molecular and genetic basis of neurological disease*, ed. R.N. Rosenberg, S.B. Prusiner, S. DiMauro, R.L. Barchi and L.M. Kunkel, pp. 753–766. Boston: Butterworth-Heinemann.

Shyu, W.-C., Lee, C.-C., Hsu, Y.-D., Lin, J.-C., Lee, J.-T., Lee, W.-H. and Tsao, W.-L. 1996. Panencephalitic Creutzfeldt–Jakob disease. Unusual presentation of magnetic resonance imaging and proton magnetic resonance spectroscopy. *Journal of Neurological Sciences*. 138: 157–160.

Squire, L.R., Knowlton, B. and Musen, G. 1993. The structure and organization of memory. *Annual Review of Psychology*. 44: 453–495.

Steele, J.C., Richardson, J.C. and Olszewski, J. 1964. Progressive supranuclear palsy: A heterogeneous degeneration involving the brain stem, basal ganglia and cerebellum, with vertical gaze and pseudobulbar palsy, buccal dystonia and dementia. *Archives of Neurology*. 10: 333–359.

Stern, Y., Mayeux, R. and Côté, L. 1984. Reaction time and vigilance in Parkinson's disease: Possible role of altered norepinephrine metabolism. *Archives of Neurology*. 41: 1086–1089.

Stern, Y., Mayeux, R., Rosen, J. and Ilson, J. 1983. Perceptual motor dysfunction in Parkinson's disease: A deficit in sequential and predictive voluntary movement. *Journal of Neurology, Neurosurgery and Psychiatry*, 46: 145–151.

Tatemichi, T.K., Sacktor, N. and Mayeux, R. 1994. Dementia associated with cerebrovascular disease, other degenerative diseases and metabolic disorders. In *Alzheimer disease*, ed. R.D. Terry, R. Katzman and K.L. Bick, pp. 123–166. New York: Raven Press.

Terry, R.D., DeTeresa, R. and Hansen, L.A. 1987. Neocortical cell counts in normal human adult aging. *Annals of Neurology*. 21: 530–556.

Terry, R.D. and Katzman, R. 1983. Senile dementia of the Alzheimer type. *Annals of Neurology*. 14: 497–506.

Terry, R.D., Masliah, E. and Hansen, L.A. 1994. Structural basis of the cognitive alterations in Alzheimer disease. In *Alzheimer disease*, ed. R.D. Terry, R. Katzman and K.L. Bick, pp. 179–196. New York: Raven Press.

Terry, R.D., Masliah, E., Salmon, D.P., Butters, N., DeTeresa, R., Hill, R., Hansen, L.A. and Katzman, R. 1991. Physical basis of cognitive alterations in Alzheimer's Disease: Synapse loss is the major correlate of cognitive impairment. *Annals of Neurology*. 30: 572–580.

Tissot, R., Constantinidis, J. and Richard, J. 1985. Pick's disease. In *Handbook of clinical neurology*, vol. 2 (46), ed. J.A.M. Frederiks, pp. 233–246. New York: Elsevier.

Tomlinson, B.E. 1992. Ageing and the dementias. In *Greenfield's neuropathology*, 5th ed., ed. J.H. Adams and L.W. Suchen, pp. 1284–1411. New York: Oxford University Press.

Tomlinson, B.E., Blessed, G. and Roth, M. 1970. Observations on the brains of demented old people. *Journal of Neurological Sciences*. 11: 205–242.

Tröster, A.I., Beatty, W.W., Staton, R.D. and Rorabaugh, A.G. 1989a. Effects of scopolamine on anterograde and remote memory in humans. *Psychobiology*. 17: 12–18.

Tröster, A.I., Salmon, D.P., McCullough, D. and Butters, N. 1989b. A comparison of the category fluency deficits associated with Alzheimer's and Huntington's disease. *Brain and Language*. 37: 500–513.

Unverzagt, F.W., Farlow, M.R., Norton, J., Dlouhy, S.R., Young, K. and Ghetti, B. 1997. Neuropsychological function in patients with Gerstmann–Sträussler–Scheinker disease from the Indiana kindred (F198S). *Journal of the International Neuropsychological Society*. 3: 169–178.

Vonsattel, J.P., Myers, R.H., Stevens, T.J., Ferrante, R.J., Bird, E.D. and Richardson, E.P. 1985. Neuropathological classification of Huntington's disease. *Journal of Neuropathology and Experimental Neurology*. 44: 559–577.

Welsh, K., Butters, N., Hughes, J., Mohs, J. and Heyman, A. 1991. Detection of abnormal memory decline in mild cases of Alzheimer's disease using CERAD neuropsychological measures. *Archives of Neurology*. 48: 278–281.

Whitehouse, P.J., Price, D.L., Struble, R.G., Clark, A.W., Coyle, J.T. and DeLong, M.R. 1982. Alzheimer's disease and senile dementia: Loss of neurons in the basal forebrain. *Science*. 215: 1297–1329.

Wisniewski, H.M. 1985. Progressive supranuclear palsy: The Steele–Richardson–Olszewski syndrome. In *Handbook of clinical neurology*, vol. 2 (46), ed. J.A.M. Frederiks, pp. 301–303. New York: Elsevier.

Yankner, B.A., Selkoe, D.J. and Cotman, C.W. 1989. Amyloid β protein enhances the survival of hippocampal neurons in vitro. *Science*. 243: 1488–1490.

Zola-Morgan, S., Squire, L.R. and Amaral, D.G. 1989.Lesions of the hippocampal formation but not lesions of the fornix or the mammillary nuclei produce long-lasting memory impairments in monkeys. *Journal of Neuroscience*. 9: 898–913.

Zubenko, G.S., Moossy, J., Martinez, A.J., Rao, G., Claassen, D., Rosen, J. and Kopp, U. 1991. Neuropathologic and neurochemical correlates of psychosis in primary dementia. *Archives of Neurology*. 46: 619–624.

4

Neurochemical aspects of memory dysfunction in neurodegenerative disease

EDISON MIYAWAKI AND WILLIAM C. KOLLER

INTRODUCTION

The relationship between 'classical' neuroanatomy and what has been termed the 'chemoarchitecture' of the brain is formidably complex, and discussions of that relationship always run the risk of oversimplification. Patterns of selective cell degeneration have been described in certain exemplary disorders (Alzheimer's, Parkinson's and Huntington's diseases), and yet such observations only inform Nieuwenhuys' important caveat that neuromediator-specified neuronal populations do not obey simple rules (Nieuwenhuys 1985).

This chapter addresses the major neurochemical changes in three archetypal degenerative disorders – Alzheimer's disease (AD), Parkinson's disease (PD) and Huntington's disease (HD) – in the context of a review of 'classical' and 'chemical' neuroanatomies pertinent to each. Some implications for a neurochemical understanding of normal memory are discussed at the chapter's conclusion.

ANATOMICAL AND NEUROTRANSMITTER CONSIDERATIONS

Alzheimer's disease

Large cholinergic neurons populate several structures in the basal forebrain that in essence form a continuum, including the nucleus basalis of Meynert, nuclei of the diagonal band of Broca and the medial septal nucleus. Mesulam divided the forebrain cholinergic neuronal population into four major groups (Mesulam et al. 1983), of which Ch4 (roughly corresponding to the nucleus basalis of Meynert, but also including cholinergic neurons

located within the internal and external medullary laminae of the globus pallidus) is of particular interest.

Cholinergic innervation of the neocortex and amygdala derives largely from Ch4 (Struble et al. 1986) and, in turn, Ch4 receives reciprocal cortical innervation from 'limbic' structures, including orbitofrontal, medial and polar temporal, prepiriform and entorhinal cortices (Mesulam and Mufson 1984). Loss of cholinergic neurons particularly in the nucleus basalis is characteristic in AD, though by no means the only hallmark of the disease (Whitehouse et al. 1981, 1982). Accordingly, cortical cholinergic 'markers,' especially the presynaptic synthetic enzyme choline acetyltransferase (ChAT) and presynaptic muscarinic ('M2') receptors, are reduced on the order of 40–90% throughout the neocortex, but particularly in those areas that represent terminal fields of basal forebrain neurons (Koo and Price 1993).

Several lines of evidence in non-AD populations suggest that manipulations of the cholinergic system interfere in some way with memory. It has been observed that patterns of deficit seen in age-related memory loss can be reproduced in younger individuals with the administration of anticholinergic medications such as scopolamine (Drachman and Leavitt 1974; Fibiger 1991); treatments that augment cholinergic function appear to have beneficial effects on memory in some models (Bartus 1979). There also appears to be a consistent relationship between loss of integrity of cholinergic neurons particularly in the medial septum and vertical limb of the diagonal band and learning impairment in animal models, perhaps as a consequence of an alteration in level of attention (Voytko et al. 1993).

Studies investigating the effects of lesions of the basal forebrain have not, however, reported consistent effects on memory. In particular, immunotoxic lesions which selectively target cholinergic forebrain neurons in animal models have not reliably produced deficits in mnemonic and learning tasks, and speculation has therefore been raised that alterations in the cholinergic system alone are not sufficient to cause disturbances in memory (Gallagher and Colombo 1995). There is an enduring interest in what precisely forebrain cholinergic neurons *do* in the brain. One speculation, variously described by different investigators, holds that the cholinergic forebrain has more to do with the 'readiness' of the brain to handle information rather than with 'memory' per se (Mesulam et al. 1986; Hasselmo and Bower 1993).

Attention has focused in recent years on the conspicuous anatomical changes (viz., senile plaques and neurofibrillary tangles) that are seen in AD and their pathogenetic role. That the severity of dementia in AD has been correlated with the degree of reduction in ChAT has fueled a 'cholinergic hypothesis' of cognitive decline, but the memory deficit has also been correlated with the number and density of senile plaques widely distributed throughout the Alzheimerian brain (Perry et al. 1978). Cholinergic neuronal loss in the basal forebrain might in fact represent a retrograde phenomenon, a consequence of degeneration affecting, albeit not exclusively, cholinergic endings in the neocortex (Price et al. 1982).

Accumulation of insoluble fibrous materials (A4–amyloid extracellularly and neurofibrillary changes such as paired helical filaments intracellularly) has been implicated in the development of senile plaques and neurofibrillary tangles (Selkoe et al. 1987; Braak and Braak 1994). These neuropathological hallmarks appear to progress in relatively stereotyped fashion, first in the limbic circuit, thence to adjoining isocortex, isocortical association areas, nonthalamic subcortical nuclei (including the nucleus basalis) and, finally, to motor centers late in the disease (Price et al. 1991; Braak and Braak 1994). The major afferent pathway from neocortical association areas to hippocampus (i.e. the projections arising from entorhinal cortex via the perforant pathway to the dentate gyrus in hippocampus) appears particularly vulnerable, such that the hippocampus, well known to be involved in memory formation, is functionally dissociated from surrounding cortical structures (Hyman et al. 1986). The disconnection does not exclusively involve cholinergic fibers, even though important forebrain cholinergic centers project heavily to and receive projections from the entorhinal cortex and other hippocampal structures.

Multiple neurotransmitter-specific populations of neurons can be represented in any given senile plaque in a way that suggests not that a specific projection system degenerates, but rather that multiple projection systems are affected in a more or less nonspecific fashion (Selkoe 1991). 'Neurites' (which derive from axons and terminals) in senile plaques may represent one or several transmitter-specific populations of neurons (Walker et al. 1988). The transmitter-specific neurites in plaques reflect normal distribution of the cells and axons expressing the transmitter phenotype (Struble et al. 1987). Such observations substantiate the general notion that in AD, anatomical pathology may be relatively focal at different phases of the disease, but not therefore selective in a way that neatly implicates an isolated neurotransmitter deficit in the pathogenesis or in the pathophysiology of its cardinal clinical manifestations.

Parkinson's disease

In contrast to AD, Parkinson's disease (PD) is the premier example of an elegant match between a neuroanatomical structural change (nigral cell loss) and an attendantly altered neurotransmitter (dopamine) system. The principal pathological finding in PD is destruction of pigmented neurons in the pars compacta of substantia nigra (SN_{pc}) and 'downstream' depletion of dopamine in the striatum. Normal aging also results in a loss of nigral cells, striatal dopamine and a decline in dopamine-synthesizing enzymes. Peculiar to PD is the observation that the ventral lateral SN_{pc} exhibits the greatest degree of cell loss, in contradistinction to the dorsal tier loss seen in normal aging (Fearnley and Lees 1991). Selective deprivation of dopaminergic input to the striatum seems to have the net effects of reducing positive feedback and increasing negative feedback to precentral motor fields (DeLong 1990).

Lewy bodies, eosinophilic cytoplasmic inclusions seen in neuromelanin-containing cells in SN_{pc} and elsewhere, are thought to be a pathological hallmark, although their role in the pathogenesis of the disorder has not been elucidated and Lewy bodies may occur in 10% of normal individuals over the age of 50 years (Gibb and Lees 1988). Lewy body disease is associated with clinical syndromes other than PD, including a dementia with fluctuating confusion and visual hallucinations (so-called 'diffuse Lewy body disease') and a variant of pure autonomic failure. In turn, a clinical variant of PD, characterized by autosomal dominant inheritance and young onset, has been described with nigral degeneration, but without Lewy bodies (Dwork et al. 1993).

In PD, a major complexity relates to the blurred distinction between cognitive and motoric domains in the disease, as suggested by several lines of evidence. First, 'bradyphrenia' in PD has been touted to be separate from, but perhaps mechanistically related to, classical motoric slowing in the disease (Rogers 1986; Revonuso et al. 1993). Second, AD-like histopathology has been observed to be six times more likely in PD than in an age matched cohort (Boller et al. 1980), which suggests that the two degenerative processes may be related in some cases. Third, as in the instance of progressive supranuclear palsy (in which the syndrome of 'subcortical dementia' was first characterized), dementia in PD can manifest differently from AD, perhaps because of pathology principally in basal ganglionic structures (Albert et al. 1974). Finally, it has become increasingly clear that cortico-basal ganglionic-cortical connections, traditionally implicated in motoric control (Denny Brown 1962), may be involved in the ongoing and long-term modifiability of both motor *and* nonmotor programs (Graybiel and Kimura 1995).

Cortical associative, sensory and motor areas project to the striatum, thence to globus pallidus and thalamus and back to the same cortical centers of origin along apparently discrete pathways or circuits (Hoover and Strick 1993). Component striatal structures have been specifically associated with one of five major circuits: dorsolateral caudate/dorsolateral prefrontal cortex; ventral striatum/cingulum; ventromedial caudate/orbitofrontal cortex; putamen/primary motor cortex, arcuate premotor area and supplementary motor area; caudate/frontal eye fields (Alexander and Crutcher 1990; Cummings 1993). At the level of the striatum, an intricate 'modular' reorganization of cortical projections occurs; cortical inputs derived from specific body part representations (e.g. from motor and sensory cortices) converge onto distributed, but overlapping zones or 'matriosomes'. The functional importance of this remapping appears to relate to the fact that in any given matriosome, several sorts of information relevant to a body part converge (Graybiel et al. 1994). It is not merely the case, however, that matriosomes allow for a convergence, for example, of sensorimotor cortical output regarding a hand or foot. Individual modules may be subject to different sorts of local neurochemical influence,

thereby increasing the possibility of ongoing and 'plastic' striatal processing.

Based on studies in awake, performing primates, Graybiel and colleagues have demonstrated that dopamine in particular may play a role in modulating the neuronal firing of a unique class of striatal neurons termed 'tonically active neurons' (TANs) in the context of motor learning. These putative interneurons, widely (though sporadically) distributed through the striatum, exhibit a pattern of firing not merely in relation to limb movement, but rather in response to reward-associated conditioning stimuli. Discharge patterns vary with the state of dopaminergic innervation: the particular pattern of firing seen in reward-based motor learning is lost after striatal infusion of 1-methyl–4-phenyl–1,2,3,6-tetrahydropyridine (MPTP), which is selectively toxic to dopaminergic fibers, but restored after administration of the mixed postsynaptic dopamine agonist, apomorphine. As the case of TANs illustrates, the dopaminergic SN_{pc} plays a 'permissive' role based on an anticipation of reward. Such observations echo an older literature which had demonstrated dopaminergic influences on saccadic eye movements specifically when generated in response to remembered and attractive targets (Hikosaka et al. 1989). Just as anatomic structures traditionally assigned to the domain of motoric control are now being implicated in higher cognitive function (Middleton and Strick 1994), dopamine's role in modulating striatal processing must now be understood as a neurotransmitter effect potentially in both motoric and cognitive domains.

Huntington's disease

AD illustrates the problems inherent in attempting to link a specific neurotransmitter deficit to a cortical disturbance that likely embraces multiple neurotransmitter functions. PD illustrates the influence of a single neurotransmitter deficit in what must increasingly be understood as contingent or interdependent rather than discrete dimensions of neural activity. Huntington's disease (HD) is a complex instance in which a known unstable expansion of a CAG trinucleotide repeat (located in an open reading frame of the 'interesting transcript 15' [or IT15] gene on chromosome 4) is associated with identifiable cell populations and anatomical pathology, striatal neurotransmitter alterations (particularly, decreases in GABA and perhaps glutamate), but *variable* phenotype affecting both motoric and cognitive domains. It is difficult to describe the modal

Huntingtonian, as the myriad neuropsychiatric manifestations may antedate, accompany or postdate the motoric
features in the disease and the motoric features themselves
may vary with age of onset, as in the instance of the 'rigid'
Westphall variant in childhood (Quarrell and Harper
1991) or in later cases in which bradykinesia appears to
accompany hallmark choreiform movements (Thompson
et al. 1988).

Such clinical heterogeneity in HD makes it difficult to
link any given phenotypic aspect with genetic markers for
the disease. Specifically in the cognitive domain, deficits in
attentional planning and learning (Rosenberg et al. 1995),
'initiation' (Paulsen et al. 1995) and psychomotor speed
(Lundervold and Reinvang 1995) have been well
characterized in both early and late HD as well as in
patients at high risk. Such abnormalities do not appear to
distinguish between gene-positive and gene-negative
presymptomatic subjects (Strauss and Brandt 1990;
Blackmore et al. 1995; Giordani et al. 1995). In general,
surprisingly few phenotypic variables correlate with HD's
genetics, save for the well-corroborated observation that
paternal inheritance 'anticipates' earlier age of onset and
greater length of triplet repeat abnormality (Claes et al.
1995).

It remains unclear how the mutant IT 15 allele or its
product results in the clinical syndrome. Anatomical
locales which bear the brunt of pathological change in HD
(tail of caudate, mediodorsal caudate and putamen) do not
differ in expression of IT 15 by in situ hybridization techniques from those areas that appear spared in the disease
(e.g. nucleus accumbens) (Landwehmeyer et al. 1995). The
gene product in question, a cytosolic 350 kDal protein
called 'huntingtin', appears to be have cytoskeletal and
membrane transport functions (Sharp et al. 1995) and may
play a role in normal basal ganglionic development (Nasir
et al. 1995), but quite apart from these considerations,
huntingtin's normal functions may undergo a 'gain-in-
function' change with the allelic mutation, such that the
new gene product is pathogenetic in some way still to be
elucidated (Albin and Tagle 1995).

In contrast to IT 15 and huntingtin's ubiquitous presence in the brain, the structural changes seen in HD follow
a stereotyped and relatively selective course during the
illness (Albin 1995). The major effect is seen in striatal projection ('spiny') neurons, which constitute the vast majority of striatal cells (Vonsattel et al. 1985); projections to
SN_{pc}, external globus pallidus (GP_e), pars reticulata of the

substantia nigra (SN_{pr}) and to internal globus pallidus
(GP_i) appear to be involved *sequentially* in the order listed.
Specific projections are associated with specific neurotransmitter and neuromodulator colocalizations: the
striato-GP_e projection, for example, expresses γ-aminobutyric acid (GABA)-enkephalin, compared to GABA-sub-
stance P (or other tachykinin) in other projection
pathways. Preferential loss of preproenkephalin striatal
neurons in HD has been elegantly demonstrated
(Richfield et al. 1995). Among striatal ('aspiny') interneurons, which represent perhaps 10% of striatal cells, a
subpopulation which coexpresses GABA and parvalbumin
degenerates preferentially late in the illness (Harrington
and Kowall 1991).

REPRESENTATIVE NEUROTRANSMITTER CHANGES AND METHODOLOGIC CONSIDERATIONS

Although by no means exhaustive, Table 4.1 summarizes
neurotransmitter changes in the three conditions discussed in the above sections. The table reflects inherent
biases in such study, in particular the tendency to focus
attention on cortical changes observed in AD and subcortical changes observed in PD and HD. Even a cursory
inspection of the literature will find that observations vary
tremendously. Methodological problems likely account for
some of the conflicting reports. Observed neurotransmitter changes may be the result of factors extraneous to
the underlying disease process – e.g. age-related change
or artifacts related to delayed autopsy (Lowe et al.
1990). Metabolite concentrations, other indices of transmitter 'turnover', presynaptic 'markers' (including synthetic enzyme concentrations) and quantification of
postsynaptic receptor populations provide useful, albeit
indirect information about neurotransmission at the
synapse, but such measures need not be specific to a
disease, e.g. reductions in homovanillic acid are seen in PD
and in other nigrostriatal degenerations (Wisser and Ratge
1989) and some degree of variation would be the result of
differing assays and other technical considerations. In PD,
exceptionally severe dopamine loss has been noted
throughout the putamen (89% to near total depletion)
and only the rostral caudate (and not other caudate subdivisions) manifested deficits of similar proportions.
GABAergic indices were noted to be unchanged in

Table 4.1. *Representative neurotransmitter changes in Alzheimer's disease, Parkinson's disease and Huntington's disease*

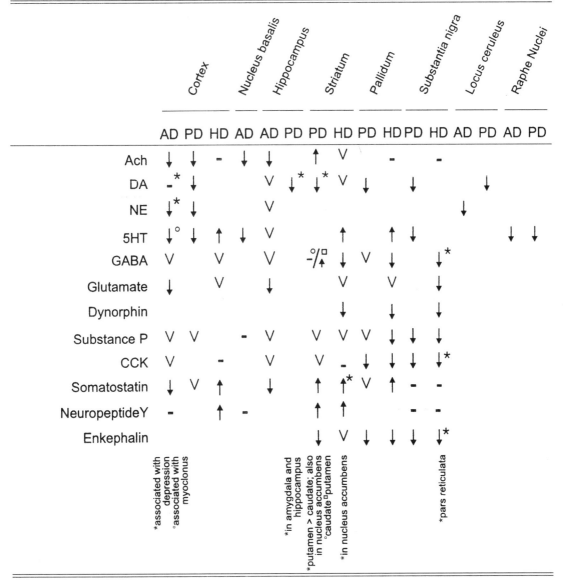

Note:
Ach: acetylcholine; AD: Alzheimer's disease; CCK: cholecystokinin; DA: dopamine; HD: Huntington's disease; PD: Parkinson's disease; NE: norepinephrine; 5HT: 5-hydroxytryptamine; GABA: γ-aminobutyric acid; ↓ = decreased; ↑ = increased; - = unchanged (all with respect to normal controls); v = variable across reports.
Sources: **AD**: Chui et al. 1985; Beal et al. 1986. D'Amato et al. 1987; Hyman et al. 1987; Sparks et al. 1988; Zweig et al. 1988; Herregodts et al 1989; Wilcox and Unnerstall 1990; Zubenko et al. 1991; Bierer et al. 1995
PD: Whitehouse et al. 1983; Chui et al. 1986; Hornykiewicz and Kish 1986; Kish et al. 1986a,b; Agid et al. 1987; Taquet et al. 1988; Torack and Morris 1988; Goto et al. 1990; Jellinger 1990; Gaspar et al. 1991.
HD: Dawbarn et al. 1985; Ellison et al. 1986, 1987; Reynolds and Pearson 1987; Beal, et al. 1988
Source: Data from Hedera and Whitehouse (1994) (with permission). Neurotransmitters in neurodegeneration. In *Neurodegenerative diseases*, ed. D. B. Calne, p. 104. Philadelphia: W.B. Saunders.

caudate, but increased in putamen (Kish et al. 1986a). Accounting for regional variation is not merely a technical concern, as cognitive deficits may be associated specifically with dopaminergic depletion in certain areas of striatum (caudate or ventral striatum) rather than others (putamen).

The issue of clinical correlation adds further complexity, because authors have observed changes associated with specific symptomatology, – e.g. AD with psychosis (Zubenko et al. 1991), AD with extrapyramidal features (Arai et al. 1984; Chui et al. 1985), or PD with dementia (Brown and Marsden 1990). Changes noted in highly specific anatomical locales may be particularly relevant to the observed clinical deficits. The significance of cholinergic reductions specific to Ch4 in AD has been addressed previously but, alternatively, a site-specific reduction in glutamate (in perforant pathway, where glutamate is a major neurotransmitter) has been thought to relate particularly to memory effects (Hyman et al. 1987). In various reports germane to all three neurodegenerations discussed in this chapter, glutamatergic/N-methyl-D-aspartate (NMDA) receptor activation has been thought potentially to be a mechanism of cell death, but conclusions regarding changes in glutamate run aground on mixed reports, e.g. reduction related to cell loss in glutamate-rich corticostriatal projections in HD (Cudkowitz and Kowall 1984) as well as evidence for glutamatergic excess (Perry and Hansen 1990).

The synapse is no longer the province exclusively of 'classical' neurotransmitters. Dale's hypothesis ('one neuron/one neurotransmitter') (Dale 1935) has been dramatically reinterpreted with the advent of colocalizing peptide neuromodulators. The clinical significance of an isolated neurotransmitter change may be as much a function of an attendant neuromodulator change, e.g. norepinephrine and neuropeptide Y in AD (Wilcox and Unnerstall 1990), GABA and metenkephalin in HD (Reiner et al. 1988), or dopamine and substance P in PD (Taquet et al. 1988). That neuromodulators appear to exert synaptic effects over longer periods of time than is the case for classical neurotransmitters suggests that they permit a further level of refinement and control in synaptic transmission.

THEORETICAL IMPLICATIONS RELATED TO NORMAL MEMORY IN THE MOTOR AND NONMOTOR DOMAINS

Anatomical or functional connections between basal ganglionic structures have begun to include a variety of neurotransmitter and neuromodulator correlations, as outlined in the above sections, but the role played by these agents in paradigms of motor learning and in other forms of memory remains unanswered. It has been observed (Graybiel 1995) that the distinction between a ventral striatum and ventral pallidum related to 'motivation' and dorsal striatum and pallidum related to 'sensorimotor' functions has been blurred by findings which suggest that dorsal striatopallidal activity is modified by nigral dopaminergic afferents in the anticipation of reward. Such observations are not entirely surprising, as the phenomenon of a neurotransmitter projection affecting a widely distributed system has been encountered before: hypotheses regarding the role played by cholinergic projections in memory formation have caused some authors to reinterpret the ascending cortical 'activating' systems postulated by Moruzzi and Magoun (1949) and Steriade and Buzsaki (1990). Dopaminergic projections appear to influence striatal activity in the setting of novel, nonautomatic actions in a context-dependent fashion, i.e. related to environmental cues related either to reward or to internal cues (Marsden and Obeso 1994), but such observations only open the debate as to how or whether the basal ganglia are involved in declarative ('explicit', subject to conscious recollection) and nondeclarative ('implicit' not subject to ongoing conscious recollection) memory in the nonmotor domain.

The striatum, and especially its ventral substructures including the nucleus accumbens, receives afferents from basolateral amygdala, the hippocampal formation and the prefrontal cortex. In turn, striatal output projects to the ventral pallidum; the major output from pallidum is directed again to the frontal cortex via mediodorsal thalamus (Mogenson et al. 1980; Robbins and Everitt 1996). Among limbic-cortical connections, the striatum holds a central (or what has been called a 'privileged') position, one which invites the possibility that striatal neurotransmitter changes may modulate hippocampal or amygdaloid activity and the forms of memory (declarative and nondeclarative, respectively) that have been linked with those structures. As has been suggested in reinforcement paradigms (Robbins et al. 1989; Robbins and Everitt 1996), glutamatergic input arising from limbic afferents can be understood to 'determine' the output of ventral striatal GABAergic medium spiny neurons projecting to ventral pallidum. The activity of spiny neurons is subject to various neurotransmitter or neuromodulator influences, both those intrinsic to striatum and those arising from other locations (particularly dopaminergic projections from SN_{pc}). Local chemical environments in the striatum may modulate limbic-ventral-striatopallidal circuits, but such modifiability does not get at the how memory is formed or whether the basal ganglia play a constitutive role. Increasingly, however, the striatum does seem to be a stage on which mechanisms of reward and motivation and mechanisms of memory will interact.

The modifiability of neural connections is by no means a new concept and chemical change seems fundamental to a molecular understanding of memory. At the turn of the century, Ramon y Cajal had advanced the notion that learning had to do with synaptic change. Later authors have postulated that for learning and memory to occur, lasting alterations in synaptic efficacy along specific neuronal pathways would need to be effected, perhaps by way of modifications in protein synthesis as a consequence of altered gene expression or by post-translational change (Squire and Davis 1981; Graybiel et al. 1990; Hyman 1993). Models of memory based on the phenomenon of long-term potentiation (LTP), a compelling model of activity-dependent synaptic 'efficacy', have attempted to link the neuromodulator-mediated changes in LTP directly to memory plasticity. Attention has focused on the activation of the NMDA class of glutamate receptor and attendant pre- and postsynaptic modifications, but induction of LTP is not solely dependent on NMDA activation. Other neurotransmitters may participate in the phenomenon (Aigner 1995; Collingridge and Bliss 1995). From the perspective of cognition in neurodegenerative disease, potentially any transmitter-related effect in a germane neuronal pathway that results in synaptic change, particularly in a less-than-immediate timeframe (as in the case of LTP), may be a clue either to pathophysiology in a given disorder or to an avenue of therapeutic intervention.

Yet, the translation of observed neurotransmitter changes to an understanding of mechanism or to an intuition of what directions therapy might take (as in the instance of acetylcholine in AD) has not been facile, nor is it likely to be. Nieuwenhuys' lament in 1985 that 'unifying concepts concerning the overall functional significance of various neuromediator-specified neuronal populations have not yet been formulated' is no less true over a decade later (Nieuwenhuys 1985). Establishing correlations between several organizational 'tiers' in the central nervous system, e.g. between transsynaptic communication among individual neurons and the domain of linked or functionally homologous anatomical structures, or the larger province embraced by 'neural networks', is problematic because synaptic neurotransmission even involving a single projection system tells only part of the story.

Dopamine, for example, is known to have short-term synaptic effects that differ from its longer-lasting effects on synaptic efficacy. This dual capacity might be understood to parallel dopamine-related short- and long-term changes in motor activity (motor activation versus reinforcement). It is tempting, but overreaching, to translate 'reinforcement' as a *behavioral* phenomenon into a transmitter-specific *physiologic* process (Wicken and Kotter 1995), just as it is tempting, but premature, to conceive of LTP as *the* molecular mechanism of memory.

In convergent neuron models involving corticostriatal, ascending dopaminergic and striatal spiny neurons, dopamine has demonstrable effects on synaptic transmission even at nondopaminergic (especially glutamatergic corticostriatal) synapses. Convergence has been thought to be an essential 'device' of the nigrostriatopallidal system (Percheron et al. 1984; Percheron and Filion 1991) which is a qualitatively different type of organization than, for example, neocortical multilayer processing. After a fashion described in network theories of learning, the arrangement of neurons in the striatum is particularly well suited for ongoing, adaptive processing among what would appear to be parallel neuronal populations (Graybiel et al. 1994). Striatal convergence sets the stage for monoamine-mediated 'heterosynaptic' plasticity (Schwartz and Greenberg 1987), akin to the phenomenon in which multiple neurotransmitter changes occur across synapses in series ('domino plasticity') (Smirnova et al. 1993; Morris and Johnston 1995). The important implication of such work is that neurotransmission does not occur in the isolation of the single synapse; the mosaic of neurotransmitter changes that may occur in a given degenerative disorder may reflect *adaptive* changes which manifest across various anatomic locales. Change in synaptic transmission may also relate to aspects that are not revealed by static changes in neurotransmitter concentrations, but rather by dynamic considerations, e.g, *phasic or timed* exposure to agonist (Wicken and Kotter 1995) or use-dependent change, as in cases of enkephalin and dynorphin release in hippocampal preparations specifically related to high-frequency stimulation of the major hippocampal afferent, the perforant pathway (Wagner et al. 1991).

CONCLUSIONS

The neurochemical underpinnings of cognition, learning and memory are currently understood at a rudimentary level, but perhaps there is enough knowledge to conspire against oversimplified or untenable presuppositions. It is unlikely, for example, that AD is a 'cholinergic' disorder quite in the way that PD is 'dopaminergic', and even in the latter case, dopaminergic effects are myriad, depending on the context in which they are studied, e.g. in motor activation, in paradigms of reward-based behavior or in long-term synaptic modification. Striatal changes in HD, presumably the result of genetically determined pathology in the medium spiny neuronal population, are stereotyped in their progression but variable in their phenotype. Adaptive or 'plastic' change in the striatal milieu may account in some degree for the heterogeneity of its clinical

manifestations. As is suggested in the variable reports of neurotransmitter changes in the three neurodegenerations discussed in this chapter, there is likely to be a diversity in neurotransmitter 'fingerprints' even among patients with the same disease. Those findings which appear consistent across investigators (reductions in acetylcholine, dopamine and GABA in AD, PD and HD, respectively) may nevertheless reflect changes far afield from etiopathogenesis. A question commonly encountered in the literature, but uniformly unanswered in any definitive way, may be paraphrased as, 'what does neurotransmitter or neuromodulator X *do* in the context of disease Y or in the normal state'? These chemicals clearly have to do with the modifiability of synaptic transmission, but it is precisely in the context of discussing modifiability or 'plasticity' in neural systems where the limits of models begin to surface. Neurochemical change provides evidence for neuronal plasticity as an ongoing phenomenon, but how the manifest adaptability of transmission across synapses actually gives rise to memory remains an open issue. In this regard it is of value to recall the comment by Collingridge and Bliss (1995), discussing the enthusiastic reception that LTP has received as a model for memory, that the epochal experiment linking neurotransmitter-mediated neuronal modifiability and learning has as yet to be published.

REFERENCES

Agid, Y., Javoy-Agid, F. and Ruberg, M. 1987. Biochemistry of neurotransmitters in Parkinson's disease. In *Movement disorders*, vol. 2, ed. C.D. Marsden and S. Fahn, pp. 166–230. London: Butterworth.

Aigner T.G. 1995. Pharmacology of memory: Cholinergic-glutaminergic interactions. *Current Opinion in Neurobiology*. 5: 155–160.

Albert M.L., Feldman, R.G. and Willis, A.L. 1974. The 'subcortical dementia' of progressive supranuclear palsy. *Journal of Neurology, Neurosurgery and Psychiatry*. 37: 121–130.

Albin R.L. 1995. Selective neurodegeneration in Huntington's disease [editorial]. *Annals of Neurology*. 38: 835–836.

Albin R.L. and Tagle, D.A. 1995. Genetics and molecular biology of Huntington's disease. *Trends in Neurosciences*. 18: 11–14.

Alexander, G.E. and Crutcher, M.D. 1990. Functional architecture of basal ganglia circuits: Neural substrates of parallel processing. *Trends in Neurosciences*. 13: 266–271.

Arai, H., Kosaka, K. and Iuzuka, A. 1984. Changes in biogenic amines and their metabolites in postmortem brains from patients with Alzheimer type dementia. *Journal of Neurochemistry*. 43: 388–393.

Bartus, R.T. 1979. Physostigmine and recent memory: Effects in young and aged non-human primates. *Science*. 206: 1087–1089.

Beal, M.F., Mazurek, M.F., Svendsen, C.N., Bird, E.D. and Martin, J.B. 1986. Widespread reduction of somatostatin-like immunoreactivity in the cerebral cortex in Alzheimer's disease. *Annals of Neurology*. 20: 489–495.

Beal, M.F., Mazurek, M.F., Ellison, D.W., Swartz, K.J., McGarvey, U., Bird, E.D. and Martin, J.B. 1988. Somatostatin and neuropeptide Y concentrations in pathologically graded cases of Huntington's disease. *Annals of Neurology*. 23: 562–569.

Bierer, L.M., Haroutunian, V., Gabriel, S., Knott, P.J., Carlin, L.S., Purohit, D.P., Perl, D.P., Schmeidler, J., Kanof, P. and Davis, K.L. 1995. Neurochemical correlates of dementia severity in Alzheimer's disease: Relative importance of the cholinergic deficits. *Journal of Neurochemistry*. 64: 749–760.

Blackmore, L., Simpson, S.A. and Crawford, J.R. 1995. Cognitive performance in UK sample of presymptomatic people carrying the gene for Huntington's disease. *Journal of Medical Genetics*. 32: 358–362.

Boller, F., Mizutani, T., Roessmann, U. and Pierluigi, G. 1980. Parkinson's disease, dementia and Alzheimer disease: Clinicopathologic correlation. *Annals of Neurology*. 7: 329–335.

Braak, H. and Braak, E. 1991. Neuropathological staging of Alzheimer-related changes. *Acta Neuropathologica*. 82: 239–259.

Braak, H. and Braak, E. 1994. Pathology of Alzheimer's disease. In *Neurodegenerative diseases*, ed. D.B. Calne, pp. 585–613. Philadelphia: W.B. Saunders Company.

Brown, R.G. and Marsden, C.D. 1990. Cognitive function in Parkinson's disease: From description to theory. *Trends in Neurosciences*. 13: 21–29.

Chui, H.C., Mortimer, J.A., Slager, V., Zarow, C., Bondareff, W. and Webster, D.D. 1986. Pathologic correlates of dementia in Parkinson's disease. *Archives of Neurology*. 43: 991–995.

Chui, H.C., Teng, E.L., Henderson, V.W. and Moy, A.C. 1985. Clinical subtypes of dementia of the Alzheimer type. *Neurology*. 35: 1544–1550.

Claes, S., VanZand, K., Legius, E., Dom, R., Malfroid, M., Baro, F., Godderis, J. and Cassiman, J.J. 1995. Correlations between triplet repeat expansion and clinical features in Huntington's disease. *Archives of Neurology*. 52: 749–753.

Collingridge, G.L. and Bliss, T.V.P. 1995. Memories of NMDA receptors and LTP. *Trends in Neurosciences*. 18: 54–56.

Cudkowitz, M. and Kowall, N.W. 1984. Degneration of pyramidal projection neurons in Huntington's disease cortex. *Annals of Neurology*. 41: 874–879.

Cummings, J.L. 1993. Frontal-subcortical circuits and human behavior. *Archives of Neurology*. 50: 873–880.

Dale, H.H. 1935. Pharmacology and nerve endings. *Proceedings of the Royal Society, London*. B28: 319–322.

D'Amato, R.J., Zweig, R.M., Whitehouse, P.J., Wenk, G.L., Singer, H.S., Mayeux, R., Price, D.L. and Snyder, S.H. 1987. Aminergic systems in Alzheimer's disease and Parkinson's disease. *Annals of Neurology*. 22: 229–236.

Dawbarn, D., DeQuidt, M.E. and Emson, P.C. 1985. Survival of basal ganglia neuropeptide Y-somatostatins in Huntington's disease. *Brain Research*. 340: 251–260.

DeLong, M.R. 1990. Primate models of movement disorders of basal ganglia origin. *Trends in Neurosciences*. 13: 281–285.

Denny Brown, D. 1962. *The basal ganglia and their relation to disorders of movement*. Oxford: Oxford University Press.

Drachman, D.A. and Leavitt, J.L. 1974. Human memory and the cholinergic system. A relationship to aging? *Archives of Neurology*. 30: 113–121.

Dwork, A.J., Balmaceda, C., Fazzini, E.A., MacCollin, M., Côté, L. and Fahn, S. 1993. Dominantly inherited, early-onset parkinsonism: neuropathology of a new form. *Neurology*. 43: 69–74.

Ellison, D.W., Beal, M.F., Mazurek, M.F., Bird, E.D. and Martin, J.B. 1986. A postmortem study of amino acid neurotransmitters in Alzheimer's disease. *Annals of Neurology*. 20: 616–621.

Ellison, D.W., Beal, M.F., Mazurek, M.F., Malloy, J.R., Bird, E.D. and Martin, J.B. 1987. Amino acid neurotransmitter abnormalities in Huntington's disease and the quinolinic acid animal model of Huntington's disease. *Brain*. 110: 1657–1673.

Fearnley, J.M. and Lees, A.J. 1991. Aging and Parkinson's disease: Substantia nigra regional selectivity. *Brain*. 114: 2283–2301.

Fibiger, H.C. 1991. Cholinergic mechanisms in learning, memory and dementia: A review of recent evidence. *Trends in Neurosciences*. 14: 220–223.

Gallagher, M. and Colombo, P.J. 1995. Ageing: The cholinergic hypothesis of cognitive decline. *Current Opinion in Neurobiology*. 5: 161–168.

Gaspar, P., Duyckaerts, C., Alvarez, C., Javoy-Agid, F. and Berger, B. 1991. Alteration of dopaminergic and noradrenergic innervations in motor cortex in Parkinson's disease. *Annals of Neurology*. 30: 365–374.

Gibb, W.R.G. and Lees, A.T. 1988. The relevance of the Lewy body to the pathogenesis of idiopathic Parkinson's disease. *Journal of Neurology, Neurosurgery and Psychiatry*. 51: 745–752.

Giordani, B., Berent, S., Boivin, M.J., Penney, J.B., Lehtinen, S., Markel, D.S., Hollingsworth, Z., Butterbaugh, G., Hichwa, R.D., Gusella, J.F. and Young, A.B. 1995. Longitudinal neuropsychological and genetic linkage analysis of persons at risk for Huntington's disease. *Archives of Neurology*. 52: 59–64.

Goto, S. Hirano, A. and Matsumoto, S. 1990. Met-enkefalin immunoreactivity in the basal ganglia in Parkinson's disease and striatonigral degeneration. *Neurology*. 40: 1051–1056.

Graybiel, A.M. 1995. The basal ganglia. *Trends in Neurosciences*. 18: 60–62.

Graybiel, A.M., Aosaki, T., Flaherty, A.W. and Kimura, M. 1994. The basal ganglia and adaptive motor control. *Science*. 265: 1826–1831.

Graybiel, A.M. and Kimura, M. 1995. Adaptive neural networks in the basal ganglia. In *Models of information processing in the basal ganglia*, ed. J.C. Houk, J.L. Davis and D.G. Beiser, pp. 103–116. Cambridge: M.I.T. Press.

Graybiel, A.M., Moratalla, R. and Robertson, H.A. 1990. Amphetamine and cocaine induce drug specific activation of the c-fos gene in striosome-matrix compartment and limbic sudivisions of the striatum. *Proceedings of the National Academy of Sciences*. 87: 6912–6916.

Harrington, K.M. and Kowall, N.W. 1991. Parvalbumin immunoreactive neurons resist degeneration in Huntington's disease striatum (abstract). *Journal of Neuropathology and Experimental Neurology*. 50: 309.

Hasselmo, M.E. and Bower, J.M. 1993. Acetylcholine and memory. *Trends in Neurosciences*. 16: 218–222.

Hedera, P. and Whitehouse, P.J. 1994. Neurotransmitters in neurodegeneration. In *Neurodegenerative diseases*, ed. D.B. Calne, pp. 97–117. Philadelphia: W.B. Saunders Company.

Herregodts, P., Bruyland, M., DeKeyser, J., Solheid, C. Michotte, Y. and Ebinger, G. 1989. Monoaminergic neurotransmitters in Alzheimer's disease: An HPLC study comparing presenile familial and sporadic senile cases. *Journal of the Neurological Sciences*. 92: 101–116.

Hikosaka, O., Sakamoto, M. and Usui, S. 1989. Functional properties of monkey caudate neurons. I. Activities related to saccadic eye movements. *Journal of Neurophysiology*. 61: 750–798.

Hoover, J.E. and Strick, P.L. 1993. Multiple output channels in the basal ganglia. *Science*. 259: 819–821.

Hornykiewicz, O. and Kish, S.J. 1986. Biochemical pathophysiology of Parkinsons's disease. *Advances in Neurology*. 45: 19–34.

Hyman, B.T., Van Hoesen, G.W. and Damasio, A.R. 1987. Alzheimer's disease: Glutamate depletion in the hippocampal perforant pathway zone. *Annals of Neurology*. 22: 37–40.

Hyman, B.T., Van Hoesen, G.W., Kromer, L.J. and Damasio, A.R. 1986. Perforant pathway changes and the memory impairment of Alzheimer's disease. *Annals of Neurology*. 20: 472–481.

Hyman, S.E. 1993. The molecular and cellular basis of addiction. *Current Opinion in Neurology and Neurosurgery*. 6: 609–613.

Jellinger, K. 1990. New developments in the pathology of Parkinson's disease. *Advances in Neurology*. 53: 1–16.

Kish, S.J., Rajput, A., Gilbert, J., Rozdilsky, B., Chang, L.J. Shannak, K. and Hornykiewicz, O. 1986b. GABA is elevated in striatal but not extrastriatal regions in Parkinson's disease: Correlations with striatal dopamine loss. *Annals of Neurology*. 20: 26–31.

Kish, S.J., Shannak, K. and Hornykiewicz, O. 1986a. Uneven pattern of dopamine loss in the striatum of patients with idiopathic Parkinson's disease. *New England Journal of Medicine*. 318: 876–880.

Koo, E.H. and Price, D.L. 1993. The neurobiology of dementia. In *Dementia*, ed. P.J. Whitehouse, pp. 55–91. Philadelphia: F.A. Davis Company.

Landwehmeyer, G.B., McNeil, S.M., Dure, L.S., Pei, G., Aizawa, H., Huang, Q., Ambrose, C., Duyao, M.P., Bird, E.D., Bonilla, E., de Young, M., Villa-Gonzales, A.J., Wexler, N.S., DiFiglia, M. B., Gusella, J.F., MacDonald, M.E., Penney, J.B., Young, A.B. and Vonsattel, J.P. 1995. Huntington's disease gene: Regional and cellular expression in brain of normal and affected individuals. *Annals of Neurology*. 37: 218–230.

Lowe, S.L., Bowen, D.M., Francis, P.T. and Neary, D. 1990. Ante mortem cerebral amino acid concentrations indicate selective degeneration of glutamate-enriched neurons in Alzheimer's disease. *Neuroscience*. 38: 571–577.

Lundervold, A.J. and Reinvang, I. 1995. Variability in cognitive function among persons at high genetic risk of Huntington's disease. *Acta Neurologica Scandinavica*. 91: 462–469.

Marsden, C.D. and Obeso, J.A. 1994. The functions of the basal ganglia and the paradox of stereotaxic surgery in Parkinson's disease. *Brain*. 117: 877–897.

Mesulam, M.M. and Mufson, E.J. 1984. Neural inputs into the nucleus basalis of the substantia innominata (Ch4) in the rhesus monkey. *Brain*. 107: 253–274.

Mesulam, M.M., Mufson, E.J., Levey, A.I. and Wainer, B.H. 1983. Cholinergic innervation of cortex by the basal forebrain: Cytochemistry and cortical connection of the septal area, diagonal band nuclei, nucleus basalis (substantia innominata) and hypothalamus in the Rhesus monkey. *Journal of Comparative Neurology*. 214: 170–197.

Mesulam, M.M., Volicer, L., Marquis, J.K., Mufson, E.J. and Green, R.C. 1986. Systematic regional differences in the cholinergic innervation of the primate cerebral cortex: Distribution of enzyme activities and some behavioral implications. *Annals of Neurology*. 19: 144–151.

Middleton, F.A. and Strick, P.L. 1994. Anatomical evidence for cerebellar and basal ganglia involvement in higher cognitive function. *Science*. 266: 458–461.

Mogenson, G.J., Jones, D.L. and Yim, C.Y. 1980. From motivation to action: functional interface between the limbic system and the motor system. *Progress in Neurobiology*. 14: 69–97.

Morris, B.J. and Johnston, H.M. 1995. A role for hippocampal opioids in long-term functional plasticity. *Trends in Neurosciences*. 18: 350–355.

Moruzzi, G. and Magoun, H.W. 1949. Brainstem reticular formation and activation of the EEG. *Electroencephalography and Clinical Neurophysiology*. 1: 455–473.

Nasir, J., Floresco, S.B., Diewert, V.M., Richman, J.M., Zeisler, J., Borowski, A., Marth, J.D., Phillips, A.B. and Hayden, M.R. 1995. Targeted disruption of the Huntington's disease gene results in embryonic lethality and behavioral and morphological changes in heterozygotes. *Cell*. 81: 811–823.

Nieuwenhuys, R. 1985. Conclusions and comments. In *Chemoarchitecture of the brain*, ed. R. Nieuwenhuys, pp. 114–176. Berlin: Springer Verlag.

Paulsen, J.S., Butters, N., Sadek, J.R., Johnson, S.A., Salmon, D.P., Swerdlow, N.R. and Swenson, M.R. 1995. Distinct cognitive profiles of cortical and subcortical dementia in advanced illness. *Neurology*. 45: 951–956.

Percheron, G. and Filion, M. 1991. Parallel processing in the basal ganglia: Up to a point [letter]. *Trends in Neurosciences*. 14: 55–59.

Percheron, G., Yelnick, J. and Francois, C. 1984. A golgi analysis of the primate globus pallidus. III. Spatial organization of the striato-pallidal complex. *Journal of Comparative Neurology*. 227: 214–227.

Perry, E.K., Tomlinson, E., Blessed, G., Bergmann, K., Gibson, P.H. and Perry, R.H. 1978. Correlation of cholinergic abnormalities with senile plaques and mental test scores in senile dementia. *British Medical Journal*. 2: 1457–1459.

Perry, T.L. and Hansen, S. 1990. What excitotoxin kills striatal neurons in Huntington's disease? Clues from neurochemical studies. *Neurology*. 40: 20–24.

Price, D.L., David, P.B., Morris, J.C. and White, D.L. 1991. The distribution of tangles, plaques and related immunohistochemical markers in healthy aging and Alzheimer's disease. *Neurobiology of Aging*. 12: 295–312.

Price, D.L., Whitehouse, P.J., Struble, R.G., Clark, A.W., Coyle, J.T., DeLong, M.R. and Hedreen, J.C. 1982. Basal forebrain cholinergic systems in Alzheimer's disease and related dementias. *Neuroscience Comment*. 1: 84–92.

Quarrell, O. and Harper, P. 1991. The clinical neurology of Huntington's disease. In *Huntington's disease*, ed. P.S. Harper, M. Morris, O.W.J. Quarrell, D.J. Shaw, A.Tyler and S. Youngman, pp. 52–57. London: W.B. Saunders Company.

Reiner, A., Albin, R.L. Anderson, K.D., D'Amato, C.J., Penney, J.B. and Young, A.B. 1988. Differential loss of striatal projection neurons in Huntington's disease. *Proceedings of the National Academy of Sciences*. 85: 5733–5737.

Revonuso, A., Portin, R., Koivikko, L., Rinne, J.O. and Rinne, U.K. 1993. Slowing of information processing in Parkinson's disease. *Brain and Cognition*. 21: 87–110.

Reynolds, G.P. and Pearson, S.J. 1987. Decreased glutamic acid and increased 5-hydroxytryptamine in Huntington's disease brain. *Neuroscience Letters*. 78: 233–238.

Richfield, E.K., Maguire-Zeiss, K.A., Vonkeman, H.E. and Voorn, P. 1995. Preferential loss of preproenkephalin versus preprotachykinin neurons from the striatum of Huntington's disease patients. *Annals of Neurology*. 38: 852–861.

Robbins, T.W., Cador, M., Taylor, J.R. and Everitt, B.J. 1989. Limbic-striatal interactions in reward-related processes. *Neuroscience and Biobehavioral Reviews*. 13: 155–162.

Robbins, T.W. and Everitt, B.J. 1996. Neurobehavioral mechanism of reward and motivation. *Current Opinion in Neurobiology*. 6: 228–236.

Rogers, D. 1986. Bradyphrenia in Parkinsonism: A historical review. *Psychological Medicine*. 16: 257–265.

Rosenberg, N.K., Sorensen, S.A. and Christensen, A.L. 1995. Neuropsychological characteristics of Huntington disease carriers: A double blind study. *Journal of Medical Genetics*. 32: 600–604.

Schwartz, J.H. and Greenberg, S.M. 1987. Molecular mechanisms for memory: Second messenger induced modification of protein kinases in nerve cells. *Annual Review of Neuroscience*. 10: 459–467.

Selkoe, D.J. 1991. The molecular pathology of Alzheimer's disease. *Neuron*. 6: 487–498.

Selkoe, D.J., Bell, D.S., Podlisny, M.B., Price, D.L. and Cork, L.C. 1987. Conservation of brain amyloid proteins in aged mammals and humans with Alzheimer's disease. *Science*. 235: 873–877.

Sharp, A.H., Loev, S.J., Schilling, G., Li, S.H., Li, X.J., Bao, J., Wagster, M.V., Kotzuk, J.A., Steiner, J.P., Lo, A., Hedreen, J., Sisodia, S., Synder, S.H., Dawson, T.M., Ryugo, D.K. and Ross, C.A. 1995. Widespread expression of Huntington's disease gene IT15 gene product. *Neuron*. 14: 1065–1074.

Smirnova, T., Laroche, S., Errington, M.L., Hicks, A.A., Bliss, T.V.P. and Mallet, J. 1993. Transsynaptic expression of presynaptic glutamate receptor during hippocampal long-term potentiation. *Science*. 262: 433–436.

Sparks, D.L., DeKosky, S.T. and Marskesbery, W.R. 1988. Alzheimer's disease: Aminergic-cholinergic alterations in hypothalamus. *Archives of Neurology*. 45: 994–999.

Squire, L.R. and Davis, H.P. 1981. The pharmacology of memory: A neuro-biological perspective. *Annual Review of Pharmacology and Toxicology*. 21: 323–356.

Steriade, M. and Buzsaki, G. 1990. Parallel activation of thalamic and cortical neurons by brainstem and basal forebrain cholinergic systems. In *Brain cholinergic systems*, ed. M. Steriade and D. Biesbold, pp. 3–64. Oxford: Oxford University Press.

Strauss, M.E. and Brandt, J. 1990. Are there neuropsychologic manifestations of the gene of Huntington's disease in asymptomatic, at-risk individuals? *Archives of Neurology*. 47: 905–908.

Struble, R.G., Lehmann, J., Mitchell, S.J., McKinney, M., Price, D.L., Coyle, J.T. and DeLong, M.R. 1986. Basal forebrain neurons provide major cholinergic innervation of primate neocortex. *Neuroscience Letters*. 66: 215–220.

Struble, R.G., Powers, R.E., Casanova, M.F., Kitt, C.A., Brown, E.C. and Price, D.L. 1987. Neuropeptidergic systems in plaques of Alzheimer's disease. *Journal of Neuropathology and Experimental Neurology*. 46: 567–584.

Taquet, H., Nomoto, M., Rose, S., Jenner, P., Javoy-Agid, F., Mauborgne, A., Benoliel, J.J., Marsden, C.D., Legrand, J.C., Agid, Y., Hamon, M. and Cesselin, F. 1988. Levels of met-enkefalin, leu-enkefalin, substance P and cholecystokinin in the brain of the common marmoset following long-term 1-methyl–4-phenyl–1,2,3,6,-tetrahydropyridine treatment. *Neuropeptides*. 12: 105–110.

Thompson, P.D., Berardelli, A., Rothwell, J.C., Day, B.L., Dick, J.P.R., Benecke, R. and Marsden, C.D. 1988. The coexistence of bradykinesia and chorea in Huntington's disease and its implications for theories of basal ganglia control of movement. *Brain*. 111: 223–244.

Torack, R.M. and Morris, J.C. 1988. The association of ventral tegumental area histopathology with adult dementia. *Archives of Neurology*. 45: 497–501.

Vonsattel, J.P., Meyers, R.H., Stevens, T.J., Ferrante, R.J., Bird, E.D. and Richardson, E.P. 1985. Neuropatho-logical classification of Huntington's disease. *Journal of Neuropathology and Experimental Neurology*. 44: 559–577.

Voytko, M.L., Olton, D.S., Richardson, R.T., Gorman, L.K., Tobin, J.R. and Price, D.L. 1993. Basal forebrain lesions in monkeys disrupt attention but not learning and memory. *Journal of Neuroscience*. 14: 167–186.

Wagner, J.J., Caudle, R.M., Neumaier, J.F. and Chavkin, C. 1991. Stimulation of endogenous opioid release displaces mu receptor binding in rat hippo-campus. *Neuroscience*. 37: 45–53.

Walker, L.C., Kitt, C.A., Cork, L.C., Struble, R.G., Dellovade, T.L. and Price, D.L. 1988. Multiple transmitter systems contribute neurites to individual senile plaques. *Journal of Neuropathology and Experimental Neurology*. 47: 138–144.

Whitehouse, P.J., Hedreen, J.C., White, C.L. and Price, D.L. 1983. Basal forebrain in the dementia of Parkinson's disease. *Annals of Neurology*. 13: 243–248.

Whitehouse, P.J., Price, D.L., Clark, A.W., Coyle, J.T and DeLong, M.R. 1981. Alzheimer disease: Evidence for selective loss of cholinergic neurons in the nucleus basalis. *Annals of Neurology*. 10: 122–126.

Whitehouse, P.J., Price, D.L., Struble, R.G., Clark, A.W., Coyle, J.T. and DeLong, M.R. 1982. Alzheimer's disease and senile dementia: Loss of neurons in the basal forebrain. *Science*. 215: 1237–1239.

Wicken, J. and Kotter, R. 1995. Cellular models of reinforcement. In *Models of information processing in the basal ganglia*, ed. J.C. Houk, J.L. Davis, D.G. Beiser, pp. 187–214. Cambridge, MA: MIT Press.

Wilcox, B.J. and Unnerstall, J.R. 1990. Identification of subpopulation of neuropeptide Y-containing locus coeruleus neurons that project to the entorhinal cortex. *Synapse*. 6: 284–291.

Wisser, H. and Ratge, D. 1989. Cate-cholamines in urine, blood and cerebrospinal fluid. In *Early diagnosis and preventive therapy in Parkinson's disease*, ed. H. Przunteck and P. Rieder, pp. 197–204. Vienna, Austria: Springer Verlag.

Zubenko, G.S., Moosy, J., Martinez, A.J., Rao, G., Claassen, D., Rosen, J. and Kopp, U. 1991. Neuropathologic and neurochemical correlates of psychosis in primary dementia. *Archives of Neurology*. 48: 619–624.

Zweig, R.M., Ross, C.A., Hedreen, J.C., Steele, C., Cardillo, J.E., Whitehouse, P.J., Folstein, M.F. and Price, D.L. 1988. The neuropathology of aminergic nuclei in Alzheimer's disease. *Annals of Neurology*. 24: 233–242.

5 Structural neuroimaging correlates of memory dysfunction in neurodegenerative disease

EDITH V. SULLIVAN, DEBORAH A. CAHN,
ROSEMARY FAMA AND PAULA K. SHEAR

INTRODUCTION

The study of in vivo brain–behavior relationships has been significantly enhanced by advances in structural neuroimaging procedures. This chapter describes the recent contributions of these technologies to our understanding of brain–behavior correlations and, in particular, the relationships between brain structures subserving memory and the memory disorders characteristic of the different etiologies of dementia. These advances are largely the result of enhanced resolution of brain images, the use of careful statistical approaches to examine imaging data and the appreciation for the influence of demographic characteristics such as age, gender and head size when considering group results.

NEUROIMAGING ISSUES

Structural brain imaging technologies provide the opportunity to determine the condition of the brain in individuals who are also given tests of cognitive, sensory and motor functioning. Even with these techniques, however, structure–function studies are difficult because these technologies are complex and there are no established conventions for acquisition, processing, analysis or statistical interpretation of neuroimaging data.

Image quality is affected by the technology chosen and the interaction of acquisition parameters that determine resolution. Structure measurements are substantially influenced by boundary definitions, which can vary across neuroanatomy atlases and by correction factors applied to account for unwanted sources of variation, such as head size, sex and age. Before reviewing the literature on the contribution of structural imaging to our understanding of the neuropathological substrates of memory impairment in neurodegenerative diseases, this chapter provides a brief overview of some essential issues to bear in mind when critically reading studies using structural imaging methods (for reviews see Jernigan and Cermak 1994; Lim et al. 1995; Raz 1996).

Influences of image acquisition on measurement
The information that can be derived from an image is first limited by the technology used for acquisition. CT is limited by the *orientation* in which images can be acquired. It was originally called computed axial tomography, referring to the fact that images could be acquired comfortably only in the axial plane (frontal to the occipital poles; see computed tomography (CT) scan in Figure 5.1 and magnetic resonance imaging (MRI) scan in Figure 5.2). This plane provides an excellent view of the lateral ventricles, basal ganglia and some cortical sulci, but is suboptimal for visualizing such structures as the frontal and temporal cortical and subcortical structures, which are better seen in the coronal plane (i.e. left to the right side of the brain; see MRI in Figure 5.2) and the corpus callosum, thalamus and mammillary bodies, which are better seen in the sagittal plane (i.e. top to the bottom of the head; see MRI in Figure 5.2).

Image *resolution* of CT is limited to distinguishing between tissue and cerebrospinal fluid (CSF) but, unlike MRI, cannot reliably distinguish tissue types, namely gray and white matter. CT is further limited by beam hardening artifact, which diminishes fluid/tissue resolution near bone and skull. Without appropriate filtering during post-image acquisition processing to minimize this artifact, cortical sulci can appear inaccurately small on CT. This

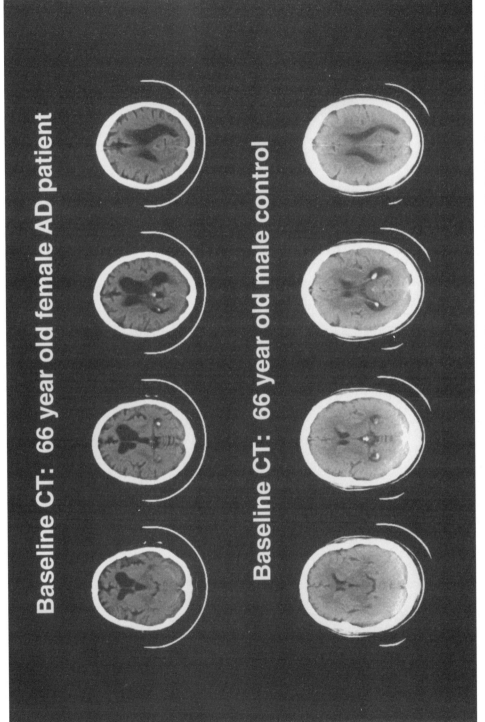

Figure 5.1. Baseline axial CT scans of a 66-year-old female patient with Alzheimer's disease and a 66-year-old male control subject. Modified from Shear et al. (1995).

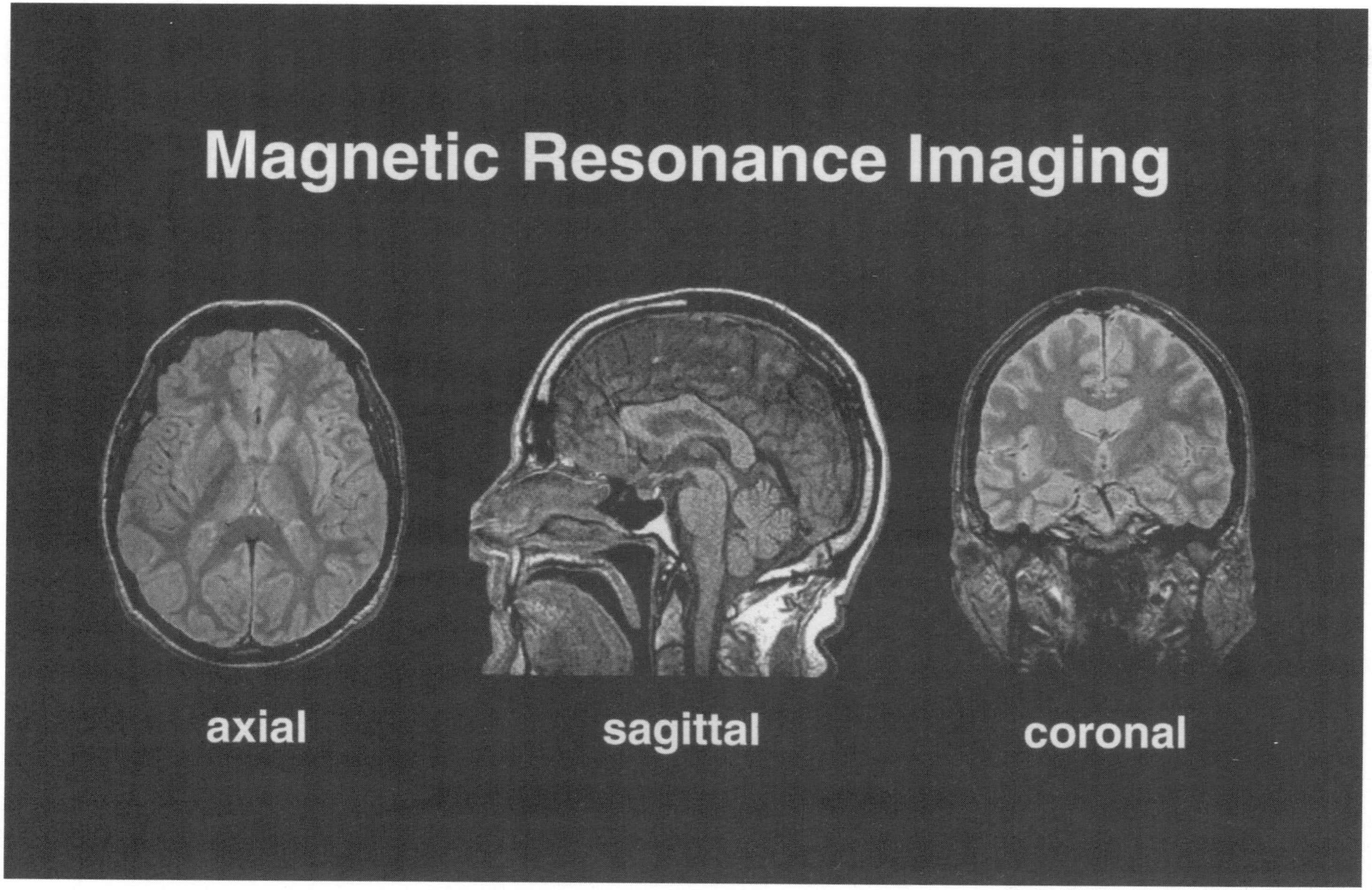

Figure 5.2. MRI scans depicting axial, sagittal and coronal views of the brain. Modified from Lim et al. (1995).

artifact also affects accurate imaging of the temporal lobes, which are encased in bone. Despite these limitations, CT has provided important data on neurodegenerative disorders that affect the ventricular system and clinically CT remains an important technology for identifying calcification and vascular rupture.

Image orientation with MRI is far more flexible than with CT. Two dimensional MR images can be acquired in any plane of section (Figure 5.2). So, for example, when using two-dimensional MRI to image the hippocampus, some researchers have chosen to acquire images in the plane that runs perpendicular to the long axis of the hippocampus. The resulting coronal images would be least affected by unwanted angulation, which could bias measurement especially of structures that are not fully volumed (Zipursky et al. 1990). Three-dimensional imaging is now possible and provides a complete picture of the brain in all planes; two-dimensional viewing planes can be oriented to an optimal plane during either acquisition or postacquisition image processing.

Structure quantification

Structure measurement is typically accomplished by boundary outlining, tissue compartmentalization, or a combination of the two. Outlining (Figure 5.3a,c) can be done by manually tracing structure borders on images displayed on a computer screen (Filipek et al. 1989; Jack et al. 1990), or digitized from film (Blatter et al. 1995). Seeding methods (Andreasen et al. 1994) can be used to detect well-defined borders automatically but usually require some manual intervention when image borders are blurred, for example, by partial voluming from adjacent structures. Partial voluming occurs when voxels are composed of more than the target tissue type, for example, when a voxel is composed of gray matter plus CSF.

Compartmentalization or segmentation is often used to categorize MRI intensities that represent different brain constituents, such as CSF, gray and white matter (Lim and Pfefferbaum 1989; Jernigan 1990). The different cranial tissue types – gray matter, white matter, CSF, blood, bones, marrow and dura – each produce somewhat different MRI signal intensities based on their biological properties, especially the amount of unbound water in each. These tissue types are said to have different relaxation times. Varying the timing of MR acquisition parameters – the excitation (repetition time, TR) and time delay before data acquisition (echo time, TE) – allows the inves-

tigator to enhance contrast between or among tissue types (Wehrli et al. 1984). To optimize this process, MR acquisition parameters that enhance signals arising from selective tissue types should be used. Thus, to achieve ideal compartmentalization of gray matter, white matter and CSF, it is best to obtain two sets of images, based on short and long echo times; the former affords good gray-white separation and the latter good CSF-tissue separation.

Manipulation of image acquisition parameters is also useful in enhancing selective brain stem nuclei, which are targeted by disease processes such as Parkinson's disease (PD) and are susceptible to partial voluming because of their small size. The presence of iron in the substantia nigra, for example, results in very little (dark) MR signal and thus makes this small structure visually salient in a surround of lighter signal intensity.

The combination of these measurement techniques can be used, for example, in outlining specific cortical gyri and then in segmenting the tissue into gray and white matter compartments (Figure 5.3b; Sullivan et al. 1995a; Marsh et al. 1996). Once identified, structures can be quantified using visual rating systems, two-dimensional areas, or three-dimensional volumes. *Ratings* (van Sweiten et al. 1990; Davila et al. 1994) are typically based on qualitative criteria of structure appearance and a categorical scale, thus limiting actual measurement precision and the possible range of scores. Area and volume measurements take advantage of the ways in which the images are acquired. CT and MR images are collected as slices through the brain in a particular plane that have a surface and a thickness. Each slice is composed of a matrix of picture elements, i.e. pixels, which refer to the surface or linear area, or voxels, which refer to the volume of the pixels. Quantification of a target brain structure, then, can be calculated by adding the pixels or voxels that are present within the borders of a selected brain region or structure.

Areas are determined from a single CT or MRI slice. Ventricle-to-brain ratios (VBR) represent a commonly used area measure. Although quantitative, area measurements are subject to bias from undersampling, which results from selecting a slice that is not adequately representative of the size of the structure as a whole. *Volumes* are determined by adding the areas of outlined structures or compartmentalized tissue or CSF measured on multiple CT or MRI slices (for CT see Jernigan 1986; Pfefferbaum et al. 1986; for MRI see Lim and Pfefferbaum 1989; Jernigan et al. 1990a; Pfefferbaum et al. 1994).

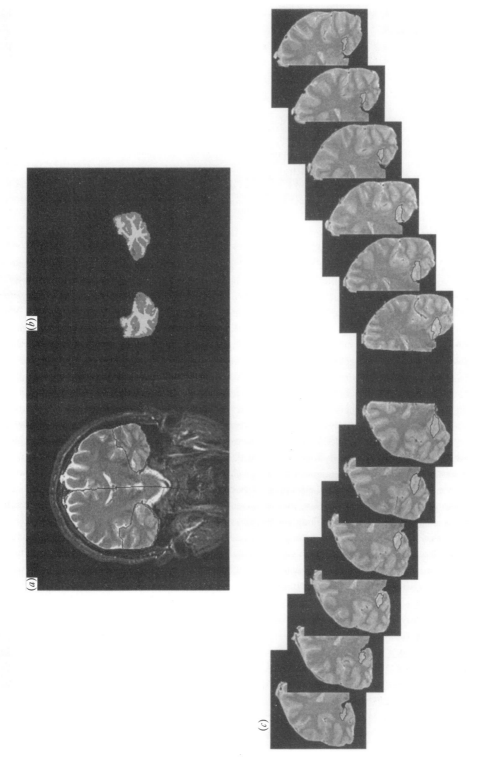

Figure 5.3. (a) The temporal lobes and hippocampus are outlined on the left and right hemispheres on this coronal MRI slice. (b) The tissue of the temporal lobes has been segmented into three compartments: gray matter in gray, white matter in light gray and CSF in black. (c) The hippocampus is measured by outlining its borders on contiguous slices. Modified from Sullivan et al. (1995a).

Measurements based on volumes are likely to provide the best estimates of actual structure size even when the volumes do not include the entire structure, in other words, when only 'partially volumed'. Stereological methods used in postmortem cell counting studies can also be applied to in vivo imaging in order to systematize the selection of slices in the sample to be used to estimate the true volume of a structure (West 1993; Keshavan et al. 1995).

Regardless of the method used, it is incumbent upon the researcher to provide quantitative data on the reliability of the measurement procedure. Furthermore, despite the obvious worth of in vivo neuroimaging, one must bear in mind the limitations of these radiological techniques, which provide only images or estimates of real structures and are susceptible to acquisition and postacquisition processing artifact affecting measurement.

Extraneous sources of variance to brain measurement and analysis

Brain imaging permits quantification of regional abnormalities present in individuals or in groups. In order to determine the extent of brain dysmorphology in disease states, however, analysis of brain imaging data must take into account unwanted sources of variance. Healthy individuals vary widely in head and brain size and some, but not all, brain structures are proportionate to overall brain size. Thus, a structure with a small absolute size may be normal in a small person. Thus *size*, in particular, intracranial volume (Mathalon et al. 1993a,b) or somatic size (Raz 1996), must be accounted for, particularly when examining gender differences or in comparing groups comprising both genders because, on average, women are inherently smaller than men.

Brain structure also varies systematically and substantially with *age* throughout the course of a lifetime. Maximal intracranial volume is not achieved until early adolescence (Dorst 1971; Dekaban and Sadowsky 1978). The increase in volume reflects a complex and dynamic interaction of increase and then decrease in cortical gray matter volume and increase in white matter volume (Pfefferbaum et al. 1994). From about age 20 years onward, cortical sulci enlarge at the expense of cortical gray matter, whereas white matter volume appears to remain relatively stable (Jernigan and Tallal 1990; Jernigan et al. 1991a; Pfefferbaum et al. 1994; Blatter et al. 1995; Raz et al. 1997). These significant normal variations in head size and age

must be taken into account before making claims about brain abnormalities associated with disease.

A number of different statistical methods have been used to account for unwanted variance. Methods to account for variation attributable to general size include ratios, proportions and regression analysis. Ratios and proportions use as their denominator, or correction factor, area of the total slice on which a structure was measured for area measurements (e.g. VBR) or intracranial volume for volume measurements. The problem with most proportional measures is that they do not fully remove the relationship between the measurement of a target structure and intracranial volume. By contrast, regression analysis can achieve such a correction (Mathalon et al. 1993a).

The approach our laboratory has taken to account for normal variation in head size and age is to adjust the brain imaging data of the patient group with respect to norms derived from large control groups spanning the adult age range (Pfefferbaum et al. 1992; Mathalon et al. 1993a; Sullivan et al. 1993b). This correction procedure involves two regression analyses and is applied separately to each brain structure measured. The first regression removes variation associated with head size in the control subjects. The residuals from this analysis are then subjected to a second regression to remove variation associated with age observed in the control subjects. The resulting volumes are expressed as Z-scores, with the expected mean *at any age*, corrected for head size differences, equaling 0 and the standard deviation equaling 1. These Z-score corrections are then applied to the data collected on individual patients and controls. The resulting Z-scores of the patients reflect disease-related brain abnormalities that are free of the normal variation attributable to head size and age (Mathalon et al. 1993b). Consequently, the head size and age-adjusted Z-score is a useful cross-sectional approach to examine relationships between age and brain volume in disease in different brain structures. The cross-sectional Z-score does not replace longitudinal study; instead it permits one to gauge the effect disease has at a given age. This capability is especially useful when examining age-related neurodegenerative diseases.

Longitudinal neuroimaging studies are, of course, ideal for tracking the progression of neurodegenerative diseases. Seldom, however, do such studies take into account two important sources of longitudinal error (for further discussion of correction methods, see Goodkin et al. 1993;

Pfefferbaum et al. 1995; Shear et al. 1995). The first type of error arises from repositioning the head in the scanner across imaging sessions. Head repositioning error is likely to be greatest for brain structure measurements based on small samples of the entire structure. The second type of error arises from the effects of normal aging. To account for these changes, a normal control group must also be studied longitudinally. Results based on longitudinal studies without the safeguards of longitudinal controls and head repositioning correction are questionable.

NEUROIMAGING AND MEMORY PERFORMANCE IN NEURODEGENERATIVE DISEASES

Normal aging

Normal aging is accompanied by selective declines in explicit memory with relative preservation of implicit memory (Monti et al. 1996; Winocur et al. 1996). Explicit memory refers to conscious retrieval of newly acquired information, while implicit memory refers to nonconscious memory such as skill learning or repetition priming (Squire and Zola-Morgan 1991; Chapter 12). This dissociation in memory decline is thought to be attributable to age-associated loss of parenchyma in the medial temporal lobes (Tomlinson 1972). In addition to loss of medial temporal lobe volume, the aging brain shows a decrease in overall cortical gray matter volume and an increase in cortical sulcal CSF volume and ventricular volume (Stafford et al. 1988; Blatter et al. 1995; Pfefferbaum et al. 1986). Thus, aging is in itself a dynamic condition of brain structure and function. Normal age-related structure – function relationships must, therefore, be taken into account before examining such relationships in neurodegenerative diseases.

In general, normal aging is associated with a modest decline in declarative memory processes (Poon 1985; Cullum et al. 1990; Petersen et al. 1992; Wiederholt et al. 1993), although the degree of impairment appears to be material-specific and related to the method of assessment (Albert 1988). Whether hippocampal volumes show a commensurate and related decline with age, however, is controversial (for a review, see Wickelgren 1996). Sullivan et al. (1995a) assessed the effect of normal aging on MRI volumes of hippocampi and temporal cortex in a cross-sectional study of 72 healthy men, aged 21–70 years. The

authors found that neither hippocampal volume nor cortical white matter volume was significantly correlated with age, whereas left and right temporal lobe gray matter volume (excluding hippocampus) did decrease with age. Furthermore, the volumes of temporal lobe sulcal CSF and temporal horn, lateral and third ventricle volumes also increased significantly with age. In order to delineate the specific brain–behavior relationships in these normal subjects, the authors conducted correlations between brain regions of interest and specific neuropsychological tests of memory. A memory deterioration index, calculated as the difference between estimated IQ and Wechsler Memory Scale (Wechsler and Stone 1945) raw scores, correlated significantly with age and left temporal lobe sulcal and bilateral ventricular volumes, but not with volumes of either hippocampus. Declines in measures of verbal and nonverbal immediate and working memory were not related to hippocampal volume but rather to the enlargement of the temporal horn and third and lateral ventricles. These results suggest that at least some component of age-related memory decline across the age range of 20–70 years is mediated more by shrinkage of extrahippocampal, medial temporal lobe volumes, than by hippocampal volume per se.

Golomb et al. (1993) investigated the relationship between hippocampal atrophy and specific memory impairments in normal elderly individuals who were designated as hippocampal atrophy-positive or hippocampal atrophy-negative based on ratings derived from films of CT, MRI or both technologies. Hippocampal atrophy was defined by the presence of perihippocampal CSF accumulation and was categorized by an experienced rater based on a four-point scale. The hippocampal atrophy positive group was defined as having at least mild to moderate perihippocampal CSF accumulation. Relative to the hippocampal atrophy-negative group, the hippocampal atrophy-positive group was significantly more impaired on tests of secondary, or delayed verbal memory, whereas the two hippocampal groups did not differ on tests of immediate memory. Thus, measures of delayed memory were more effective than measures of initial memory in distinguishing hippocampal atrophy-negative from hippocampal atrophy-positive subjects. In addition, the results demonstrate an association of hippocampal atrophy with impaired verbal memory in normal elderly adults. While this study employed measures of increased perihippocampal CSF as indirect markers of hippocampal atrophy, these authors have argued that CSF markers are more easily detectable and may more accurately reflect atrophy of the hippocampal formation, including the subiculum and entorhinal cortex of the parahippocampal gyrus than hippocampal volume per se (De Leon et al. 1995). Other volumetric studies do not provide support for substituting CSF measures, such as the temporal horns, as markers of hippocampal shrinkage because of the lack of relationship between measured hippocampal volumes and temporal horn or sulcal volumes (Sullivan et al. 1995a).

Another MRI study examined the differential contribution of limbic neocortical regions of the temporal lobes to declarative memory processes in normal elderly individuals, ranging in age from 55 to 88 years (Golomb et al. 1994). The volumes of the hippocampal formation, superior temporal gyrus and subarachnoid CSF compartment (reflecting generalized temporal, perisylvian and frontoparietal gyral atrophy) were adjusted for intersubject head size variability with multiple linear regression. The volumes were measured on digitized images by manually tracing the anatomical regions of interest. Accompanying MRI, all subjects received an extensive battery of neuropsychological tests, allowing for calculation of Initial and Delayed memory composite scores and investigation of short-term memory and language skills. A series of linear regressions revealed a dissociation in that hippocampal volume significantly predicted delayed memory performance while the volume of the superior temporal gyrus did not. Furthermore, the hippocampal volume did not correlate significantly with the measures of non-delayed memory. The authors interpreted these findings as suggesting anatomical specificity for the relationship between hippocampal volume and delayed memory performance, but cautioned that this interpretation was limited by the absence of a double-dissociation; namely, they did not test the associations between superior temporal gyrus and nondelayed memory performance.

Age-associated memory impairment

The term 'age-associated memory impairment' (AAMI) (Chapter 18) has remained controversial since its proposal by the National Institute of Mental Health (Caine 1993; Barker et al. 1995). AAMI refers to mild memory impairment related to normal aging that is distinct from the memory deficits observed in dementia. It is identified by subjective memory complaint, absence of memory-impairing medical conditions and memory test scores greater than 1 standard deviation below the mean for young adults (Crook et al. 1986). Neuropsychological studies which aim to distinguish subjects with AAMI from normal elderly and from demented patients have been largely equivocal and have contributed to the continuing debate regarding the utility of this diagnostic entity (Smith et al. 1991; O'Brien and Levy 1992; Malec et al. 1993). Given the disputes regarding the specificity and reliability of the diagnosis, it is not surprising to find only a limited number of studies regarding brain–behavior relationships in AAMI.

In an effort to characterize AAMI and its clinical course, Soininen et al. (1994) conducted a study of memory functioning in normal elderly subjects and subjects classified as having AAMI. Although normal subjects had larger right hippocampi than left, as has been observed by others (Jack et al. 1988; Cook et al. 1992), the AAMI subjects showed abnormally small volumetric asymmetry. The AAMI subjects and normal elderly subjects did not differ in terms of brain-size normalized volumes of hippocampus or amygdala. Nonetheless, brain-size normalized MRI volumes of the hippocampus and amygdala based on proportions were correlated with performance on tests of visual and verbal memory. In both normal individuals and individuals with AAMI, the degree of hippocampal asymmetry was found to correlate with performance on the Benton Visual Retention Test (Benton 1974), while amygdala volumes correlated with visual but not verbal memory performance. These findings suggest that individuals with AAMI have mild structural abnormalities in both the amygdala and hippocampus relative to normal elderly individuals. Additionally, the authors proposed that the relationship between amygdala volume and visual memory may reflect disruption of connections between the amygdala and frontal lobes, rather than damage to the amygdala alone. Follow-up studies are needed to determine if the presence of mild structural abnormalities represents a risk for future development of AD, or if it is a reflection of increased variability in cognitive functioning in normal elderly adults.

Alcoholism

Chronic alcoholism.

Chronic alcoholism is associated with a well-established constellation of cognitive impairments involving problem solving, abstract reasoning, visuospatial abilities, short-term memory, perceptual motor integration and new learning (see Parsons 1987; Fein et al. 1990; Oscar-Berman and Hutner 1993). These deficits, especially those involving mnemonic processes, are subtle (Butters and Brandt 1985) and can show significant recovery with sobriety and continued abstinence from alcohol (Brandt et al. 1983; Reed et al. 1992). Although the effects of duration of alcoholism and of lifetime alcohol consumption on cognitive status have been difficult to establish, age is an important determinant of extent of cognitive impairment. Unlike brain structure studies, most neuropsychological studies have failed to show that age accelerates the adverse effects of alcohol on cognitive functions (Becker et al. 1983; Grant et al. 1984; Ryan and Butters 1984; Shelton et al. 1984; Ellis and Oscar-Berman 1989).

Early CT studies in chronic alcoholics revealed a significantly dilated ventricular system and enlarged cortical sulci throughout the cortex (Haubek and Lee 1979; Wilkinson 1985; Pfefferbaum et al. 1988; Lishman 1990). Later, MRI studies provided convincing evidence that the increases in CSF-filled spaces occur at the expense of the two major brain tissue types, gray matter and white matter (Jernigan et al. 1991b). The effect of age on brain structure is critically important in alcoholism because older alcoholics (that is, from about age 45 years onward) appear to be especially vulnerable to the adverse effects of alcohol consumption (Wilkinson and Carlen 1980; Ron et al. 1982; Sullivan et al. 1995b; Pfefferbaum et al. 1996). Furthermore, the age-alcohol interaction persists even when duration of alcoholism is taken into account (Pfefferbaum et al. 1992). Although the cortical gray matter and white matter volume loss in alcoholics is widespread, the volume loss in the frontal lobes is relatively greater than that detected in the more posterior reaches of the cortex in older (more than 45 years of age) relative to younger alcoholics (Sullivan et al. 1996c). This observation supports postmortem studies, which identified the frontal lobes as being particularly damaged in alcoholics (Courville 1955; Harper and Kril 1990).

A number of CT studies of chronic alcoholics described the neuropsychological status of the patients but did not provide direct correlations between the radiological and neuropsychological measures. Several studies presenting such correlations had mixed results. Some observed no significant correlations between brain morphology and memory (Ron 1983; Pfefferbaum et al. 1988). Those that did report significant correlations were based on rather gross indices of brain integrity. Such correlations

were observed between Luria-Nebraska Memory scores and ventricle-to-brain ratios (Zelazowski et al. 1981); verbal recognition and lateral ventricular area as well as third ventricular to brain ratio; and recall and recognition of verbal and nonverbal material (Acker et al. 1987).

One of the clearest finding of selective brain–memory relationships in alcoholics using CT employed tissue density measures and third ventricle-to-intracranial width ratios in conjunction with memory as well as non-mnemonic tests (Gebhardt et al. 1984). This study showed that in nonamnesic alcoholics density measures of the thalamus were correlated with performance on a long-term memory test but not on short-term memory or digit symbol substitution tests. Importantly, none of the cognitive test measures correlated significantly with CT density measures from frontal or parietal regions.

MRI provides a superior opportunity to investigate the relationship between the volume of circumscribed brain regions and test performance on specific component processes of memory. A study from our laboratory used anatomically based MRI measures and observed significant volume deficits in the hippocampus and temporal lobe bilaterally in 47 alcoholics compared with 72 controls (Sullivan et al. 1995b); however, this study was unsuccessful in identifying significant correlations between the extent of hippocampal volume loss and explicit memory test performance.

Korsakoff's syndrome.

In contrast to 'uncomplicated' chronic alcoholism, Korsakoff's syndrome is marked by severe and relatively circumscribed global amnesia (Butters and Cermak 1980; Victor et al. 1989). The amnesia is thought to arise from thiamine deficiency, which can occur with the malnourishment commonly experienced by chronic alcoholics. Although the amnesia is a salient clinical feature, patients with alcoholic Korsakoff's syndrome also suffer the throes of 'uncomplicated' alcoholism and thus display the impairments in executive, visuospatial, learning and short-term memory functioning affecting nonamnesic alcoholics (for a review, see Oscar-Berman and Hutner 1993). The rigorous study of Korsakoff's syndrome has contributed immeasurably to current theories of memory (Butters and Cermak 1980; Squire and Butters 1992). Despite the resulting extensive body of literature, however, the neuropathology underlying the amnesia of Korsakoff's syndrome remains controversial. Consequently, clues gleaned from in vivo neuroimaging studies of amnesic and non-amnesic alcoholics can contribute substantially to the identification of compromised brain structural systems producing global amnesia.

Some in vivo CT and MRI studies have successfully identified patterns of brain dysmorphology distinguishing amnesic and nonamnesic alcoholics. An early CT study of relatively large groups of nonamnesic ($N = 68$) and amnesic ($N = 25$) alcoholics found significant correlations between a number of memory measures and CT measures of sulcal and ventricular evidence of atrophy, but these correlations were not unique to memory measures (Wilkinson and Carlen 1980). A later CT study (Shimamura et al. 1988) reported that Korsakoff's syndrome patients had lower signal density values in the thalamus and tissue in the region of the third ventricle than did nonamnesic alcoholics and controls. By contrast, both alcoholic groups had cortical atrophy in the frontal and perisylvian areas. Within the Korsakoff's syndrome patients, memory test performance was correlated with condition of the thalamus and frontal cortex, whereas performance on nonmnemonic cognitive measures was not correlated with any brain region examined. Analogous correlations for the alcoholic group were not reported. These authors concluded that the combined diencephalic and frontal lobe pathology contributes to the amnesia and cognitive impairment of Korsakoff's syndrome.

Degeneration of the mammillary nuclei has been considered, although not with firm foundation (Victor et al. 1989), to be a principal site of pathology for alcohol-related amnesia. Mammillary body atrophy may be a neuropathological marker for Wernicke's encephalopathy (Torvik et al. 1982; Charness and DeLaPaz 1987; Harper and Krill 1993), which is a common albeit not omnipresent precursor of Korsakoff's syndrome (Bigler et al. 1989; Blansjaar et al. 1992), but such atrophy appears to be neither necessary nor sufficient to produce amnesia in alcoholics. Two complementary studies, each using a three-point rating scale of mammillary body shrinkage, support this supposition. In the first study, Davila et al. (1994) demonstrated a significant incidence of mammillary body shrinkage in older, nonamnesic alcoholics compared with age-matched control subjects. In the second study, Shear et al. (1996) observed that, relative to the nonamnesic alcoholics in the Davila et al. study, amnesic alcoholics had a similar incidence of mammillary body shrinkage. The frequency of abnormality in the amnesic

patients was the same whether or not the patients were also diagnosed as having dementia and, furthermore, several amnesic patients had normal mammillary body ratings.

Using anatomically determined MRI measurement of brain structures, Squire et al. (1990) observed significantly smaller area measures of the mammillary nuclei but not of the hippocampal formation in four alcoholic Korsakoff's syndrome patients relative to four non-Korsakoff's syndrome amnesic patients, whereas the non-Korsakoff's syndrome amnesics showed the opposite pattern of regional sparing and loss. There is a suggestion that these abnormalities were selective because the area measures of other brain regions, in this case the temporal lobes and parahippocampal gyrus, did not differ significantly among the two amnesic groups and a group of six control subjects. The small sample sizes precluded direct examination of correlations between the extent of brain structure area deficits and memory impairments. Nonetheless, these authors concluded that the insignificantly and inconsistently smaller hippocampal size of the Korsakoff's syndrome patients relative to the controls cannot contribute importantly to the amnesic syndrome. In contrast to the later findings of Shear et al. and Davila et al., these authors further concluded that the amnesia is more likely to be associated with the shrinkage observed in the mammillary nuclei possibly combined with thalamic abnormalities observed with CT in these same patients (Shimamura et al. 1988).

An MRI study by Jernigan et al. (1991d) reported geometrically determined volume measurements of cortical and subcortical gray matter regions in eight Korsakoff's syndrome compared with 12 nonamnesic alcoholics and 13 age-matched controls. Both alcoholic groups had significant cortical sulcal enlargement, which occurred at the expense of cortical gray matter loss. The Korsakoff's syndrome group, however, showed even greater volume loss than the nonamnesic alcoholics in regions that, like the study by Squire et al. (1990), also included the anterior diencephalon and orbitofrontal cortex, but unlike the Squire et al. study, included the medial temporal lobes. A reasonable conclusion is that neuropathology in some combination of these three brain regions underlies or at least contributes importantly to the amnesia of alcoholic Korsakoff's syndrome.

Consistent with the findings of Jernigan et al. (1991d), an MRI study by Sullivan et al. (1996b) reported that relative to an age-range matched control group, Korsakoff's syndrome patients and nonamnesic alcoholics had significantly and comparably smaller gray matter volumes throughout the cortex; an observed white matter volume deficit was confined to the prefrontal region. In addition, both alcoholic groups had similarly enlarged cortical sulci and third ventricles. Although both alcoholic groups had significantly smaller anterior hippocampi than the control group, these structures were significantly smaller (by 1 standard deviation) in the Korsakoff's syndrome relative to the nonamnesic alcoholics. Together with the earlier observations from our laboratory (Davila et al. 1994; Shear et al. 1996) that amnesic and nonamnesic alcoholics share a similar degree of clinically detectable mammillary body shrinkage, these results suggest that extensive hippocampal volume deficits contribute to alcohol-related amnesia.

In a departure from research in explicit memory, a recent study of alcoholic patients with and without Korsakoff's syndrome, examined a form of implicit, or procedural, memory with a classical conditioning paradigm involving acquisition of an eye blink conditioned response. Unexpectedly, both alcoholic groups were significantly impaired relative to controls in response acquisition (McGlinchey-Berroth et al. 1995). Although MRI data were not acquired on these subjects, converging evidence from other studies suggests a cerebellar substrate for this conditioned response deficit, especially in light of the burgeoning literature supporting the role of the cerebellum in motor and conditioned learning (for reviews, see Ghez 1991; Leiner et al. 1993; Kim et al. 1995). The MRI studies by Davila et al. (1994) and Shear et al. (1996), which used a three-point rating system, observed significant atrophy in cerebellar vermis and hemispheres in both nonamnesic and amnesic alcoholics. A quantitative MRI study confirmed and extended these findings and revealed significant tissue volume loss in the anterior superior vermis, which may contribute to residual ataxia in detoxified alcoholic patients (Davila et al. 1994) and in the gray matter of both cerebellar hemispheres (Sullivan et al. 1996a), which may underlie the impairment in eye blink conditioning.

Alzheimer's disease

Copious studies have documented the severe decline in various components of declarative, or explicit, memory in AD (Chapters 10, 11 and 18). Likewise, imaging studies have identified significant structural changes in patients

with AD relative to normal elderly subjects (Sullivan et al. 1993b; Shear et al. 1995; Seab et al. 1988; Pfefferbaum et al. 1990; Jernigan et al. 1991c). On CT, the most prominent dysmorphic feature in AD is an increased volume of CSF in the lateral ventricles and cortical sulci (De Leon et al. 1989a; De Carli et al. 1990; Erkinjuntti et al. 1993; Sullivan et al. 1993b; Shear et al. 1995). CT and MRI studies report gray matter volume deficits (Jernigan et al. 1990b, 1991c) and significant shrinkage of hippocampal volumes in these patients relative to normal elderly controls (De Leon et al. 1989b, 1993; Kesslak et al. 1991; Jack et al. 1992). Despite the vast number of neuropsychological and neuroimaging studies published, few studies have employed both careful quantitative imaging methods and tests of selective memory functions to verify the implications of the separate imaging and behavioral studies.

A large body of literature documents relationships between the extent of sulcal and ventricular enlargement and dementia severity, as measured by dementia screening tests (De Leon et al. 1980; Eslinger et al. 1984; Bigler et al. 1985; Förstl et al. 1995). Additional relationships between demographic variables, such as age-related increases in brain volume variability (Zatz et al. 1982; Jernigan et al. 1990b; Pfefferbaum et al. 1994), age of onset (Albert et al. 1984; Brandt et al. 1989) and age (Shear et al. 1995), have also been reported, indicating that these factors act as potential sources of heterogeneity and must be taken into account when considering brain–behavior relationships.

The relationship between quantified medial temporal lobe changes observed with MRI and the memory deficits commonly observed in AD patients have only just recently been reported. Deweer et al. (1995) analysed the relationship between volumetric measures of the hippocampal formation, amygdala and caudate nucleus and quantitative and qualitative indices of explicit memory. Patients in the mild to moderate stage of AD were found to have pronounced atrophy of the hippocampal formation and amygdala relative to age-matched normal control subjects. Brain–behavior relationships were investigated using regression analyses and revealed that the volume of the hippocampal formation correlated significantly with both quantitative measures of memory, such as the memory quotient from the Wechsler Memory Scale (Wechsler and Stone 1945), as well as with qualitative indices of memory performance, including extra list intrusions on the Grober and Buschke test (Grober and Buschke 1987) and the California Verbal Learning Test (CVLT; Delis et al. 1987).

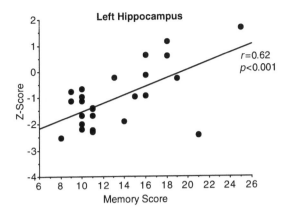
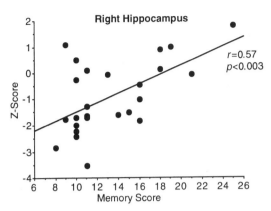

Figure 5.4. Correlations between left and right hippocampal
volumes and Memory subtest scores from the DRS in 25 patients
with AD. Modified from Fama et al. (1997).

The hippocampal formation showed a strong relationship to memory subtests of dementia screening tests, such as the Mini Mental State Examination (MMSE) and the Mattis Dementia Rating Scale (DRS; Mattis 1988). Furthermore, the authors found that hippocampal volume was more strongly related to measures of delayed memory than to measures of short-term, or immediate memory. By contrast, the hippocampal volume did not correlate significantly with any of the nonmnemonic, or 'executive function' tests administered, such as the Wisconsin Card Sorting Test (WCST) or verbal fluency tests. Based on this dissociation, the authors concluded that early in the course of AD, significant atrophy of the hippocampal formation is present and is implicated in the memory disorders these patients exhibit, thus supporting years of speculation from a mixture of in vivo and postmortem observations that the extent of memory loss in AD is directly related to the extent of hippocampal volume loss. The volumes of neither the amygdala nor the caudate nucleus correlated significantly with measures of explicit memory performance. Taken together, these results indicate that the hippocampus is a selective and independent predictor of memory functioning in AD. These authors did not test the relative contributions of these different structures to memory performance, however, so it is unclear if the hippocampal formation was the sole predictor, after taking into account the variance accounted for by the other brain structures.

Fama et al. (1997) examined the relationships between

regional brain volume measures derived from MRI and cognitive performance on the five subtests of the DRS in AD patients to determine whether the DRS subtest scores were predictably related to volumes of specific brain regions. Six geometrically defined brain regions were measured. In addition, anatomically defined volumes of hippocampus, temporal horn and temporal cortex were obtained. All MRI volumes were corrected for normal variation in head size and age. Memory performance was significantly and selectively related to hippocampal volume (Figure 5.4). Temporal horn volume was significantly, but not selectively associated with memory performance. The remaining DRS subscales, with the exception of the Conceptualization subscale, showed significant relationships with other regional brain volumes, but not with hippocampal volumes.

The degree of dementia as measured by the DRS also correlates with abnormal white matter volume in AD patients. Stout et al. (1996) conducted multiple regression analyses to determine the relative contributions of cortical gray matter and abnormal white matter volume to performance on the DRS. Cortical gray matter volume shrinkage and abnormal white matter volume made significant independent contributions to dementia severity and were associated with all subtests of the DRS except Initiation/Perseveration, which correlated only with abnormal white matter volume. These findings emphasize the relationship between neocortical volume abnormalities and cognitive decline in AD and also suggest that abnormal white matter volume makes an independent contribution to the prediction of dementia severity. Like Fama et al. (1997), these authors found a significant independent contribution of limbic cortical gray matter volume to performance on the memory subscale of the DRS.

Although several studies have demonstrated that the extent of hippocampal atrophy correlates with memory impairment in patients with AD, material-specific lateralization of this structure–function relationship has been inconsistent. We recently examined the relationships between selected temporal lobe structures and recognition memory in a group of 20 AD patients using the Warrington Recognition Memory Test (Cahn et al. 1998). The results showed that right hippocampal volume made a significant independent contribution to face recognition, after accounting for left hippocampal volume. Furthermore, right hippocampal volume contributed significantly and independently to the prediction of face recognition after accounting for right temporal horn volume. The absence of a relationship between left temporal region volumes and word recognition may indicate that other variables (i.e. verbal processing deficits, verbal IQ) may be mediating, or masking, a similar relationship (Golomb et al. 1993, 1994).

Frontal lobe dementias: Pick's disease

Pick's disease, considered a subtype of frontal dementia, is characterized by diffuse atrophy of the frontal and temporal neocortex. Patients with Pick's disease often present with deficits in executive functioning, changes in personality and language impairment. Pick's, which is often clinically indistinguishable from other cortical dementias (Katzman 1986; Mendez et al. 1993), is identified upon autopsy by the presence of intracytoplasmic inclusions, or Pick's bodies (Chapter 3). Imaging and neuropsychological studies of frontal lobe dementia have been largely limited to case studies, in part because the diagnosis often remains elusive until autopsy (Cappa et al. 1995). Inspection of CT usually reveals dilation of the frontal horns and Sylvian fissures, atrophy of the frontal and temporal lobes and subcortical structures, such as the caudate nucleus and widening of frontal sulci (McGreachie et al. 1979; Wechsler et al. 1982; Knopman et al. 1989).

Few studies have investigated the relationship between the structural changes seen in Pick's disease and behavioral abnormalities. Knopman et al. (1989) reviewed the ante-

mortem imaging studies of six patients with autopsy-confirmed diagnoses of Pick's disease. The authors qualitatively defined two dominant patterns of atrophy in reviewing the CT films of these patients. The first was marked atrophy of the frontal lobes, characterized by enlargement of the frontal horns of the lateral ventricles, decreased width of the frontal polar cortical mantle, atrophy of the caudate nucleus and enlargement of the third ventricle. The second pattern comprised temporal pole atrophy. One of the six Pick's patients had a nondistinctive profile of CT findings. Neuropsychological test data were available for only two of the patients. The first patient's CT films revealed the pattern of frontal atrophy and enlargement of the ventricular system and the neuropsychological profile was significant for impairment of tests of executive function but relative sparing of recent memory functions. The second patient, also with a pattern of frontal atrophy, did not show striking impairments on tests of executive function or recent memory but did show impaired nonverbal memory. These findings suggest notable variability in the clinical presentation as well as neuroimaging findings in this disorder. Clearly, larger studies with more comprehensive test batteries and more refined quantification of structural abnormalities are needed to better characterize brain–behavior relationships in Pick's disease.

Parkinson's disease

Parkinson's disease (PD) is an idiopathic, neurodegenerative condition characterized by motor abnormalities of tremor, rigidity and bradykinesia. Cognitive impairments in memory, executive functions and visuospatial processing are common (for reviews, see Brown and Marsden 1990; Huber and Cummings 1992). Symptom onset occurs typically after age 50 years, with a prevalence rate of 1% for individuals over the age of 60 years. A clear dementing condition is observed in only a subset of PD cases, with prevalence rates ranging from less than 10% to greater than 90% (Cummings 1988).

PD results from degeneration of the pigmented cells in the pars compacta of the substantia nigra and often in other brain stem nuclei (i.e. locus coeruleus) (Drayer 1988; Freedman 1990; Adams and Victor 1993). The degeneration of these neurons results in dopamine depletion in the nigrostriatal, mesolimbic and mesofrontal pathways (Growdon et al. 1990). The dopamine depletion in the nigrostriatal pathway may be primarily responsible for the motor symptoms, but dysfunction in the mesolimbic and mesofrontal pathways may be primarily responsible for the PD-associated cognitive deficits (Lees and Smith 1983; Sagar and Sullivan 1988; Levin et al. 1989). Although the predominant pathophysiological findings implicate sub-cortical structures, cortical changes similar to those in AD (i.e. neurofibrillary tangles and senile plaques) also occur in PD (Boller et al. 1980; Ross et al. 1992).

Memory complaints are common but not pervasive in PD patients (El-Awar et al. 1987). The pattern of PD memory impairment is similar to that observed in patients with frontal lobe lesions (Taylor et al. 1986a; Gabrieli et al. 1996). Free recall of newly presented information (episodic memory) is generally more impaired than recognition memory (Breen 1993). Deficits in short-term (working) memory relative to long-term memory occur in medicated (Sagar et al. 1988a; Huber et al. 1989b; Levin et al. 1989; Sullivan and Sagar 1989, 1991; Sullivan et al. 1989; Massman et al. 1990; Taylor et al. 1990) and unmedicated (Cooper et al. 1991; Sullivan et al. 1993a) PD patients. The underlying causes of the short-term memory impairment in PD have been attributed to disruption of corticostriatal connections or deafferentation of basal ganglia cortical projections (Bowen 1975; Taylor et al. 1986b; Sagar et al. 1988b; Robbins 1996). Remote memory for events is gener-ally intact but the ability to date remote events is impaired even in nondemented PD patients (Sagar et al. 1988a). Impairments in contextual memory for recently presented information (Sagar et al. 1985, 1988b) and procedural memory (Saint-Cyr et al. 1988; Heindel et al. 1989; Robbins 1996) have also been observed in PD. Given the neuro-psychological performance of PD patients and dissociations between memory abilities in PD and other neurodegener-ative diseases, the PD memory impairment may reflect frontal-striatal rather than medial temporal or diencephalic dysfunction (Pillon et al. 1993; Daum et al. 1995).

CT and MRI studies of PD reveal regional brain atrophy, ventricular and sulcal enlargement and periven-tricular white matter abnormalities (Starkstein and Leiguarda 1993; Mathalon et al. 1995). Steiner et al. (1985) compared 85 PD patients to 149 normal controls (ages 24–84 years) with CT and found significant atrophy, using region-to-brain ratio measures, in the periventricular area surrounding the third ventricle and the medial frontal lobes. Atrophic changes were observed primarily in the younger PD group (24–49 years) compared to age-matched controls for both subcortical and cortical mea-

sures. Greater cortical atrophy was also found in the 60–79 year old PD group than in their age-matched controls. Gender, disease duration and amount of time on anti-parkinsonian medication did not significantly relate to the degree of brain atrophy in these patients. These authors concluded that PD is heterogeneous and that the variety of PD that strikes younger individuals may result in a greater degree of structural brain changes.

Using CT, Mathalon et al. (1995) compared the profiles of regional sulcal and ventricular volumes in PD and AD patients. Although the AD group generally had signifi-cantly greater CSF volumes than the PD group, the two groups displayed different patterns of abnormalities. Within the AD group, the lateral ventricles, sylvian fissures and temporal sulci were equally abnormal and more enlarged than the frontal and parieto-occipital sulci and third ventricle. By contrast, within the PD group, the cortical sulci and third ventricle regions had greater CSF volumes than the lateral ventricles, with sylvian and tem-poral volumes comparable to those in the remaining corti-cal regions, unlike the pattern seen in the AD group.

Basal ganglia structures and the small brain nuclei, which are targeted by disease processes such as PD, are best visualized with MRI. Duguid et al. (1986) reported a narrow range of MR signal intensities, possibly arising from high iron deposition, representing the pars compacta in PD patients. Asymmetry in the width of the pars com-pacta, most evident in the early stages of PD, and a reduc-tion in the average width of the pars compacta in later stage PD, have also been observed with MRI (Huber et al. 1990). Signal hypointensities in the globus pallidus, red nucleus, dentate nucleus and putamen are evident on MRI and are believed to be a result of iron deposition in these areas (Drayer 1988). Hippocampal atrophy has also been observed with MRI in demented and nondemented PD patients (Laakso et al. 1996).

Overall cognitive abilities in PD have been associated with atrophic changes in regional brain areas and ventricu-lar enlargement observed with CT (Portin et al. 1984; Inzelberg et al. 1987), although such relationships have not been found in all studies (Schneider et al. 1979; Huber et al. 1989a). Increased dementia severity in PD was associated with CT-derived measures of central (e.g. caudate) atrophy but not generalized cortical abnormalities (Korczyn et al. 1986; Inzelberg et al. 1987), providing evidence that the cognitive impairments associated with PD may be primar-ily subcortical in nature.

Surprisingly few PD studies, however, report specific brain–behavior relationships in memory functions. Using CT, Starkstein and Leiguarda (1993) did observe that verbal memory deficits, assessed with the Rey Auditory Verbal Learning Test, were significantly correlated with large ventricle-brain ratios, while visual memory deficits, assessed with the Benton Visual Retention Test, were associated with greater frontal-temporal atrophy in the region of the sylvian fissure (i.e. measured as the area of the sylvian cistern at the level of the pineal gland, divided by the whole brain area). Verbal fluency performance, assessed with FAS, correlated with measures of cortical and left frontal-temporal atrophy. Executive functioning, assessed with the WCST, revealed correlations between number of perseverations and all derived cortical and sub-cortical measures used in this study, whereas number of categories was associated with atrophy in diencephalic regions.

In summary, general dementia severity in PD has been inconsistently associated with generalized cortical and subcortical atrophy. Although the mesolimbic and meso-frontal pathways involved in PD have been implicated in the cognitive deficits associated with this disease, no clear pattern of brain–behavior associations has been documented with neuroimaging techniques as yet. The dearth of brain–behavior relationships may be due to the difficulty of imaging and quantifying the small subcortical and striatal structures (e.g. substantia nigra, pars compacta) primarily involved in PD. Additionally, although structural brain abnormalities have been observed in PD, it may be that the cognitive deficits associated with this disease are primarily the result of the underlying neuro-chemical dysfunction, which would be observed with functional imaging techniques (Chapter 6).

Huntington's disease

Huntington's disease (HD) is an inherited (autosomal dominant transmission) progressive neurodegenerative disorder characterized by cognitive, motor and personality abnormalities (Folstein et al. 1990). Symptom onset is generally in the fourth or fifth decade, although cases of juvenile onset HD exist (Adams and Victor 1993). Patients with HD often have difficulty maintaining concentration (e.g. serial 7's) (Brandt et al. 1988) and have deficits in executive functioning (e.g. mental flexibility) (Sax et al. 1983) and visuospatial processing (Butters et al. 1978). Although dysarthria and dysprosody may be present, severe aphasia,

as is observed in AD, rarely occurs in HD (Brandt and Bylsma 1993).

Memory impairment, particularly impairment of short-term declarative memory, is often one of the first documented neuropsychological deficits in HD (Butters et al. 1978; Crosson 1992). Component processes of procedural learning (implicit memory) are also impaired (Martone et al. 1984; Heindel et al. 1988). As in other neurodegenerative disorders thought to affect subcortical structures primarily (e.g. PD), patients with HD often perform markedly better on recognition than free recall memory tests, implying that a retrieval rather than an encoding deficit characterizes the memory impairment in HD (Butters et al. 1986). Crosson (1992) notes, however, that HD patients are still generally impaired on recognition memory tasks relative to control subjects, which suggests that factors in addition to a retrieval deficit (e.g. impairment in initial registration of information) may underlie the memory dysfunction observed in HD.

The most striking structural abnormalities in HD as observed with MRI are in the striatum, particularly the caudate nucleus (Simmons et al. 1986; Jernigan and Butters 1989). In the very early stages of this disease, however, the putamen may show greater atrophy than the caudate (Harris et al. 1992). Caudate atrophy, measured as a ratio of the shortest distance between the heads of the caudate nuclei divided by the distance between the outer (Sax et al. 1983) or inner (Starkstein et al. 1989) tables of the skull, has been consistently observed in vivo with CT and MRI (Harris et al. 1992) and in postmortem study (Brandt and Bylsma 1993) and correlates with disease duration (Starkstein et al. 1989) and the level of functional impairment (Shoulson et al. 1982; Bamford et al. 1989).

Nonspecific abnormalities, including enlargement of the sulci, lateral ventricles and third ventricle and cortical atrophy occur in HD (Simmons et al. 1986; Starkstein et al. 1989). Cortical atrophy generally follows structural changes in the striatum and initially involves the frontal cortex (Starkstein et al. 1989) and then proceeds to more posterior cortical regions as the disease progresses (Sax et al. 1983). Additional structural volume deficits, expressed as a proportion of total intracerebral volume, occur in the diencephalic and mesial temporal lobe (e.g. hippocampus, parahippocampal gyrus) regions (Jernigan and Butters 1989).

Several studies have examined brain–behavior relationships in HD with CT- or MRI- derived brain measures. Using CT images, Sax et al. (1983) examined 26 definite or probable HD patients and found significant correlations between a linear ratio measure of caudate atrophy and measures of WAIS Verbal (Comprehension and Digit Span) and Performance IQ (Block Design, Object Assembly, Digit Symbol, Picture Arrangement) subscale scores and WMS scores (Digit Span, Memory for Paragraphs, Visual Reproduction, Associative Learning). Severity of chorea was also significantly associated with caudate atrophy. Comparisons between patients with minimal and patients with advanced caudate atrophy revealed statistically significant differences on cognitive measures (particularly memory and visuospatial abilities), which suggests an association between greater caudate atrophy and poorer cognitive abilities. Furthermore, multiple regression analyses indicated that caudate atrophy had a stronger correlation with cognitive deficits than did frontal horn enlargement or age. Motor abnormalities (i.e. chorea) did not account for the relationships between cognitive measures and caudate atrophy, thus raising the possibility that independent motor and cognitive dysfunctions occur in HD. Subsequent studies confirmed the findings of Sax et al. (1983) and reported significant correlations between CT-derived measures of caudate atrophy and cognitive measures (Starkstein et al. 1988; Bamford et al. 1989). Relationships between CT-derived measures of frontal lobe atrophy and cognition have been observed in some (Bamford et al. 1989; Starkstein et al. 1992) but not all (Starkstein et al. 1988) studies of HD.

Structure–function relationships which speak directly to the memory impairment in HD include a study by Bamford et al. (1989) who examined 60 mild to moderate HD patients (Stages I and II according to the Total Functional Capacity score). CT measures of frontal lobe atrophy (expressed as the ratio of the linear distance between the frontal horns over the linear distance between the outer table of the skull) and caudate atrophy (expressed as the ratio of the linear distance between the heads of the caudate nuclei over the distance between the outer table of the skull) were both significantly associated with a verbal memory factor derived from a principal components analysis of a neuropsychological battery, which included verbal learning, delayed recall and recognition and selective reminding, consistency of recall and mean number of words recalled. In another study, Starkstein et al. (1992) examined 29 patients with mild to moderate HD using a

variety of neuropsychological measures and MRI. The memory/speed factor (a composite score derived from measures of the Stroop, CERAD Verbal Learning Test, Benton Visual Retention Test and Trail Making Test) was significantly related to MRI-derived measures of caudate and frontal region atrophy and to the left (but not right) sylvian cistern. These authors concluded that atrophic changes in both subcortical and cortical regions are associated with mnemonic and nonmnemonic cognitive deficits observed in HD.

Multiple sclerosis

Multiple sclerosis is a disorder characterized by recurrent central nervous system demyelination. Multiple sclerosis brain lesions are most prevalent in periventricular white matter regions or the gray-white juncture and frequently encroach on the corpus callosum, with callosal atrophy being a common finding (Goodkin et al. 1994; Francis et al. 1995; Sobel 1995). The neurological symptoms in this disorder most often have an abrupt onset and are focal in nature, although more diffuse behavioral symptoms may occur also. It has been estimated that nearly 80% of multiple sclerosis patients show evidence of white matter abnormalities on MRI brain scan (for a review, see Rolak 1996). Furthermore, the incidence of these abnormalities in patients with definite multiple sclerosis exceeds that seen in patients with clinically isolated syndromes characteristic of multiple sclerosis (i.e. optic neuritis, brain stem syndrome or spinal cord syndrome), many of whom go on to develop the full-blown disease (Ron et al. 1991; Feinstein et al. 1992).

Neuropsychological deficits are observed in approximately half of the patients with multiple sclerosis (for reviews, see Beatty 1993; Rao 1995) and a proportion of these patients develop a frank dementia (Huber et al. 1987; Filley et al. 1989). Memory impairments are common in this population as are deficits in executive functioning, attention, visuospatial functioning and speed of information processing. Implicit learning appears to be intact for both linguistic information and motor skills (Beatty 1993). This pattern of cognitive deficits has led several authors to describe multiple sclerosis as being a prototypical subcortical dementia (Filley et al. 1989). Patients with the chronic-progressive form of the disease have more severe cognitive deficits than do those with relapsing-remitting illness (Franklin et al. 1988; Feinstein et al. 1992) and may be more likely to develop features characteristic of cortical dementia (Beatty et al. 1989). It is important, then, to classify patients as having relapsing-remitting or chronic-progressive forms of the disease or to document whether the study participants are experiencing acute exacerbations of their symptoms.

In multiple sclerosis, several factors complicate efforts to establish meaningful associations between cognitive ability and structural brain measures. Multiple sclerosis plaques may change in size over time (Koopmans et al. 1989) and MRI changes can occur in the absence of new neurological symptomatology (Isaac et al. 1988; Willoughby et al. 1989). Also, as Goodkin et al. (1993, 1994) have described, the position of the patient's head in the scanner may significantly affect measured volumes of small and irregularly shaped areas such as multiple sclerosis plaques, which would be expected to reduce the magnitude of brain–behavior correlations by increasing error variance. Measurement difficulty has led to a reliance on visual ratings of plaque volume, which provide less sensitive estimates of morphological change than do volumetric analyses. Studies by Rao et al. (1989) and Swirsky-Sacchetti et al. (1992) use two-dimensional area measurements of lesions rather than visual ratings and indicate that total plaque volume is the best correlate of cognitive impairment.

Increased numbers of or size of multiple sclerosis plaques on MRI are associated with reduced cognitive ability (Rao et al. 1989; Pozzilli et al. 1991), although other authors have found few significant brain–behavior correlations (Feinstein et al. 1992; Maurelli et al. 1992). In addition, callosal atrophy appears to be related to behavioral measures of interhemispheric transfer and speed of information processing (Huber et al. 1992; but see Brainin et al. 1988).

Several authors have speculated that the periventricular lesions characteristic of multiple sclerosis cause cognitive deficits by disconnecting prefrontal pathways from limbic structures (Filley et al. 1989). In addition, however, variability among individual patients in the extent and pattern of cognitive dysfunction may reflect heterogeneous neuropathology. For example, while neuropathological case reports provide evidence that extensive frontal plaques may be present in multiple sclerosis patients who develop clear dementia (Mendez and Frey 1992), callosal atrophy observed on MRI may differentiate patients who do and do not meet dementia criteria (Huber et al. 1987). A provocative study reported that patients with severe memory impairment, but not those with intact memory,

have bilateral medial temporal lesions visualizable on MRI (Brainin et al. 1988), which is consistent with a neuropathological case report of plaques in the hippocampus and columns of the fornix in two multiple sclerosis patients (Fontaine et al. 1994). Thus, it is unlikely that the hypothesized frontal disconnection syndrome explains in full the cognitive deficits that these patients display, particularly those with more marked memory disorders.

Acquired immunodeficiency syndrome (AIDS)

Human immunodeficiency virus (HIV)-associated dementia) produces a behavioral syndrome of cognitive, behavioral and motor disturbances that develops as the immune system fails and AIDS-related complications arise (Navia et al. 1986; Price et al. 1988). The neuropsychological deficits seen in HIV-associated dementia are often referred to as comprising a 'subcortical dementia' and consist of inattention, mental slowing, reduced spontaneity and motor performance and poor coordination (Tross et al. 1988; Miller et al. 1990). Furthermore, concomitant alcohol abuse has been shown to exacerbate cortical dysfunction, as shown by increased latency of the P300A waveform of an event related potential in alcohol-abusing patients with HIV (Fein et al. 1995). Neuropsychological findings have not been consistent, however and may vary relative to disease stage (Poutiainen et al. 1993).

Neuropathological findings at autopsy usually include mild to moderate cerebral atrophy and marked degeneration of subcortical structures, particularly the basal ganglia and thalamus (Navia 1990). These neuropathological findings are associated with quantitative brain measures of AIDS patients with postmortem MRI (Heindel et al. 1994). Consistent with neuropathological findings, neuroimaging studies have shown atrophy to be more prominent in subcortical structures relative to cortical regions (Aylward et al. 1995) and CSF volume increases to be greater in the lateral ventricles than in the cortical sulci (Gelman and Guinto 1992). Loss of white matter volume also occurs (Jernigan et al. 1993; Aylward et al. 1995).

Few studies have examined the relationship between memory impairment and brain atrophy in AIDS, although several studies report correlations between extent of brain atrophy and response speed (Jacobsen et al. 1989). Poutiainen et al. (1993) investigated the relationship between memory performance and MRI and CT ratings in patients with AIDS-related complex (ARC) and AIDS without opportunistic infections or unusual neoplasms of the central nervous system. Patients with peripheral atrophy (enlargement of sulci in frontal, temporal, parietal or occipital lobes), central atrophy (enlargement of lateral ventricles, third ventricle, or both), or infratentorial atrophy (enlargement of fourth ventricle) were more impaired on a memory factor score than subjects without such atrophic changes. Patients with advanced stages of infection who had central or infratentorial atrophy also showed greater memory impairment than patients without similar atrophy. In patients with asymptomatic seropositivity and patients with persistent generalized lymphadenopathy, the relationships between brain measures and memory performance were not significant. The memory impairment observed in AIDS therefore, may well be related to incipient brain alterations that accompany this progressive disorder. One study (Kieburtz et al. 1996) specifically examined the relationship between hippocampal volume and memory performance but did not find a significant correlation. The findings of this study were limited, however, by small sample size.

CONCLUSIONS

Quantitative neuroradiological studies in combination with careful neuropsychological testing and questioning provide invaluable information about the neuropathology of amnesia and dementia. The very nature of dementia implies that multiple brain systems are involved, thus making it likely that multiple memory components and systems also become compromised. Normal age-related memory decline (to be distinguished from AAMI) may be more associated with the well-documented loss of cortical gray matter volume, which may be most prominent in the prefrontal cortex, than to hippocampal shrinkage, which does not appear to be a necessary correlate of normal aging. By contrast, AD is characterized by severe loss of hippocampal volume and, importantly, the extent of the loss is selectively related to extent of impairment in explicit

memory functioning and may also contribute to AAMI. The memory impairment of the so-called subcortical dementias, PD, HD, and multiple sclerosis, is different from that observed in AD, which has traditionally been classified as a cortical dementia. Mnemonic deficits associated with these diseases involve working, contextual and strategic memory systems subserved principally by striatofrontal brain systems. In addition, procedural or skill learning is also affected and may be attributable to compromised basal ganglia observed postmortem in these diseases. Little evidence from direct correlations between in vivo brain measures and memory test performance, however, is available to support this contention. In chronic alcoholism and alcoholic Korsakoff's syndrome, diencephalic, thalamic and possibly hippocampal atrophy may contribute to explicit memory impairment, frontal cortical loss to contextual and working memory and cerebellar tissue loss to motor learning and classical conditioning impairment, although these selective relationships have not been firmly established. In multiple sclerosis and HIV-associated dementia, marked white matter abnormalities and their change during the disease course may provide an important contribution to the fluctuating memory impairments of these diseases. Yet, hippocampal pathology may underlie explicit memory loss in multiple sclerosis but not in HIV-associated dementia.

ACKNOWLEDGMENTS

We thank Adolf Pfefferbaum, MD and Kelvin O. Lim, MD for support and their longstanding and continuing efforts in mentoring us in all aspects of structural neuroimaging. We also thank Laura Marsh, MD, for the hippocampus figures and Margaret J. Rosenbloom, MA for invaluable help with this manuscript. Support for this chapter was provided by AA 05965, AA 10723, AG 11427, MH 30854, MH 40041, MH 18905 and the Norris Foundation.

REFERENCES

Acker, C., Jacobson, R.R. and Lishman, W.A. 1987. Memory and ventricular size in alcoholics. *Psychological Medicine.* 17: 343–348.

Adams, R.D. and Victor, M. 1993. *Principles of neurology.* New York: McGraw-Hill.

Albert, M., Naeser, M.A., Levine, H.L. and Garvey, A.J. 1984. Ventricular size in patients with presenile dementia of the Alzheimer's type. *Archives of Neurology.* 41: 1258–1263.

Albert, M.S. 1988. Cognitive function. In *Geriatric neuropsychology*, ed. M.S. Albert and M.B. Moss, pp. 33–53. New York: Guilford Press.

Andreasen, N.C., Harris, G., Cizadlo, T., Arndt, S., O'Leary, D.S., Swayze, V. and Flaum, M. 1994. Techniques for measuring sulcal/gyral patterns in the brain as visualized through magnetic resonance scanning: BRAINPLOT and BRAINMAP. *Proceedings of the National Academy of Sciences, USA.* 90: 93–97.

Aylward, E.H., Brettschneider, P.D., Mcarthur, J.C., Harris, G.J., Schlaepfer, T.E., Henderer, J.D., Barta, P.E., Tien, A.Y. and Pearlson, G.D. 1995. Magnetic resonance imaging measurement of gray matter volume reductions in HIV dementia. *American Journal of Psychiatry.* 152: 987–994.

Bamford, K.A., Caine, E.D., Kido, D.K., Plassche, W.M. and Shoulson, I. 1989. Clinical-pathologic correlation in Huntington's disease: A neuropsychological and computed tomography study. *Neurology.* 39: 796–801.

Barker, A., Jones, R. and Jennison, C. 1995. A prevalence study of Age-Associated Memory Impairment. *British Journal of Psychiatry.* 167: 642–648.

Beatty, W.W. 1993. Memory and 'frontal lobe' dysfunction in multiple sclerosis. *Journal of Neurological Sciences.* 115 (Suppl.): S38–S41.

Beatty, W.W., Goodkin, D.E., Monson, N. and Beatty, P.A. 1989. Cognitive disturbances in patients with relapsing remitting multiple sclerosis. *Archives of Neurology.* 46: 1113–1119.

Becker, J.T., Butters, N., Hermann, A. and D'Angelo, N. 1983. A comparison of the effects of long-term alcohol abuse and aging on the performance of verbal and nonverbal divided attention tasks. *Alcoholism: Clinical and Experimental Research.* 7: 213–219.

Benton, A.L. 1974. *Revised Visual Retention Test: Clinical and Experimental Applications,* 4th ed. New York: The Psychological Corporation.

Bigler, E.D., Hubler, D.W., Cullum, C.M. and Turkheimer, E. 1985. Intellectual and memory impairment in dementia: computerized axial tomography volume correlations. *Journal of Nervous and Mental Disease.* 173: 347–352.

Bigler, E.D., Nelson, J.E. and Schmidt, R.D. 1989. Mammillary body atrophy identified by magnetic resonance imaging in alcohol amnestic (Korsakoff's) syndrome. *Neuropsychiatry, Neuropsychology and Behavioral Neurology.* 2: 189–201.

Blansjaar, B., Vielvoye, G., van Dijk, J. and Rijnders, R. 1992. Similar brain lesions in alcoholics and Korsakoff patients: MRI, psychometric and clinical findings. *Clinical Neurology and Neurosurgery.* 93: 197–203.

Blatter, D.D., Bigler, E.D., Gale, S.D., Johnson, S.C. Anderson, C., Burnett, B.M., Parker, N., Kurth, S. and Horn, S. 1995. Quantitative volumetric analysis of brain MRI: Normative database spanning five decades of life. *American Journal of Neuroradiology.* 16: 241–245.

Boller, F., Mizutani, T., Roessman, U. and Gambetti, P. 1980. Parkinson's disease, dementia and Alzheimer's disease: Clinicopathological correlations. *Annals of Neurology.* 7: 329–335.

Bowen, F.P., Kamienny, R.S., Burns, M.M. and Yahr, M.D. 1975. Parkinsonism: Effects of levodopa treatment on concept formation. *Neurology.* 25: 701–704.

Brainin, M., Goldenberg, G., Ahlers, C., Reisner, T., Neuhold, A. and Deecke, L. 1988. Structural brain correlates of anterograde memory deficits in multiple sclerosis. *Journal of Neurology.* 235: 362–365.

Brandt, J., Butters, N., Ryan, C. and Bayog, R. 1983. Cognitive loss and recovery in long-term alcohol abusers. *Archives of General Psychiatry.* 40: 435–442.

Brandt, J., Folstein, S.E. and Folstein, M. 1988. Differential cognitive impairment in Alzheimer's and Huntington's disease. *Annals of Neurology.* 23: 555–561.

Brandt, J., Mellits, E.D., Rovner, B., Gordon, B., Selnes, O.A. and Folstein, M.F. 1989. Relation of age at onset and duration of illness to cognitive functioning in Alzheimer's disease. *Neuropsychiatry, Neuropsychology and Behavioral Neurology.* 2: 93–101.

Brandt, J.A. and Bylsma, F.W. 1993. The dementia of Huntington's disease. In *Neuropsychology of Alzheimer's disease and other dementias*, ed. R.W. Parks, R.F. Zec and R.S. Wilson, pp. 265–282. New York: Oxford University Press.

Breen, E.K. 1993. Recall and recognition memory in Parkinson's disease. *Cortex.* 29: 91–102.

Brown, R.G. and Marsden, C.D. 1990. Cognitive function in Parkinsons disease – From description to theory. *Trends in Neurosciences.* 13: 21–29.

Butters, N. and Brandt, J. 1985. The continuity hypothesis: the relationship of long-term alcoholism to the Wernicke–Korsakoff syndrome. In *Recent developments in alcoholism*, vol. 3, ed. M. Galanter, pp. 207–226. New York: Plenum Publishing.

Butters, N. and Cermak, L.S. 1980. *Alcoholic Korsakoff's syndrome.* New York: Academic Press.

Butters, N., Sax, D., Montgomery, K. and Tarlow, S. 1978. Comparison of the neuropsychological deficits associated with early and advanced Huntington's disease. *Archives of Neurology.* 35: 585–589.

Butters, N., Wolfe, J., Granholm, E. and Martone, M. 1986. An assessment of verbal recall, recognition and fluency abilities in patients with Huntington's disease. *Cortex.* 22: 11–32.

Cahn, D.A., Sullivan, E.V., Shear, P.K., Marsh, L., Fama, R., Tinklenberg, J.R., Yesavage, J.A., Lim, K.O. and Pfefferbaum, A. 1998. Neuroanatomical correlates of verbal and nonverbal recognition memory. *Journal of the International Neuropsychological Society.* In press.

Caine, E.D. 1993. Should aging-associated cognitive decline be included in the DSM-IV? *Journal of Neuropsychiatry and Clinical Neurosciences.* 5: 1–5.

Cappa, S.F., Perani, D., Messa, C., Miozzo, A. and Fazio, F. 1995. Varieties of progressive non-fluent aphasia. *Annals of the New York Academy of Sciences.* 777: 243–248.

Charness, M.E. and DeLaPaz, R.L. 1987. Mammillary body atrophy in Wernicke's encephalopathy: Antemortem identification using magnetic resonance imaging. *Annals of Neurology.* 22: 595–600.

Cook, M.J., Fish, D.R., Shorvon, S.D., Straughan, K. and Stevens, J.M. 1992. Hippocampal volumetric and morphometric studies in frontal and temporal lobe epilepsy. *Brain.* 115: 1001–1015.

Cooper, J.A., Sagar, H.J., Jordan, N., Harvey, N. and Sullivan, E.V. 1991. Cognitive impairment in early, untreated Parkinson's disease and its dissociation from motor disability. *Brain.* 114: 2095–2122.

Courville, C.B. 1955. *Effects of alcohol on the nervous system in man.* Los Angeles: San Lucas Press.

Crook, T., Bartus, R.T., Ferris, S.H., Whitehouse, P., Cohen, G.D. and Gershon, S. 1986. Age-associated memory impairment: Proposed diagnostic criteria and measures of clinical change – Report of a National Institute of Mental Health work group. *Developmental Neuropsychology.* 2: 261–276.

Crosson, B. 1992. *Subcortical functions in language and memory.* New York: Guilford Press.

Cullum, C.M., Butters, N., Tröster, A.I. and Salmon, D.P. 1990. Normal aging and forgetting rates on the Wechsler Memory Scale – Revised. *Archives of Clinical Neuropsychology.* 5: 23–30.

Cummings, J.L. 1988. Intellectual impairment in Parkinson's disease: Clinical, pathologic and biochemical correlates. *Journal of Geriatric Psychiatry and Neurology.* 1: 24–36.

Daum, I., Schugens, M.M., Spieker, S., Poser, U., Schonle, P.W. and Birbaumer, N. 1995. Memory and skill acquisition in Parkinson's disease and frontal lobe dysfunction. *Cortex.* 31: 413–432.

Davila, M.D., Shear, P.K., Lane, B., Sullivan, E.V. and Pfefferbaum, A. 1994. Mammillary body and cerebellar shrinkage in chronic alcoholics: An MRI and neuropsychological study. *Neuropsychology.* 8: 433–444.

De Carli, C., Kaye, J.A., Horwitz, B. and Rapoport, S.I. 1990. Critical analysis of the use of computer-assisted transverse axial tomography to study human brain in aging and dementia of the Alzheimer type. *Neurology.* 40: 872–883.

Dekaban, A. and Sadowsky, D. 1978. Changes in brain weights during the span of human life: Relation of brain weights to body heights and body weights. *Annals of Neurology.* 14: 345–356.

De Leon, M.J., Convit, A., DeSanti, S., Golomb, J., Tarshish, C., Rusinek, H., Bobinski, M., Ince, C., Miller, D.C., Wisniewski, H.M. and George, A.E. 1995. The hippocampus in aging and Alzheimer's disease. *Neuroimaging Clinics of North America.* 5: 1–17.

De Leon, M.J., Ferris, S.G. and George, A.E. 1980. Computed tomography evaluations of brain–behavior relationships in senile dementia of the Alzheimer's type. *Neurobiology of Aging.* 1: 69–79.

De Leon, M.J., George, A.E., Reisberg, B., Ferris, S.H., Kluger, A., Stylopoulos, L.A., Miller, J.D., La Regina, M.E., Chen, C. and Cohen, J. 1989a. Alzheimer's disease: Longitudinal CT studies of ventricular change. *American Journal of Neuroradiology.* 10: 371–376.

De Leon, M.J., George, A.E., Stylopoulos, L.A., Smith, G. and Miller, D.C. 1989b. Early marker for Alzheimer's disease: The atrophic hippocampus. *Lancet.* ii: 672–673.

De Leon, M.J., Golomb, J., George, A.E., Convit, A., Tarshish, C.Y., McRae, T., De Santi, S., Smith, G., Ferris, S.H., Noz, M. and Rusinek, H. 1993. The radiologic prediction of Alzheimer disease: the atrophic hippocampal formation. *American Journal of Neuroradiology.* 14: 897–906.

Delis, D.C., Kramer, J.H., Kaplan, E. and Ober, B.A. 1987. *The California Verbal Learning Test.* New York: Psychological Corporation.

Deweer, B., Lehericy, S., Pillon, B., Baulac, M., Chiras, J., Marsault, C., Agid, Y. and Dubois, B. 1995. Memory disorders in probable Alzheimer's disease: the role of hippocampal atrophy as shown with MRI. *Journal of Neurology, Neurosurgery and Psychiatry.* 58: 590–597.

Dorst, J.P. 1971. Changes of the skull during childhood. In *Radiology of the skull and brain: The skull,* ed. T.H. Newton and D.G. Potts, pp. 118–131. St. Louis: C.V. Mosby Co.

Drayer, B.P. 1988. Imaging of the aging brain part II. Pathologic conditions. *Radiology.* 166: 797–806.

Duguid, J.R., De La Paz, R. and DeGroot, J. 1986. Magnetic resonance imaging of the midbrain in Parkinson's disease. *Annals of Neurology.* 20: 744–747.

El-Awar, M., Becker, J.T., Hammond, K.M., Nebes, R.D. and Boller, F. 1987. Learning deficit in Parkinson's disease: comparison with Alzheimer's disease and normal aging. *Archives of Neurology.* 44: 180–184.

Ellis, R.J. and Oscar-Berman, M. 1989. Alcoholism, aging and functional cerebral asymmetries. *Psychological Bulletin.* 106: 128–147.

Erkinjuntti, T., Lee, D.H., Gao, F.Q., Steenhuis, R., Eliasziw, M., Fry, R., Merskey, H. and Hachinski, V.C. 1993. Temporal lobe atrophy on magnetic resonance imaging in the diagnosis of early Alzheimer's disease. *Archives of Neurology.* 50: 305–310.

Eslinger, P.J., Damasio, H., Graff-Radford, N. and Damasio, A. 1984. Examining the relationship between computed tomography and neuropsychological measures in normal and demented elderly. *Journal of Neurology, Neurosurgery and Psychiatry.* 47: 1319–1325.

Fama, R., Sullivan, E.V., Shear, P.K., Marsh, L., Yesavage, J.A., Tinklenberg, J.R., Lim, K.O. and Pfefferbaum, A. 1997. Selective cortical and hippocampal volume correlates of Mattis Dementia Rating subscales in Alzheimer's disease. *Archives of Neurology.* 54: 719–728.

Fein, G., Bachman, L., Fisher, S. and Davenport, L. 1990. Cognitive impairments in abstinent alcoholics. *Western Journal of Medicine.* 152: 531–537.

Fein, G., Biggins, C.A. and MacKay, S. 1995. Delayed latency of the event-related brain potential P3A component in HIV disease: progressive effects with increasing cognitive impairment. *Archives of Neurology.* 52: 1109–1118.

Feinstein, A., Kartsounis, L.D., Miller, D.H., Youl, B.D. and Ron, M.A. 1992. Clinically isolated lesions of the type seen in multiple sclerosis: A cognitive, psychiatric and MRI follow up study. *Journal of Neurology, Neurosurgery and Psychiatry.* 55: 869–876.

Filipek, P.A., Kennedy, D.N., Caviness, V.S., Rossnick, S.L., Spraggins, T.A. and Starewicz, P.M. 1989. Magnetic resonance imaging-based brain morphometry: development and application to normal subjects. *Annals of Neurology.* 25: 61–67.

Filley, C.M., Heaton, R.K., Nelson, L.M., Burks, J.S. and Franklin, G.M. 1989. A comparison of dementia in Alzheimer's disease and multiple sclerosis. *Archives of Neurology.* 46: 157–161.

Folstein, S.E., Brandt, J. and Folstein, M.F. 1990. Huntington's disease. In *Subcortical dementia,* ed. J.L. Cummings, pp. 87–107. New York: Oxford University Press.

Fontaine, B., Seilhean, D., Tourbah, A., Daumas-Duport, C., Duyckaerts, C., Benoit, N., Devaux, B., Hauw, J.-J., Rancurel, G. and Lyon-Caen, O. 1994. Dementia in two histologically confirmed cases of multiple sclerosis: One case with isolated dementia and one case associated with psychiatric symptoms. *Journal of Neurology, Neurosurgery and Psychiatry.* 57: 353–359.

Förstl, H., Zerfab, R., Geiger-Kabisch, C., Sattel, H., Besthorn, C. and Hentschel, R. 1995. Brain atrophy in normal ageing and Alzheimer's disease: Volumetric discrimination and clinical correlations. *British Journal of Psychiatry.* 167: 739–746.

Francis, G.S., Evans, A.C. and Arnold, D. 1995. Neuroimaging in multiple sclerosis. *Neurologic Clinics.* 13: 145–171.

Franklin, G.M., Heaton, R.K., Nelson, L.M., Filley, C.M. and Seibert, C. 1988. Correlation of neuropsychological and MRI findings in chronic/progressive multiple sclerosis. *Neurology.* 38: 1826–1829.

Freedman, M. 1990. Parkinson's disease. In *Subcortical dementia*, ed. J.L. Cummings, pp. 108–122. New York: Oxford University Press.

Gabrieli, J.D.E., Singh, J., Stebbins, G.T. and Goetz, C.G. 1996. Reduced working memory span in Parkinson's disease: Evidence for the role of a frontostriatal system in working and strategic memory. *Neuropsychology.* 10: 322–332.

Gebhardt, C.A., Naeser, M.A. and Butters, N. 1984. Computerized measures of CT scans of alcoholics: Thalamic region related to memory. *Alcohol.* 1: 133–140.

Gelman, B.B. and Guinto, F.C. 1992. Morphometry, histopathology and tomography of cerebral atrophy in the acquired immunodeficiency syndrome. *Annals of Neurology.* 32: 31–40.

Ghez, C. 1991. The cerebellum. In *Principles of neural science*, 3rd ed., ed. E.R. Kandel, J.H. Schwartz and T.M. Jessell, pp. 626–646. New York: Elsevier.

Golomb, J., De Leon, M.J., Kluger, A., George, A.E., Tarshish, C. and Ferris, S.H. 1993. Hippocampal atrophy in normal aging: An association with recent memory impairment. *Archives of Neurology.* 50: 967–973.

Golomb, J., Kluger, A., De Leon, M.J., Ferris, S.H., Convit, A., Mittelman, M.S., Cohen, J., Rusinek, H., De Santi, S. and George, A.E. 1994. Hippocampal formation size in normal human aging: A correlate of delayed secondary memory performance. *Learning and Memory.* 1: 45–54.

Goodkin, D.E., Rudnick, R.A. and Ross, J.S. 1994. The use of brain magnetic resonance imaging in multiple sclerosis. *Archives of Neurology.* 51: 505–518.

Goodkin, D.E., Vanderburg-Medendorp, S. and Ross, J. 1993. The effect of repositioning error on serial magnetic resonance imaging scans. *Archives of Neurology.* 50: 569–570.

Grant, I., Adams, K.M. and Reed, R. 1984. Aging, abstinence and medical risk factors in the prediction of neuropsychologic deficit among long-term alcoholics. *Archives of General Psychiatry.* 41: 710–718.

Grober, E. and Buschke, H. 1987. Genuine memory deficits in dementia. *Developmental Neuropsychology.* 3: 13–36.

Growdon, J.H., Corkin, S. and Rosen, T.J. 1990. Distinctive aspects of cognitive dysfunction in Parkinson's disease. In *Parkinson's disease: Anatomy, pathology and therapy – Advances in neurology*, vol. 53. ed. M.B. Streifler, A.D. Korczyn, E. Melamed and M.B.H. Youdim, pp. 365–376. New York: Raven Press.

Harper, C.G. and Kril, J.J. 1990. Neuropathology of alcoholism. *Alcohol and Alcoholism.* 25: 207–216.

Harper, C.G. and Krill, J.J. 1993. Neuropathological changes in alcoholics. In *Alcohol induced brain damage: NIAAA Research Monograph No. 22*, ed. W.A. Hunt and S.J. Nixon, pp. 39–69. Rockville, MD: National Institute of Health.

Harris, G.J., Pearlson, G.D., Peyser, C.E., Aylward, E.H., Roberts, J., Barta, P.E., Chase, G.A. and Folstein, S.E. 1992. Putamen volume reduction on magnetic resonance imaging exceeds caudate changes in mild Huntington's disease. *Annals of Neurology.* 31: 69–75.

Haubek, A. and Lee, K. 1979. Computed tomography in alcoholic cerebellar atrophy. *Neuroradiology.* 18: 77–79.

Heindel, W.C., Butters, N. and Salmon, D.P. 1988. Impaired learning of a motor skill in patients with Huntington's disease. *Behavioral Neuroscience.* 102: 141–147.

Heindel, W.C., Jernigan, T.L., Archibald, S.L., Achim, C.L., Masliah, E. and Wiley, C.A. 1994. The relationship of quantitative brain magnetic resonance imaging measures to neuropathologic indexes of human immunodeficiency virus infection. *Archives of Neurology.* 51: 1129–1135.

Heindel, W.C., Salmon, D.P., Shults, C.W., Walicke, P.A. and Butters, N. 1989. Neuropsychological evidence for multiple implicit memory systems: A comparison of Alzheimer's, Huntington's and Parkinson's disease patients. *Journal of Neuroscience.* 9: 582–587.

Huber, S.J., Bornstein, R.A., Rammohan, K.W., Christy, J.E., Chakeres, D.W. and McGhee, R.B. 1992. Magnetic resonance imaging correlates of neuropsychological impairment in multiple sclerosis. *Journal of Neuropsychiatry and Clinical Neurosciences.* 4: 152–158.

Huber, S.J., Chakeres, D.W., Paulson, G.W. and Khanna, R. 1990. Magnetic resonance imaging in Parkinson's disease. *Archives of Neurology.* 47: 735–737.

Huber, S.J. and Cummings, J.L. ed. 1992. *Parkinson's disease: Behavioral and neuropsychological aspects.* New York: Oxford University Press.

Huber, S.J., Paulson, G.W., Shuttleworth, E.C., Chakeres, D., Clapp, L.E., Pakalnis, A., Weiss, K. and Rammohan, K. 1987. Magnetic resonance imaging correlates of dementia in multiple sclerosis. *Archives of Neurology.* 44: 732–736.

Huber, S.J., Shuttleworth, E.C., Christy, J.A., Chakeres, D.W., Curtin, A. and Paulson, G.W. 1989a. Magnetic resonance imaging in dementia of Parkinson's disease. *Journal of Neurology, Neurosurgery and Psychiatry*. 52: 1221–1227.

Huber, S.J., Shuttleworth, E.C. and Freidenberg, D.L. 1989b. Neuropsychological differences between the dementias of Alzheimer's disease and Parkinson's disease. *Archives of Neurology*. 46: 1287–1291.

Inzelberg, R., Treves, T., Reider, I., Gerlenter, I. and Korczyn, A.D. 1987. Computed tomography brain changes in Parkinsonian dementia. *Neuroradiology*. 29: 535–539.

Isaac, C., Li, D.K.B., Genton, M., Jardine, C., Grochowski, E., Palmer, M., Kastrukoff, L.F., Oger, J. and Paty, D.W. 1988. Multiple sclerosis: a serial study using MRI in relapsing patients. *Neurology*. 38: 1511–1515.

Jack, C.R., Bentley, M.D., Twomey, C.K. and Zinsmeister, A.R. 1990. MR Imaging-based volume measurements of the hippocampal formation and anterior temporal lobe: Validation studies. *Radiology*. 176: 205–209.

Jack, C.R., Petersen, R.C., O'Brien, P.C. and Tangalos, E.G. 1992. MR-based hippocampal volumetry in the diagnosis of Alzheimer's disease. *Neurology*. 42: 183–188.

Jack, C.R., Sharbrough, F.W., Twomey, C.K., Cascino, G.D., Hirschorn, K.A., Marsh, W.R., Zinsmeister, A.R. and Scheithauer, B. 1988. Temporal lobe seizures: Lateralization with MR volume measurements of the hippocampal formation. *Radiology*. 175: 423–429.

Jacobsen, J., Gyldensted, C., Brun, B., Bruhn, P., Helweg-Larsen, S. and Arlien-Soborg, P. 1989. Cerebral ventricular enlargement related to neuropsychological measures in unselected AIDS patients. *Acta Psychiatrica Scandinavica*. 79: 59–62.

Jernigan, T.L. 1986. Anatomical validators: Issues in the use of computed tomography. In *Clinical memory assessment of older adults*, ed. L.W. Poon, pp. 353–358. Washington DC: American Psychological Association.

Jernigan, T.L. 1990. Techniques for imaging brain structure – Neuropsychological applications. *Neuropsychology. Neuromethods*. vol. 17. ed. A.A. Boulton, G.B. Baker and M. Hiscock, pp. 81–105. Clifton, NJ: Humana Press.

Jernigan, T.L. and Butters, N. 1989. Neuropsychological and neuroradiological distinctions between Alzheimer's and Huntington's disease. *Neuropsychology*. 3: 283–290.

Jernigan, T.L. and Cermak, L.S. 1994. Structural basis of memory. In *Localization and neuroimaging in neuropsychology*, ed. A. Kertesz, pp. 599–620. New York: Academic Press.

Jernigan, T.L. and Tallal, P. 1990. Late childhood changes in brain morphology observable with MRI. *Developmental Medicine and Child Neurology*. 32: 379–385.

Jernigan, T.L., Archibald, S.L., Berhow, M.T., Sowell, E.R., Foster, D.S. and Hesselink, J.R. 1991a. Cerebral structure on MRI. 1. Localization of age-related changes. *Biological Psychiatry*. 29: 55–67.

Jernigan, T.L., Archibald, S., Hesselink, J.R., Atkinson, J.H., Velin, R.A., McCutchan, J.A., Chandler, J. and Grant, I. 1993. Magnetic resonance imaging morphometric analysis of cerebral volume loss in human immunodeficiency virus infection. *Archives of Neurology*. 50: 250–255.

Jernigan, T.L., Butters, N., DiTraglia, G., Schafer, K., Smith, T., Irwin, M., Grant, I., Schuckit, M. and Cermak, L. 1991b. Reduced cerebral grey matter observed in alcoholics using magnetic resonance imaging. *Alcoholism: Clinical and Experimental Research*. 15: 418–427.

Jernigan, T.L., Press, G.A. and Hesselink, J.R. 1990a. Methods for measuring brain morphologic features on magnetic resonance images: Validation and normal aging. *Archives of Neurology*. 47: 27–32.

Jernigan, T.L., Salmon, D.P., Butters, N. and Hesselink, J.R. 1991c. Cerebral structure on MRI. 2. Specific changes in Alzheimer's and Huntington's diseases. *Biological Psychiatry*. 29: 68–81.

Jernigan, T.L., Salmon, D.P., Butters, N., Shults, C.W. and Hesselink, J.R. 1990b. Specificity of brain–structural changes in Alzheimer's, Huntington's and Parkinson's diseases [abstract]. *Journal of Clinical and Experimental Neuropsychology*. 12: 410.

Jernigan, T.L., Schafer, K., Butters, N. and Cermak, L.S. 1991d. Magnetic resonance imaging of alcoholic Korsakoff patients. *Neuropsychopharmacology*. 4: 175–186.

Katzman, R. 1986. Differential diagnosis of dementing illness. *Neurologic Clinics*. 4: 329–340.

Keshavan, M.S. Anderson, S., Beckwith, C., Nash, K., Pettegrew, J.W. and Krishnan, K.R.R. 1995. A comparison of stereology and segmentation techniques for volumetric measurements of lateral ventricles in magnetic resonance imaging. *Psychiatry Research: Neuroimaging*. 61: 53–60.

Kesslak, J.P., Nalcioglu, O. and Cotman, C.W. 1991. Quantification of magnetic resonance scans for hippocampal and parahippocampal atrophy in Alzheimer's disease. *Neurology*. 41: 51–54.

Kieburtz, K., Ketonen, L., Cox, C., Grossman, H., Holloway, R., Booth, H., Hickey, C., Feigin, A. and Caine, E.D. 1996. Cognitive performance and regional brain volume in Human Immunodeficiency Virus Type 1 infection. *Archives of Neurology.* 53: 155–158.

Kim, J.J., Clark, R.E. and Thompson, R.F. 1995. Hippocampectomy impairs the memory of recently, but not remotely, acquired trace eyeblink conditioned responses. *Behavioral Neuroscience.* 109: 195–203.

Knopman, D.S., Christensen, K.J., Schut, L.J., Harbaugh, R.E., Reeder, T., Ngo, T. and Frey, W. 1989. The spectrum of imaging and neuropsychological findings in Pick's disease. *Neurology.* 39: 362–368.

Koopmans, R.A., Grochowski, E., Cutler, P.J. and Paty, D.W. 1989. Benign versus chronic progressive multiple sclerosis: magnetic resonance imaging features. *Annals of Neurology.* 25: 76–81.

Korczyn, A.D., Inzelberg, R., Treves, T., Neufeld, M., Reider, I. and Rabey, P.M. 1986. Dementia of Parkinson's disease. In *Advances in neurology,* vol. 45, ed. M.D. Yahr and K.J. Bergmann, pp. 399–403. New York: Raven Press.

Laakso, M.P., Partanen, K., Riekkinen, P., Lehtovirta, M., Helkala, E.L., Hallikainen, M., Hanninen, T., Vainio, P. and Soininen, H. 1996. Hippocampal volumes in Alzheimer's disease, Parkinson's disease with and without dementia and in vascular dementia: an MRI study. *Neurology.* 46: 678–681.

Lees, A.J. and Smith, E. 1983. Cognitive deficits in the early stages of Parkinson's disease. *Brain.* 106: 257–270.

Leiner, H.C., Leiner, A.L. and Dow, R.S. 1993. Cognitive and language functions of the human cerebellum. *Trends in Neurosciences.* 16: 444–447.

Levin, B.E., Llabre, M.M. and Weiner, W.J. 1989. Cognitive impairments associated with early Parkinson's disease. *Neurology.* 39: 557–561.

Lim, K.O. and Pfefferbaum, A. 1989. Segmentation of MR brain images into cerebrospinal fluid spaces, white and gray matter. *Journal of Computer Assisted Tomography.* 13: 588–593.

Lim, K.O., Rosenbloom, M.J. and Pfefferbaum, A. 1995. In vivo structural brain assessment. In *Psychopharmacology: The fourth generation of progress,* ed. F.E. Bloom and D.J. Kupfer, pp. 881–894. New York: Raven Press.

Lishman, W.A. 1990. Alcohol and the brain. *British Journal of Psychiatry.* 156: 635–644.

Malec, J.F., Ivnik, R.J. and Smith, G.E. 1993. Neuropsychology and normal aging: The clinician's perspective. In *Neuropsychology of Alzheimer's disease and other dementias,* ed. R.W. Parks, R.F. Zec and R.S. Wilson, pp. 81–111. New York: Oxford University Press.

Marsh, L., Lauriello, J., Sullivan, E. and Pfefferbaum, A. 1996. Neuroimaging in neuropsychiatric disorders. In *Handbook of human brain function: Neuroimaging,* vol. 2, ed. E. Bigler, 73–125. New York: Plenum Press.

Martone, M., Butters, N., Payne, M., Becker, J.T. and Sax, D.S. 1984. Dissociations between skill learning and verbal recognition in amnesia and dementia. *Archives of Neurology.* 41: 965–970.

Massman, P.J., Delis, D.C., Butters, N., Levin, B.E. and Salmon, D.P. 1990. Are all subcortical dementias alike? Verbal learning and memory in Parkinson's and Huntington's disease patients. *Journal of Clinical and Experimental Neuropsychology.* 12: 729–744.

Mathalon, D.H., Sullivan, E.V., Rawles, J.M. and Pfefferbaum, A. 1993a. Correction for head size in brain-imaging measurements. *Psychiatry Research: Neuroimaging.* 50: 121–139.

Mathalon, D.H., Sullivan, E.V., Rawles, J.M. and Pfefferbaum, A. 1993b. Correction for head size in brain-imaging measurements [letter]. *Psychiatry Research: Neuroimaging.* 50: 284.

Mathalon, D., Sullivan, E.V., Shear, P.K., Lim, K.O., Sagar, J.A., Yesavage, J., Tinklenberg, J.R. and Pfefferbaum, A. 1995. Discrimination of Alzheimer's and Parkinson's disease by analysis of regional CSF profiles using quantitative CT brain imaging [abstract]. *Abstracts: Society for Neuroscience 25th Annual Meeting.* 31(Part 2): 1488.

Mattis, S. 1988. *Dementia Rating Scale (DRS) Professional Manual.* Odessa, FL: Psychological Assessment Resources, Inc.

Maurelli, M., Marchioni, E., Cerretano, R., Bosone, D., Bergamaschi, R., Citterio, A., Martelli, A., Sibilla, L. and Savoldi, F. 1992. Neuropsychological assessment in MS: Clinical, neuropsychological and neuroradiological relationships. *Acta Neurologica Scandinavica.* 86: 124–128.

McGlinchey-Berroth, R., Cermak, L.S., Carrillo, M.C., Armfield, S., Gabrieli, J.D.E. and Disterhoft, J.F. 1995. Impaired delay eyeblink conditioning in amnesic Korsakoff's patients and recovered alcoholics. *Alcoholism: Clinical and Experimental Research.* 19: 1127–1132.

McGreachie, R.E., Flemming, J.O., Sharer, R. and Hyman, R.A. 1979. Diagnosis of Pick's disease by computed tomography. *Journal of Computer Assisted Tomography.* 3: 113–115.

Mendez, M.F. and Frey, W.H. 1992. Multiple sclerosis dementia (abstract). *Neurology.* 42: 696.

Mendez, M.F., Selwood, A., Mastri, A.R. and Frey, W.H. 1993. Pick's disease versus Alzheimer's disease: a comparison of clinical characteristics. *Neurology.* 43: 289–292.

Miller, E.N., Selnes, O.A., McArthur, J.C., Satz, P., Becker, J.T., Cohen, B.A., Sheridan, K., Machado, A.M., VanGorp, W.G. and Visscher, B. 1990. Neuropsychological performance in HIV–1 infected homosexual men – The multicenter AIDS cohort study (MACS). *Neurology.* 40: 197–203.

Monti, L.A., Gabrieli, J.D.E., Reminger, S.L., Rinaldi, J.A., Wilson, R.S. and Fleischman, D.A. 1996. Differential effects of aging and Alzheimer's disease on conceptual implicit and explicit memory. *Neuropsychology.* 10: 101–112.

Navia, B. 1990. The AIDS dementia complex. In *Subcortical dementia,* ed. J.L. Cummings, pp. 181–198. New York: Oxford University Press.

Navia, B.A., Jordan, B.D. and Price, R.W. 1986. The AIDS dementia complex, I: Clinical features. *Annals of Neurology.* 19: 517–524.

O'Brien, J.T. and Levy, R. 1992. Age-associated memory impairment: Too broad an entity to justify drug treatment yet. *British Medical Journal.* 49: 839–845.

Oscar-Berman, M. and Hutner, N. 1993. Frontal lobe changes after chronic alcohol ingestion. In *Alcohol-induced brain damage, NIAAA Research Monographs No. 22,* ed. W.A. Hunt and S.J. Nixon, pp. 121–156. Rockville, MD: Government Printing Office.

Parsons, O.A. 1987. Do neuropsychological deficits predict alcoholics treatment course and recovery? In *Neuropsychology of alcoholism: Implications for diagnosis and treatment,* ed. O.A. Parsons, N. Butters and P.E. Nathan, pp. 273–290. New York: Guilford Press.

Petersen, R.C., Smith, G., Kokmen, E., Ivnik, R.J. and Tangalos, E.G. 1992. Memory function in normal aging. *Neurology.* 42: 396–401.

Pfefferbaum, A., Lim, K.O., Desmond, J. and Sullivan, E.V. 1996. Thinning of the corpus callosum in older alcoholic men: A magnetic resonance imaging study. *Alcoholism: Clinical and Experimental Research.* 20: 752–757.

Pfefferbaum, A., Lim, K.O., Zipursky, R.B., Mathalon, D.H., Lane, B., Ha, C.N., Rosenbloom, M.J. and Sullivan, E.V. 1992. Brain gray and white matter volume loss accelerates with aging in chronic alcoholics: A quantitative MRI study. *Alcoholism: Clinical and Experimental Research.* 16: 1078–1089.

Pfefferbaum, A., Mathalon, D.H., Sullivan, E.V., Rawles, J.M., Zipursky, R.B. and Lim, K.O. 1994. A quantitative magnetic resonance imaging study of changes in brain morphology from infancy to late adulthood. *Archives of Neurology.* 51: 874–887.

Pfefferbaum, A., Rosenbloom, M.J., Crusan, K. and Jernigan, T.L. 1988. Brain CT changes in alcoholics: the effects of age and alcohol consumption. *Alcoholism: Clinical and Experimental Research.* 12: 81–87.

Pfefferbaum, A., Sullivan, E.V., Jernigan, T.L., Zipursky, R.B., Rosenbloom, M.J., Yesavage, J.A. and Tinklenberg, J.R. 1990. A quantitative analysis of CT and cognitive measures in normal aging and Alzheimer's disease. *Psychiatry Research: Neuroimaging.* 35: 115–136.

Pfefferbaum, A., Sullivan, E.V., Mathalon, D.H., Shear, P.K., Rosenbloom, M.J. and Lim, K.O. 1995. Longitudinal changes in magnetic resonance imaging brain volumes in abstinent and relapsed alcoholics. *Alcoholism: Clinical and Experimental Research.* 19: 1177–1191.

Pfefferbaum, A., Zatz, L. and Jernigan, T.L. 1986. Computer-interactive method for quantifying cerebrospinal fluid and tissue in brain CT scans: Effects of aging. *Journal of Computer Assisted Tomography.* 10: 571–578.

Pillon, B., Deweer, B., Agid, Y. and Dubois, B. 1993. Explicit memory in Alzheimer's, Huntington's and Parkinson's diseases. *Archives of Neurology.* 50: 374–379.

Poon, L.W. 1985. *Differences in human memory with aging: Nature, causes and clinical implications.* New York: Van Nostrand Reinhold.

Portin, R., Raininko, R. and Rinne, U.K. 1984. Neuropsychological disturbances and cerebral atrophy determined by computed tomography in parkinsonian patients with long-term levodopa treatment. In *Advances in neurology,* vol. 40. ed. R.G. Hassler and J.F. Christ, pp. 219–227. New York: Raven Press.

Poutiainen, E., Elovaara, I., Raininko, R., Hokkanen, L., Valle, S.-L., Lahdevirta, J. and Iivanianen, M. 1993. Cognitive performance in HIV–1 infection: Relationship to severity of disease and brain atrophy. *Acta Neurologica Scandinavica.* 87: 88–94.

Pozzilli, C., Passafiume, D., Bernardi, S., Pantano, P., Incocci, C., Bastiannello, S., Bozzano, L., Lenzi, G.L. and Fieschi, C. 1991. SPECT, MRI and cognitive functions in multiple sclerosis. *Journal of Neurology, Neurosurgery and Psychiatry.* 54: 110–115.

Price, R.W., Brew, B.J., Sidtis, J., Rosenblum, M., Scheck, A.C. and Cleary, P. 1988. The brain in AIDS: Central nervous system HIV–1 infection and AIDS dementia complex. *Science*. 239: 586–592.

Rao, S.M. 1995. Neuropsychology of multiple sclerosis. *Current Opinion in Neurology*. 8: 216–220.

Rao, S.M., Leo, G.J., Haughton, V.M., Aubin-Baugert, P.S. and Bernadin, L. 1989. Correlation of magnetic resonance imaging with neuropsychological testing in multiple sclerosis. *Neurology*. 39: 161–166.

Raz, N. 1996. Neuroanatomy of the aging brain observed in vivo: a review of structural MRI findings. In *Handbook of human brain functioning: Neuroimaging*, vol. 2, ed. E. D. Bigler, pp. 153–182. New York: Plenum Press.

Raz, N., Gunning, F.M., Head, D., Dupuis, J.H., McQuain, J.H., Briggs, S.D., Loken, W.J., Thornton, A.E. and Acker, J.D. 1997. Selective aging of the human cerebral cortex observed in vivo: Differential vulnerability of the prefrontal gray matter. *Cerebral Cortex*. 7: 268–282.

Reed, R.J., Grant, I. and Rourke, S.B. 1992. Long-term abstinent alcoholics have normal memory. *Alcoholism: Clinical and Experimental Research*. 16: 677–683.

Robbins, T.W. 1996. Refining the taxonomy of memory. *Science*. 273: 1353–1354.

Rolak, L.A. 1996. The diagnosis of multiple sclerosis. *Neurologic Clinics*. 14: 27–43.

Ron, M.A. 1983. *The alcoholic brain: CT scan and psychological findings*. Cambridge: Cambridge University Press.

Ron, M.A., Acker, R.W., Shaw, G.K. and Lishman, W.A. 1982. Computerized tomography of the brain in chronic alcoholism: A survey and follow-up study. *Brain*. 105: 497–514.

Ron, M.A., Callanan, M.M. and Warrington, E.K. 1991. Cognitive abnormalities in multiple sclerosis – A psychometric and MRI study. *Psychological Medicine*. 21: 59–68.

Ross, G.W., Mahler, M.E. and Cummings, J.L. 1992. The dementia syndromes of Parkinson's disease: Cortical and subcortical features. In *Parkinson's disease: Behavioral and neuropsychological aspects*, ed. S.J. Huber and J.L. Cummings, pp. 132–148. New York: Oxford University Press.

Ryan, C. and Butters, N. 1984. Alcohol consumption and premature aging: A critical review. In *Recent developments in alcoholism*, vol. 2, ed. M. Galanter, pp. 223–250. New York: Plenum Press.

Sagar, H.J. and Sullivan, E.V. 1988. Patterns of cognitive impairment in dementia. In *Recent advances in clinical neurology*, vol. 5, ed. C. Kennard, pp. 47–86. Edinburgh: Churchill Livingstone.

Sagar, H.J., Cohen, N.J., Corkin, S. and Growdon, J.H. 1985 . Dissociations among processes in remote memory. *Annals of the New York Academy of Sciences*. 444: 533–535.

Sagar, H.J., Cohen, N.J., Sullivan, E.V., Corkin, S. and Growdon, J.H. 1988a. Remote memory function in Alzheimer's disease and Parkinson's disease. *Brain*. 111: 201–222.

Sagar, H.J., Sullivan, E.V., Gabrieli, J.D.E., Corkin, S. and Growdon, J.H. 1988b. Temporal ordering and short-term memory deficits in Parkinson's disease. *Brain*. 111: 525–539.

Saint-Cyr, J.A., Taylor, A.E. and Lang, A.E. 1988. Procedural learning and neostriatal dysfunction in man. *Brain*. 111: 941–959.

Sax, D.S., O' Donnell, B., Butters, N., Menzer, L., Montgomery, K. and Kayne, H.L. 1983. Computed tomographic, neurologic and neuropsychological correlates of Huntington's disease. *International Journal of Neuroscience*. 18: 21–36.

Schneider, E., Fischer, P.A., Jacobi, P., Becker, H. and Hacker, H. 1979. The significance of cerebral atrophy for the symptomatology of Parkinson's disease. *Journal of Neurological Sciences*. 42: 187–197.

Seab, J.P., Jagust, W.J., Wong, S.T.S., Roos, M.S., Reed, B.R. and Budinger, T.F. 1988. Quantitative NMR measurements of hippocampal atrophy in Alzheimer's disease. *Magnetic Resonance in Medicine*. 8: 200–208.

Shear, P.K., Sullivan, E.V., Lane, B. and Pfefferbaum, A. 1996. Mammillary body and cerebellar shrinkage in chronic alcoholics with and without amnesia. *Alcoholism: Clinical and Experimental Research*. 20: 1489–1495.

Shear, P.K., Sullivan, E.V., Mathalon, D.H., Lim, K.O., Davis, L.F., Yesavage, J.A., Tinklenberg, J.R. and Pfefferbaum, A. 1995. Longitudinal volumetric computed tomographic analysis of regional brain changes in normal aging and Alzheimer's disease. *Archives of Neurology*. 52: 340–392.

Shelton, M.D., Parsons, O.A. and Leber, W.R. 1984. Verbal and visuospatial performance in male alcoholics: A test of the premature-aging hypothesis. *Journal of Consulting and Clinical Psychology*. 52: 200–206.

Shimamura, A.P., Jernigan, T.L. and Squire, L.R. 1988. Korsakoff's syndrome: Radiological (CT) findings and neuropsychological correlates. *Journal of Neuroscience*. 8: 4400–4410.

Shoulson, I., Plassche, W. and Odoroff, C. 1982. Huntington's disease: Caudate atrophy parallels functional impairment. *Neurology*. 32: 143–150.

Simmons, J.T., Pastakia, B., Chase, T.N. and Shults, C.W. 1986. Magnetic resonance imaging in Huntington's disease. *American Journal of Neuroradiology.* 7: 25–28.

Smith, G., Ivnik, R.J., Petersen, R.C., Malec, J.F., Kokmen, E. and Tangalos, E. 1991. Age-associated memory impairment diagnoses: Problems of reliability and concerns for terminology. *Psychology and Aging.* 6: 551–558.

Sobel, R.A. 1995. The pathology of multiple sclerosis. *Neurologic Clinics.* 13: 1–21.

Soininen, H.S., Partanen, K., Pitkanen, A., Vainio, P., Hanninen, T., Hallikainen, M., Koivisto, K. and Riekkinen, P.J. 1994. Volumetric MRI analysis of the amygdala and the hippocampus in subjects with age-associated memory impairment: Correlation to visual and verbal memory. *Neurology.* 44: 1660–1668.

Squire, L. and Butters, N. (ed.) 1992. *Neuropsychology of memory,* 2nd ed. New York: Guilford Press.

Squire, L.R. and Zola-Morgan, S. 1991. The medial temporal lobe memory system. *Science.* 253: 1380–1386.

Squire, L.R., Amaral, D.G. and Press, G.A. 1990. Magnetic resonance imaging of the hippocampal formation and mammillary nuclei distinguish medial temporal lobe and diencephalic amnesia. *Journal of Neuroscience.* 10: 3106–3117.

Stafford, J.L., Albert, M.S., Naeser, M.A., Sandor, T. and Garvey, A.J. 1988. Age-related differences in computed tomographic scan measurements. *Archives of Neurology.* 45: 409–415.

Starkstein, S., Folstein, S.E., Brandt, J., Pearlson G.D., McDonnell, A. and Folstein, M. 1989. Brain atrophy in Huntington's disease – A CT-scan study. *Neuroradiology.* 31: 156–159.

Starkstein, S.E., Brandt, J., Bylsma, F., Peyser, C., Folstein, M. and Folstein, S.E. 1992. Neuropsychological correlates of brain atrophy in Huntington's disease: A magnetic resonance imaging study. *Neuroradiology.* 34: 487–489.

Starkstein, S.E., Brandt, J., Folstein, S., Strauss, M., Berthier, M.L., Pearlson, G.D., Wong, D., McDonnell, A. and Folstein, M. 1988. Neuropsychological and neuroradiological correlates in Huntington's disease. *Journal of Neurology, Neurosurgery and Psychiatry.* 51: 1259–1263.

Starkstein, S.E. and Leiguarda, R. 1993. Neuropsychological correlates of brain atrophy in Parkinson's disease: A CT scan study. *Movement Disorders.* 8: 51–55.

Steiner, I., Gomori, J.M. and Melamed, E. 1985. Features of brain atrophy in Parkinson's disease. *Neuroradiology.* 27: 158–160.

Stout, J., Jernigan, T., Archibald, S.L. and Salmon, D.P. 1996. Association of dementia severity with cortical gray matter and abnormal white matter volumes in dementia of the Alzheimer type. *Archives of Neurology.* 53: 742–749.

Sullivan, E.V. and Sagar, H.J. 1989. Nonverbal recognition and recency discrimination deficits in Parkinson's disease and Alzheimer's disease. *Brain.* 112: 1503–1517.

Sullivan, E.V. and Sagar, H.J. 1991. Double dissociation of short-term and long-term memory for non-verbal material in Parkinson's disease and global amnesia: A further analysis. *Brain.* 114: 893–906.

Sullivan, E.V., Deshmukh, A., Desmond, J.E., Lane, B.J., Shear, P.K. and Pfefferbaum, A. 1996a. Volumetric MRI analysis of cerebellar hemispheres and vermis in chronic alcoholics: Relationship to ataxia [abstract]. *Journal of the International Neuropsychological Society.* 2: 34.

Sullivan, E.V., Marsh, L., Mathalon, D.H., Lim, K.O. and Pfefferbaum, A. 1995a. Age-related decline in MRI volumes of temporal lobe gray matter but not hippocampus. *Neurobiology of Aging.* 16: 591–606.

Sullivan, E.V., Marsh, L., Mathalon, D.H., Lim, K.O. and Pfefferbaum, A. 1995b. Anterior hippocampal volume deficits in nonamnesic, aging chronic alcoholics. *Alcoholism: Clinical and Experimental Research.* 19: 110–122.

Sullivan, E.V., Marsh, L., Shear, P.K., Lim, K.O. and Pfefferbaum, A. 1996b. Hippocampal but not cortical volumes distinguish amnesic and nonamnesic alcoholics [abstract]. *Abstracts: Society for Neuroscience,* 22: 1865.

Sullivan, E.V., Mathalon, D.H., Lim, K.O. and Pfefferbaum, A. 1996c. Frontal lobe volume deficits in older alcoholic men [abstract]. *Alcoholism: Clinical and Experimental Research.* 20: 33A.

Sullivan, E.V., Sagar, H.J., Cooper, J.A. and Jordan, N. 1993a. Verbal and non-verbal short-term memory impairments in untreated Parkinson's disease. *Neuropsychology.* 7: 396–405.

Sullivan, E.V., Sagar, H.J., Gabrieli, J.D.E., Corkin, S. and Growdon, J.H. 1989. Different cognitive profiles on standard behavioral tests in Parkinson's disease and Alzheimer's disease. *Journal of Clinical and Experimental Neuropsychology.* 11: 799–820.

Sullivan, E.V., Shear, P.K., Mathalon, D.H., Lim, K.O., Yesavage, J.A., Tinklenberg, J.R. and Pfefferbaum, A. 1993b. Greater abnormalities of brain cerebrospinal fluid volumes in younger than older patients with Alzheimer's disease. *Archives of Neurology*. 50: 359–373.

Swirsky-Sacchetti, T., Mitchell, D.R., Seward, J., Gonzales, C., Lublin, F., Knobler, R. and Field, H.L. 1992. Neuropsychological and structural brain lesions in multiple sclerosis – A regional analysis. *Neurology*. 42: 1291–1295.

Taylor, A.E., Saint-Cyr, J.A. and Lang, A.E. 1986a. Frontal lobe dysfunction in Parkinson's disease. *Brain*. 109: 845–883.

Taylor, A.E., Saint-Cyr, J.A. and Lang, A.E. 1990. Memory and learning in early Parkinson's disease: Evidence for a frontal lobe syndrome. *Brain and Cognition*. 13: 211–232.

Taylor, A.E., Saint-Cyr, J.A., Lang, A.E. and Kenny, F.T. 1986b. Parkinson's disease and depression: A critical re-evaluation. *Brain*. 109: 279–292.

Tomlinson, B.E. 1972. Morphological brain changes in nondemented old people. In *Ageing of the central nervous system: Biological and psychological aspects*, ed. H.M. VanPraag and A.F. Kalverbove, pp. 38–57. Haarlem, The Netherlands: DeErven F. Bohn NV.

Torvik, A., Lindboe, C.F. and Rodge, S. 1982. Brain lesions in alcoholics: A neuropathological study with clinical correlations. *Journal of Neurological Sciences*. 56: 233–248.

Tross, S., Price, R., Navia, B., Thaler, H., Gold, J. and Sidtis, J. 1988. Neuropsychological characterization of the AIDS dementia complex: A preliminary report. *Acquired Immune Deficiency Syndromes*. 2: 81–88.

Van Sweiten, J.C., Hijdra, A., Koudstaal, P.J. and van Gijn, J. 1990. Grading white matter lesions on CT and MRI: a simple scale. *Journal of Neurology, Neurosurgery and Psychiatry*. 53: 1080–1083.

Victor, M., Adams, R.D. and Collins, G.H. 1989. *The Wernicke–Korsakoff syndrome and related neurologic disorders due to alcoholism and malnutrition*, 2nd ed. Philadelphia: FA. Davis Co.

Wechsler, A.F., Verity, M.A., Rosenschein, S., Fried, I. and Scheibel, A.B. 1982. Pick's disease: A clinical, computed tomographic and histologic study with Golgi impregnation observations. *Archives of Neurology*. 39: 287–290.

Wechsler, D. and Stone, J. 1945. *Wechsler Memory Scale*. New York: Psychological Corporation.

Wehrli, R.W., MacFall, J.R., Shutts, D., Breger, R. and Herfkens, R.J. 1984. Mechanisms of contrast in NMR imaging. *Journal of Computer Assisted Tomography*. 8: 369–380.

West, M.J. 1993. New stereological methods for counting neurons. *Neurobiology of Aging*. 14: 275–285.

Wickelgren, I. 1996. Is hippocampal cell death a myth? *Science*. 271: 1229–1230.

Wiederholt, W.C., Cahn, D.A., Salmon, D.P., Butters, N., Kritz-Silverstein, D. and Barrett-Connor, E. 1993. The effects of age, education and gender in an elderly community cohort. *Journal of the American Geriatrics Society*. 41: 639–647.

Wilkinson, D.A. 1985. Neuroradiologic investigations of alcoholism. In *Alcohol and the brain: Chronic effects*, ed. R. Tarter and D.H. Van Thiel, pp. 183–215. New York: Plenum.

Wilkinson, D.A. and Carlen, P.L. 1980. Relationship of neuropsychological test performance to brain morphology in amnesic and non-amnesic chronic alcoholics. *Acta Psychiatrica Scandinavica*. 62 (Suppl. 286): 89–101.

Willoughby, E.W., Grochowski, E., Li, D.K., Oger, J., Kastrukoff, L.F. and Paty, D.W. 1989. Serial magnetic resonance scanning in multiple sclerosis: A second prospective study in relapsing patients. *Annals of Neurology*. 25: 43–49.

Winocur, G., Moscovitch, M. and Stuss, D.T. 1996. Explicit and implicit memory in the elderly: Evidence for a double dissociation involving medial temporal- and frontal-lobe functions. *Neuropsychology*. 10: 57–65.

Zatz, L., Jernigan, T.L. and Ahumada, A.J. 1982. Changes on computed cranial tomography with aging: Intracranial fluid volume. *American Journal of Neuroradiology*. 3: 1–11.

Zelazowski, R., Golden, C.J., Graber, B., Blose, I.L., Bloch, S., Moses, J.A., Jr., Zatz, L.M., Stahl, S.M., Osmon, D.C. and Pfefferbaum, A. 1981. Relationship of cerebral ventricular size to alcoholic's performance on the Luria-Nebraska neuropsychological battery. *Journal of Studies on Alcohol*. 42: 749–756.

Zipursky, R.B., Lim, K.O. and Pfefferbaum, A. 1990. Volumetric assessment of cerebral asymmetry from CT scans. *Psychiatry Research: Neuroimaging*. 35: 71–89.

6

Functional neuroimaging correlates of memory dysfunction in neurodegenerative disease

STANLEY BERENT AND BRUNO GIORDANI

INTRODUCTION

Although this chapter is concerned primarily with memory, it is important to note that behavior and its relationship to the central nervous system are multifaceted and interactive. An effective understanding of neuropsychological dysfunction in one area carries the requirement that one also consider perception, sensation, motor performance, motivation, psychosocial factors and other aspects of behavior. In addition to the individual's personal history, five broad areas of neuropsychological functioning can be identified as important to consider in any study of brain and behavior – intelligence, cognition, sensory/motor function, affect (including coping or adaptation) and language (Berent 1990). These functional areas are interactive as well as independent. While good science necessitates reduction and simplification in order to account for intervening and experimental variables, it is also important to bear in mind that an organism of interest is the product of multiple internal and external forces and that behavior is multiply determined as a result.

Memory

The concept of memory, itself, is not unitary. Modern science has produced a complex categorization of memory that includes such classes as declarative (an image or proposition), its episodic and semantic subtypes, and procedural (e.g. implicit memory and skill learning) (Roskies 1994; Chapters 11 and 12). A well-established taxonomy of memory also divides memory into short- and long-term processes, and there is considerable literature that provides validating evidence for these conceptual distinctions (Martinez and Kesner 1986). As reviewed by Roskies (1994), it is believed that specific classes of memory are mediated by different brain networks. For example, declarative memories are said to reside short-term in cortical areas and then at some point in the process, hippocampal as well as other structures become involved. Temporal regions of the brain are crucially involved in episodic memory, but other brain regions seem also to be important for the formation of this class of memories. From his review of the literature, Roskies concludes that the neurological substrates of memory are heterogeneous and widely distributed.

NEUROIMAGING TECHNIQUES

Techniques for imaging the brain were at first limited to angiography and encephalography; however, methods and devices for brain imaging have made substantial advances since the introduction of computerized tomography (CT) in the mid-1970s (Housenfield 1974). While there are a number of problems yet to overcome in the application of these methods to the study of brain and behavior, some of which are discussed more fully later on, we now have the tools needed to simultaneously study both sides of the brain–behavior coin. In addition to CT, some of the more important techniques for brain imaging include magnetic resonance imaging (MRI; Chapter 5), functional magnetic resonance imaging (fMRI), spectroscopic MRI, single photon emission computed tomography (SPECT) and positron emission tomography (PET).

These imaging techniques produce data that are either primarily functional or structural in nature. The functional or structural nature of the resulting data derives from the way in which the particular device obtains its information. For example, the MRI is considered to produce an image that represents a structural reconstruction of the organ under study. The phenomenon upon which this technique rests was first described by Bloch (1946) and Purcell (1946) and their colleagues. To produce the image, the MRI capitalizes on the principle that certain nuclei (e.g. protons) have a magnetic moment that is arranged randomly in the resting condition (i.e. when the only influence on these nuclei is the Earth's magnetic field). By systematically exposing these nuclei to a magnetic field of specified strength (e.g. 0.02–1.5 Tesla), they are caused to align along this field. A radio wave displaces the magnetic moment and when the nuclei are allowed to return to their original state, measurement is made in several parameters that then are used to reconstruct an image of whatever structure these nuclei represent (i.e. the brain) (Young 1984; Freer 1994).

fMRI is still a relatively new but promising technique for brain imaging (Bandettini et al. 1992). Like PET, fMRI produces a functional picture of the brain and allows, therefore, for studies of brain activation in response to stimulus presentation. A potential advantage to the use of fMRI over PET lies in its greater magnitude of spatial resolution. This difference in resolution could be critical when questions necessitate the imaging of neuronal structures that may be no larger than 2–4 mm in size. It is important to keep in mind, however, that a resolution capacity of 2 mm may still be two or more times greater than the physiological mechanism of interest (Ungerleider 1995). As pointed out by Ungerleider (1995), it is also important to recognize that both PET and fMRI provide only indirect measures of neuronal activity, e.g. blood flow and metabolism in the case of PET and blood oxygenation in fMRI. To this observation, one might caution that functional images in general have only an indirect relationship to neuroanatomy as defined by commonly employed structural mapping.

As elucidated by Frackowiak (1986), imaging techniques such as MRI and CT provide images of structure, either by measuring the density of protons, as in the case of MRI, or through indirect measurement of density through quantification of X-ray stopping power, as in CT. In contrast to the MRI, PET produces a functional image. Information is obtained regarding metabolism or function, with only coincidental correspondence to structure. Although its foundations are older, much of the modern approach with PET rests on the pioneering work regarding the theoretical basis of the radioactive deoxyglucose method for the measurement of local cerebral glucose utilization carried out by Sokoloff et al. (1977). This method is based on an autoradiographic technique and uses a radio labeled ligand such as [^{14}C]- or [^{18}F]deoxyglucose. Deoxyglucose mimics glucose in cell transport, but differs in that deoxyglucose does not undergo glycolysis. A multicompartment model is employed to describe the measurement of the tagged ligand in terms of its uptake and metabolism within the brain. The resulting data are applied against a model to produce an image of greater and lesser metabolic activity in terms of relative brain location (Sokoloff et al. 1977; Frackowiak et al. 1980; Sokoloff and Smith 1983; Freer 1994).

The development of brain imaging techniques in recent times has provided science with a collection of important tools that might be used to increase our understanding of the relationships that exist between experience and physiology. Development of these techniques in recent years has been described by Ungerleider (1995) as 'explosive'. Like Roskies (1994), Ungerleider reviews recent work that employed functional neuroimaging and concludes that findings from these efforts indicate that memory in humans involves cortical regions that are involved in motor control and sensory processing. Like Roskies too, Ungerleider suggests that memory is a complex process, involving various stages of encoding, storage and retrieval as well as multiple areas of cortical representation.

Imaging methodology

There are two primary ways in which neuroimaging can be applied to the study of behavior and to the study of memory specifically. One of these approaches involves the presentation of behavioral stimuli and simultaneous measurement of brain activity, referred to usually as an 'activation study'. The second approach can be termed a 'resting state' study, wherein activity of the brain is determined for specified regions of interest (ROIs) and then is correlated with some characteristic aspect of the person's behavior. In the former technique, it is presumed that changes in neuronal activity in response to task demands will be accompanied by changes in blood flow or metabolism that are then measurable by the imaging technique at hand (e.g. PET, SPECT, etc.). The latter approach rests on the assumption that relatively enduring aspects of the individual's behavior (e.g. traits in the case of normality and symptoms in the face of abnormality) will likewise be mirrored in the individual's status of neuronal activity.

There are practical research considerations associated with both activation and resting state approaches. For example, the expense of the PET procedure might restrict sample size. This can serve to seriously limit the power of statistical analyses, masking potentially significant effects, or giving undue weighting to outliers (Duara et al. 1990). As PET does not provide a direct structural image, thus region identification may be complicated (e.g. by super-imposing MRI or CT images whose spatial orientations might differ from PET). In this respect, fMRI may have an advantage over PET in that the fMRI technique allows for direct correlation of measures of function to structure within a single imaging event (Le Bihan 1996). The fMRI is yet new enough, however, that possible limitations to the technique cannot be completely evaluated.

The chosen chemical ligand in PET activation studies can influence the results of behavioral measurement as well. Fatigue during testing may result, for example, when a ligand with a long half-life is chosen, requiring behavioral measurement over an extended period of time. In addition, with the successive task trials often required over longer scan times, cognitive demands for the subjects may change significantly as persons become more proficient with the task, affecting potential areas of cerebral activation. Choice of a short half-life ligand, on the other hand, could result in too short a time period for adequate measurement of a more complex behavioral paradigm or for the introduction of undue variance related to scanning during short normal fluctuations in subjects' attention (Duara et al. 1990).

In functional imaging studies with humans, agitated patients may require sedation in order to complete scans and this pharmacological intervention could confound the results. The use of activation procedures (e.g. learning paradigms) with dementia patients presents particular challenges, which suggests perhaps why so few of these studies have been completed (Miller et al. 1987; Riddle et al. 1993). If the same task were presented to both patients and controls, to give an example, task demands might differ dramatically between the two groups and result in differences in patterns of cerebral activation which are not directly related to the experimental variable. To elaborate, in a study that involves patients with a diagnosis of Alzheimer's disease (AD), a difficult learning procedure might result in little or no metabolic activation in the patients, not because these patients were neurologically incapable of learning the task, but because they were unable to understand the directions initially. Conversely, a task that is sufficiently easy for the AD patient might be overly simple and incapable of challenging a metabolic reaction in the normal person.

Activation and resting state studies both tend to be localizationistic in nature. They rest on the assumption that stimulus–activated areas within the brain bear functional relationships to the behavioral stimuli, or similar to brain lesion studies, that level of task performance will correlate with neuronal activity in functionally dependent neuroanatomical areas. There are philosophical cautions implied by either of these approaches. Roskies (1994) has listed three of these as the following: (1) care must be taken to correctly identify the cognitive demands of a given task, (2) it is difficult to know which cognitive component of a given task is specifically related to changes in, or chronically altered, measured brain activity, and (3) an understanding of the true nature of the relationship between the measured brain activity and underlying neuronal activity remains incomplete. One must add to these cautions the general understanding that correlation does not imply causality. Observed changes in blood flow in a given region of interest might reflect changes in neuronal circuitry far removed from the area observed.

With regard to the general problem of determining causal relationships from correlational studies, Sarter et al. (1996) have suggested a need to approach the question from convergent directions. These authors term the correlational investigation, as employed in brain imaging studies, a 'top-down' approach, and they attempt to alert the reader to the dangers inherent in inferences derived from this approach. To concretely complete their argument, Sarter et al. provide the very effective metaphor of a LED 'on-off' indicator in a heating system. If only a top-down approach were used to determine the cause of failure in the system, one might never discover a malfunction in the furnace as opposed to the indicator itself. By combining various strategies to address the scientific question at hand, one can overcome this potential limitation. These general limitations have been visited by Ungerleider (1995), as well, who criticized imaging studies that limited inquiry to *map* the brain in terms of assigning specific functions to structural areas without attempting to understand underlying neural mechanisms. For Ungerleider, the most powerful approach would be to use data derived from imaging technology to test specific hypotheses derived from animal as well as human physiological studies and theories of cognition. The use of imaging technology in combination with other approaches to the study of memory would enhance the effectiveness of a given study. Such studies might employ premortem (e.g. genetic and/or behavioral markers for individuals who are 'at risk' for specified diseases) as well as postmortem approaches (e.g. correlation studies between neuropathological findings and measures of learning and memory completed before death).

PSYCHOMETRICS

Objective and quantitative measurement of behavior is achieved through one or a combination of three primary approaches. These include formal psychometrics (psychological testing), structured interview with objective history, and the application of sound scientific principles in the conduct of the research (e.g. as when presenting a carefully designed task to subjects in a controlled experiment). In regard to formal psychometric procedures, testing has become increasingly sophisticated since the latter part of the last century. Techniques that meet scientifically published and acceptable criteria for validity and reliability presently exist (American Psychological Association 1985) and consensus agreement on definitions has been achieved for a number of key behavioral phenomena, e.g. intelligence (Berent 1990).

As can be seen from the above discussions, both psychometric and imaging techniques present challenges that must be recognized and resolved when employing these approaches in scientific investigations and/or in attempting to interpret their results. Both are less than perfect in measurement accuracy, for instance. In both, however, a standard error of measurement can usually be determined. The variability of PET measured cerebral metabolic rate of glucose has been calculated at 15–30%, a value within the range of other standard physiological measures with clinical utility, but relatively low sensitivity (Duara 1990). Specific psychological test measures vary in measurement variability, but some standard tests (e.g. WAIS-R, WMS-R) show variability in measurement that reflects relatively high sensitivity, in the less than 20% range (Matarazzo 1972). Issues of validity (i.e. Does the technique measure what it purports to measure?) as well as reliability (i.e. To what extent does variability in measurement reflect device versus subject variability?) pertain to

both psychometric and imaging techniques. Reliability is especially important in longitudinal studies where test-retest designs are intended to measure subject changes over time. Procedures associated with both types of techniques should be carefully standardized and normative data (currently often less than ideal) should be available (Chapter 16). With regard to imaging techniques specifically, there are the problems posed by cortical atrophy and what has been termed 'partial volume effect'. Freer (1994) describes partial volume effect as being common to all imaging devices, wherein the border between ventricles and adjacent brain tissue appears to be well defined but in actuality reflects areas which contain unknown amounts of fluid and tissue.

Aging and the problem of normal versus abnormal decline

There are other problems that are deserving of mention in any discussion of imaging studies of behavior because of their cautionary importance. There is the problem of normative baseline for instance. In both imaging and psychometric results, individual differences are relatively substantial. In terms of memory, specifically, people vary in their capacity to learn and recall what they have learned. This problem holds special relevance in the study of memory decline and neurodegenerative disease because memory decline often occurs during the usual course of aging. Whether such decline is due to disease or is an inevitable consequence of aging remains controversial (Chapters 18 and 21). This concern has in itself become an important scientific question. Kral (1962), for example, introduced the term, 'benign senescent forgetfulness' (BSF), to differentiate what he believed to be the phenomenon of 'normal' decline in cognitive function from the malignant conditions of dementia. Other terms used to describe the occurrence of memory decline with age have included 'late life forgetfulness' (LLF) (Smith et. al. 1991) and 'age associated memory impairment' (AAMI) (Crook et al. 1986).

Imaging studies have generally yielded inconsistent findings with regard to changes in cerebral structure and function as a result of 'normal' aging (Friedland and Jagust 1990; Davis et al. 1994; Freer 1994; Jagust 1994). Even when cognition remains within normal limits, there may be age-associated changes in brain volume, weight, cortical thickness and other aspects of brain morphology (Terry et al. 1987; Tomlinson 1992; Davis et al. 1994). Senile plaques, considered the hallmark of AD (Chapter 3), a disorder with special relevance to the study of memory, have been observed in nonsymptomatic elderly persons as well (Berg et al. 1993). Grady (1996), using PET to measure regional cerebral blood flow (rCBF), has demonstrated that although younger and older subjects may not differ in the success with which they perform certain cognitive (e.g. visual or spatial perception) tasks, or in the apparent primary cortical pathways involved in such performance, overall regional cerebral blood flow patterns may differ significantly between the two age groups, suggesting that older subjects must employ more widespread areas of cortical activation in order to maintain performance.

There is evidence, on the other hand, to suggest that cognitive impairment is not solely due to aging alone and that indices of cognitive dysfunction can identify persons who are specifically at risk for developing dementia (Hanninen et al. 1994; Masur et al. 1994; Chapter 17). Hanninen et al. (1994) reported that a relatively large number of patients with age-associated memory impairment (about 30%) developed a diagnosable disorder (9% specifically developing AD) within 3 years of initial study and Treves et al. (1994) reported that persons with AAMI are at twofold risk than are comparably aged persons without AAMI. Masur and colleagues (1994) were able to accurately identify a subgroup of nondemented persons aged 75–85 years with an 85% likelihood of developing dementia within 4 years of initial study and another subgroup with a 95% probability of remaining dementia free during the same period.

In addition to strictly psychometric approaches, there have been attempts to relate PET findings to behavioral indices and/or to the clinical diagnosis of AD in patients at the earliest possible point in their symptom picture (Friedland et al. 1983; Kuhl et al. 1983, 1987; Foster et al. 1984; Grady et al. 1988; Haxby et al. 1990). Haxby and colleagues (1990) indicated that cerebral metabolic changes might precede detectable cognitive decline in some neurodegenerative conditions, thus presenting the possibility that glucose utilization might serve as a very early marker for AD. Earlier, Kuhl et al. (1987) had shown that abnormalities of glucose metabolism in parietal regions of the brain were present in AD before global cerebral hypometabolism of glucose was detectable. More importantly, Kuhl and colleagues reported that PET could be used to identify mildly demented AD patients before the diagnosis could be confirmed on clinical grounds. Others have

also examined this question, however, with mixed results (Pietrini et al. 1993; Small et al. 1994).

NEUROLOGICAL DISEASES

Neurodegeneration may relate to multiple underlying factors (e.g. disease, diminished blood supply), but it frequently involves deterioration of neural structures and/or functions in areas that are believed to subserve learning and memory. As a result of this, neurodegenerative conditions present a serendipitous opportunity to investigate and model brain–memory relationships. To take substantial advantage of the neurological model in the study of memory, methods and techniques are required that allow for acceptably accurate measurement of brain as well as behavior.

To date, a number of diseases have been studied with imaging techniques. Some of these disorders clearly compromise aspects of memory at some point during the degenerative course. Human immunodeficiency virus (HIV)-positive individuals with and without demonstrable cognitive impairment (Sacktor et al. 1995) and patients with AIDS-related dementia, or HIV-associated dementia (Brunetti et al. 1991), for example, have been studied using a variety of imaging techniques. Individuals with HIV related disorders represent a very heterogeneous group in terms of psychological and social make-up as well as medical complications they experience. It is perhaps for this reason that imaging studies to date have yielded inconsistent results. There are other neurological disorders, however, that appear more homogeneous from a number of perspectives. As such, these disorders might represent better models for studying relationships between the cognitive symptoms with which they are associated and the disease-induced, underlying neural changes. Parkinson's disease (PD) with dementia (PDD), Huntington's disease (HD), multiple system atrophy (MSA), progressive supranuclear palsy (PSP), olivopontocerebellar atrophy (OPCA), Pick's disease and Alzheimer's disease (AD) are some of these disorders to which imaging studies have been applied.

Dementia is estimated to occur in approximately 20% of patients with PD (Salmon and Franck 1989). The dementia of PD is typically classified as a subcortical one; however, the possibility that AD coexists with PD in these PDD cases is yet to be resolved as some PDD patients have been found on PET to have metabolic dysfunction similar in distribution to that observed in AD (Kuhl et al. 1984). Giordani et al. (1995) have shown, further, that PD patients without dementia evidence PET-measured regional glucose metabolism lower than that in normal individuals, but higher than in PDD patients. Furthermore, metabolic rates correlated with neuropsychological task performance. Plate 6.1 illustrates the differences in cerebral glucose metabolism among these various categories of PD.

Subcortical degeneration predominates in a number of other diseases, including HD, multisystem atrophy, olivopontocerebellar atrophy and progressive supranuclear palsy. It is believed that many of these disorders progress to include involvement of frontal regions of the brain, either directly or through disruption of cortical-subcortical pathways (Salmon and Franck 1989). Dementia has been identified consistently as a feature of HD, but only inconsistently or rarely in other subcortical degenerations (e.g. olivopontocerebellar atrophy). A precise neuropsychological description of some of these dementias is often lacking. In some cases (e.g. olivopontocerebellar atrophy), the identification of memory deficits as a symptom of a specific disease has remained controversial (Kish et al. 1988; Berent et al. 1990). In HD, neuropsychological measures of verbal learning and memory have been found to correlate significantly with cerebral metabolic activity in the caudate nuclei (Berent et al. 1988).

The cortical dementias studied with functional imaging techniques include Pick's disease and AD. With regard to Pick's disease, structural (i.e. CT and MRI) imaging studies have revealed findings that are consistent with the known neuropathology of the disease (i.e. atrophy in frontal and temporal regions and widening of the interhemispheric fissure anteriorly). PET studies of patients with Pick's disease reveal decreases in metabolism in frontal regions of interest (Davis et al. 1994). Pick's disease is a relatively rare dementing illness and perhaps because of its rarity, there remains much to learn about the neuropsychological impairment in the disorder, especially the precise nature of memory impairments, as well as the relationship between these impairments and underlying cerebral structural and metabolic changes.

Many of the studies cited have been descriptive and, as such, have contributed importantly to our understanding of the course and symptomatology of the disorder. Most have placed more emphasis on the disease than on the cognitive phenomena, however. This has limited the increase in understanding of functional neuroanatomical relationships as might otherwise have resulted from such inquiry. Of the many neurological diseases, AD may present the memory researcher with the best model in terms of its predictable, pronounced and relatively specific and early involvement of memory dysfunction.

AD is the most common cause of dementia, accounting for over half of all diagnosed dementias in the USA and Europe (Ebly et al. 1994). AD is generally regarded as a disease of the elderly and its incidence continues to rise with increasing age. The incidence of AD is said to double in the population approximately every 5 years between the ages of 65 and 85 (Drachman 1994). While it is necessary to exclude a variety of dementing conditions, the clinical diagnosis of even mild AD is highly reliable using NINCDS/ADRDA criteria (McKhann et al. 1984). Forette et al. (1989) reported 95% reliability of the AD clinical diagnosis and Friedland (1993) a reliability rate of 85%.

The neuropathology of AD has been well studied and multiple studies have revealed that certain changes in neuronal tissue accompany the disorder (Chapter 3). These include neurofibrillary tangles and senile plaques with amyloid deposits. In later stages of the disease, tissue abnormality is widespread, primarily involving cortical structures ranging from parietal and temporal regions to frontal lobes. From a behavioral perspective, the disease progresses from at first subtle alterations in memory to a more general decline in intellectual function and eventual severe disruption of most cognitive functions. It would be valuable to study patients over the course of AD, comparing alterations in behavior with changes in image-derived data. These data could be used to prospectively test hypotheses derived from physiological studies and cognitive theory. To accomplish this most effectively, one would wish to have a marker for individuals who are at risk for later onset of progressive cognitive deterioration. Recent works have shown promise for the development of both behavioral as well as genetic markers for at least some individuals.

While many studies employing a variety of biochemical and neuroimaging approaches to identify individuals at risk have yielded conflicting results, apolipoprotein E (APOE), and the APOE type 4 allele (APOE ε4) more specifically, linked to chromosome 19, has been fairly consistently related to some forms of AD (Small et al. 1995; Chapters 17 and 18). In a study by Small and colleagues (1995), it was shown that inheritance of APOE $\varepsilon 4$ was associated with reduced cerebral parietal metabolism in subjects who were genetically 'at risk' for developing AD. Patients with dementia were found to have even lower metabolic rates than the APOE $\varepsilon 4$ subjects. Evidence that the type 4 allele of APOE is a risk factor for AD comes also from a study by Reiman et al. (1996), who showed that even in cognitively normal, middle-aged subjects, the presence of this allele was associated with reduced glucose metabolism in the same brain regions as in patients diagnosed with probable AD. Combining a genetic marker such as APOE status with an index of behavioral decline would represent a powerful addition to our ability to use neurological disease models in the study of learning and memory.

In a study conducted at our institution (Berent et al. 1995), it was hypothesized that patients with psychometrically determined isolated memory impairment would show progression of neuropsychological symptoms over time and a pattern of [18F]–2–fluoro–2-deoxy-D-glucose utilization similar to that observed in AD (i.e. glucose hypometabolism in parietal regions of the brain). Isolated memory impairment patients were found to initially perform similarly to normal control subjects on measures of intellect, language, attention, psychomotor performance, affect, recall of previously over-learned material and general mental status. However, the isolated memory impairment subjects' immediate and delayed recall and recognition were comparable to that in the AD group. Glucose metabolism was analysed as a ratio of metabolism in specific cerebral cortical regions (i.e. frontal, temporal, parietal and occipital) to thalamus. Data were transformed from images using a stereotactic anatomical standardization and z-score method (Minoshima et al. 1995). The AD group's metabolism differed significantly from that of normal control and isolated memory impairment groups in all but the occipital region. Thirty-eight per cent of the isolated memory impairment group evidenced abnormality in their initial parietal/thalamic ratio; however, 75% of 11 isolated memory impairment subjects re-evaluated 2 years later were found to evidence abnormal PET findings. Of the isolated memory impairment subjects with initially abnormal PET findings at baseline, 88% converted to AD within 2 years. In contrast, 31% of those subjects with initially normal PET findings developed AD 2 years later. In total, 55% of the 11 isolated memory impairment patients re-tested after 2 years were found to have converted to

probable AD and at the present time, 39% of the entire sample of 23 isolated memory impairment patients have progressed to probable AD. Plate 6.2 reflects the differences in scans between AD, normal control and isolated memory impairment patients, the last with and without abnormal PET findings, as discussed in more detail above.

The observation that a substantial minority of the isolated memory impairment subjects had cerebral hypometabolism in a regional pattern similar to AD suggests that isolated memory impairment represents an early stage in progressive dementia. The fact that the memory deficit in isolated memory impairment was as pronounced as it was in the patients with a clinical diagnosis of probable AD is consistent with the notion that memory is a domain of cognition affected in the earliest stages of AD. That such a large percentage of isolated memory impairment subjects converted to AD within 2 years of initial study suggests that memory declines profoundly before a clinical diagnosis of AD can be made. The isolated memory impairment subjects had impaired memory despite demonstrating normal cerebral metabolism in many cases and because of this, isolated memory impairment presents an exciting opportunity to study memory in relation to brain chemistry at a time when the biological changes in disease progression are first occurring.

When these isolated memory impairment findings are contrasted to results from studies discussed earlier that used other approaches to similar problems, e.g. the research with APOE by Reiman et al. (1996), new questions emerge. For instance, Reiman et al. found that individuals positive for the APOE $\varepsilon 4$ allele evidenced abnormal cerebral metabolism in regions similar to those affected in patients with AD. In the studies on isolated memory impairment, it was found that some persons with abnormal cognition demonstrated normal levels of glucose metabolism. Is there a population difference between the two studies? It would be interesting to know the genetic variations between these two samples. Also, while the majority of the isolated memory impairment patients appear to eventually progress to AD, there is the need to wait for the completion of longitudinal phases of the cited APOE studies to learn if these patients do eventually develop the disease. As mentioned earlier, future studies that combine various approaches, e.g. genetic and behavioral, will likely contribute greatly to our understanding of the neural substrates of learning and memory.

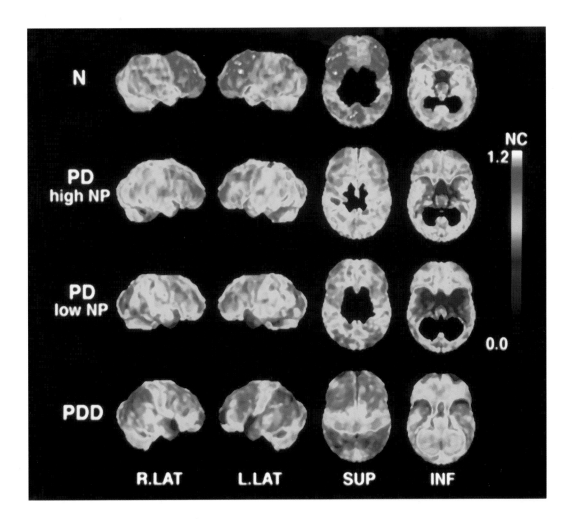

Plate 6.1. Right lateral (R.LAT), left lateral (L.LAT), superior (SUP) and inferior (INF) three-dimensional stereotactic surface projections of [^{18}F]FDG PET results normalized to the cerebellum for four subjects of equivalent age: normal control (N), Parkinson's disease with memory and visual-spatial ability within the upper 25th percentile of the sample of patients without dementia (PD/high NP), Parkinson's disease with memory and visual-spatial ability within the lower 25th percentile of the sample (PD/low NP) and Parkinson's disease with dementia (PDD).

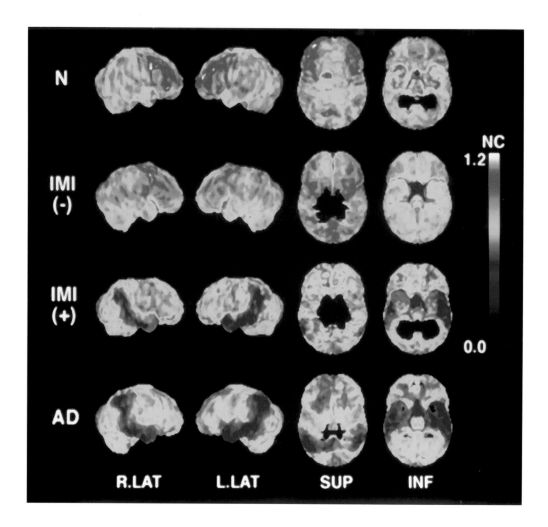

Plate 6.2. Right lateral (R.LAT), left lateral (L.LAT), superior (SUP) and inferior (INF) three–dimensional stereotactic surface projections of [¹⁸F]FDG PET results normalized to the thalamus for four subjects of equivalent age: normal control (N), isolated memory impairment with normal parietal/thalamic ratio (IMI–), IMI with abnormal parietal/thalamic ratio (IMI+), Alzheimer's disease (AD).

CONCLUSIONS

Neuroimaging studies of neurodegenerative diseases have generally yielded findings about loci of neuropathology consistent with those derived from neuropathological studies (Davis et. al. 1994). In this respect, imaging studies can be said to have some specificity, at least to the extent that the neurodegenerative disease under study is specific. This latter observation is especially relevant for cognitive studies that seek to employ a disease model, as many neurological disorders overlap pathologically during their course. AD represents one disorder, however, that appears to have specificity in terms of metabolic alterations that are mainly in temporal-parietal cortex, at least early in the course of the disease and this represents a situation that is not shared by other dementing illnesses (Friedland and Jagust 1990). AD also appears to have specificity in behavioral manifestations that are primarily limited to learning and memory, also early in the course of the disease (Berent et al. 1995). It may also become increasingly possible to identify variants of AD, through genetic (e.g. APOE) and other markers (e.g. behavioral), that follow a regular and predictable course over the course of disease progression. These subtypes of AD may thus become important models to guide studies of cognitive decline seeking to elucidate the relationship of such decline to changes in neural substrates.

Functional imaging studies have produced false negative and false positive findings in addition to verifying expected brain–behavior relationships in some instances. Functional neuroimaging studies of memory deficits have yielded provocative if not definitive findings. For example, as Fletcher et al. (1997) point out in their review, imaging studies have been surprisingly useful and even instrumental, in highlighting the role of the prefrontal cortex in episodic memory encoding and retrieval processes. Surprisingly, however, functional imaging studies have had little success in clarifying the role of the hippocampus and medial temporal lobes in memory. It may be that the correct regions of cerebral metabolic change have not yet been identified, that a technically fine enough resolution has not yet been achieved, or that the right ligand has not yet been employed. As mentioned earlier, imaging data are but analogs to the neural mechanisms which are of ultimate interest. Furthermore, resolution of functional images remains problematic in that the finest resolution presently available is not fine enough to detect certain brain structures. The power of imaging technology will also be greatly enhanced as more ligands become available for safe and effective use. For instance, most studies to date have employed glucose. While glucose provides for an informative picture of brain activity in general, it may lack specificity for a given neurochemical system. In a study by Holthoff et al. (1994), to give a specific example, PD subjects were found to have a significant reduction of striatal [^{18}F]dopa uptake despite a finding of normal metabolic rate for regional glucose. These researchers were able to correlate the [^{18}F]dopa metabolism with performance on a verbal selective reminding task, adding to information about the role of dopaminergic pathways in memory processing. It was mentioned earlier that fMRI appears to have some advantages over PET, e.g. in terms of image resolution and the capacity to obtain structural and functional data in a single setting. PET, however, remains the technique of choice in the area of neuropharmacological imaging. In this respect, PET possesses the greatest technical capacity to effectively image receptor binding (Le Bihan 1996). It is at this level of neuronal activity that much can be discovered about the processes of learning and memory.

Findings from studies of memory that have employed functional imaging technology to date have produced findings consistent with much that was previously believed to be true. In some cases, new insights have resulted. In most instances, findings have, hopefully heuristically, raised more questions than they have answered. What can be said about the state of knowledge that has resulted from scientific inquiry with functional imaging technology? Some general conclusions might include the following:

1. Human memory involves brain regions believed to be involved in motor control and sensory processing.

2. Memory encoding, storage and retrieval processes are likely mediated by different brain regions.

3. Distinctions between declarative, procedural and other types of memory have utility in cognitive research and these various classes of memory appear to be mediated by different neural networks.

4. The normal brain may work differently than the diseased brain and the young brain may work differently than the old brain in how each changes physiologically in response to experiential stimuli.

5. Short-term memory traces appear to be represented differently than are long-term memories and these differences may be systematically dynamic.
6. Memory may be mediated simultaneously by different brain regions.
7. A localizing model that consists solely of brain mapping will not suffice to answer the complex questions involved in understanding how the brain responds to experience.
8. Structural imaging alone is likely to be of limited value in furthering our understanding of how the brain processes and stores learned information.
9. The value of functional imaging techniques is limited by the value of the questions asked.
10. Several techniques used together (e.g. imaging and neuropathology) may be more powerful than any alone.
11. Memory subtypes may be mediated by different neurochemical systems and these distinctions may prove to be more important than are differences in structural regions.
12. Neural substrates of memory are heterogeneous and distributed widely in the brain.

Through systematic, objective and quantitative measurement of both behavior and cerebral physiology, the future promise of functional neuroimaging remains very bright. In addition to direct experiments on learning and memory, attention should also be paid to the careful psychometric description of the nature and progression of cognitive deficits in neurological diseases. Both activation and resting state studies have a place in these inquiries and such states would be most effectively used in conjunction with other techniques and methods, as well as through systematic testing of hypotheses that are thoughtfully derived from empirically based theory and knowledge. Attention will need to be given to the differences that probably exist between normal and diseased brain function, and methods will need to be employed that allow for imaging of various neurochemical systems. Imaging remains an important tool that is almost certain to aid in unraveling the mysteries that remain regarding where and how the brain learns and recalls what it has learned.

ACKNOWLEDGMENTS

This work supported in part by Grants from US Public Health Service (5 RO1 NS 24896, 5 P50 AG 08671-07) and National Institutes of Health (NS 15655, AG 08671 and AG 07378). This support is gratefully acknowledged. The authors acknowledge the assistance of Carol Persad, Andrea Miller and Pat Bohland in the preparation of this manuscript and Dr Satoshi Minoshima in preparing the illustrative figures.

REFERENCES

American Psychological Association. 1985. *Standards for educational and psychological testing*. Washington, DC: Author.

Bandettini, P.A., Wong, E.C., Hinks, R.S., Tikofsky, R.S. and Hyde, J.S. 1992. Time course EPI of human brain function during task activation. *Magnetic Resonance in Medicine*. 25: 390–397.

Berent, S. 1990. Modern approaches to neuropsychological testing. In *Advances in neurology*, vol. 55, ed. D. Smith, D. Treiman and M. Trimble, pp. 423–437. New York: Raven Press.

Berent, S., Giordani, B., Gilman, S., Junck, L., Lehtinen, S., Markel, D.S., Boivin, M., Kluin, K.J., Parks, R. and Koeppe, R.A. 1990. Neuropsychological changes in olivopontocerebellar atrophy. *Archives of Neurology*. 47: 997–1001.

Berent, S., Giordani, B., Lehtinen, S., Markel, D., Penney, J.B., Buchtel, H.A., Starosta-Rubenstein, S., Hichwa, R. and Young, A.B. 1988. Positron emission tomographic scan investigations of Huntington's disease: Cerebral metabolic correlates of cognitive function. *Annals of Neurology*. 23: 541–546.

Berent, S., Giordani, B., Minoshima, S., Foster, N.L., Koeppe, R.A. and Kuhl, D.E. 1995. Isolated memory impairment (IMI): Relationship to cognition, brain metabolism and Alzheimer's disease. *Journal of Cerebral Blood Flow and Metabolism*. 15: S102.

Berg, L., McKeel, D.W., Miller, J.P., Baty, J. and Morris, J.C. 1993. Neuropathological indexes of Alzheimer's disease in demented and nondemented persons aged 80 years and older. *Archives of Neurology*. 50: 349–358.

Bloch, F., Hansen, W.W. and Packard, M.E. 1946. Nuclear induction. *Physical Review*. 69: 127.

Brunetti, A., Soricelli, A., Mansi, L. and Salvatore, M. 1991. Functional brain imaging in AIDS-related dementia: A review. In *Biochemical and social developments in AIDS and associated tumors*, ed. G. Giraldo, M. Salvatore, M. Piazza, D. Zarrilli and E. Beth-Geraldo, pp. 227–234. Basel: Karger.

Crook, T., Bartus, R.T., Ferris, S.H., Whitehouse, P., Cohen, G.D. and Gershon, S. 1986. Age associated memory impairment: Proposed diagnostic criteria and measures of clinical change – Report of a National Institute of Mental Health work group. *Developmental Neuropsychology*. 2: 261–276.

Davis, P.C., Mirra, S.S. and Alazraki, N. 1994. The brain in older persons with and without dementia: Findings on MR, PET and SPECT images. *American Journal of Radiology*. 162: 1267–1278.

Drachman, A. 1994. If we live long enough, will we all be demented? *Neurology*. 44: 1563–1565.

Duara, R. 1990. Utilization of positron emission tomography for research and clinical application in dementia. In *Positron emission tomography in dementia*, ed. R. Duara, pp.1–12. New York: Wiley-Liss.

Duara, R., Loewenstein, D.A. and Barker, W.W. 1990. Utilization of behavioral activation paradigms for positron emission tomography studies in normal young and elderly subjects and in dementia. In *Positron emission tomography in dementia*, ed. R. Duara, pp. 131–148. New York: Wiley-Liss.

Ebly, E.M., Parhad, I.M., Hogan, D.B. and Fung, T.S. 1994. Prevalence and types of dementia in the very old. *Neurology*. 44: 1593–1600.

Fletcher, P.C., Frith, C.D. and Rugg, M.D. 1997. The functional neuroanatomy of episodic memory. *Trends in Neurosciences*. 20: 213–218.

Forette, F., Henry, J.F., Orgogozo, J.M., Dartigues, J.F., Pere, J.J., Hugonot, L., Isreal, L., Loria, Y., Goulley, F., Lallemand, A. and Boller, F. 1989. Reliability of clinical criteria for the diagnosis of dementia. *Archives of Neurology*. 46: 646–648.

Foster, N.L., Chase, T.N., Mansi, L. Brooks, R. Fedio, P., Patronas, N.J. and DiChiro, G. 1984. Cortical abnormalities in Alzheimer's disease. *Annals of Neurology*. 16: 649–654.

Frackowiak, R.S.J. 1986. An introduction to positron emission tomography and its applications to clinical investigation. In *New brain imaging techniques and psychopharmacology*, ed. M.R. Trimble, pp. 25–34. Oxford: Oxford University Press.

Frackowiak, R.S.J., Lenzi, G.-L., Jones, T. and Heather, J.D. 1980. Quantitative measurement of regional cerebral blood flow and oxygen metabolism in man using ^{15}O and positron emission tomography. *Journal of Computer Assisted Tomography* 4: 727–736.

Freer, C.E.L. 1994. Imaging and the brain. In *Dementia and normal aging,* ed. F.A.Huppert, C. Brayne and D.W. O'Connor, pp.131–163. New York: Cambridge University Press.

Friedland, R.P. 1993. Alzheimer's disease: Clinical features and differential diagnosis. *Neurology*, 43 (Suppl. 4): S45-S51.

Friedland, R.P. and Jagust, W.J. 1990. Positron and single photon emission tomography in the differential diagnosis of dementia. In *Positron emission tomography in dementia*, ed. R. Duara, pp. 161–177. New York: Wiley-Liss.

Friedland, R.P., Budinger, T.F., Gantz, E., Yano, Y., Mathis, C.A., Koss, E., Ober, B.A., Heusman, R.H. and Derenzo, A.E. 1983. Regional cerebral metabolic alterations in dementia of the Alzheimer's type: Positron emission tomography with [18F]fluorodeoxyglucose. *Journal of Computer Assisted Tomography*. 7: 590–598.

Giordani, B., Berent, S., Minoshima, S., Boivin, M.J., Frey, K.A., Guire, K.E., Koeppe, R.A. and Kuhl, D.E. 1995. Cortical and subcortical [^{18}F] FDG hypometabolism in nondemented and demented Parkinson's patients. *Journal of Cerebral Blood Flow and Metabolism*. 15: S762.

Grady, C.L. 1996. Age-related changes in cortical blood flow activation during perception and memory. *Annals of the New York Academy of Sciences*. 777: 14–21.

Grady, C.L., Haxby, J.V., Horwitz, B., Sundaram, M., Berg, B., Shapiro, M.B., Friedland, R.P. and Rapoport, S.I. 1988. Longitudinal study of the early neuropsychological and cerebral metabolic changes in dementia of the Alzheimer's type. *Journal of Clinical and Experimental Neuropsychology*. 5: 576–596.

Hanninen, T., Hallikainen, M., Koivisto, K., Helkala, E-L, Reinkainen, K.J., Mykkanen, L., Laakso, M., Pyorala, K. and Reikkinen, Sr., P.J. 1994. A follow-up study of subjects with age-associated memory impairment. *Neurology.* 44 (Suppl. 2): A143.

Haxby, J.V., Grady, C.L., Koss, E., Horwitz, B., Heston, L., Shapiro, M.B., Friedland, R.P. and Rapoport, S.I. 1990. Longitudinal study of cerebral metabolic asymmetries and associated neuropsychological patterns in early dementia of the Alzheimer's type. *Archives of Neurology.* 47: 753–760.

Holthoff, V.A., Vieregge, P., Kessler, J., Pietrzyk, U., Herholtz, K., Bönner, J., Wagner, R., Wienhard, K., Pawlik, G and Heiss, W.-D. 1994. Discordant twins with Parkinson's disease: Early signs of impaired cognitive circuits. *Annals of Neurology.* 36: 176–182.

Housenfield, G.N. 1974. Computerized transverse axial scanning (tomography). I. Description of system. *British Journal of Radiology.* 46: 1023–1047.

Jagust, W.J. 1994. Functional imaging in dementia: An overview. *Journal of Clinical Psychiatry.* 55: 5–11.

Kish, S.J., El-Awar, M., Leach, L., Oscar-Berman, M., Schut, L. and Freedman, M. 1988. Cognitive deficits in dominantly-inherited olivoponto-cerebellar atrophy: Implications for the cholinergic hypothesis of Alzheimer's dementia. *Annals of Neurology.* 24: 200–206.

Kral, V.A. 1962. Senescent forgetfulness: Benign and malignant. *Canadian Medical Association Journal.* 86: 257–260.

Kuhl, D.E., Metter, E.J., Riege, W.H., Hawkins, R.A., Mazziotta, J.C., Phelps, M.E. and Kling, A.S. 1983. Local cerebral glucose utilization in elderly patients with depression, multiple infarct dementia and Alzheimer's disease. *Journal of Nuclear Medicine.* 24: P21.

Kuhl, D.E., Metter, E.J. and Riege, W.H. 1984. Pattern of local cerebral utilization determined in Parkinson's disease by the (18F) fluorodeoxy-glucose method. *Annals of Neurology.* 15: 419–424.

Kuhl, D.E., Small, G.W., Riege, W.H., Fujikawa, D.G., Metter, E.J., Benson, D.F., Ashford, J.W., Mazziotta, J.C., Maltese, A. and Dorsey, D.A. 1987. Abnormal PET-FDG scans in early Alzheimer's disease. *Journal of Nuclear Medicine.* 28: 645.

Le Bihan, D. 1996. Functional MRI of the brain: Principles, applications and limitations. *Journal of Neuroradiology.* 23: 1–5.

Martinez, J.L. and Kesner, R.P. 1986. *Learning and memory: A biological view.* New York: Academic Press.

Masur, D.M., Sliwinski, M., Lipton, R.B., Blau, A.D. and Crystal, H.A. 1994. Neuropsychological prediction of dementia and the absence of dementia in healthy elderly persons. *Neurology.* 44: 1427–1432.

Matarazzo, J.D. 1972. *Wechsler's measurement and appraisal of adult intelligence*, 5th ed. New York: Oxford University Press.

McKhann, G., Drachman, D., Folstein, M., Katzman, R., Price, D. and Stadlan, E.M. 1984. Clinical diagnosis of Alzheimer's disease. Report of the NINCDS-ADRDA Work Group under the auspices of the Department of Health and Human Services Task Force on Alzheimer's disease. *Neurology.* 34: 939–944.

Miller, J.D., de Leon, M.J., Ferris, S.H., Kluger, A., George, A.E., Reisberg, B., Sachs, J.H. and Wolf, A.P 1987. Abnormal temporal lobe response in Alzheimer's disease during cognitive processing as measured by ^{11}C–2-Deoxy-D-Glucose and PET. *Journal of Cerebral Blood Flow and Metabolism.* 7: 248–251.

Minoshima, S., Frey, K.A., Koeppe, R.A., Foster, N.L. and Kuhl, D.E. 1995. A diagnostic approach in Alzheimer's disease using three-dimensional stereotactic surface projections of Fluoxide–^{18} FDG PET. *Journal of Nuclear Medicine.* 36: 1238–1248.

Pietrini, P., Azari, N.P., Grady, C.L., Salerno, J.A., Gonzales-Aviles, A., Heston, L.L., Pettigrew, K.D., Horwitz, B., Haxby, J.V. and Schapiro, M.B. 1993. Pattern of cerebral metabolic interactions in a subject with isolated amnesia at risk for Alzheimer's disease: A Longitudinal evaluation. *Dementia.* 4: 94–101.

Purcell, E.M., Taurry, H.C. and Pound, R.V. 1946. Resonance absorption by nuclear magnetic moments in a solid. *Physical Review.* 69: 37.

Reiman, E.M., Caselli, R.J., Yun, L.S., Kewei Chen, M.S., Bandy, D., Minoshima, S., Thibodeau, S.N. and Osborne, D. 1996. Preclinical evidence of Alzheimer's disease in persons homozygous for the e4 allele for apolipoprotein E. *New England Journal of Medicine.* 334: 752–758.

Riddle, W., O'Carroll, R.E., Dougall, N., VanBeck, M., Curran, S.M., Ebmeier, K.P. and Goodwin, G.M. 1993. A single photon emission computerised tomography study of regional brain function underlying verbal memory in patients with Alzheimer-type dementia. *British Journal of Psychiatry.* 163: 166–172.

Roskies, A.L. 1994. Mapping memory with positron emission tomography. *Proceedings of the National Academy of Sciences*. 91: 1989–1991.

Sacktor, N., Van Heertum, R.L., Dooneief, G., Gorman, J., Khandji, A., Marder, K., Nour, R., Todak, G., Stern, Y. and Mayeux, R. 1995. A comparison of cerebral SPECT abnormalities in HIV-positive homosexual men with and without cognitive impairment. *Archives of Neurology*. 52: 1170–1173.

Salmon, E. and Franck, G. 1989. Positron emission tomography in degenerative dementias. *Acta Neurologica Belgica*. 89: 150–155.

Sarter, M., Berntson, G.G. and Cacioppo, J.T. 1996. Brain imaging and cognitive neuroscience: Toward strong inference in attributing function to structure. *American Psychologist*. 51: 13–21.

Small, G.W., Mazziotta, J.C., Collins, M.T., Baxter, L.R., Phelps, M.E., Mandelkern, M.A., Kaplan, A., La Rue, A., Adamson, C.F., Chang, L., Guze, B.H., Corder, E.H., Saunders, A.M., Haines, J.L., Pericak-Vance, M.A. and Roses, A.D. 1995. Apolipoprotein E type 4 allele and cerebral glucose metabolism in relatives at risk for Alzheimer disease. *Journal of the American Medical Association*. 273: 942–947.

Small, G.W., Okonek, A., Mandelkern, M.A., La Rue, A., Chang, L., Khonsary, A., Ropchan, J.R. and Blahd, W.H. 1994. Age-associated memory loss: Initial neuropsychological and cerebral metabolic findings of a longitudinal study. *International Journal of Psychogeriatrics*. 6: 23–44.

Smith, G., Ivnik, R.J., Petersen, R.C., Malec, J.F., Kokmen, E. and Tangalos, E. 1991. Age-associated memory impairment diagnoses: Problems of reliability and concerns for terminology. *Psychology and Aging*. 6: 551–558.

Sokoloff, L. and Smith, C. 1983. Biological principles for the measurement of metabolic rates in vivo. In *Positron emission tomography of the brain*, ed. W.-D. Heiss and M.E. Phelps, pp. 2–18. New York: Springer-Verlag.

Sokoloff, L., Reivich, M., Kennedy, C., Des Rosiers, M.H., Patlak, C.S., Pettigrew, K.D., Sakurada, O. and Shinohara, M. 1977. The [^{14}C]deoxy-glucose method for the measurement of local cerebral glucose utilization: Theory, procedure and normal values in the conscious and anesthetized albino rat. *Journal of Neurochemistry*. 28: 897–916.

Terry, R.D., DeTeresa, R. and Hansen, L.A. 1987. Neocortical cell counts in normal human adult aging. *Annals of Neurology*. 21: 530–539.

Tomlinson, B.E. 1992. Ageing and the dementias. In *Greenfield's neuropathology*, 5th ed., ed. J.H. Adams and L.W. Duchen, pp. 1284–1410. New York: Oxford University Press.

Treves, T.A., Kertzman, S., Verchovsky, R. and Korczyn, A.D. 1994. Incidence of dementia in age-associated memory impairment (AAMI). *Neurology*. 44 (Suppl. 2): A238.

Ungerleider, L.G. 1995. Functional brain imaging studies of cortical mechanisms for memory. *Science*. 270: 769–775.

Young, S.W. 1984. *Nuclear magnetic resonance imaging: Basic principles*. New York: Raven Press.

7

The biology of neurodegenerative disease

HANS J. MARKOWITSCH

INTRODUCTION

The 'Biological Perspectives' represented in the first part of this book point to the tremendous advances made in the understanding of neurodegenerative conditions since their early descriptions. Many of these advances would not have been possible without animal research and several chapters highlight the importance of studying the behavior of animals with surgical or 'chemical' brain lesions in order to gain insights into basic mechanisms of neurodegenerative diseases. The chapters also discuss methodological approaches, such as neurochemical and neuroanatomical ones, to elucidate structure–function relations in patients with neurodegenerative diseases. In the sections that follow, the utility of animal models of neurodegenerative diseases is discussed. This is followed by an analysis of studies with humans examining the neurochemical and neuroanatomical correlates of memory in neurodegenerative diseases.

ANIMALS AS MODELS OF NEURODEGENERATIVE DISEASES IN HUMANS

While specific etiologies have been discovered for some neurodegenerative diseases, the causes of others remain the object of scientific curiosity and fascination. Oscar-Berman and Bardenhagen (Chapter 1) dealt with one approach to unravel some of the many questions accompanying neurodegenerative diseases, namely the conduct of animal research – especially with regard to memory disturbances. These authors strongly argue for the feasibility of extrapolating from animal data to human conditions and provide numerous examples of both animal studies with implications for human behavior and of 'animal' tasks used in studies of patients with neurodegenerative diseases. Nevertheless, the authors acknowledge that the sensitivity of 'animal' tests to human memory dysfunction has still to be determined and that methodological limitations, including an improper mimicking of human neurodegenerative diseases in animal models, may hinder proper inferences and outcomes. Furthermore, the network character of information processing in the brain which, for example, strongly links prefrontal and limbic circuits, impedes the making of unidimensional, straightforward inferences about brain–behavior relationships.

Oscar-Berman and Bardenhagen stressed the importance of using different memory tests (e.g. declarative versus working memory, or declarative versus procedural memory tests) to study the effects of brain damage on memory. It might, however, also be noted that it seems particularly difficult (if not impossible) to mimic free recall and episodic memory conditions in animals (Tulving and Markowitsch 1994), yet these very forms of memory are those most sensitive to amnesia in humans.

The mimicking of the motor and cognitive dysfunctions in Huntington's disease (HD) by using nonprimate animal models was the target of Kesner and Filoteo (Chapter 2). These authors, like Oscar-Berman and Bardenhagen, point out some of the limitations of animal models for the study of neurodegenerative diseases. Animal models seem to have great difficulty complying with especially the multitude of behavioral effects and the time course of neurodegenerative diseases. On the other hand, chemical lesioning techniques which started with the application of kainic acid (now known to have convulsive properties) and ibotenic acid (Divac et al. 1978; Guldin and Markowitsch 1981, 1982) and which allow selective neuronal damage while leaving axons of passage unaffected, have given a new impetus to investigate human neurodegenerative diseases in animals. Intracranial injections of quinolinic acid, an N–methyl-D-aspartate (NMDA) antagonist, are now considered to most closely mimic the effects of HD on neurons (Chapter 2).

Brain damage versus brain dysfunction

In discussing the time course of HD, Kesner and Filoteo stress an important finding obtained in human patients at the beginning of the disease process: Here, structural lesions may still be absent or not detectable by static (structural) imaging methods such as magnetic resonance imaging (MRI), while dynamic (functional) imaging methods, e.g. positron emission tomography (PET), may already reveal reduced metabolic activity in the striatum. This finding implies that abnormal neuronal metabolism (i.e. brain dysfunction) may be a precursor of later morphological brain damage. Reduced neuronal metabolism appears to be a quite general observation in patients with suspected neurodegeneration. It is known, for example, that nearly 80% of the nigral dopaminergic cells might be lost before parkinsonian symptoms manifest themselves overtly.

The availability of dynamic imaging methods (e.g. single photon emission computed tomography (SPECT), PET and functional magnetic resonance imaging (fMRI)) has allowed a number of new insights into the course of neurodegenerative diseases. Dynamic imaging techniques also permit a much better correlation between behavioral outcomes and underlying neuronal damage than may be available even from post mortem microscopical inspection of brain slices.

Two cases we have had the opportunity to study in detail (one with cognitive deficits after a heart attack and one with presumably stress-induced cognitive deterioration) illustrate how functional (dynamic) imaging techniques might reveal cerebral dysfunction in the apparent absence of radiologically verifiable structural brain changes. Markowitsch et al. (1997b) studied a 36-year-old office clerk who had lost his position as a consequence of hypoxic brain damage following a heart attack and 14 days of coma. The patient was studied neuropsychologically and with static and dynamic imaging methods (MRI, PET) 6–9 months after his heart attack. He had severe and persistent anterograde and retrograde amnesias, as well as other cognitive deficits. MRI indicated only nonspecific cortical atrophy. Imaging with PET, on the other hand, revealed severe and significant bilateral affectations of the thalamus, of both medial and lateral temporal cortices, as well as occipito-parietal hypometabolism. This case illustrates that dynamic, but not static brain imaging analyses may reveal quite severe and widespread brain dysfunction which corresponds well to observed cognitive alterations.

Even more spectacular is the case studied by Markowitsch et al. (1998). A 23-year-old employee of an insurance company with 11 years of education discovered the outbreak of a fire in his house. Although the fire was successfully extinguished during the ensuing hours, the patient the next morning appeared to have sustained a major loss of cognitive abilities and underwent psychiatric hospitalization. While all neurological and structural neuroradiological examinations failed to reveal evidence of brain damage, PET imaging provided striking evidence of major hypometabolism especially in the memory-sensitive regions of the brain. This hypometabolism was unusually profound, amounting to metabolism values which were two to three standard deviations below those of age and gender-matched controls and fell even below the values for the severely amnesic patient described earlier.

The case of this patient is remarkable because it indicates that a stressful event (the house fire) can ecphorize remembrance of a similarly stressful scene experienced during childhood and thereby induce not only severe, enduring and widespread cognitive disturbances, but also alter the brain's metabolism to a significant degree. Psychic mechanisms thus may induce a blocking, inhibition or alteration of the normal activity of cognitive neuronal networks with the consequence of widespread reductions in the interaction between neuronal assemblies. Apparently even sporadic environmental stress can induce long-lasting brain dysfunction with subsequent massive cognitive deterioration. Excessive release of glucocorticoids, the adrenal steroids secreted during stress, might induce such brain changes (Bremner et al. 1995a,b; Sapolsky 1996a,b). Figure 7.1 illustrates the effect of re-exposure to a stressful situation on cerebral metabolism in a patient without any evidence of organic brain damage as visible by high-resolution MRI.

Time and content-based subdivisions of memory distinguish among neurodegenerative diseases

Chapters 1 and 2 in this volume both emphasize the differential applicability of various animal models to the study of distinct forms of learning and memory. While the subdivision of memory into short-term and long-term forms and the attribution of short-term or working memory processes to cortical structures, in particular within the frontal lobe, has long been stressed (Jacobsen 1935; Goldman-Rakic and Friedman 1991), much less is known about the final form of memory representations and the

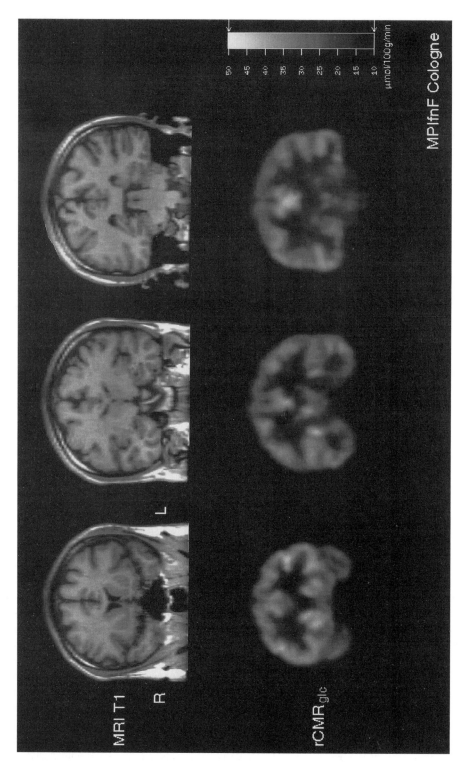

Figure 7.1. Magnetic resonance imaging (MRI) and FDG-positron–emission–tomography (FDG-PET) based coronal sections from anterior to posterior (left to right) through the brain of a patient with cognitive dysfunction after re-exposure to a very stressful situation. While there are no changes to be seen in MRI, FDG-PET revealed a major metabolic reduction in widespread cortical and subcortical areas, most particularly in the memory-processing medial temporal lobe (notice the black 'holes' in the bottom middle section). Data from H.J. Markowitsch, Josef Kessler, Christian van der Ven, Gerald Weber–Luxenburger, Manfred Albers and Wolf-Dieter Heiss.

Table 7.1. *Important terms in mnestic information processing*

Time sequence of information processing	
Information registration	Perception of stimuli via the sensory channels (eye/retina, ear/cochlea, skin/mechanoreceptors) and immediately adjoining specific nuclear and cortical structures
Information encoding	Further processing of information aimed at identifying, classifying and sorting perceived stimuli
Information consolidation	Integrating and embedding of processed information in the existing framework
Information storage	'Final placing' of information, engram formation
Information retrieval	(Re-)ecphorizing of stored information
Ecphory	The process by which retrieval cues interact with stored information so that an image or a representation of the target information appears
Time-dependent subdivisions of memory	
Sensory memory (also echoic or iconic memory)	The persistence of observed stimuli within the sensory input channels (range of milliseconds)
Short-term or working memory	Remembrance of perceived stimuli for seconds or at best 1, 2 minutes (5–7 independent units)
Long-term memory	Principally life-long preservation of information
Single terms	
Engram	Memory trace in the brain
Forgetting	Loss of information or blocking of retrieval (via decay or interference processes).
Free recall	Recall of learned information without cuing or other aids
Cued recall	Recall of learned information with cuing (partial information presentation, categorization, etc.)
Recognition	Selection of a target stimulus from among a number of usually related stimuli
Anterograde amnesia	Inability to acquire information after a certain event (brain damage) so that it cannot be recalled at a later time point
Retrograde amnesia	Inability, to recall/retrieve previously acquired information after a certain event (brain damage; psychic shock)
Source memory	Knowledge about the specific circumstances during which a particular event was acquired
Prospective memory	Memory of the future; knowledge of what is intended to be done in the future

anatomical substrates of content-specific memories. Tables 7.1 and 7.2 and Figure 7.2 give an overview of classifications of memory systems and their potential neural substrates.

Although the distinctions among different memory systems are still not universally accepted (Roediger 1990; Roediger et al. 1990), they have advanced our understanding of the relationship between focal brain damage and memory disturbances and provided a basis for the formulation of specific hypotheses with respect to the memory processing abilities of patients with different neurodegenerative diseases (Haupts et al. 1994; Rieger and Markowitsch 1996). As Kesner and Filoteo described in Chapter 2, there seems – at least with respect to HD

patients – to be progress in supporting a differentiation of memory along both content and time-based dimensions. HD patients seem to be particularly deficient in learning motor-based procedural memory tasks, yet less so in other tasks. Such a dissociation would support a classification of memory systems based on the contents of such systems. In addition, these patients have major problems in initiating systematic strategies to retrieve information from remote memory and consequently have a retrograde amnesia characterized by a flat temporal gradient (i.e. an equal impairment for all past decades) (Chapter 10). The observation that there is only a weak correlation between retrograde and anterograde amnesia would support time-based

Table 7.2. *Content-based memory systems*

System	Description, other terms	Retrieval
Episodic memory	Autobiographical events, personal memory	Explicit
Knowledge	Facts of the world, semantic memory	Implicit
Short-term memory	Working memory, primary memory	Explicit
Procedural system	Motor related, sensory, and cognitive skills	Implicit
(Perceptual) Priming system	Perceptual representation, quasi-memory	Implicit
Other systems or forms	Conditioning procedures, habituation, sensitization	Implicit

Note:
Episodic memory refers to individual-specific (or autobiographical) memory, i.e. information specific with respect to time and place. Knowledge refers to information of a more general nature which cannot be traced back to a specific point in time and place. This kind of information includes knowledge of the world and will consequently be referred to as knowledge system. Squire (1987) subsumes episodic and semantic memory under declarative memory. For Tulving (1993) a major difference between the two is that episodic memory is explicitly ('consciously') retrieved, while the knowledge system is an implicit one.
Source: This classification is largely based on Table 1 of Tulving (1993, 1994, 1995).

memory classification systems. As is lucidly explained by Kesner and Filoteo, there are numerous parallels between the memory performance of rodents with caudate nucleus damage and patients with HD; these parallels appear to a great extent to be due to the motor demands of the tasks and tests employed.

BRAIN'S CHEMISTRY IN NEURODEGENERATIVE DISEASE

Miyawaki and Koller in Chapter 4 rightly point out what Nieuwenhuys (1985) observed, namely that the relationship between the brain's anatomy and its neurochemistry is extremely complex and that inferences about anatomical–chemical relationships are full of hindrances.

In the case of Alzheimer's disease (AD), the 'cholinergic hypothesis' of memory dysfunction has enjoyed a longstanding, if perhaps undeserved, position of privilege; however, as Miyawaki and Koller point out, the results of animal models at least in part de-emphasize a memory-related role of the cholinergic forebrain and instead indicate that this structural forebrain complex might have to do more with the 'readiness' of the brain to handle information. Blokland (1996), in a recent and quite exhaustive review, came to rather similar conclusions. He concluded that acetylcholine is more specifically involved in attentional than in learning and memory processes. Miyawaki and Koller also rekindle Price and colleagues'

hypothesis that cholinergic neuronal loss in the basal forebrain in AD patients might be a phenomenon not of anterograde, but rather retrograde degeneration (Price et al. 1982; Price 1986). This hypothesis is still controversial. Neary and co-workers (1986a,b), for example, found that Alzheimer's dementia is primarily associated with loss of large cortical, but not subcortical neurons (Pearson and Powell 1987). The opposite view – that changes on the subcortical level are the cause of cortical degenerations – was emphasized by de la Monte (1989) (see also Fibiger 1991). Regardless of the outcome of this debate, the cholinergic hypothesis per se cannot fully account for a disease as complex as AD or the full spectrum of behavioral changes that occur at different stages of this disease (see Table 4.1 in Chapter 4 by Miyawaki and Koller).

Present-day knowledge of neuroanatomy and of neurotransmitter/neuromodulator interactions speaks for widespread interactions between neural systems and among cognitive functions (e.g. attention and memory). As Miyawaki and Koller delineated, dorsal and ventral portions of the striatum interact to a much greater extent than previously thought, an observation which raises the issue to what degree the striatum may be involved in explicit memory processing in the nonmotor domain. Recent work already strongly favors the view that the striatum has a role in nonmotor learning and memory. Irle et al. (1992) compared memory performance in five patient groups with damage to: (1) the basal forebrain *and* the striatum, (2) the basal forebrain only, (3) the striatum only, (4) the ventral

Registration, encoding, consolidation, storage, and retrieval of information

Registration

Sensory systems

Encoding

Short-term memory Priming	Sensory cortex	Working memory

Procedural memory (probably also storage places) | Cerebellum, basal ganglia

Encoding, consolidation, transfer to long-term memory

Bottleneck structures of the limbic system

- medial temporal lobe region — hippocampal formation, ento-, peri- and parahippocampal region; amygdala (for emotional flavoring of memory)

- medial diencephalon — anterior and mediodorsal thalamic region, mammillary bodies

- basal forebrain — medial septum, basal nucleus of Meynert, diagonal band of Broca

- fiber systems —
  Papez circuit
  -fornix
  -mammillo-thalamic tract
  -anterior thalamic peduncles (to cingulate cortex and subiculum)
  -cingulum
  basolateral limbic circuit
  -ventral amygdalofugal tract
  -anterior thalamic peduncle (from mediodorsal thalamus to the sub-callosal area of the medial prefrontal cortex)
  -bandeletta diagonalis (from the subcallosal area to the amygdala)

Storage

Engrams	Cerebral cortex (primarily non-primary cortical regions)
(Recall from the priming system)	*left:* mainly engrams of the knowledge system *right:* mainly engrams of episodic memories

Recall

Recall from the knowledge system Left basal prefrontal and left latero-polar region	Recall from the episodic memory system Right basal prefrontal and right latero-temporal polar temporal lobe region

Figure 7.2. Possible brain structures involved in the processes from information registration to information recall. For the memory-related terminology, see Table 7.1. It is assumed that the temporo-frontal region implicated in recall is necessary for triggering, i.e. for gaining access to stored engrams which are distributed in network-fashion within the cerebral cortex.

frontal cortex only, or (5) the ventral frontal cortex, the striatum and the basal forebrain. These researchers found considerable and persistent explicit memory deficits only in patients with damage to both the basal forebrain *and* the striatum, leading them to conclude that either system might be able to counterbalance dysfunction in the other. Rousseaux et al. (1996) also strongly emphasized striatal damage as the source of many cognitive disorders and, similarly, Rieger and Markowitsch (1996), who compared explicit and implicit memory in groups with early Parkinson's disease (PD) and either prefrontal or medial temporal damage, found that patients with PD had the most widespread disturbance of both explicit and implicit memory.

Taken together, such findings argue for a still more intervowen network in long-term information processing than has been assumed on the basis of results using modern neuroimaging techniques (Buckner and Tulving 1995). As has been suggested from the outcome of single case studies using large test batteries, components of attention, motivation and emotion may influence memory performance quite substantially after damage to some 'bottleneck' or strategic brain loci (Markowitsch et al. 1994; Markowitsch and Calabrese 1996), while damage to other brain regions may lead to more focal deficits (Babinsky et al. 1997; Reinkemeier et al. 1997). It has still to be found out, however, whether members of the first class of loci are more likely to be nodal convergence zones, both hodologically and by their transmitter influx, than are members of the second class.

STRUCTURAL AND FUNCTIONAL NEUROIMAGING AND INTERINDIVIDUAL DIFFERENCES

While both neuroanatomical and neurochemical atlases of the brain usually refer to an average brain, Sullivan, Cahn, Fama and Shear in Chapter 5 (on structural neuroimaging correlates of memory dysfunction) emphasize inter- and intraindividual differences. Interindividual differences are most obvious between the sexes, with males having more voluminous brains on average and brains which show some subtle deviations in anatomy from those of females (Pritzel and Markowitsch 1997). Numerous other variables could be listed which show interindividual differences as well (Markowitsch 1988b). Intraindividually, we know that age affects brain size and, perhaps more importantly, that age differentially affects various brain regions.

Age not only influences the brain, but also cognitive functions. Thus, some domains of memory are vulnerable to age as evident from AAMI (age-associated memory impairment; Chapters 18 and 21). Although certain factors such as cognitive training and a background in high-level intellectual functioning may protect against such an age-related decline in memory (Shimamura et al. 1995; Chapter 14), consumption of alcohol and other potentially toxic substances may accelerate it (Kessler et al. 1986, 1987). Indeed, prolonged heavy alcohol consumption may induce alcoholic dementia or Korsakoff's syndrome (Markowitsch 1988a, 1992, 1994). As Sullivan et al. (Chapter 5) discuss, it is probable that alcohol-related neuropathology, in addition to involving the diencephalon, also involves the cerebral cortex (including hippocampus) and cerebellum.

The riddle of the prefrontal cortex

The example of alcohol-related brain damage returns us to the discussion of the multifocal involvement of brain structures in specific diseases. Here, one structural complex, the prefrontal cortex, has to be listed with high priority. While the prefrontal cortex is not as directly involved in some neurodegenerative diseases as are, for example, the basal ganglia in PD, it still seems to play a quite ubiquitous role in many disease-related forms of cognitive decline. Being an especially extensive and subdivisible area of the human brain (Markowitsch 1988c), the prefrontal cortex is currently of interest for a variety of reasons. It is the cortical region containing most dopaminergic afferents; dynamic brain imaging studies implicate

the prefrontal cortex in memory retrieval (Markowitsch 1995a); and it is affected by the aging process probably more extensively and earlier on than are other brain structures (Craik et al. 1990).

Several neurodegenerative diseases provide the opportunity to elucidate the functions of prefrontal cortex. Frontal dementia, Pick's disease and semantic dementia (Groen and Endtz 1982; Hodges et al. 1992; Graham and Hodges 1997) share as a common feature the central involvement in the disease of the prefrontal cortex. The memory deficits of PD patients also resemble those of patients with prefrontal damage (Rieger and Markowitsch 1996; Chapter 5). Unfortunately, while the behavioral and cognitive consequences of PD have been widely studied, those of Pick's disease have rarely been studied with formal and sound psychometric instruments. One issue raised by previous studies is whether memory deficits are attributable to frontal pathology, or to some disconnection or deafferentation of one region from another.

Several observations make plausible fronto-temporolimbic disconnection hypotheses of behavioral changes. Due to the strong interconnectivity of the orbitofrontal cortex with the anterior temporal cortex (e.g. via the uncinate fasciculus) (Ebeling and von Cramon 1992) and due to their common thalamic and other afferents (Markowitsch et al. 1985), these two cortical regions demonstrate a considerable degree of functional relatedness. This is evident from studies in nonhuman primates (Myers 1972; Franzen and Myers 1973) and from the similarity of the behavioral sequelae of damage to either the temporopolar (Markowitsch et al. 1985) or the orbitofrontal cortex (Röhrenbach and Markowitsch 1997). The similarity of major personality deviations after white matter lesions in these regions (Haupts et al. 1994) are further indicators of the functional relatedness of these regions. In principle, one might also infer a functional relationship between these cortical structures that is mediated via the adjacent basal forebrain nuclei and the nucleus accumbens. These structures might represent an interface between the motor and limbic systems and may be of particular relevance in PD (Calabrese et al. 1997). In addition, pathology of the amygdala, another limbic system component, has been related to cognitive and behavioral changes in PD (Braak et al. 1994; 1995). Nevertheless, as is stressed by Sullivan and co-workers, a disconnection hypothesis (based on disruption of the pathways interconnecting prefrontal and limbic systems) cannot fully account for the

range of cognitive deficits observed in patients with neuro-degenerative diseases such as multiple sclerosis.

Insights from special subgroups

Studies of patients at different stages of a given disease, or of groups with different ages at disease onset, can yield further insights into the neurobehavioral consequences of neurodegenerative changes and their mechanisms. For example, it has been reported that working memory (Law et al. 1994), as well as numerous other cognitive functions (Selnes et al. 1995) are intact in the early stage of human immunodeficiency virus (HIV)-infection, but that severe cognitive declines occur in the more advanced stages of the disease (McArthur et al. 1993; Hall et al. 1996; Hinkin et al. 1996; Kieburtz et al. 1996). Peavy et al. (1994) found that HIV-infected patients' verbal memory problems resemble those of HD rather than AD patients, thus suggesting that subcortical neuropathological changes probably underlie this memory dysfunction. This interpretation is consistent with findings from structural imaging studies indicating greater subcortical than cortical damage.

The time course of neurodegenerative diseases has been largely neglected up to now. While some studies lead one to believe that the order in which a disease affects given brain regions follows a reliable and predictable course, recent work indicates that there may be qualitative differences in disease progression dependant upon age of disease onset. Giannakopoulos et al. (1996) found that neuronal loss and lesion distribution differ significantly in AD patients beyond the age of 90 years and those of younger age. While the subiculum and the CA1 field of the hippocampus sustain the severest neuronal loss in younger patients, very old Alzheimer's patients demonstrate neuronal losses principally in the entorhinal, prefrontal (area 9) and inferotemporal (area 20) regions. Furthermore, the very old patients have relatively few neurofibrillary tangles in areas 9 and 20. These findings suggest that some brain regions might have a genetically determined resistance to AD pathology, but that even selective neuronal loss may be sufficient for centarians to manifest AD symptoms. The findings of Giannakopoulos et al. (1996) also raise the issue whether probably genetically (or biochemically) determined factors might retard the pathological progression of AD, or whether a homogeneous disease progression accompanied by severe mental deterioration is inevitable (Figure 7.3). In the near future both structural and functional neuroimaging will likely improve the predictability of whether

neuroanatomical alterations will ultimately lead to benign or malignant cognitive and behavioral changes.

Functional neuroimaging and memory dysfunction

Despite its brief existence, functional neuroimaging has led to an enormous knowledge base relating memory to brain metabolic activity, as indexed by cerebral blood flow and blood oxygenation changes (Figure 7.1 provides an example of PET-visualized changes in regional glucose metabolism). Many functional neuroimaging studies deal with the neural correlates of memory functions in non-brain damaged subjects. Insights gained from such studies are only sometimes compatible with the findings derived from studies of brain-damaged subjects (Buckner and Tulving 1995; Markowitsch 1995a). Consequently new efforts and hypotheses are needed to integrate these apparently method-related discrepancies concerning the cerebral correlates of memory.

Berent and Giordani in Chapter 6 on functional neuroimaging correlates of memory deficits in neurodegenerative disease address these methodological and conceptual problems and incongruities. These authors hypothesize that differences in the functional imaging correlates of memory observed in healthy and diseased subjects might reflect the simple fact that the normal brain works differently than the diseased brain. For example, certain areas activated in subjects with neurodegenerative disease might represent areas recruited by a given task so as to compensate for neural dysfunction in the areas activated in healthy subjects. Berent and Giordani pay much attention to the discussion of the potential usefulness and limitations of the different imaging techniques. For example, they refer to the discussion of Sarter et al. (1996) who offered numerous suggestions and cautions about the application and usefulness of dynamic imaging techniques in cognitive neuroscience.

As the course of neurodegenerative diseases frequently spans years and sometimes decades (see Figure 3.2), the cerebral dysfunction in the initial stage of a disease may not be visible with static (structural) neuroimaging techniques. Such brain changes may, however, be apparent on dynamic (functional) neuroimaging. The frequent use of SPECT to detect neuronal dysfunction in early probable AD demonstrates the value of functional imaging in differential diagnosis.

Magnetoencephalography and dynamic brain imaging

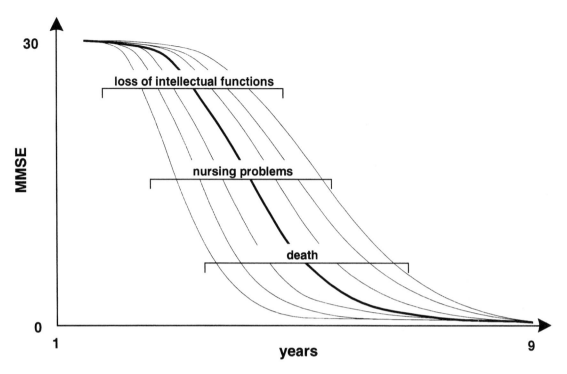

Figure 7.3. An idealized curve of the possible intellectual decline in
Alzheimer's disease. MMSE: Mini-Mental State Exam score
(maximum = 30).

techniques also are excellent methods to study interacting
networks in the brain and – what is particularly important
for neurodegenerative diseases – they allow for the detection of remote lesion effects. The use of PET in particular
has already borne fruit by pointing out loci of brain dysfunction remote from the apparent main focus of dysfunction (Goldenberg et al. 1991) and such distant changes in
brain dysfunction have been interpreted as a consequence
of long-term diaschisis effects (Jacobs et al. 1996). PET
studies, unlike structural imaging studies, also allow for
the determination of specific circumstances of long-term
degenerative processes of a disease such as focal temporal
lobe epilepsy, which sometimes will lead to additional
frontal hypometabolism (Jokeit et al. 1997).

The conclusions drawn by Berent and Giordani that
memory encoding, storage and retrieval processes may be
mediated by different brain regions and that different forms
of content-varying memories (e.g. episodic as opposed to
procedural memories) are mediated by different neural networks, are well supported by recent dynamic imaging
studies (Fink et al. 1996; Tulving et al. 1996; Markowitsch

et al. 1997a), as well as by reports based on other methods
(Markowitsch 1995b; Wilding and Rugg 1996) (see Figure
7.2).

While Berent and Giordani point out that the higher
resolution of fMRI in comparison to PET is a main advantage of fMRI, this difference in resolution is minimized
in new generation PET scanners (Wienhard et al. 1994).
Functional MRI does seem, however, to possess greater
flexibility and versatility in cognitive neuroscience studies
as it can, for instance, be used repeatedly within short
intervals, while the radioactive tracing required by PET
and SPECT restricts these techniques' repeated application within a short time.

NEUROPATHOLOGY AND COGNITIVE
DETERIORATION

An invaluable resource for specialists as well as nonspecial-
ists is the very scholarly chapter on neuropathology and
cognitive dysfunction provided by Testa and colleagues

(Chapter 3). The chapter provides valuable facts, substantial background information, as well as a state of the art review of probable causes, concomitants and consequences of neurodegenerative disease. Instructive figures enhance the clarity and broad perspective of the presentation. Tables 3.1–3.3, in particular, are a useful resource as they list the clinical and neuropathological criteria for various neurodegenerative diseases.

Testa and colleagues point to the common distinction between cortical and subcortical dementias as a convenient method for classifying and measuring clinical symptoms. Their description of AD, as well of other common cortical and subcortical degenerative diseases, makes obvious that different pathological changes or processes within a given disease contribute to different cognitive disturbances. At the same time, anatomical links existing among different diseases are elucidated.

During the next years it is likely that the debate initiated by Alzheimer (1907) and Kraepelin (1910) and largely discounted by Testa et al., namely that there are at least two forms (presenile, senile) of AD, might be rekindled. This debate might expand to a discussion of the possibility that additional disease types can be postulated given our increased knowledge gained from anatomical, biochemical, genetic and behavioral studies of neurodegenerative diseases.

Another line of potential research might involve elucidation of the anatomical, biochemical and possibly genetic, relationships between forms of PD and forms of AD. Braak et al. (1995, 1996) repeatedly emphasized that important components of the limbic system are damaged during the disease process in both AD and PD. Almost certainly the search for the best predictors of AD both from structural and behavioral perspectives will also continue.

BIOLOGICAL PERSPECTIVE OF NEURODEGENERATIVE DISEASES

Technical progress and the interaction of modern computer science and refined anatomical, genetic and pathological methodologies have resulted in a tremendous increase in knowledge about causes and consequences of neurodegenerative diseases. Studies using animals have helped to model disease onset, disease course and specific structure–function relations. Despite these advances we still do not know the underlying causes of most of the prevalent neurodegenerative diseases and our inferences, as far as they are based on dynamic imaging techniques, are indirect. The progress in neurodegenerative disease diagnosis continues to outstrip that made in treatment. Although the development of treatments can be more rational than in the past given our greater understanding of the biology of neurodegenerative disease (Chapter 21), current treatments for many, if not most, neurodegenerative diseases still lead to only a retardation in disease progression. Thus, many issues remain to be resolved before the biological basis of neurodegenerative diseases and cognitive impairment can be conceived as fundamentally understood.

REFERENCES

Alzheimer, A. 1907. Ueber eine eigenartige Erkrankung der Hirnrinde. *Allgemeine Zeitschrift für Psychiatrie.* 4: 146–148.

Babinsky, R., Spiske, K., Neufert, C., Engel, H. and Markowitsch, H.J. 1997. Attentional dysfunctions following left parietal infarction. *Neurology, Psychiatry and Brain Research.* 4: 139–142.

Blokland, A. 1996. Acetylcholine: A neurotransmitter for learning and memory? *Brain Research Reviews.* 21: 285–290.

Braak, H., Braak, E., Yilmazer, D., de Vos, R.A.I., Jansen, E.N.H., Bohl, J. and Jellinger, K. 1994. Amygdala pathology in Parkinson's disease. *Acta Neuropathologica.* 88: 493–500.

Braak, H., Braak, E., Yilmazer, D., Schultz, C., de Vos, R.A.I. and Jansen, E.N.H. 1995. Nigral and extranigral pathology in Parkinson's disease. *Journal of Neural Transmission.* 46: 15–31.

Braak, H., Braak, E., Yilmazer, D., de Vos, R.A.I., Jansen, E.N.H. and Bohl, J. 1996. Pattern of brain destruction in Parkinson's and Alzheimer's diseases. *Journal of Neural Transmission.* 103: 455–490.

Bremner, J.D., Krystal, J.H., Southwick, S.M. and Charney, D.S. 1995a. Functional neuroanatomical correlates of the effects of stress on memory. *Journal of Traumatic Stress*. 8: 527–553.

Bremner, J.D., Randall, P., Scott, T.M., Bronen, R.A., Seibyl, J.P., Southwick, S.M., Delaney, R.C., McCarthy, G., Charney, D.S. and Innis, R.B. 1995b. MRI-based measurement of hippo-campal volume in patients with combat-related posttraumatic stress disorder. *American Journal of Psychiatry*. 152: 973–981.

Buckner, R.L. and Tulving, E. 1995. Neuroimaging studies of memory: Theory and recent PET results. In *Handbook of Neuropsychology*, vol. 10, ed. F. Boller and J. Grafman, pp. 439–466. Amsterdam: Elsevier.

Calabrese, P., Holinka, B., Durwen, H.F., Haupts, M., Markowitsch, H.J. and Gehlen, W. 1997. Die Neuropsychologie des Parkinson Syndroms. In *Psychologie und Morbus Parkinson*, ed. P. Fuchs and D. Emmans pp. 15–41. Göttingen: Vandenhoek & Ruprecht.

Craik, F.I.M., Morris, L.W., Morris, R.G. and Loewen, E.R. 1990. Relations between source amnesia and frontal lobe functioning in older adults. *Psychology of Aging*. 5: 148–151.

De la Monte, S.M. 1989. Quantitation of cerebral atrophy in preclinical and end-stage Alzheimer's disease. *Annals of Neurology*. 25: 450–459.

Divac, I., Markowitsch, H.J. and Pritzel, M. 1978. Behavioral and anatomical consequences of small intrastriatal injections of kainic acid in the rat. *Brain Research*. 151: 523–532.

Ebeling, U. and von Cramon, D. 1992. Topography of the uncinate fascicle and adjacent temporal fiber tracts. *Acta Neurochirurgica*. 115: 143–148.

Fibiger, H.C. 1991. Cholinergic mechanisms in learning, memory and dementia: A review of recent evidence. *Trends in Neurosciences*. 14: 220–223.

Fink, G.R., Markowitsch, H.J., Reinkemeier, M., Bruckbauer, T., Kessler, J. and Heiss, W.-D. 1996. Cerebral representation of one's own past: Neural networks involved in autobiographical memory. *Journal of Neuroscience*. 16: 4275–4282.

Franzen, E.A. and Myers, R.E. 1973. Neural control of social behavior: Prefrontal and anterior temporal cortex. *Neuropsychologia*. 11: 141–157.

Giannakopoulos, P., Hof, P.R., Savioz, A., Guimon, J., Antonarakis, S.E. and Bouras, C. 1996. Early-onset dementias: Clinical, neuropathological and genetic characteristics. *Acta Neuropathologica*. 91: 451–465.

Goldenberg, G., Podreka, I., Pfaffelmeyer, N., Wessely, P. and Deecke, L. 1991. Thalamic ischemia in transient global amnesia: A SPECT study. *Neurology*. 41: 1748–1752.

Goldman-Rakic, P.S. and Friedman, H.R. 1991. The circuitry of working memory revealed by anatomy and metabolic imaging. In *Frontal lobe function and dysfunction*, ed. H.S. Levin, H.M. Eisenberg and A.L. Benton, pp. 72–91. New York: Oxford University Press.

Graham, K.S. and Hodges, J.R. 1997. Differentiating the roles of the hippocampal complex and the neocortex in long-term memory storage: Evidence from the study of semantic dementia and Alzheimer's disease. *Neuropsychology*. 11: 1–13.

Groen, J.J. and Endtz, L.J. 1982. Hereditary Pick's disease: Second re-examination of a large family and discussion of other hereditary cases, with particular reference to electroen-cephalography and computerized tomography. *Brain*. 105: 443–459.

Guldin, W.O. and Markowitsch, H.J. 1981. No detectable remote lesions following massive intrastriatal injections of ibotenic acid. *Brain Research*. 225: 446–451.

Guldin, W.O. and Markowitsch, H.J. 1982. Epidural kainate, but not ibotenate, produces lesions in local and distant regions of the brain. A comparison of the intracerebral actions of kainic acid and ibotenic acid. *Journal of Neuroscience Methods*. 5: 351–380.

Hall, M., Whaley, R., Robertson, K., Hamby, S., Wilkins, J. and Hall, C. 1996. The correlation between neuropsychological and neuroanatomic changes over time in asymptomatic and symptomatic HIV–1-infected individuals. *Neurology*. 46: 1697–1702.

Haupts, M., Calabrese, P., Babinsky, R., Markowitsch, H.J. and Gehlen, W. 1994. Everyday memory impairment, neuropsychological findings and physical disability in multiple sclerosis. *European Journal of Neurology*. 1: 159–163.

Hinkin, C.H., van Gorp, W.G., Satz, P., Marcotte, T., Durvasula, R.S., Wood, S., Campbell, L. and Baluda, M.R. 1996. Actual versus self-reported cognitive dysfunction in HIV–1 infection: Memory-metamemory dissociations. *Journal of Clinical and Experimental Neuropsychology*. 18: 431–443.

Hodges, J.R., Patterson, K., Oxbury, S. and Funnell, E. 1992. Semantic dementia: Progressive fluent aphasia with temporal lobe atrophy. *Brain*. 115: 1783–1806.

Irle, E., Wowra, B., Kunert, H.J., Hampl, J. and Kunze, S. 1992. Memory disturbances following anterior communicating artery rupture. *Annals of Neurology*. 31: 473–480.

Jacobs, A., Herholz, K., Pietrzyk, U., Würker, M., Wienhard, K. and Heiss, W-D. 1996. Diaschisis of specific cerebellar lobules: Pontine haematoma studies with high-resolution PET and MRI. *Journal of Neurology*. 243: 131–136.

Jacobsen, C.F. 1935. Functions of the frontal association area in primates. *A.M.A. Archives of Neurology and Psychiatry*. 33: 558–569.

Jokeit, H., Seitz, R., Markowitsch, H.J., Neumann, N., Ebner, A. and Witte, O.W. 1997. Prefrontal asymmetric interictal glucose hypometabolism and cognitive impairment in patients with temporal lobe epilepsy. *Brain*. 120: 2283–2294.

Kessler, J., Irle, E. and Markowitsch, H.J. 1986. Korsakoff and alcoholic subjects are severely impaired in animal tasks of association memory. *Neuropsychologia*. 24: 671–680.

Kessler, J., Markowitsch, H.J. and Bast-Kessler, C. 1987. Memory of alcoholic patients, including Korsakoff's, tested with a Brown-Peterson paradigm. *Archives of Psychology*. 101: 115–132.

Kieburtz, K., Ketonen, L., Cox, C., Grossman, H., Holloway, R., Booth, H., Hickey, C., Feigin, A. and Caine, E.D. 1996. Cognitive performance and regional brain volume in human immunodeficiency virus type 1 infection. *Archives of Neurology*. 53: 155–158.

Kraepelin, E. 1910. *Das senile und präsenile Irresein*. Leipzig: Barth.

Law, W.A., Martin, A., Mapou, R.L., Roller, T.L., Salazar, A.M., Temoshok, L.R. and Rundell, J.R. 1994. Working memory in individuals with HIV infection. *Journal of Clinical and Experimental Neuropsychology*. 16: 173–182.

Markowitsch, H.J. 1988a. Diencephalic amnesia: A reorientation towards tracts? *Brain Research Reviews*. 13: 351–370.

Markowitsch, H.J. 1988b. Individual differences in memory performance and the brain. In *Information processing by the brain*, ed. H.J. Markowitsch, pp. 125–148. Toronto: H. Huber.

Markowitsch, H.J. 1988c. Anatomical and functional organization of the primate prefrontal cortical system. In *Comparative primate biology*, vol. IV, *Neurosciences*, ed. H.D. Steklis and J. Erwin, pp. 99–153. New York: Alan R. Liss.

Markowitsch, H.J. 1992. Diencephalic amnesia. In *Trastornos de la Memoria*, ed. D. Barcia Salorio, pp. 269–336. Barcelona: Editorial MCR.

Markowitsch, H.J. 1994. The thalamus and memory. In *Fatal familial insomnia. inherited prion diseases, sleep and the thalamus*, ed. C. Guilleminault, E. Lugaresi, P. Montagnu and P.-L. Gambetti, pp. 117–127. New York: Raven Press.

Markowitsch, H.J. 1995a. Which brain regions are critically involved in the retrieval of old episodic memory? *Brain Research Reviews*. 21: 117–127.

Markowitsch, H.J. 1995b. Anatomical basis of memory disorders. In *The cognitive neurosciences*, ed. M.S. Gazzaniga, pp. 665–679. Cambridge, MA: MIT Press.

Markowitsch, H.J. and Calabrese, P. 1996. Commonalities and discrepancies in the relationship between behavioural outcome and the results of neuroimaging in brain-damaged patients. *Behavioural Neurology*. 9: 45–55.

Markowitsch, H.J., Calabrese, P., Würker, M. Durwen, H.F., Kessler, J., Babinsky, R., Brechtelsbauer, D., Heuser, L. and Gehlen, W. 1994. The amygdala's contribution to memory – A PET-study on two patients with Urbach-Wiethe disease. *NeuroReport*. 5: 1349–1352.

Markowitsch, H.J., Emmans, D., Irle, E., Streicher, M. and Preilowski, B. 1985. Cortical and subcortical afferent connections of the primate's temporal pole: A study of rhesus monkeys, squirrel monkeys and marmosets. *Journal of Comparative Neurology*. 242: 425–458.

Markowitsch, H.J., Fink, G.R., Thöne, A.I.M., Kessler, J. and Heiss, W.-D. 1997a. Persistent psychogenic amnesia with a PET-proven organic basis. *Cognitive Neuropsychiatry*. 2: 135–158.

Markowitsch, H.J., Kessler, J., Van der Ven, C., Weber-Luxenburger, G. and Heiss, W.-D. 1998. Psychic trauma causing grossly reduced brain metabolism and cognitive deterioration. *Neuropsychologia*. 36: 77–82.

Markowitsch, H.J., Weber-Luxenburger, G., Ewald, K., Kessler, J. and Heiss, W.-D. 1997b. Patients with heart attacks are no valid models for medial temporal lobe amnesia. A neuropsychological and FDG-PET study with consequences for memory research. *European Journal of Neurology*. 4: 178–184.

McArthur, J.C., Hoover, D.R., Bacellar, H., Miller, E.N., Cohen, B.A., Becker, J.T., Graham, N.M.H., McArthur, J.H., Selnes, O.A., Jacobson, L.P., Visscher, B., Concha, M. and Saah, A. for the Multicenter AIDS Cohort Study. 1993. Dementia in AIDS patients: Incidence and risk factors. *Neurology*. 43: 2245–2252.

Myers, R.E. 1972. Role of prefrontal and anterior temporal cortex in social behavior and affect in monkeys. *Acta Neurobiologica Experimentalis*. 32: 567–579.

Neary, D., Snowden, J.S., Bowen, D.A., Sims, N.R., Mann, D.M.A., Benton, J.S., Northen, B., Yates, P.O. and Davison, A.N. 1986a. Neuropsychological syndromes in presenile dementia due to cerebral atrophy. *Journal of Neurology, Neurosurgery and Psychiatry*. 49: 163–174.

Neary, D., Snowden, J.S., Mann, D.M.A., Bowen, D.M., Sims, N.R., Northen, B., Yates, P.O. and Davison, A.N. 1986b. Alzheimer's disease: A correlative study. *Journal of Neurology, Neurosurgery and Psychiatry*. 49: 229–237.

Nieuwenhuys, R. 1985. *Chemoarchitecture of the brain*. Berlin: Springer Verlag.

Parkinson, J. 1817. *An essay on the shaking palsy*. London: Nelly and Jones.

Pearson, R.C.A. and Powell, T.P.S. 1987. Anterograde vs. retrograde degeneration of the nucleus basalis medialis in Alzheimer's disease. *Journal of Neural Transmission*. Suppl. 24: 139–146.

Peavy, G., Jacobs, D., Salmon, D.P., Butters, N. Delis DC, Taylor, M., Massman, P., Stout, J.C., Heindel, W.C., Kirson, D., Atkinson, J.H., Chandler, J.L., Grant, I. and the HNRC Group. 1994. Verbal memory performance of patients with human immunodeficiency virus infection: Evidence of subcortical dysfunction. *Journal of Clinical and Experimental Neuropsychology*. 16: 508–523.

Price, D.L. 1986. New perspectives on Alzheimer's disease. *Annual Review of Neuroscience*. 9: 489–512.

Price, D.L., Whitehouse P.J., Struble, R.G., Clark, A.W., Coyle, J.T., DeLong, M.D. and Hedreen, J.C. 1982. Basal forebrain cholinergic systems in Alzheimer's disease and related dementias. *Neuroscience Commentaries*. 1: 84–92.

Pritzel, M. and Markowitsch, H.J. 1997. Sexueller Dimorphismus: Inwieweit bedingen Unterschiede im Aufbau des Gehirns zwischen Mann und Frau auch Unterschiede im Verhalten? *Psychologische Rundschau*. 48: 16–31.

Reinkemeier, M., Markowitsch, H.J., Rauch, B. and Kessler, J. 1997. Memory systems for people's names: A case study of a patient with deficits in recalling, but not learning people's names. *Neuropsychologia*. 35: 677–684.

Rieger, B. and Markowitsch, H.J. 1996. Implicit and explicit mnestic performance of patients with prefrontal, medial temporal and basal ganglia damage. *Neurology, Psychiatry and Brain Research*. 4: 53–74.

Roediger, H.L., III 1990. Implicit memory: A commentary. *Bulletin of the Psychonomic Society*. 28: 373–380.

Roediger, H.L., Rajaram, S. and Srinivas, K. 1990. Specifying criteria for postulating memory systems. *Annals of the New York Academy of Sciences*. 608: 572–595.

Röhrenbach, C. and Markowitsch, H.J. 1997. Störungen im Bereich exekutiver und überwachender Funktionen: der Präfrontalbereich. In *Enzyklopädie der Psychologie,* Themenbereich C, Serie I, Bd 2: Klinische Neuropsychologie, ed. H.J. Markowitsch, pp. 329–493. Göttingen: Hogrefe.

Rousseaux, M., Godefroy, O., Cabaret, M. and Bernati, T. 1996. Syndrome dysexécutif et troubles du contrôle moteur dans les lésions préfrontales médio-basales et cingulaires. *Revue Neurologique*. 152: 517–527.

Sapolsky, R.M. 1996a. Why stress is bad for your brain. *Science*. 273: 749–750.

Sapolsky, R.M. 1996b. Stress, glucocorticoids and damage to the nervous system: The current state of confusion. *Stress*. 1: 1–19.

Sarter, M., Berntson, G.G. and Cacioppo, J.T. 1996. Brain imaging and cognitive neuroscience: Toward strong inference in attributing function to structure. *American Psychologist*. 51: 13–21.

Selnes, O.A., Galai, N., Bacellar, H., Miller, E.N., Becker, J.T., Wesch, J., Van Gorp, W. and McArthur, J.C. 1995. Cognitive performance after progression to AIDS: A longitudinal study from the Multicenter AIDS cohort study. *Neurology*. 45: 267–275.

Shimamura, A.P., Berry, J.M., Mangels, J.A., Rusting, C.L. and Jurica, P.J. 1995. Memory and cognitive abilities in university professors: Evidence for successful aging. *Psychological Science*. 6: 271–277.

Squire, L.R. 1987. *Memory and brain*. New York: Oxford University Press.

Tulving, E. 1993. Varieties of consciousness and levels of awareness in memory. In *Attention: Selection, awareness and control. A tribute to Donald Broadbent*, ed. A. Baddeley and L. Weiskrantz, pp. 283–299. Oxford: Oxford University Press.

Tulving, E. 1994. What are the memory systems of 1994? In *Memory systems 1994*, ed. D.L. Schacter and E. Tulving, pp. 1–38. Cambridge: MIT Press.

Tulving, E. 1995. Organization of memory: Quo vadis? In *The cognitive neurosciences*, ed. M.S. Gazzaniga, pp. 839–847. Cambridge: MIT Press.

Tulving, E. and Markowitsch, H.J. 1994. Why should animal models of memory model human memory? *Behavioral Brain Sciences*. 17: 498–499.

Tulving, E., Markowitsch, H.J., Craik, F.I.M., Habib, R. and Houle, S. 1996. Novelty and familiarity activations in PET studies of memory encoding and retrieval. *Cerebral Cortex*. 6: 71–79.

Wienhard, K., Dahlborn, M., Eriksson, L., Michel, C., Bruckbauer, T., Pietrzyk, U. and Heiss, W.D. 1994. The ECAT EXACT HR: Performance of a new high resolution positron scanner. *Journal of Computer Assisted Tomography*. 18: 110–118.

Wilding, E.L. and Rugg, M.D. 1996. An event-related potential study of recognition memory with and without retrieval of source. *Brain*. 119: 889–905.

PART II

Cognitive perspectives

8 The role of executive deficits in memory disorders in neurodegenerative disease

ADRIAN M. OWEN, BARBARA J. SAHAKIAN
AND TREVOR W. ROBBINS

INTRODUCTION

There is now overwhelming evidence that patients with neurodegenerative disorders, including Parkinson's disease (PD), Huntington's disease (HD), progressive supranuclear palsy (also known as Steele-Richardson-Olszewski syndrome), multiple system atrophy, Alzheimer's disease (AD), Korsakoff's syndrome and fronto-striatal dementia exhibit diverse patterns of cognitive impairment that can include deficits of 'executive function'. The term 'executive function' generally refers to those mechanisms by which performance is optimized in situations requiring the simultaneous operation of a number of different cognitive processes (Baddeley 1986). Executive functioning is required, therefore, when sequences of responses must be generated and scheduled and when novel plans of action must be formulated and carried out. The frontal lobes have long been known to play an important role in executive functioning, although the fact that the 'dysexecutive syndrome' may be observed in patients with damage to other brain regions (Morris et al. 1990), suggests that an equivalence between the prefrontal cortex and executive functioning cannot be assumed. In addition, much of the research on executive deficits in neurodegenerative groups has focused on broad descriptions of individual patient groups and how their behaviour might best be characterized using standard clinical neuropsychological tools. For example, impairments on the Wisconsin Card Sorting Test (Grant and Berg 1948), a classic test of executive function, have been described in many neurodegenerative groups including PD (Lees and Smith 1983), progressive supranuclear palsy (Pillon et al. 1986) and HD (Josiassen et al. 1983). Tasks such as the Wisconsin Card Sorting Test place significant demands on many different aspects of cognitive

function some, or all, of which may be impaired in a given patient and performance is ultimately determined, therefore, by a complex interaction between multiple dysfunctional processes. In recent years, however, improved methods of assessment combined with a theory-driven approach to task design has led to great advances in our understanding of the fundamental mechanisms which mediate these higher-order cognitive processes. As a direct result, it has been possible to define impairments of executive function in neurodegenerative diseases more precisely, in terms of the specific neuropsychological mechanisms involved.

FUNCTIONAL ANATOMY OF EXECUTIVE FUNCTION: WORKING MEMORY

One aspect of executive function that has received much attention in recent years is working memory. The term 'working memory' was introduced into the experimental psychology literature by Baddeley (1986) to replace the existing concept of a passive short-term memory store and to emphasize, within a single model, both the temporary storage and the 'on-line' manipulation of information that occurs during a wide variety of cognitive activities. Since then, considerable evidence has accumulated to suggest that the lateral surface of the frontal-lobe plays a critical role in certain aspects of working memory. This evidence comes from the study of patients with excisions of frontal cortex (Petrides and Milner 1982; Owen et al. 1990, 1995a, 1996c; for a review, see Petrides 1989), from lesion and electrophysiological recording work in nonhuman primates (Goldman-Rakic 1987; Petrides 1994) and more recently, from functional neuroimaging studies in humans

Figure 8.1. Schematic drawing of
the lateral surface of the human
brain to indicate the location of the
dorsolateral frontal cortex (areas 9,
46 and 9/46), and the ventrolateral
frontal cortex (areas 45 and 47/12).
The numbering scheme is taken
from the recent cytoarchitectonic
reparcellation of the human frontal
cortex by Petrides and Pandya
(1994). ifs: inferior frontal sulcus;
sfs: superior frontal sulcus.

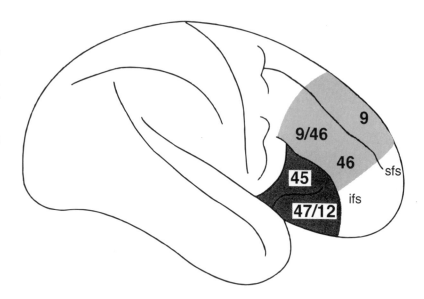

(Jonides et al. 1993; Petrides et al. 1993a,b; McCarthy et al. 1994; Smith et al. 1995, 1996; Courtney et al. 1996; Gold et al. 1996; Goldberg et al. 1996; Owen et al. 1996a,b; Sweeney et al. 1996). In the monkey it has been shown that lesions confined to one part of the dorsolateral frontal cortex, namely the cortex lining the sulcus principalis (i.e. area 46) result in severe impairments on tests of spatial working memory, such as spatial delayed alternation and delayed response (Goldman-Rakic 1987; Fuster 1989; Chapter 1). Similarly, monkeys with lesions limited to the mid-dorsal part of the lateral frontal cortex are severely impaired on certain nonspatial working memory tasks (Petrides 1988, 1991, 1994). On the basis of this and related evidence, a general theoretical framework regarding the role of the different regions of the lateral frontal cortex in working memory processing has recently been described (Petrides 1994). According to this view, there are two executive processing systems within the lateral frontal cortex which mediate different aspects of working memory through reciprocal connections to modality specific posterior cortical association areas. The first stage of interaction between these posterior association areas and frontal regions occurs primarily within the ventrolateral frontal cortex (i.e. areas 45 and 47). Thus, these areas (see Figure 8.1) are concerned primarily with the active organization of sequences of responses based on conscious, explicit retrieval of information from short-term memory. By contrast, the mid-dorsolateral frontal cortex

(dorsal area 46 and area 9) is assumed to constitute a second level of interaction of executive processes with memory and is recruited only when the active manipulation and monitoring of information within working memory is required (Figure 8.1). This two-stage model of lateral frontal cortical function, by which two anatomically and cytoarchitectonically distinct regions of the frontal lobe are linked with different aspects of executive processing, describes how information is both retained and manipulated within working memory to optimize performance on a variety of tasks.

While the human and animal studies described above support the view that different regions of the prefrontal cortex play distinct roles in working memory, this involvement appears to depend critically on reciprocal connections with more posterior neural structures. Goldman-Rakic (1990) has described several multisynaptic connections between the prefrontal cortex and the hippocampal formation and has speculated that these connections imply a reciprocal functional relationship in working memory (Goldman-Rakic et al. 1984). In keeping with this suggestion, it is well established that damage to the hippocampus and related structures in rats produces severe and enduring deficits in spatial working memory tasks (Olton et al. 1978; Olton and Papas 1979; Rawlins and Olton 1982; Rawlins and Tsaltas 1983; Aggleton et al. 1986; Sziklas and Petrides 1993). Thus, contemporary accounts view working memory as a distributed process that critically depends on a close functional interaction between regions of the lateral frontal cortex and more posterior cortical structures (including the hippocampus).

WORKING MEMORY AND NEURODEGENERATIVE DISEASE: AN OVERVIEW

In recent years, a number of studies have assessed working memory in patients with PD (Gotham et al. 1988; Morris et al. 1988; Bradley et al. 1989; Cooper et al. 1991, 1993; Singh et al. 1991; Owen et al. 1992, 1993, 1995b; Postle et al. 1993). Although methodological differences preclude direct comparisons between studies, in general the results lend support to the notion that deterioration of working memory processes in these patients progresses in parallel with the degeneration of motor functions that characterizes this disorder. For example, while nonmedicated patients with mild clinical symptoms have been repeatedly shown to be unimpaired on a test of spatial working memory (Morris et al. 1988; Owen et al. 1992), deficits on the same task have been observed in medicated patients and particularly in those with severe clinical symptoms (Owen et al. 1992). Further comparisons between studies also suggest that some aspects of working memory may be affected earlier in the course of PD than others. For example, Bradley et al. (1989) found that patients with mild to moderate PD were impaired on a test of visuospatial working memory, whilst performance on an analogous test of verbal working memory was unaffected. Similarly, Postle et al. (1993) and Owen et al. (1997) have demonstrated that, while spatial working memory is impaired in medicated patients with mild PD, working memory for visual shapes is relatively preserved.

Working memory performance has also been investigated in HD using a variety of spatial (Orsini et al. 1987; Lange et al. 1995; Lawrence et al. 1996), visual (Orsini et al. 1987; Rich et al. 1996) and verbal (Orsini et al. 1987), tasks. For example, Rich et al. (1996) have shown that HD patients perform significantly worse than controls on all versions of the self-ordered pointing task devised by Petrides and Milner (1982), making more returns to pictures or abstract designs that have already been selected. Polymodal deficits were also observed by Orsini et al. (1987), who demonstrated that both spatial span and digit span were similarly impaired in HD. In addition, on both tasks the HD patients performed more poorly than a group of patients with PD.

Deficits have also been described in other neurodegenerative groups, including patients with AD (Baddeley et al. 1986) on a variety of executive tasks that could be said to involve working memory. The results of cross-sectional comparisons between such studies or between different neurodegenerative groups are difficult to evaluate in terms the likely neuropathological mechanisms underlying the deficits observed, for a number of reasons. Principally, many different tasks have been employed which vary, both in terms of the modality of the stimuli used and in terms of the relative emphasis on different executive processes. Given the theoretical and anatomical arguments outlined above, such tasks are likely to depend on different components of a widely distributed neural system. Second, the different neurodegenerative groups studied often differ markedly in terms of their clinical characteristics such as age of onset, illness duration, rates of cognitive decline and medication regimes. Third, many of the standard clinical neuropsychological tasks that have been employed to test executive function in elderly neurodegenerative groups have not been adequately validated in a normal ageing population. Executive functions such as working memory appear to be particularly vulnerable to the effects of normal ageing (van Gorp and Mahler 1990), a pattern which may reflect the disproportionate reduction in neuron density in the prefrontal cortex and basal-ganglia (Haug and Eggers 1991).

TOWARDS A THEORETICALLY DRIVEN APPROACH

In recent years, some of these issues have been addressed directly in a series of studies that have attempted to use a standardized battery of computerized tasks (The Cambridge Neuropsychological Test Automated Battery: CANTAB), including test of executive function, to assess a broad range of neurodegenerative groups (Sahakian et al. 1988, 1990; Lange et al. 1992, 1995; Owen et al. 1992, 1993; Robbins et al. 1992; Lawrence et al. 1996). Two of these tests, which assess different aspects of spatial memory, are of particular relevance to the subject of this chapter as they can be related directly to contemporary accounts of working memory. Thus, broadly speaking, they map directly onto the two frontal lobe (ventrolateral and dorsolateral), executive systems proposed by Petrides (1994), emphasizing the short-term retention and execution of sequences of spatial responses on the one hand and active, 'on-line' manipulation of spatial information within a spatial search task on the other. Moreover, the functional architecture subserving performance on these tasks has been investigated using positron emission tomography (PET) (Owen et al. 1996b), the results of which concur fully with the findings from comparisons between groups of neurosurgical patients with frontal lobe or temporal lobe excisions (Owen et al. 1990, 1995a). Finally, standardization studies using large samples ($N>340$) of healthy volunteers have provided important information about the effects of normal ageing on task performance (Robbins, 1996).

The first of these two tasks, is a computerized version of the block tapping test devised by Corsi (described in Milner 1971). Each trial begins with the same arrangement of nine squares, presented on the screen in a pseudo random pattern. Subjects are instructed to observe the boxes because some will change color, one after the other. Their task is to remember the location and the sequential order of the boxes that change. During each series, one box changes color for three seconds and then returns to white before the next in the sequence changes to the same color. The subject is then prompted by a tone to repeat the sequence by touching the boxes in the same order. After each successful trial, the number of boxes changing in the next sequence is increased, from two up to a maximum of nine boxes. Performance is scored according to the *highest* level at which the subject successfully recalls the sequence of boxes. Clearly, this task emphasizes the short-term retention and reproduction of spatial information within working memory but requires little manipulation of that information and, in this sense, is likely to involve ventro-lateral frontal areas according to the model proposed by Petrides (1994). A recent functional imaging study combining both PET and magnetic resonance imaging (MRI) has verified that this is the case (Owen et al. 1996b). When normal volunteer subjects performed a modified version of this computerized task, a significant region of increased cerebral blood flow (CBF) was observed in ventrolateral frontal cortex (area 47) in the right hemisphere. No significant changes were observed in more dorsolateral areas of frontal cortex, even when subjects were required to learn and reproduce a 'supra-span' sequence of eight boxes.

In terms of the absolute measure of spatial span, this task is not sensitive to unilateral temporal lobe damage, or amygdalo–hippocampectomy (Owen et al. 1995a). Patients with frontal lobe damage are also unimpaired according to this gross measure (Owen et al. 1990), although deficits are observed when one considers the number of trials required to reach maximum span.

The second test of frontal executive function is essentially a modification of a task used by Passingham (1985) to examine the effects of prefrontal cortex lesions in primates and is conceptually similar to the 'radial arm maze' which has been successfully used to assess working memory in rats (Olton 1982). Subjects are required to 'search through' a number of colored boxes presented on a computer screen (by touching each one) in order to find blue 'tokens' which are hidden inside by the computer. The object is to avoid those boxes in which a token has already been found. Like the span task described above, this test places a significant load on memory for spatial information, although unlike that test, it also requires the active reorganization and manipulation of information within working memory, factors which interact closely with the more fundamental mnemonic requirements to affect performance. Thus, control subjects often adopt a search strategy which involves retracing a systematic 'route' and 'editing' or 'monitoring' those locations where tokens have been found previously. This searching strategy can be captured by an index which is demonstrably uncontaminated by overall mnemonic performance (Owen et al. 1990, 1996c) and yet which correlates highly with such performance (Robbins 1996). This strategy, which has been described in detail elsewhere (Owen et al. 1990, 1997), is illustrated in Figure 8.2.

The emphasis on 'strategy' in this task clearly implicates the dorsolateral frontal executive processing system according to the model proposed recently by Petrides (1994). It is important to note, therefore, that in a recent PET study, significant changes in CBF were clearly observed in the right mid-dorsolateral frontal cortex (areas 46 and 9), when subjects performed a slightly modified version of this task (Owen et al. 1996b). In addition, as in the spatial span task, the ventrolateral frontal cortex was also activated, confirming that more basic mnemonic factors also contribute to overall performance on this test. Thus, the spatial search appears to be governed by two major factors, one related to short-term spatial memory and the other to strategic processes, which depend upon ventrolateral and dorsolateral regions of the frontal cortex, respectively. The possibility that these two levels of exec-

Spatial working memory; 'frontal' strategy

Protocol of AW

```
SET 15 (6 boxes)
8   5   1
8   3
5   8   2
8   4
8
2   5

SET 16 (6 boxes)
10   6   12
10   0    1
10   6
0    1   10
8
1    0

SET 19 (8 boxes)
13  12   8   9
12   8   2
1
13  12
9    6   4
2    1   9   12  13   4   9   8
1    9   6
12   8   2    4   6   9   8   12   4   2   13

SET 20 (8 boxes)
11  10
6   11   1
14   2   4    6
11   5   4
2   14   1   11   6    5
14   2
0   11
4    6   1   14
```

Spatial working memory; 'perfect' use of strategy

Protocol of HM

```
SET 15 (6 boxes)
1   3   2
1   3
1   4   5
1   4
1
8

SET 16 (6 boxes)
1   6   10
1   6    0
1   6
1   8
1
12
```

Spatial arrangement of boxes; key

```
        1           1 4                 2
                                0    4
                3
                            1 1           5
                       1 3
        6                                8
                                  7
        9   1 0                         1 2
```

```
SET 19 (8 boxes)
1   6   9   13
1   6   9
1
6   12
6   8
6   4
6
2

SET 20 (8 boxes)
1   6
1   10  14
1   10  11   5
1   10  11
1   10   4   2
1   10
1
4
```

Figure 8.2. Left: a typical response pattern from one of the frontal lobe patients (AW), illustrating how the 'strategy' score is calculated. Right: corresponding normal response pattern from a typical healthy control subject (HM). On the right hand side, the spatial arrangement of boxes as they appear on the screen is illustrated schematically. For each subject, four example trials ('sets') are shown. Horizontal rows represent the choices (boxes) made during each search through the array and vertical columns represent the total number of searches made during each problem. The strategy score is estimated by totalling the number of novel boxes used to initiate a search sequence (all such boxes are underlined). In this example the strategy scores for the patient and for the control are 18 and 9, respectively. Numbers in bold represent 'between search' errors. Numbers in outline represent 'within search' errors. For a full description, see Owen et al. 1990; 1992; 1993; 1995 ; 1997.

utive processing constitute distinct functional systems which are differentially involved in these two tasks is suggested further by a recent large-sample factor analysis of normal control performance which has identified separate mnemonic and strategic factors in performance (Robbins 1996).

Neurosurgical patients with frontal lobe damage are significantly impaired on this 'strategic' spatial searching task and make more returns to boxes in which a token has previously been found ('between search' errors) even at the simplest levels of task difficulty (Owen et al. 1990, 1995a). In addition, these patients are less efficient in the use of the repetitive searching strategy described above, confirming that at least some of their impairment in spatial working memory may arise secondarily from a more fundamental deficit in the use of organizational strategies. A typical response pattern from one of the frontal lobe patients is presented in Figure 8.2 (left), along with the corresponding normal response pattern from a typical healthy control subject (Figure 8.2, right). This task is also sensitive to deficits in patients with temporal lobe damage and in patients with selective amygdalo-hippocampectomy (Owen et al. 1995a, 1997), although only at the most extreme level of task difficulty (i.e. eight boxes). Moreover, unlike the frontal lobe patients, the temporal lobe groups utilize a normal and effective searching strategy.

In recent years, these two tasks have been used to draw theoretically driven comparisons between groups of

Figure 8.3. Performance on the
spatial span task for the **(a)** non
medicated PD patients with mild
clinical symptoms (NMED PD),
medicated PD patients with mild
clinical symptoms (MED PD
(mild)) and medicated PD patients
with severe clinical symptoms
(MED PD (severe)) (from Owen et
al. 1992). **(b)** Medicated patients
with severe clinical symptoms tested
both 'on' and 'off' levodopa
medication (from Lange et al. 1992).
(c) Patients with MSA and PSP
(SRO) (from Robbins et al., 1994).
(d) Patients with mild HD (from
Lawrence et al. 1996), and patients
with severe HD or AD matched for
severity of dementia (from Lange et
al. 1995). Bars represent standard
error of the mean (s.e.m.)

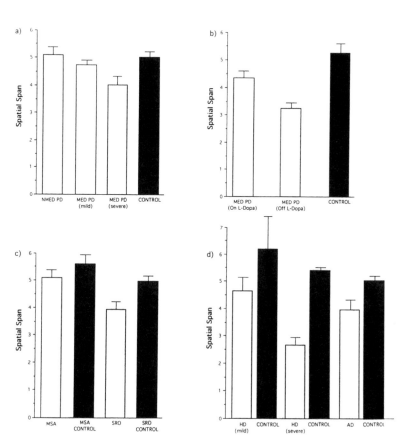

patients at different stages of PD (Owen et al. 1992, 1993), between patients with PD, progressive supranuclear palsy and multiple system atrophy (Robbins et al. 1992, 1994) and between groups of patients with HD and AD matched for degree of dementia (Lange et al. 1995).

WORKING MEMORY IN PARKINSON'S DISEASE: THE EFFECTS OF DISEASE SEVERITY

Several recent studies have compared the performance of different groups of patients with PD on these two spatial memory tests which tap demonstrably different aspects of executive function (Morris et al. 1988; Lange et al. 1992; Owen et al. 1992; Robbins et al. 1994). A central model for much of this work has been the concept of cortico-striatal loops (Alexander et al. 1986), which emphasizes the functional inter-relationships between the neocortex and the striatum. Of particular interest is the fact that the princi-

pal target of basal ganglia outflow appears to be the frontal lobes. Furthermore, different sectors of the striatum project to specific premotor regions such as the supplementary motor area or to discrete regions within dorsal and ventral regions of the frontal cortex which have been implicated in higher cognitive functions. A cross-sectional study of patients with PD clearly demonstrated that levodopa medicated and nonmedicated patients at different stages of the disease can be differentiated in terms of their performance on the test of spatial span (Owen et al. 1992) that is known to involve regions of the ventrolateral frontal lobe (Owen et al. 1996b). Thus, a significant impairment was only observed in a subgroup of patients who were medicated and had severe clinical symptoms (Figure 8.3a). This effect was relatively specific as none of the three PD groups was impaired on a test of pattern recognition memory known to be sensitive to temporal lobe, but not frontal lobe, damage (Owen et al. 1995a). It is also unlikely that high doses of dopaminergic medication adversely affect performance in this group as a parallel study of 10

Figure 8.4. Performance on the Self-Ordered Spatial Search task for **(a)** non-medicated PD patients with mild clinical symptoms (NMED PD), medicated PD patients with mild clinical symptoms (MED PD (mild)) and medicated PD patients with severe clinical symptoms (MED PD (severe)) (from Owen et al. 1992). **(b)** Medicated patients with severe clinical symptoms tested both 'on' and 'off' levodopa medication (from Lange et al. 1992) **(c)** Patients with MSA and PSP (SRO) (from Robbins et al. 1994) **(d)** Patients with mild HD (from Lawrence et al. 1996), and patients with severe HD or AD matched for severity of dementia (from Lange et al. 1995). Bars represent standard error of the mean (s.e.m.)

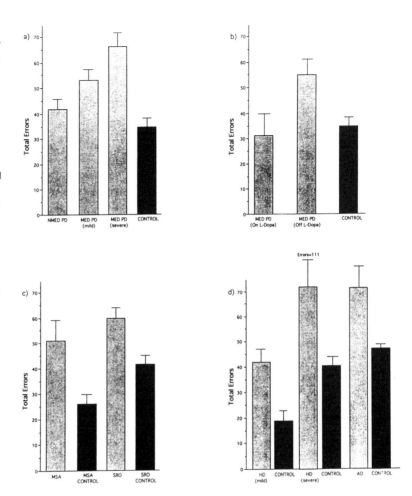

patients with severe PD has demonstrated that levodopa withdrawal severely disrupts performance on the spatial span task (Figure 8.3b) but does not affect pattern recognition memory (Lange et al. 1992).

In general, patients with PD are more impaired on the strategic searching task (Figure 8.4a) which emphasizes functions known to involve dorsolateral regions of the frontal cortex (Owen et al. 1996b). Thus, like the frontal lobe group, medicated PD patients with both mild and severe clinical symptoms made more errors than matched controls and a non-significant trend towards impairment was observed in the nonmedicated PD group (Owen et al. 1992, 1993). Unlike the frontal lobe patients however, none of the three PD groups was significantly impaired on the measure of task strategy when assessed independently, although subsequently when the same two medicated PD groups were combined for matched comparisons with

other basal ganglia groups (see Robbins et al. 1994), 'frontal like' strategic deficits were suggested. Again, it is unlikely that dopaminergic medication plays any detrimental role in the performance of the medicated PD groups on this spatial self-ordered searching task because controlled withdrawal of levodopa results in a twofold increase in the total number of errors made (Lange et al. 1992; Figure 8.4b).

The results of these studies clearly demonstrate that patients at different stages of PD can be differentiated in terms of their performance on two tests of spatial memory known to involve different regions of the frontal lobe. Among the patients with PD, there is an apparent increase in severity and broadening of spatial memory impairments as patients show increasing clinical disability. Thus, when the task simply involved the retention and recall of a spatial sequence within working memory, deficits were only observed in a subgroup of patients with severe clinical symptoms. By contrast, when the task required the active manipulation of spatial information within working memory, deficits were observed in medicated patients with both mild and severe clinical symptoms. These differences cannot simply be explained in terms of the concurrent deterioration of motor function in these patients because of the controlled nature and design of these tests. The results do, in fact, concur fully with more extensive neuropsychological evaluations of these same patient groups which suggest that the pattern of cognitive impairment in PD emerges and subsequently progresses according to a defined sequence which evolves in parallel with the motor deficits that characterize the disorder (Owen et al. 1992, 1993). This apparent 'progression' on tests which are known to emphasize different aspects of executive function and appear to depend critically on different regions within the lateral frontal cortex could simply reflect a global difference in cognitive capacity between patients with mild and severe PD. This seems unlikely, however, as the three PD groups could not be distinguished in terms of their performance on a test of pattern recognition memory. This test is not sensitive to frontal lobe excisions, although significant deficits have been observed in patients with temporal lobe lesions (Owen et al. 1995a) and with both mild and moderate dementia of the Alzheimer type (Sahakian et al. 1990; Sahgal et al. 1991). Furthermore, in the series of studies described here, the PD patients were clinically diagnosed as nondemented and were screened for dementia using both the Mini Mental State Examination (Folstein et al. 1975) and the Kendrick Object Learning Test (Kendrick 1985). The possibility that concomitant depression in PD may play a significant role in the progressive pattern of deficits observed can also be discounted because clinical measures of depression did not correlate with performance on either of the spatial memory tests (Owen et al. 1992). In addition, a quite distinct pattern of deficits on these and other tests of cognitive function, has been reported recently for a population of clinically depressed subjects (Elliot et al. 1996).

The question therefore arises as to whether a plausible neural account might be formulated for this progressive sequence of working memory deficits in patients with PD. Nondopaminergic forms of pathology, including noradrenergic, serotonergic and cholinergic deafferentation of the cortex (Agid et al. 1987), may play a significant role in

some of the cognitive deficits observed (Chapters 3 and 4). Similarly, cortical Lewy bodies, which may occur even in the early stages of PD, may play a contributory role (Byrne et al. 1989; Gibb et al. 1989). The fact that both tasks are extremely sensitive to the effects of controlled levodopa withdrawal in a group of patients with severe PD (Lange et al. 1992) suggests a predominantly dopaminergic substrate for both deficits. Moreover, recent anatomical and neuropathological evidence suggests that this evolving pattern of impairments may be linked to what is known about the likely spatiotemporal progression of dopamine depletion within the striatum in relation to the terminal distribution of its cortical afferents. This is highlighted by a detailed postmortem neurochemical analysis which shows uneven patterns of striatal dopamine loss in patients dying with idiopathic PD (Kish et al. 1988). The study confirms the well-documented finding that the putamen is more severely depleted than the caudate nucleus and extends the analysis to show that the caudal putamen is more affected than the more rostral portions. In view of anatomical and electrophysiological evidence, the putamen is generally implicated in the motor deficits associated with PD.

Dopamine levels in the caudate nucleus, which appear to be a more serious candidate for mediating the cognitive sequelae of PD, are also substantially depleted. This depletion is greatest (to a maximum of about 90%) in the most rostrodorsal extent of the head of this structure, an area which is heavily connected with dorsolateral regions of the frontal lobe (Yeterian and Pandya 1991). It seems likely, therefore, that these rostrodorsal regions of the caudate nucleus are subjected to greater disruption by the disease and probably at an earlier stage of its progression. By contrast, ventral regions of the caudate, which are preferentially connected with more ventral regions of the frontal lobe (Yeterian and Pandya 1991), are relatively spared in early PD, which may leave functions which are maximally dependent on this neural circuitry relatively intact.

PD is also characterized by dopamine depletion within the frontal cortex itself (Scatton et al. 1983) and degeneration of the mesocortical dopamine system, which projects to the frontal lobes and other cortical areas, may also play a significant role in the apparent progressive deterioration of 'frontal' working memory deficits in PD. This system however, is known to be less severely affected (50% depletion) than the nigrostriatal dopamine system in PD (Agid et al. 1987) and possibly at a later stage of the disease process. It may therefore contribute to the more global pattern of frontal lobe deficits observed in patients with severe PD.

A COMPARATIVE STUDY OF MEMORY IN PARKINSON'S DISEASE, PROGRESSIVE SUPRANUCLEAR PALSY AND MULTIPLE SYSTEM ATROPHY

A recent comparative study of patients with PD, progressive supranuclear palsy and multiple system atrophy has demonstrated that these patients can also be differentiated in terms of their performance on these two spatial memory tasks. The latter group of patients are particularly interesting because, unlike PD and progressive supranuclear palsy, relatively few studies have specifically investigated the nature of cognitive deficits in multiple system atrophy. In addition to the intrinsic striatal (caudate plus putamen) pathology, damage to the nigrostriatal dopamine pathway in multiple system atrophy is at least equal to, or even greater than, that seen in PD. Like patients with severe PD, a group of patients with progressive supranuclear palsy were significantly impaired, compared to a matched control group, on the test of spatial span, while normal performance was observed in a group of patients with multiple system atrophy (Robbins et al. 1994; Figure 8.3c). The progressive supranuclear palsy patients also made significantly more errors on the spatial search task, although unlike the PD patients, this deficit was quite clearly related to the inappropriate use of the repetitive search strategy, a pattern that is known to characterize the performance of patients with frontal lobe damage (Owen et al. 1990, 1997). In the multiple system atrophy patient group, deficits were also observed in terms of errors (Figure 8.3c), although, unlike the progressive supranuclear palsy group, the strategic element of task performance was preserved (Robbins et al. 1992, 1994).

Thus, like the PD group, the progressive supranuclear palsy patients were significantly impaired on both of the spatial memory tasks, implicating both dorsal and ventral regions of the lateral frontal cortex (Petrides 1994; Owen et al. 1996b). In addition, these patients showed some impairment in a measure of the efficient use of a strategy for mediating the spatial search task, similar to that observed in frontal lobe patients. Together, these findings suggest a profound frontal lobe involvement in progressive supranuclear palsy, a pattern that is maintained when other frontal lobe tasks are considered (Robbins et al. 1994). They also concur, in a general sense, with the findings of other behavioral (Dubois et al. 1988; Grafman et al. 1990) and neuroimaging (Blin et al. 1990) studies. For example, in the latter PET study, the frontal-like cognitive impairments in patients with progressive supranuclear palsy were found to be correlated with frontal metabolic activity rather than activity in the caudate nucleus.

The fact that performance on the spatial search task was severely impaired in the multiple system atrophy group, while performance on the spatial span task was largely intact, also suggests some similarities between these patients and the neurosurgical group with circumscribed frontal lobe damage, although in general, this pattern is rather less consistent than in the patient group with progressive supranuclear palsy. This general pattern is maintained across a broad range of neuropsychological tasks (Robbins et al. 1992, 1994). The fact that these patients were only impaired on the mnemonic and not the strategic, aspect of task performance on the spatial search test suggests that the deficit observed cannot simply be explained in terms of high level executive dysfunction and may reflect additional deficiencies of spatial memory capacity that are dependent on posterior cortical and subcortical systems.

COMPARATIVE STUDIES OF MEMORY IN ALZHEIMER'S AND HUNTINGTON'S DISEASES

It seems likely that striatal dysfunction, as occurs in both PD and HD, would lead to a similar pattern of executive deficits, given the functional inter-relationship that exists between different parts of the frontal cortex and the basal ganglia described above (Alexander et al. 1986). Of particular significance for HD, in view of the primary site of its striatal neuropathology, may be the anatomical and functional relations that exist between the caudate nucleus and the prefrontal cortex.

Lawrence et al. (1996), assessed 18 patients with early HD on tests of executive and mnemonic function, including the two spatial memory tasks of interest here. At this stage of the disease, damage is thought to be restricted primarily to the caudate nucleus and the putamen (Vonsattel et al. 1985; Chapter 3). The HD group had significantly shorter spatial spans than a matched control group (Figure 8.3d), but performance on this task was far superior to that of a group of patients with more severe clinical symptoms (Lange et al. 1995). Although the deficit in spatial span observed in the mild HD patients reached significance, it is notable that their performance, unlike that of the severe HD group, was relatively good compared to other patient groups who are impaired on this task (see Figure 8.3). The mild HD cases were also significantly impaired in terms of the number of errors committed on the spatial search task (Lawrence et al. 1996; Figure 8.4d) and this group also made significantly less use of the efficient searching strategy, known to improve performance on this task. This pattern of deficit is similar to that observed in neurosurgical patients with frontal lobe damage. In the more severe HD group, deficits on the spatial search task (errors), were far greater than in any other group that has been assessed on this test (Figure 8.4d). In addition, this group showed a tendency to make a very high number of within search errors, i.e. to make repeated, incorrect responses within a given search. This severe impairment in basic mnemonic processing was not observed in the more mildly affected HD patients and is consistent with increased ventrolateral frontal lobe and/or medial temporal lobe involvement late in the course of HD. Together, these findings may suggest a similar pattern of functional degeneration in HD to that observed previously in PD (Owen et al. 1992), by which functions of the dorsolateral frontal cortex are affected at an earlier stage of the disease process than functions of either the ventrolateral frontal cortex or the medial temporal lobe structures. This functional similarity fits with what is known about the neuropathological progression of HD in which neuronal loss begins with the striosome compartment of the head of the caudate nucleus and progresses in a dorsal-to-ventral direction (Hedreen and Folstein 1995). Striosomes in the dorsal regions of the caudate nucleus are connected primarily with the dorsolateral frontal cortex, while those in ventral regions of the caudate nucleus receive input from limbic-related areas. Importantly, however, unlike patients with mild PD, the patients with mild HD studied by Lawrence et al. (1996), were also impaired on a test of visual pattern recognition memory which is known not to involve the frontal lobe, but rather, the temporal lobe and medial temporal lobe structures (Owen et al. 1995a). Connections from the inferotemporal cortex project heavily to the ventrocaudal striatum (ventral putamen and

tail of the caudate nucleus) (Yeterian and Pandya 1995), which has important implications for the pattern of deficits observed in HD, because, unlike PD, some of the earliest neuropathological changes in HD have been reported to occur in the tail of the caudate nucleus (Vonsattel et al. 1985). Thus, it seems likely that the additional impairment in pattern recognition memory in early HD is a result of damage to the ventrocaudal striatum.

Like patients with HD, patients with AD can be expected to be impaired in tests of executive function as the disease progresses, although both neuroimaging and neuropsychological evidence supports the hypothesis that anterior cortical functions are relatively more immune to disruption in this disease (Parks et al. 1993). Sahgal et al. (1991, 1995) have reported spatial span to be impaired in patients with both mild and moderate AD, with the moderate group being significantly more impaired than those with mild AD. Both groups were also impaired on the spatial search task, but not differentially and strategic deficits of the type seen following frontal lobe damage were not evident.

Lange et al. (1995) compared performance in patients with mild to moderate AD and HD matched for level of clinical dementia on these, and other tests of executive function, in order that any differences in specific cognitive functions could not be attributed simply to nonspecific intellectual deterioration. Patients with HD had considerably shorter spatial span scores than patients with AD (Figure 8.3d), although both groups were impaired relative to control subjects matched for age and premorbid IQ. In addition, the HD group made more errors on the spatial search task than the AD group, particularly at more extreme levels of task difficulty (Figure 8.4d). The results clearly demonstrate that, when matched for level of dementia, patients with HD are significantly inferior to patients with AD on the two spatial memory tests that are know to be sensitive to frontal lobe damage and basal ganglia dysfunction. In fact, this general pattern of deficit was maintained across a range of tests of executive function (Lange et al. 1995) and in this sense, the findings are consistent with the existence of greater fronto-striatal pathology in HD than in AD (Berent et al. 1988; Weinberger et al. 1988; Starkstein et al. 1992). It is important to note, however, like patients in the later stages of PD, the deficits in the HD group were not limited to tests clearly requiring executive function. This suggests that the entire pattern of cognitive deficits in HD cannot be explained by a fronto-striatal hypothesis and may include impairments arising from additional pathology which affects cortical regions other than the prefrontal cortex, such as the temporal lobe. The results are consistent, therefore, with the hypothesis that the neural substrates of many of the cognitive deficits in HD are centered on the caudate nucleus (Berent et al. 1988; Weinberger et al. 1988; Starkstein et al. 1992), but that additional cortical atrophy may also be significant (Berent et al. 1988).

EXECUTIVE FUNCTION AND NEURODEGENERATIVE DISEASE: FUTURE DIRECTIONS

The studies described above clearly demonstrate how neuropsychological models of working memory function, developed largely through animal lesion studies and tested using sophisticated functional neuroimaging techniques, have led directly to a marked reappraisal of the status of cognitive deficits in neurodegenerative disease. Much of this work has sought to verify the 'frontal' nature of cognitive deficits in neurodegenerative groups, such as PD and HD and, on the whole, experimental results have supported such a model; however, that is not to say that cognitive impairments resulting from striatal dysfunction are identical to those seen following damage to associated frontal regions. In fact, the studies reported here demonstrate quite clearly that when task demands are subjected to a careful process analysis, subtle but important differences emerge between frontal lobe patients and patients with various neurodegenerative diseases. For example, the deficit in 'strategic' aspects of task performance, which is central to the pattern of impairment observed in patients with frontal lobe damage, is clearly present in patients with HD and progressive supranuclear palsy, but less obvious in PD and markedly absent in multiple system atrophy. Future studies should seek to investigate these potentially important functional differences further by relating them to what is known about the differential neuropathology in each condition.

In drawing comparisons both within and between groups of patients, it is also important to consider the possibility that other 'nonfrontal' aspects of cognitive function may be affected. For example, in some respects, the pattern of deficits observed on the spatial search task in patients with severe PD is similar to that observed in

patients with temporal lobe excisions who make more errors than controls, but exhibited no deficit in task strategy (Owen et al., 1997). This observation is consistent with recent cross-sectional studies which have demonstrated that, while cognitive deficits in early PD are predominantly 'frontal like', performance on tasks which depend preferentially on the medial temporal lobe structures is also affected in the later stages of the disease process (Owen et al. 1992, 1993).

Finally, the majority of studies that have investigated executive processes in neurodegenerative disease in recent years have concentrated on patients with PD and this presumably reflects greater patient availability in this group and the fact that the underlying neuropathology of PD is relatively well established. Future studies, however, should seek to make more direct comparisons between groups of patients with different neurodegenerative disorders including PD, multiple system atrophy, progressive supranuclear palsy and HD and, wherever possible, match across groups for the severity of clinical symptoms. In addition, increasingly sophisticated functional imaging techniques such as functional MRI and PET (Chapter 6) may supplement such comparisons and provide a mechanism by which the neural underpinnings of some of the deficits described above can be more clearly defined. For example, a recent blood flow activation study using PET in patients with PD has demonstrated normal changes in regional cerebral blood in the prefrontal cortex during two tests of executive function involving planning and spatial working memory (Owen et al. 1996a). In contrast, abnormal blood flow in the internal segment of the globus pallidus was observed during both tasks suggesting that striatal dopamine depletion in PD may affect the expression of frontal lobe functions in PD by disrupting the normal pattern of basal ganglia outflow to this region.

Such investigations, when combined with information derived from cognitive psychology, clinical neuropsychology and neurobiology should certainly provide a significant focus for future research and may lead ultimately to a better understanding of the distinctive roles played by the frontal cortex and the striatum in the operation of the 'fronto-striatal' functional loops (Alexander et al. 1986).

ACKNOWLEDGMENTS

During the preparation of this manuscript, A. M. Owen was supported by a Pinsent-Darwin Research Scholarship at the University of Cambridge, UK. Much of the work presented in this chapter was supported by a Program Grant from the Wellcome Trust to T.W. Robbins, B.J. Everitt, A. C. Roberts and B.J. Sahakian.

REFERENCES

Aggleton, J.P., Hunt, P.R. and Rawlins, J.N.P. 1986. The effects of hippocampal lesions upon spatial and non-spatial tests of working memory. *Behavioural Brain Research*. 19: 133–146.

Agid, Y., Javoy-Agid, F. and Ruberg, M. 1987. Biochemistry of neurotransmitters in Parkinson's disease. In *Movement disorders*, vol. 2, ed. C.D. Marsden and S. Fahn, pp. 166–230. London: Butterworth.

Alexander, G.E., Delong, M.R. and Strick, P.L. 1986. Parallel organization of functionally segregated circuits linking basal ganglia and cortex. *Annual Review of Neuroscience*. 9: 357–381.

Baddeley, A.D. 1986. *Working memory*. New York: Oxford University Press.

Baddeley, A.D., Logie, R., Bressi, S., Della Sala, S. and Spinnler, H. 1986. Dementia and working memory. *Quarterly Journal of Experimental Psychology*. 38A: 603–618.

Berent, S., Giordani, B., Lehtinen, S., Markel, D., Penney, J.B., Buchtel, H.A., StarostaRubinstein, S., Hichwa, R. and Young, A.B. 1988. Positron emission tomographic scan investigations of Huntington's disease: Cerebral correlates of cognitive function. *Annals of Neurology*. 23: 541–546.

Blin, J., Baron, J., Dubois, B., Pillon, B., Cambon, H., Cambier, J. and Agid, Y. 1990. Positron emission tomography study in progressive supranuclear palsy: Brain hypometabolic pattern and clinicometabolic correlation. *Archives of Neurology*. 47: 747–752.

Bradley, V.A., Welch, J.L. and Dick, D.J. 1989. Visuospatial working memory in Parkinson's disease. *Journal of Neurology, Neurosurgery and Psychiatry*. 52: 1228–1235.

Byrne, E.J., Lennox, G., Lowe, J. and Godwin-Austin, R.B. 1989. Diffuse Lewy body disease: Clinical features in 15 cases. *Journal of Neurology, Neurosurgery and Psychiatry*. 52: 709–717.

Cooper, J.A., Sagar, H.J., Jordan, N., Harvey N.S. and Sullivan, E.V. 1991. Cognitive impairment in early, untreated Parkinson's disease and its relationship to motor disability. *Brain*. 114: 2095–2122.

Cooper, J.A., Sagar., H.J. and Sullivan, E.V. 1993. Short-term memory and temporal ordering in early Parkinson's disease: Effects of disease chronicity and medication. *Neuropsychologia*. 31: 933–949.

Courtney, S.M., Ungerleider, L.G., Keil, K. and Haxby, J.V. 1996. Object and spatial visual working memory activate separate neural systems in human cortex. *Cerebral Cortex*. 6: 39–49

Dubois, B., Pillon, B., Legault, F., Agid, Y. and L'Hermitte, F. 1988. Slowing of cognitive processing in progressive supranuclear palsy: A comparison with Parkinson's disease. *Archives of Neurology*. 45: 1194–1199.

Elliot, R., Sahakian, B.J., McKay, A.P., Herrod, J.J., Robbins, T.W. and Paykel, E.S. 1996. Neuropsychological impairments in unipolar depression: The influence of perceived failure on subsequent performance. *Psychological Medicine*. 26: 975–989.

Folstein, M.F., Folstein, S.E. and McHugh, P.R. 1975. 'Mini-Mental State': A practical method for grading the cognitive state of patients for the clinician. *Journal of Psychiatric Research*. 12: 189–198.

Fuster, J.M. 1989. *The prefrontal cortex: Anatomy, physiology and neuropsychology of the frontal lobe*. New York: Raven Press.

Gibb, W.R.G., Luthert, P.J., Janota, I. and Lantos, P.L. 1989. Cortical Lewy body dementia: Clinical features and classification. *Journal of Neurology, Neurosurgery and Psychiatry*. 52: 185–192.

Gold, J.M., Berman, K.F., Randolph, C., Goldberg, T.E. and Weinberger, D.R. 1996. PET validation of a novel prefrontal task: Delayed response alternation. *Neuropsychology*. 10: 3–10.

Goldberg, T.E., Berman, K.F., Randolph, C., Gold, J.M. and Weinberger, D.R. 1996. Isolating the mnemonic component in spatial delayed response: A controlled PET ^{15}O-labelled water regional cerebral blood flow study in normal humans. *Neuroimage*. 3: 69–78.

Goldman-Rakic, P.S. 1987. Circuitry of primate prefrontal cortex and the regulation of behavior by representational memory. In *Handbook of physiology, section 1: The nervous system*, vol. V, ed. F. Plum and V. Mountcastle, pp. 373–417. Bethesda: American Physiological Society

Goldman-Rakic, P.S. 1990. Cellular and circuit basis of working memory in prefrontal cortex of nonhuman primates. In *Progress in Brain Research*, vol. 85., ed. H.B.M. Uylings, C.G. Van Eden, J.P.C. De Bruin, M.A. Corner and M.G.P. Feenstra, pp. 325–336. Amsterdam: Elsevier.

Goldman-Rakic, P.S., Selemon, L.D. and Schwartz, M.L. 1984. Dual pathways connecting the dorsolateral prefrontal cortex with the hippocampal formation and parahippocampal cortex in the rhesus monkey. *Neuroscience*. 12: 719–743.

Gotham, A.M., Brown, R.G. and Marsden, C.D. 1988. 'Frontal' cognitive functions in patients with Parkinson's disease 'on' and 'off' levodopa. *Brain*. 111: 299–321.

Grafman, J., Litvan, I., Gomez, C. and Chase, T.N. 1990. Frontal lobe function in progressive supranuclear palsy. *Archives of Neurology*. 47: 553–558.

Grant, D.A. and Berg, E.A. 1948. A behavioural analysis of degree of reinforcement and ease of shifting to new responses in a Weigl-type card sorting problem. *Journal of Experimental Psychology*. 38: 404–411.

Haug, H. and Eggers, R. 1991. Morphometry of the human cortex cerebri and corpus striatum during aging. *Neurobiology of Aging*. 12: 336–338.

Hedreen, J.C. and Folstein, M.F. 1995. Early loss of neostriatal striosome neurons in Huntington's disease. *Journal of Neuropathology and Experimental Neurology*. 54: 105–120.

Jonides, J., Smith, E.E., Koeppe, R.A., Awh, E., Minoshima, S. and Mintun, M.A. 1993. Spatial working memory in humans as revealed by PET. *Nature*. 363: 623–625.

Josiassen, R.C., Curry, L.M. and Mancall, E.L., 1983. Development of neuropsychological deficits in Huntington's disease. *Archives of Neurology*. 40: 791–796.

Kendrick, D.C. 1985. *Kendrick Cognitive Tests For The Elderly*. Windsor, Berks.: NFER-NELSON Publishing Company Ltd.

Kish, S.J., Shannak, K. and Hornykiewicz, O. 1988. Uneven patterns of dopamine loss in the striatum of patients with idiopathic Parkinson's disease: Pathophysiologic and clinical implications. *New England Journal of Medicine*. 318: 876–880.

Lange, K.W, Robbins, T.W., Marsden, C.D., James, M., Owen, A.M. and Paul, G.M. 1992. L-Dopa withdrawal in Parkinson's disease selectively impairs cognitive performance in tests sensitive to frontal lobe dysfunction. *Psychopharmacology*. 107: 394–404.

Lange, K.W., Sahakian, B.J., Quinn, N.P., Marsden, C.D. and Robbins, T.W. 1995. Comparison of executive and visuospatial memory function in Huntington's disease and dementia of Alzheimer type matched for degree of dementia. *Journal of Neurology, Neurosurgery and Neuropsychiatry*. 58: 598–606.

Lawrence, A.D., Sahakian, B.J., Hodges, J.R., Rosser, A.E., Lange, K.W. and Robbins, T.W. 1996. Executive and mnemonic functions in early Huntington's disease. *Brain* 119: 1633–1645.

Lees, A.J. and Smith, E. 1983. Cognitive deficits in the early stages of Parkinson's disease. *Brain*. 106: 257–270.

McCarthy, G., Blamire, A.M., Puce, A., Nobre, A.C., Bloch, G., Hyder, F., Goldman-Rakic, P. and Shulman, R.G. 1994. Functional magnetic resonance imaging of human prefrontal cortex activation during a spatial working memory task. *Proceedings of the National Academy of Sciences*. 91: 8690–8694.

Milner, B. 1971. Interhemispheric differences in the localization of psychological processes in man. *British Medical Bulletin*. 27: 272–277.

Morris, R.G., Downes, J.J. and Robbins, T.W. 1990. The nature of the dysexecutive syndrome in Parkinson's disease. In *Lines of thinking*, vol. 2., ed. K.J. Gilhooly, M.T.G. Keane, R.H. Loge and G. Erdos, pp. 247–258. London: Wiley and Sons.

Morris, R.G., Downes, J.J., Sahakian, B.J., Evenden, J.L., Heald, A. and Robbins, T.W. 1988. Planning and spatial working memory in Parkinson's disease. *Journal of Neurology, Neurosurgery and Psychiatry*. 51: 757–766.

Olton, DS. 1982. Spatially organized behaviors of animals: Behavioral and neurological studies. In *Spatial abilities*, ed. M. Potegal, pp. 325–360. New York: Academic Press.

Olton, D.S. and Papas, B.C. 1979. Spatial memory and hippocampal function. *Neuropsychologia*. 17: 669–682.

Olton, D.S., Walker, J.A. and Gage, F.H. 1978. Hippocampal connections and spatial discrimination. *Brain Research*. 139: 295–308.

Orsini, A., Fragaasi, N.A., Chiacchio, L., Falanga, A.M., Cocchiaro, C. and Grossi, D. 1987. Verbal and spatial memory span in patients with extrapyramidal disease. *Perceptual and Motor Skills*. 65: 555–558.

Owen A.M., Beksinska, M., James, M., Leigh, P.N., Summers, B.A., Marsden, C.D., Quinn, N.P., Sahakian, B.J. and Robbins T.W. 1993. Visuo-spatial memory deficits at different stages of Parkinson's disease. *Neuropsychologia*. 31: 627–644.

Owen A.M., Downes, J.D., Sahakian, B.J., Polkey, C.E. and Robbins T.W. 1990. Planning and spatial working memory following frontal lobe lesions in man. *Neuropsychologia*. 28: 1021–1034.

Owen A.M., Doyon, J., Petrides, M. and Evans, A.C. 1996a. Planning and spatial working memory examined with positron emission tomography (PET). *European Journal of Neuroscience*. 8: 353–364.

Owen A.M., Evans, A.C. and Petrides, M. 1996b. Evidence for a two-stage model of spatial working memory processing within the lateral frontal cortex: A positron emission tomography study. *Cerebral Cortex*. 6: 31–38.

Owen, A.M., Iddon, J.L., Hodges, J. R. and Robbins T.W. 1997. Spatial and non-spatial working memory at different stages of Parkinson's disease. *Neuropsychologia*. 35: 519–532.

Owen A.M., James, M., Leigh, P.N., Summers, B.A., Quinn, N.P., Marsden, C.D. and Robbins,T.W. 1992. Fronto-striatal cognitive deficits at different stages of Parkinson's disease. *Brain*. 115: 1727–1751.

Owen, A.M., Morris, R.G., Sahakian, B.J., Polkey, C.E. and Robbins, T.W. 1996c. Double dissociations of memory and executive functions in working memory tasks following frontal lobe excisions, temporal lobe excisions or amygdalo–hippocampectomy in man. *Brain* 119: 1597–1615.

Owen, A.M., Sahakian, B.J., Hodges, J.R., Summers, B.A., Polkey, C.E. and Robbins, T.W. 1995b. Dopamine-dependent fronto-striatal planning deficits in early Parkinson's disease. *Neuropsychology*. 9: 126–140.

Owen, A.M., Sahakian, B.J., Semple, J., Polkey, C.E. and Robbins, T.W. 1995a. Visuo-spatial short term recognition memory and learning after temporal lobe excisions, frontal lobe excisions or amygdalo-hippocampectomy in man. *Neuropsychologia*. 33: 1–24.

Parks, R.W., Haxby, J.F. and Grady, C.L. 1993. Positron emission tomography in Alzheimer's disease. In *Neuropsychology of Alzheimer's disease and other dementias*, ed. R.W. Parks, R.F. Zec and R.S. Wilson, pp. 459–488. New York: Oxford University Press.

Passingham, R.E. 1985. Memory of monkeys (*Macaca mulatta*) with lesions in prefrontal cortex. *Behavioural Neuroscience*. 99: 3–21.

Petrides, M. 1988. Performance on a non-spatial self-ordered task after selective lesions of the primate frontal cortex [abstract]. *Society for Neuroscience Abstracts*. 14: 2.

Petrides, M. 1989. Frontal lobes and memory. In *Handbook of neuropsychology*, vol. 3, ed. F. Boller and J. Grafman, pp. 75–90, Amsterdam: Elsevier.

Petrides, M. 1991. Monitoring of selections of visual stimuli and the primate frontal cortex. *Proceedings of the Royal Society of London*. 246B: 293–298.

Petrides, M. 1994. Frontal lobes and working memory: Evidence from investigations of the effects of cortical excisions in nonhuman primates. In *Handbook of neuropsychology*, vol. 9., ed. F. Boller and J. Grafman, pp. 59–82. Amsterdam: Elsevier.

Petrides, M. and Milner, B. 1982. Deficits on subject-ordered tasks after frontal-and temporal-lobe lesions in man. *Neuropsychologia*. 20: 249–262.

Petrides, M. and Pandya, D.N. 1994. Comparative architectonic analysis of the human and the macaque frontal cortex. In *Handbook of neuropsychology*, vol. 9, ed. F. Boller and J. Grafman, pp. 17–58. Amsterdam: Elsevier.

Petrides, M., Alivisatos, B., Evans, A.C. and Meyer, E. 1993a. Dissociation of human mid-dorsolateral from posterior dorsolateral frontal cortex in memory processing. *Proceedings of the National Academy of Sciences*. 90: 873–877.

Petrides, M., Alivisatos, B., Evans, A.C. and Meyer, E. 1993b. Functional activation of the human frontal cortex during the performance of verbal working memory tasks. *Proceedings of the National Academy of Sciences*. 90: 878–882.

Pillon, B., Dubois, B., L'Hermitte, F. and Agid, Y. 1986. Heterogeneity of cognitive impairment in progressive supranuclear palsy, Parkinson's disease and Alzheimer's disease. *Neurology*. 36: 1179–1185.

Postle, B.R., Corkin, S. and Growdon, J.H. 1993. Dissociation between two kinds of visual working memory in Parkinson's disease [abstract]. *Society for Neuroscience Abstracts*. 10: 1002.

Rawlins, J.N.P. and Olton, D.S. 1982. The septo-hippocampal system and cognitive mapping. *Behavioural Brain Research*. 5: 331–358

Rawlins, J.N.P. and Tsaltas, E. 1983. The hippocampus, time and working memory. *Behavioural Brain Research*. 10: 233–262.

Rich, J.B., Bylsma, F.W. and Brandt, J. 1996. Self-ordered pointing performance in Huntington's disease patients. *Neuropsychiatry, Neuropsychology and Behavioral Neurology*. 9: 99–106.

Robbins, T.W. 1996. Dissociating executive functions of the prefrontal cortex. *Philosophical Transactions of the Royal Society, B* 351: 1463–1471.

Robbins T.W., James M., Lange K.W., Owen A.M., Quinn N.P. and Marsden C.D. 1992. Cognitive performance in multiple system atrophy. *Brain*. 115: 271–291.

Robbins, T.W., James, M., Owen, A.M., Lange, K.W, Lees, A.J., Leigh, P.N., Marsden, C.D., Quinn, N.P. and Summers, B.A. 1994. Cognitive deficits in progressive supranuclear palsy, Parkinson's disease and multiple system atrophy in tests sensitive to frontal lobe dysfunction. *Journal of Neurology, Neurosurgery and Psychiatry*. 57: 79–88.

Sahakian, B.J., Downes, J.J., Eagger, S., Evenden, J.L., Levy, R, Philpot, M.P., Roberts, A.C. and Robbins, T.W. 1990. Sparing of attentional relative to mnemonic function in a subgroup of patients with dementia of the Alzheimer type. *Neuropsychologia*. 28: 1197–1213.

Sahakian, B.J., Morris, R.G., Evenden, J.L., Heald, A., Levy, R., Philpot, M.P. and Robbins, T.W. 1988. A comparative study of visuo-spatial learning and memory in Alzheimer-type dementia and Parkinson's disease. *Brain*. 111: 695–718.

Sahgal, A., McKeith, I.G., Galloway, P.H., Tasker, N. and Steckler, T. 1995. Do differences in visuospatial ability between senile dementias of the Alzheimer's and Lewy body types reflect differences solely in mnemonic function? *Journal of Clinical and Experimental Neuropsychology*. 17: 35–43.

Sahgal, A., Sahakian, B.J., Robbins T.W., Wray, C.J., Lloyd, S., Cook, J.H., McKeith, I.G., Disley, J.C.A., Eagger, S., Boddington, S. and Edwardson, J.A. 1991. Detection of visual memory and learning deficits in Alzheimer's disease using the Cambridge Neuropsychological Test Automated Battery. *Dementia*. 2: 150–158.

Scatton, B., Javoy-Agid, F., Rouqier, L., Dubois, B. and Agid, Y. 1983. Reduction of cortical dopamine, noradrenaline, serotonin and their metabolites in Parkinson's disease. *Brain Research*. 275: 321–328.

Singh, J., Gabrieli, J.D.E. and Goetz, C.G. 1991. Impaired working memory in unmedicated Parkinson's disease. *Society for Neuroscience Abstracts*, 17.

Smith, E.E., Jonides, J.J. and Koeppe, R.A. 1996. Dissociating verbal and spatial working memory using PET. *Cerebral Cortex*. 6: 11–20.

Smith, E.E., Jonides, J.J., Koeppe, R.A., Awh, E., Schumacher, E.H. and Minoshima, S. 1995. Spatial versus object working memory: PET investigations. *Journal of Cognitive Neuroscience*. 7: 337–356.

Starkstein, S.E., Brandt, J., Bylsma, F., Peyser, C., Folstein, M. and Folstein, S.E. 1992. Neuropsychological correlates of brain atrophy in Huntington's disease: A magnetic resonance imaging study. *Neuroradiology*. 34: 487–489.

Sweeney, J.A., Minutun, M.A., Kwee, S., Wiseman, M.B., Brown, D.L., Rosenberg, D.R. and Carl, J.R. 1996. Positron emission tomography study of voluntary saccadic eye movements and spatial working memory. *Journal of Neurophysiology*. 75: 454–468.

Sziklas, V. and Petrides, M. 1993. Memory impairments following lesions to the mamillary region of the rat. *European Journal of Neuroscience*. 5: 525–540.

Van Gorp, W.G. and Mahler, M. 1990. Subcortical features of normal aging. In *Subcortical dementia*, ed. J.L. Cummings, pp. 231–250. New York: Oxford University Press.

Vonsattel, J.P., Myers, R.H., Stevens, T.J., Ferrante, R.J., Bird, E.D. and Richardson, E.P. 1985. Neuropathological classification of Huntington's disease. *Journal of Neuropathology and Experimental Neurology*. 44: 559–577.

Weinberger, D.R., Beran, K.E., Iadrola, M., Driesen, N. and Zec, R. 1988. Prefrontal cortical blood flow and cognitive function in Huntington's disease. *Journal of Neurology, Neurosurgery and Psychiatry*. 51: 94–104.

Yeterian, E.H. and Pandya, D.N. 1991. Prefrontostriatal connections in relation to cortical architectonic organization in rhesus monkeys. *Journal of Comparative Neurology*. 312: 43–67.

Yeterian, E.H and Pandya, D.N. 1995. Corticostriatal connections of extrastriate visual areas in rhesus monkeys. *Journal of Comparative Neurology*. 352: 436–457.

9

Prospective memory in aging and neurodegenerative disease

ROBERT G. KNIGHT

INTRODUCTION

In everyday life the experience of remembering takes two forms. One is *retrospective* memory, which is concerned with the reconstruction of past events, the other is *prospective* memory, i.e. remembering to carry out an intended action in the future (Wilkins and Baddeley 1978; Meacham and Leiman 1982; Winograd 1988). In this chapter the focus is on prospective memory, which is the complex process of remembering to remember. In questionnaire studies, self-perception of prospective memory is assessed with items such as: 'Do you find you forget appointments?' or 'Do you sometimes forget to give a message to someone?' (Hermann and Neisser 1978; Bennett-Levy and Powell 1980). For most of us, lapses of memory of this kind occur from time to time, but there is evidence that prospective memory failure can be a profound problem following brain injury or dementia (Cockburn 1995; Kinsella et al. 1996). For example, in a test of practical memory skills, Knight and Godfrey (1985) found that a group of amnesic patients with Korsakoff's syndrome were never able to complete a task in which they had to follow a set of three instructions involving a visit to a clinic secretary. In practice, amnesic and demented patients have considerable problems executing any kind of prospective memory task.

Despite its obvious relevance to understanding memory functioning in our daily lives, prospective memory has been little studied in the experimental literature. In both clinical and experimental research, the primary focus has been on retrospective recall. To a large extent, this is the consequence of the difficulties inherent in the specification and measurement of the component processes required to complete a prospective memory task. These cognitive processes include planning to remember a future action, executing the plan (e.g. recognizing the retrieval cue) and recalling the encoded intention. Thus, executing even the simplest prospective memory tasks necessitates some amount of self-initiated problem solving, the integration of component memory processes and the retrospective retrieval of an intention to act. There are signs, however, of an increasing interest in prospective memory. This has been stimulated not only by a concern with the construction of ecologically valid measures of memory for use in neuropsychological practice, but also by the search for a better understanding of how regions of the brain work together in learning and memory. An example of the research with the latter emphasis is the study of the effects of focal frontal lobe damage on memory (e.g. Milner et al. 1985; Janowsky et al. 1989b; Bisiacchi 1996). Before discussing issues that arise from this research, however, it is instructive to consider more closely the characteristics of prospective memory function.

MEASURING PROSPECTIVE MEMORY

Instances of prospective memory abound in the routines of daily living. Remembering to take pills at meal times, to collect the children after a music class or to send an anniversary card are all tasks that require prospective memory. Most prospective memory tasks also involve some degree of retrospective recall. For example, remembering to pass on a telephone message to a colleague is prospective memory; recalling the substance of the message is retrospective recall. An important feature of prospective tasks is the way in which they are located in a network of concurrent activities. As this paragraph is being written, for example, I am aware that in an hour I have a colloquium to attend. Concentration on the effort of writing may compete with my ability to attend to the appropriate time cues; in this sense, prospective remembering typically takes place in a dual-task paradigm. The everyday performance of intended actions is also compounded by other noncognitive considerations. I may remember the time for the seminar, but be so engrossed in my current activity that I decide not to attend. In this case, it can be seen that 'prospective remembering is a goal-oriented activity embedded in a hierarchy of activities' (Winograd 1988, p.350). An intention may not be performed and hence memory may appear to fail, because it is a less desirable activity than the one currently under action.

There is also a social dimension to the execution of intentions in everyday life: prospective memory can imply a commitment to act that individuals may take more or less seriously. The conscientious person displays this attribute by honoring the expression of their intentions, an unreliable person may forget an implied promise as soon as it is uttered. Furthermore, actions are more likely to be carried out in some circumstances (i.e. when the commitment is to a high status person in public) than in others. Thus, the execution of prospective memory tasks depends to some extent on noncognitive motivation and personality factors and these need to be taken into account in the practical assessment of impaired patients.

Prospective memory tasks differ in a variety of ways. For example, some are carried out on an *habitual* basis (i.e. taking a tablet after every meal). Others are *episodic* and irregular, such as remembering to collect airline tickets before a flight or to attend a dental appointment (Meacham and Leiman 1982). Another important distinction is between *event-* and *time-* based tasks (Einstein and McDaniel 1990). In an event-based test, an external stimulus provides a cue for action; a post office, for example, cues the posting of a letter. Time-based tasks require that the action is performed after a specified time interval (Harris and Wilkins 1982). Planning to take a tablet after 4 hours is an instance of this type of prospective memory. Here the action occurs after some monitoring of the passage of time and is driven primarily by internal cues. Time-based tasks require self-initiated monitoring and retrieval, thus they are generally more sensitive to memory deficits than event-based tasks (Einstein et al. 1995). Another dichotomy was proposed by Ellis (1988) between 'pulses', such as 'attend a seminar at 3 pm' which have a narrow time frame and 'steps', such as 'phone a colleague tomorrow', which have a broader time constraint.

The above considerations add up to noting that prospective memory is not a simple unitary concept. Tasks used to assess prospective memory may vary in both difficulty level and the component processes they draw

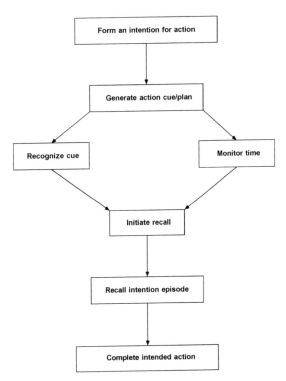

Figure 9.1. A Component Model of Prospective Memory

upon for their execution (Dalla Barba 1993). In the laboratory these processes may be investigated under controlled circumstances and significant deficits determined. The execution of intention in everyday life, however, maybe complicated by contextual and noncognitive considerations.

MODELS OF PROSPECTIVE MEMORY

Several authors have advanced a theoretical structure for the operation of prospective memory, recognizing the features of its operation introduced above (Levy and Loftus 1984; Huppert and Beardsall 1993). The components of a general model for completing both time- and event-based actions is presented in Figure 9.1. The initial stage of this model is the development of plan for action that may be expressed in a variety of ways. Event-based plans typically involve a cue that may be internal ('when I feel anxious, I will use my relaxation cues') or external ('when I get to the sports goods store, I will buy some tennis balls'). The range of possible cues is immense and limited only by the ingenuity of the person constructing the plan. In tests of prospective memory where the experimenter provides the cue for action, the distinctiveness of the cue is important. Cockburn (1996) in a study of 18 brain injured patients with a mild degree of amnesia found that an action signaled by a physical change in stimuli was performed but that many subjects forgot what to do when they finished the task, a cue that may be less salient in the testing situation. In some situations it may be desirable to initiate an external mnemonic, for example, set an alarm clock or write a diary note. Relying on such an external cue generally enhances the ability to remember to carry out intentions (Maylor 1990). The ability to self-initiate strategies for future action is not a unique requisite of prospective memory. This skill may be more generally classified as an instance of *executive control*; failure in such strategic thinking, often termed *dysexecutive syndrome*, is seen in many patients with frontal lobe damage (Daum and Ackermann 1994; Cockburn 1995; Glisky 1996). Time-based tasks involve constructing an internal plan to monitor the passage of time, which again may necessitate considerable initiative to complete successfully.

The next stage involves the execution of the action plan. This is perhaps the unique feature of prospective memory: the use of the cue or knowledge of the passing of time to self-initiate a retrospective memory search. In the typical retrospective memory study the experimenter provides the cue for recall; in contrast, prospective memory compels the individual to initiate their own search for the meaning of the cuing stimulus ('what was I supposed to do after 4 hours?' or 'what did I mean to say when I saw the doctor?'). Furthermore, such self-initiated retrieval strategies require effortful and controlled processing, making them especially vulnerable to any form of cerebral dysfunction. The process of retrieval of information when a cue is recognized is a form of retrospective memory. Thus failure of controlled or explicit memory search will inhibit the execution of prospective memory tasks.

The model in Figure 9.1 implies that a prospective memory task may be failed for more than one reason. A person with dysexecutive syndrome as a result of frontal damage and normal memory function will perform poorly because they are unable to organize an appropriate action plan and to self initiate appropriate retrieval strategies (Glisky 1996). This is illustrated in the case study of a

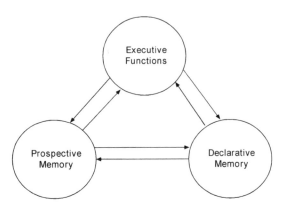

Figure 9.2. A representation of the possible interactions among Executive, Declarative and Prospective Memory Functions. From Tröster and Fields, 1995. Frontal cognitive function and memory in Parkinson's disease. *Behavioural Neurology, 8*, 59–74 (figure 1). Reprinted by permission. Copyright ©1995, Rapid Sciences Publishers.

patient with frontal-type memory loss following a thalamic lesion (Daum and Ackermann 1994), where the patient was able to remember what to do if prompted by the researcher, but never responded to a cue by himself. Similarly, Bisiacchi (1996) has reported results from three single case studies of patients with frontal deficits that illustrate the contribution that impairment in planning abilities may play in the prospective memory failure of nonamnesic patients. In contrast, a person with profound amnesia but normal executive and intellectual functioning may not recognize the cue and if it is drawn to their attention, will not recall its meaning. Viewed in this way, prospective memory is a complex cognitive operation, which draws on explicit or declarative memory and is controlled by frontal-based executive processes (Glisky 1996). This conceptualization is made explicit in the tripartite schema presented by Tröster and Fields (1995), which describes a series of reciprocal interactions between declarative memory, prospective memory and executive functions (Figure 9.2).

This dissociable contribution of executive functioning and declarative memory to prospective memory proposed by the model in Figure 9.2 is supported by the study of memory impairment in patients with frontal lobe deficits. In a series of studies involving patients with circumscribed frontal lesions, Shimamura and colleagues (Shimamura et al. 1991; Mangels et al. 1996) have shown that there are some memory-related tasks that are impaired in non-

Table 9.1. *Impairments in memory and cognition in patients with frontal lobe damage, alcoholic Korsakoff's syndrome, and amnesic disorders*

Task	Outcome		
	FL	AK	AM
Free recall of word lists (Rey AVLT)[a]	−	−	−
Wechsler Memory Scale-Revised Delayed Memory[d]	+	−	−
Paired associate learning[a]	+	−	−
Story and Diagram Recall[a]	+	−	−
Short-term memory (Digit Span)[d]	−	−	+
Release from proactive interference[a,c]	+	−	+
Feeling of knowing: Metamemory[b,f]	−	−	+
Source memory[c]			
Memory for temporal order[e,g]	−	−	−
Wisconsin Card Sorting Test[d]	−	−	+
Verbal Fluency[d]	−	−	+
Dementia Rating Scale Initiation[d]	−	−	+

Note:

FL: Frontal lobe damage; AK: Alcoholic Korsakoff's syndrome; AM: Amnesic disorders; AVLT: Auditory verbal learning test; +: No deficit; −: Deficit.

Sources: [a] Janowsky et al. 1989a; [b] Janowsky et al. 1989b; [c] Janowsky et al. 1989c; [d] Shimamura et al. 1991; [e] Squire, 1982; [f] Shimamura and Squire, 1986; [g] Shimamura et al. 1990.

amnesic frontal damaged patients. Table 9.1 presents a summary of their findings concerning patients with circumscribed anterograde amnesia, alcoholic Korsakoff's syndrome (with presumed diencephalic and frontal deficits) and circumscribed frontal lobe damage. The results in the summary table suggest that on those tests of memory typically sensitive to severe amnesia, patients with frontal lobe damage perform normally. For example, on the delayed recall tests of the Wechsler Memory Scale – Revised, which resulted in severe deficits for amnesic patients, the frontal patients performed normally. On the Rey Auditory Verbal Learning Test, a test that requires free recall of a list of unrelated words and is more sensitive to memory dysfunction, deficits emerged in the performance of the frontal patients. This is explained by recent findings demonstrating that the frontal lobes are important in the organization of retrieval and encoding strategies in free recall tasks (Gershberg and Shimamura 1995; Fletcher et al. 1997). Thus, as memory tasks become more dependent on strategic processing for accurate recall, it becomes more likely that frontal lobe patients will show deficits. This is exemplified by the finding that

frontal patients are impaired on recall tests of remote memory, but not when the test involves recognition (Mangels et al. 1996; Chapter 10).

On some memory related tasks both frontal and amnesic deficits are necessary to produce disorders. One such task involves release from proactive interference. Proactive interference tasks are those where learning a list of stimuli is inhibited by having just learned a list of similar stimuli. For example, proactive interference builds up and recall declines as subjects learn successive lists of animal names; however, if four lists of animal names are followed by a list of vegetable names, performance on the fifth list will return to normal, an effect known as release from proactive interference. Amnesic patients with concurrent frontal damage such as those with Korsakoff's syndrome do not release normally; amnesics with more specific deficits typically do (Squire 1982). There is also a group of tests, generally regarded as measures of executive function, on which amnesic patients perform normally, but frontal patients do not. These include tasks involving planning, initiation, set shifting and problem-solving (Cockburn 1995; Glisky 1996). The significance of this research with frontal patients for the study of prospective memory in the neurodegenerative disorders is that it reinforces the validity of the component model of memory in Figure 9.1 and its relationship to declarative memory and executive functions as described in Figure 9.2. It suggests an underlying biological basis for the multiple components of prospective memory operation and provides an explanation for the failure of prospective memory in nonamnesic patients.

Indeed, on the basis of their work with frontal patients, Shimamura et al. (1991) have proposed that 'the definition of prospective memory could justifiably be broadened to include processes and strategies involved in planning, monitoring and organizing *memory*, not just actions. Like a prospector searching for gold, prospective memory concerns self-initiated searches and retrieval of information in memory' (p.191). Although this definition is useful in that it draws attention to the common features of all memory tasks that require controlled strategic processing for their execution, it does minimize the significance of the intention of future action implicit in more specific denotations. Not all tasks involving self-initiated retrieval are a consequence of a previously formed intention. For this reason a narrower definition of prospective memory may be more valuable.

AGING AND PROSPECTIVE MEMORY

The most substantial literature on prospective memory is concerned with the effects of age on the performance of prospective memory tasks (for a review, see Maylor 1995). A stimulus for this work was Craik's (1986) observation that aging is detrimental to self-initiated cognitive processes and that the operation of prospective memory would therefore be unduly sensitive to aging. This research is of significance not only because of the intrinsic interest in understanding changes consequent on aging, but also because this work has helped clarify the dimensions of prospective memory. Furthermore, as many neurodegenerative diseases have an onset late in life, it is important to separate disease-related changes from the normal effects of aging.

Many of the early research reports concluded that aging had little impact on prospective memory but caused substantial changes in retrospective memory in both naturalistic and laboratory-based investigations (Sinnott 1986;

Dobbs and Rule 1987; West 1988; Einstein and McDaniel 1990; Maylor 1990). Subsequent research has highlighted the fact that negative findings may have been the result of using tests of prospective memory that made insufficient demands on the resources of participants to reveal changes due to aging; when the tests were made more difficult, age effects occurred (Einstein et al. 1992, 1995; Maylor 1993; Mäntylä 1994; Hannon et al. 1995). For example, Einstein et al. (1995) employed a time-based test in which participants were asked to press a computer key every 10 minutes while concurrently performing two different background tasks. A clock that they could monitor to check the elapsed times was located in the experimental room. They found that younger participants (aged 18–21 years) performed the key press closer to the target times and maintained a more efficient time monitoring strategy than did the older group (aged 61–78 years). On an event-based prospective memory task, however, in which subjects were asked to press a key whenever a particular word or class of words appeared during the presentation of stimuli for concurrent information processing, Einstein et al. 1992 confirmed their previous findings. Specifically, there was no significant age effect, leading them to conclude that the degree to which self-initiated processes were required determined whether prospective memory deficits were observed. As time-based tasks place greater reliance on self-initiated retrieval strategies than do event-based tasks, they are more likely to reveal deficits.

A study by Mäntylä (1994), however, has demonstrated that younger subjects do display superior prospective memory on event-based tests that require substantial processing resources. In this study, participants read a list of words and were instructed to respond with a particular action whenever a category instance appeared. For any category (e.g. *vehicle*), the words could have high typicality (e.g. *car*) or low typicality (e.g. *rocket*). They found that the older participants were not only less likely to respond when an atypical item appeared (prospective memory) but also less likely to recall the correct act to perform (retrospective memory) when they did respond. Aging effects can therefore be elicited on those event-based tasks that require complex processing.

An important outcome of this research is the manner in which the psychometric features of prospective memory tasks have been shown to influence findings. In particular, task difficulty level has been found to be a significant factor; if a test is too easy then differences between groups may not emerge. A related problem concerns task matching. Frequently, an aim of a particular investigation is to demonstrate a dissociation in performance between two groups on two contrasted tasks (e.g. prospective versus retrospective memory tests). This will only be valid where the reliability and difficulty levels of the two tests are comparable (Chapman and Chapman 1973; Haist et al. 1992). This is an important factor to consider in the design of comparative studies of prospective memory impairment.

PROSPECTIVE MEMORY AND DEMENTING DISORDERS

Alzheimer's disease
Caregivers' accounts suggest that in about 50% of cases, the first sign of dysfunction in persons with dementia of the Alzheimer's type (AD) is memory loss (Oppenheim 1994). As the disorder progresses, amnesia becomes a pronounced feature of the clinical presentation, until eventually most forms of learning and retention are compromised. Experimental studies have demonstrated that on any memory task that requires conscious or controlled retrieval, persons with AD will be severely impaired (e.g. Weingartner et al. 1981; Simon et al. 1994). Thus, on any memory task that involves explicit and retrospective free or cued recall, persons with AD are impaired. There is evidence that even on tasks requiring implicit or automatic processes, which profoundly amnesic patients perform normally, mildly to moderately impaired AD patients will show significant deficits (Salmon et al. 1988; Burke et al. 1994).

Deficits in retaining material held in primary or short-term memory for periods of up to about 30 seconds have been demonstrated in AD using a variety of well-known tests (Morris 1994). Patients with AD display pervasive impairments on measures of memory span, tests using the Peterson-Brown distractor technique and indices of recency effects in free recall tasks, which have an impact on their ability to perform many activities in their everyday lives (Morris and Baddeley 1988; Knight 1992). A productive way to conceptualize these deficits is in terms of the working memory model of Baddeley and Hitch (1974). A series of studies by Baddeley, Morris and colleagues (Morris 1994) have found that it is a dysfunction of the central executive processes of working memory that is responsible for the short-term memory deficit (Chapter 8). In this model the central executive system has a limited capacity and functions to initiate and coordinate cognitive processes. The operation of the central executive has primarily been explored in dual task paradigms and its relevance to the execution of prospective memory tasks, which are characteristically also studied in divided attention experiments, requiring complex resource allocation, will be apparent.

Failure of the executive functions in working memory in AD appears to be part of a more generalized disruption in processing on any task that requires executive function. On tasks which assess executive abilities such set-shifting, sequencing and self-monitoring of performance, AD patients show deficits that are most apparent when task demands involve concurrent manipulation of information (Lafleche and Albert 1995). For example, in a test of executive control functions in AD, Mack and Patterson (1995) found that Porteus Maze performance, which requires strategic planning and monitoring of performance, was deficient in many of these patients. Thus, many patients with AD show features of the dysexecutive syndrome that are seen in many patients with predominantly frontal lobe damage. Indeed, Becker et al. (1992) have proposed that patients in the initial stages of the disorder AD can be divided into two groups, those that show the distinctive features of dysexecutive syndrome without severe amnesia (presumably because of greater generalized frontal lobe deficit) and those that have a circumscribed amnesic deficit (resulting from more prominent temporal lobe degeneration).

The foregoing suggests that AD patients will have specific difficulties with prospective memory tests. In terms of the model presented in Figure 9.1, there is evidence that at most (if not all) of the processing stages in prospective memory AD patients will show deficits. It can be expected therefore that failure to carry out prospective memory tasks in everyday life will be an early and important marker for the onset of dementia. This is in fact the case. Huppert and Beardsall (1993) tested 12 minimally demented and nine mildly/moderately demented patients, together with two groups of normal controls, on the Rivermead Behavioural Memory Test (RBMT; Wilson et al. 1985), which contains practical tests of both prospective and retrospective memory. The three prospective tests involved remembering: (1) to ask the experimenter to telephone for a taxi, (2) to deliver a message and (3) to ask for the return of a personal belonging. There were also several retrospective memory tests that required recall of objects, a name, a word list and a route around a room.

Huppert and Beardsall found that the prospective memory tests were particularly sensitive to the effects of dementia. Both dementia groups showed significant impairments and there was no difference between the minimally and mildly/moderately demented groups. So even at the very earliest stages of the disorder, where the disorder could not be detected using a clinical mental status examination, decline in prospective memory was detected. This was in contrast to scores on the retrospective memory tests where the less impaired group scored at a level intermediate to the controls and the more demented group. Normal subjects did slightly better on the prospective memory tests than the retrospective tests, which suggests that the sensitivity of the prospective tasks was not due to their greater difficulty levels. The authors suggest that prospective memory deficits may be dissociable from retrospective recall deficits because they found no correlation between scores on the two tasks for the demented patients. Covariance analyses also showed that when the variance due to retrospective deficits was partialed out, significant group differences on the prospective tests remained. Although, as the authors acknowledge, this study did not use tasks where the cognitive processes could be precisely measured and that it was therefore difficult to discern the underlying basis for the prospective memory deficit, their results established the susceptibility of demented patients to dysfunctions of prospective memory.

Parkinson's disease

Idiopathic Parkinson's disease (PD) is the most common disorder of abnormal movement occurring in later life and has been the subject of intense scrutiny by neuropsychologists over the past decade (Brown and Marsden 1990; Bondi et al. 1993; Taylor and Saint-Cyr 1995; Bondi and Tröster 1997). Characterizing the pattern of cognitive deficits in PD has, however, remained controversial and the research effort has been hampered by a variety of methodological issues. In particular, establishing the diagnosis of PD is problematic. In a study of PD patients with clinical signs of dementia, about half were found to have neuropathological signs of AD or diffuse cortical Lewy body disease (Hughes et al. 1993). The classification of Lewy body diseases is undergoing refinement and revision at the present time, but it is apparent that many patients

diagnosed as having PD might have other concomitant degenerative disorders. This makes it difficult to establish even fundamental epidemiological information about the disorder such as the prevalence of concurrent dementia or depression. Practical problems in the testing of patients also arise when taking account of PD patients' variable response to medication (Taylor and Saint-Cyr 1995).

With respect to memory, despite the problems created by issues of diagnosis and ongoing treatment, there is some convergence in the literature on the nature of deficits seen in PD and possible explanations for their occurrence. It is generally acknowledged that memory impairment is seen in PD, although the occurrence is not invariable and severity tends to be less than that seen in AD. Deficits are primarily seen on tests that require conscious control of processing and retrieval, such as traditional free recall tests of word lists (Beatty et al. 1989) and on tests of procedural learning (Saint-Cyr et al. 1988; Harrington et al. 1990). On recognition tests (Lees and Smith 1983; Flowers et al. 1989; Pillon et al. 1993) and semantic priming tasks, their performance is typically normal. Thus, on explicit tests of declarative memory requiring conscious control of encoding or retrieval, persons with PD display some deficits. It is also apparent that the most pervasive deficits that PD groups show on neuropsychological testing are revealed on tests of executive functioning. On tests that require adapting to new situations, self-initiation of cognitive processes, or self-monitoring of performance, PD patients are impaired. An example of this is provided by the accumulated evidence that PD patients perform poorly on the Wisconsin Card Sorting Test and other measures of self-initiated set-shifting (e.g. Taylor et al. 1986; Owen et al. 1993; Van Spaendonck et al. 1995). Taylor and Saint-Cyr (1995) concluded that 'Any task or situation for which no prior experience exists, which lacks explicit guidelines, which is highly effort demanding (i.e. extends beyond normal attentional resources) and which "forces" the subject to develop his own plans or action (formulate and switch novel mental sets and/or established sets in novel combinations) will be difficult' (p.283).

Theoretical accounts of memory deficits in PD are divided on whether memory failure is caused by retrieval failure (possibly mediated in part by basal ganglia functioning) or whether it is part of a more general dysexecutive syndrome (resulting from frontal or frontal-striatal circuit lesions). A model of cognitive failure in PD is provided by Brown and Marsden (1990), who postulate that the dysfunction of a Supervisory Attentional System is responsible for the failure to allocate resources for the completion of complex strategic tasks. This system can be regarded as an executive system, which controls the performance of tasks that require the integration of more than one cognitive process for their execution. The biological basis for this system is the cortical-subcortical circuitry of the frontal lobes. A detailed review of these contrasting views is provided by Tröster and Fields (1995) and is beyond the scope of this chapter. Although the assertion that PD causes failure on tasks generally regarded as measures of executive function is not controversial, at issue is whether this failure can be ascribed to frontal lobe pathology and whether the range of memory deficits seen in PD is best explained by a generalized dysexecutive syndrome.

There are no studies of prospective memory in PD. This is unfortunate because it would appear that the issues raised by the study of memory impairment in PD might be clarified by the detailed examination of prospective memory in this disorder. It is likely that persons with PD will have considerable difficulties with all aspects of tasks that require the formulation and self-initiated retrieval of action plans. These components of prospective memory require the kind of effortful and self-controlled processing that PD patients find most demanding. They may well have less difficulty however, on the retrospective component of those event-based tasks that have highly congruent retrieval cues than will persons with AD, i.e. their retrospective memory functioning is likely to be relatively intact under some circumstances and dissociable from their executive system-based functioning deficits.

Other neurodegenerative disorders

There are no studies available that directly examine prospective memory in other neurodegenerative diseases. There is good reason to believe, however, that prospective memory dysfunction is likely to be an early and disabling symptom of these diseases. In Huntington's disease (HD), a progressive neurological disease resulting in degeneration of neostriatal neurons, particularly of the caudate nucleus (Chapter 3), cognitive loss including memory failure is an almost invariable consequence (Beatty and Butters 1986; Wilson et al. 1987). Although on average the degree of retrospective memory loss is less than that seen in patients with severe amnesia, as in AD, it is more pronounced than in PD (Butters et al. 1985). The ability to learn new skills also is impaired in HD, while generally being preserved in many other forms of dementia (Martone et al. 1984). Patients with HD have also been found to have marked impairments on tasks that are sensitive to frontal damage and dysexecutive syndrome. For example, Brandt et al. (1995) found failures in source memory in a group of early-stage HD patients with minimal impairments in declarative memory. Thus, in terms of our model in Figure 9.2, both failure in declarative and executive function appear likely to contribute to prospective memory loss in HD.

Recently, a small group of elderly patients with Lewy bodies predominating in cortical regions has been identified and distinguished from patients with PD, who have subcortical Lewy body degeneration and persons with AD, who have cortical degeneration characterized by the presence of neurofibrillary tangles. Persons with Lewy body dementia have deficits in higher cognitive functioning accompanied by mild parkinsonism, psychosis and a fluctuating confusional state (Filley 1995). The precise taxonomy of disorders associated with Lewy bodies remains a matter of debate and there has been little neuropsychological research focused on this disorder. The particular vulnerability of the frontal cortex to degenerative changes in Lewy body dementia is reflected, however, in dissociations between their performance and that of AD patients. For example, set-shifting ability is more impaired in the early stages of Lewy body dementia than in AD (Owen et al. 1991). On a self-initiated search task, Sahgal et al. (1995) found that Lewy body dementia and AD groups did not differ in their memory skills, but that cognitive processes thought to be dependent on frontal-subcortical function were more impaired in patients with Lewy body dementia. Thus, like patients with specific frontal damage, it is probable that patients with Lewy body dementia will fail prospective memory tasks primarily on the basis of their executive impairments.

IMPLICATIONS FOR CLINICAL PRACTICE

The research to date clearly demonstrates that prospective memory impairment is an early sign of memory failure and that prospective memory tests are particularly sensitive to the onset of dementia. This is illustrated by the sensitivity of the prospective memory tests in the Rivermead Behavioural Memory Test. Prospective memory tasks are, however, complex and there is little in the way of systematic study of the cognitive processes involved in this form of memory failure in dementia. This is of some significance in planning rehabilitation strategies. For example, it is possible that nonamnesic patients with frontal damage, who display features of a dysexecutive syndrome, would benefit from training in the planning of strategies for remembering intended actions. The specifically amnesic patient, however, may have the ability to organize future cues, but not the ability to recognize the cue or retrieve its meaning. In this case rehabilitation may involve training the patient to use a universal cue for action (i.e. set a timer and check a diary when it sounds). The more diffusely damaged and severely demented Alzheimer patients are only likely to be able to use prospective memory in very limited circumstances.

Evidence that demented Alzheimer patients can benefit from interventions designed to enhance their prospective memory skills comes from McKitrick et al. (1992). They taught four women with AD to perform a prospective memory task using a spaced-retrieval technique. The task required the women to select a colored coupon from amongst several differently colored coupons and offer it to the therapist in exchange for a dollar after a week's delay.

The spaced-retrieval method involved gradually expanding the time between giving the instruction to remember and cuing the recall from a few seconds to several minutes during the hour-long training sessions. Using this method, the participants were able to learn the prospective memory task and were able to adapt to changes in the color of the target coupon. Similar forms of prospective memory training have been employed with patients who were severely amnesic following head trauma (Sohlberg et al. 1992a,b).

Finally, it should be noted that the study of prospective memory offers the opportunity to study component cognitive processes in models of controlled memory processing by contrasting the deficits of specific neurological groups. There recently has been a surge of interest in this type of research (Filoteo et al. 1995). Prospective memory requires the coherent operation of a number of processing stages that are likely to be differentially affected by the different cortical and subcortical dementias. Comparative studies of this kind represent a considerable challenge but offer the prospect of a better understanding of the nature of future memory failure.

REFERENCES

Baddeley, A.D. and Hitch, G.J. 1974. Working memory. In *The psychology of learning and motivation,* vol. 8, ed. G.H. Bower, pp. 47–88. New York: Academic Press.

Beatty, W.W. and Butters, N. 1986. Further analysis of encoding in patients with Huntington's disease. *Brain and Cognition.* 5: 387–398.

Beatty, W.W., Staton, R.D., Weir, W.S., Monson, N. and Whitaker, H.A. 1989. Cognitive disturbances in Parkinson's disease. *Journal of Geriatric Psychiatry and Neurology.* 2: 22–33.

Becker, J.T., Bajulaiye, O. and Smith, C. 1992. Longitudinal analysis of a two-component model of the memory deficit in Alzheimer's disease. *Psychological Medicine.* 22: 437–455.

Bennett-Levy, J. and Powell, G.E. 1980. The subjective memory questionnaire SMQ: An investigation into the reporting of 'real life' memory skills. *British Journal of Clinical Psychology.* 19: 177–188.

Bisiacchi, P.S. 1996. The neuropsychological approach in the study of prospective memory. In *Prospective memory: Theories and applications,* ed. M. Brandimonte, G.O. Einstein and M.A. McDaniel, pp. 297–317. Mahwah, NJ: Lawrence Erlbaum.

Bondi, M.W., Kaszniak, A.W., Bayles, K.A. and Vance, K.T. 1993. Contributions of frontal system dysfunction to memory and perceptual abilities in Parkinson's disease. *Neuropsychology.* 7: 89–102.

Bondi, M.W. and Tröster, A.I. 1997. Parkinson's disease: Neurobehavioral consequences of basal ganglia dysfunction. In *Handbook of neuropsychology and aging,* ed. P.D. Nussbaum, pp. 216–245. New York: Plenum Press.

Brandt, J., Bylsma, W., Aylward, E.H., Rothlind, J. and Gow, C.A. 1995. Impaired source memory in Huntington's disease and its relation to basal ganglia atrophy. *Journal of Clinical and Experimental Neuropsychology.* 17: 868–877.

Brown, R.G. and Marsden, C.D. 1990. Cognitive function in Parkinson's disease. *Trends in Neurosciences.* 13: 21–29.

Burke, J., Knight, R.G. and Partridge, F.M. 1994. Priming deficits in patients with dementia of the Alzheimer's type. *Psychological Medicine*. 24: 987–993.

Butters, N., Wolfe, J., Martone, M., Granholm, E. and Cermak, L.S. 1985. Memory disorders associated with Huntington's disease: Verbal recall, verbal recognition and procedural memory. *Neuropsychologia*. 23: 729–743.

Chapman, L.J. and Chapman, J.P. 1973. Problems in the measurement of cognitive deficit. *Psychological Bulletin*. 79: 380–385.

Cockburn, J. 1995. Task interruption in prospective memory: A frontal lobe function? *Cortex*. 31: 87–97.

Cockburn, J. 1996. Failure of prospective memory after acquired brain damage: Preliminary investigation and suggestions for future directions. *Journal of Clinical and Experimental Neuropsychology*. 18: 304–309.

Craik, F.M. 1986. A functional account of age differences in memory. In *Human memory and cognitive capabilities: Mechanisms and performances*, ed. F. Klix and H. Hagendorf, pp. 409–422. Amsterdam: Elsevier.

Dalla Barba, G. 1993. Prospective memory: A new memory system? In *Handbook of neuropsychology*, vol. 8, ed. F. Boller and J. Grafman, pp. 239–251. Amsterdam: Elsevier.

Daum, I. and Ackermann, H. 1994. Frontal-type memory impairment associated with thalamic damage. *International Journal of Neuroscience*. 77: 187–198.

Dobbs, A.R. and Rule, B.G. 1987. Prospective memory and self-reports of memory abilities in older adults. *Canadian Journal of Psychology*. 41: 209–222.

Einstein, G.O. and McDaniel, M.A. 1990. Normal aging and prospective memory. *Journal of Experimental Psychology (Learning, Memory and Cognition)*. 16: 717–726.

Einstein, G.O., Holland, L.J., McDaniel, M.A. and Guynn, M.J. 1992. Age-related deficits in prospective memory: The influence of task complexity. *Psychology and Aging*. 7: 471–478.

Einstein, G.O., McDaniel, M.A., Richardson, S., Guynn, M.J. and Cunfer, A.R. 1995. Aging and prospective memory: Examining the influences of self-initiated retrieval processes. *Journal of Experimental Psychology (Learning, Memory and Cognition)*. 21: 996–1007.

Ellis, J.A. 1988. Memory for future-intentions: Investigating pulses and steps. In *Practical aspects of memory: Current research and issues*, vol. 1, ed. M.M. Gruneberg, P.E. Morris and R.N. Sykes, pp. 132–136. Chichester: Wiley.

Filley, C.M. 1995. Neuropsychiatric features of Lewy Body Disease. *Brain and Cognition*. 28: 229–239.

Filoteo, J.V., Delis, D.C., Roman, M.J., Demadura, T., Ford, E., Butters, N., Salmon, D.P., Paulsen, J., Shults, C.W., Swanson, M. and Swerdlow, N. 1995. Visual attention and perception in patients with Huntington's disease: Comparisons with other subcortical and cortical dementias. *Journal of Clinical and Experimental Neuropsychology*. 17: 656–667.

Fletcher, P.C., Frith, C.D. and Rugg, M.D. 1997. The functional neuroanatomy of episodic memory. *Trends in Neurosciences*. 20: 213–218.

Flowers, K.A., Pearce, I. and Pearce, J.M.S. 1989. Recognition memory in Parkinson's disease. *Journal of Neurology, Neurosurgery and Psychiatry*. 47: 1174–1181.

Gershberg, F.B. and Shimamura, A.P. 1995. Serial position effects in implicit and explicit tests of memory. *Journal of Experimental Psychology (Learning, Memory and Cognition)*. 20: 1370–1378.

Glisky, E. L. 1996. Prospective memory and the frontal lobes. In *Prospective memory: Theories and applications*, ed. M. Brandimonte, G.O. Einstein and M.A. McDaniel, pp.249–266. Mahwah, NJ: Lawrence Erlbaum.

Haist, F., Shimamura, A.P. and Squire, L.R. 1992. On the relationship between recall and recognition memory. *Journal of Experimental Psychology (Learning, Memory and Cognition)*. 18: 691–702.

Hannon, R., Adams, P., Harrington, S., Fries-Dias, C. and Gipson, M.T. 1995. Effects of brain injury and age on prospective memory self-rating and performance. *Rehabilitation Psychology*. 40: 289–297.

Harrington, D.L., Haaland, K.Y., Yeo, R.A. and Marder, E. 1990. Procedural memory in Parkinson's disease: Impaired motor but not visuopercep-tual learning. *Journal of Clinical and Experimental Neuropsychology*. 12: 323–339.

Harris, J.E. and Wilkins, A.J. 1982. Remembering to do things: A theoretical framework and illustrative experiment. *Human Learning*. 1: 123–136.

Hermann, D.J. and Neisser, U. 1978. An inventory of everyday memory experiences. In *Practical aspects of memory*, ed. M.M. Gruneberg, P.E. Morris and R.N. Sykes, pp. 35–51. London: Academic Press.

Hughes, A.J., Daniel, S.E., Blankson, S. and Lees, A.J. 1993. A clinicopatho-logic study of 100 cases of Parkinson's disease. *Archives of Neurology*. 50: 140–148.

Huppert, F.A. and Beardsall, L. 1993. Prospective memory impairment as an early indicator of dementia. *Journal of Clinical and Experimental Neuropsychology*. 15: 805–821.

Janowsky, J.S., Shimamura, A.P., Kritchevsky, M. and Squire, L.R. 1989a. Cognitive impairment following frontal lobe damage and its relevance to human amnesia. *Behavioural Neuroscience*. 103: 548–560.

Janowsky, J.S., Shimamura, A.P. and Squire, L.R. 1989b. Memory and meta memory: Comparisons between patients with frontal lobe lesions and amnesic patients. *Psychobiology*. 17: 3–11.

Janowsky, J.S., Shimamura, A.P. and Squire, L.R. 1989c. Source memory impairment in patients with frontal lesions. *Neuropsychologia*. 27: 1043–1056.

Kinsella, G., Murtagh, D., Landry, A., Homfray, K., Hammond, M., O'Breine, L., Dwyer, L., Lamont, M. and Ponsford, J. 1996. Everyday memory following traumatic brain injury. *Brain Injury*. 10: 499–507.

Knight, R.G. 1992. *The neuropsychology of degenerative brain diseases*. Hillsdale, NJ: Lawrence Erlbaum.

Knight, R.G. and Godfrey, H.P.D. 1985. The assessment of memory impairment: The relationship between different methods of evaluating dysamnesic deficits. *British Journal of Clinical Psychology*. 24: 125–131.

Lafleche, G. and Albert, M.S. 1995. Executive function deficits in mild Alzheimer's disease. *Neuropsychology*. 9: 313–320.

Lees, A.J. and Smith, E. 1983. Cognitive deficits in the early stages of Parkinson's disease. *Brain*. 106: 257–270.

Levy, R.L. and Loftus, G.R. 1984. Compliance and memory. In *Everyday memory: Actions and absent mindedness*, ed. J.E. Harris and P.E. Morris, pp. 93–112. New York: Academic Press.

Mack, J.L. and Patterson, M.B. 1995. Executive dysfunction and Alzheimer's disease: Performance on a test of planning ability, the Porteus Maze test. *Neuropsychology*. 9: 556–564.

Mangels, J.A., Gershberg, F.B., Shimamura, A.P. and Knight, R.T. 1996. Impaired retrieval from remote memory in patients with frontal lobe damage. *Neuropsychology*. 10: 32–41.

Mäntylä, T. 1994. Remembering to remember: Adult age difference in prospective memory. *Journals of Gerontology*. 49: 276–282.

Martone, M., Butters, N., Payne, M., Becker, J. and Sax, D. 1984. Dissociations between skill learning and verbal recognition in amnesia and dementia. *Archives of Neurology*. 41: 965–970.

Maylor, E.A. 1990. Age and prospective memory. *Quarterly Journal of Experimental Psychology*. 42A: 471–493.

Maylor, E.A. 1993. Aging and forgetting in prospective and retrospective memory tasks. *Psychology and Aging*. 8: 420–428.

Maylor, E.A. 1995 Prospective memory in normal aging and dementia. *Neurocase*. 1: 285–289.

McKitrick, L.A., Camp, C.J. and Black, F.W. 1992. Prospective memory intervention in Alzheimer's disease. *Journal of Gerontology: Psychological Sciences*. 47: 337–343.

Meacham, J.A. and Leiman, B. 1982. Remembering to perform future actions. In *Memory observed: Remembering in natural contexts*, ed. U. Neisser, pp. 327–336. San Francisco: Freeman.

Milner, B., Petrides, M. and Smith, M.L. 1985. Frontal lobes and the temporal organization of memory. *Human Neurobiology*. 4: 137–142.

Morris, R.G. 1994. Working memory in Alzheimer-type dementia. *Neuropsychology*. 8: 544–554.

Morris, R.G. and Baddeley, A.D. 1988. Primary and working memory functioning in Alzheimer-type dementia. *Journal of Clinical and Experimental Neuropsychology*. 10: 279–296.

Oppenheim, G. 1994. The earliest signs of Alzheimer's disease. *Journal of Geriatric Psychiatry and Neurology*. 7: 116–120.

Owen, A.M., Roberts, A.C., Hodges, J.R., Simmers, B.A., Polkey, C.E. and Robins and T.W. 1993. Contrasting mechanisms of impaired attentional set-shifting in patients with frontal lobe damage or Parkinson's disease. *Brain*. 116: 1159–1175.

Owen, A.M., Roberts, A.C., Polkey, C.E., Sahakian, B.J. and Robbins, T.W. 1991. Extra-dimensional versus intra-dimensional set shifting performance following frontal lobe excisions, temporal lobe excisions or amygdalo-hippocampectomy in man. *Neuropsychologia*. 29: 993–1006.

Pillon, B., Deweer, B., Agid, Y. and DuBois, B. 1993. Explicit memory in Alzheimer's, Huntington's and Parkinson's diseases. *Archives of Neurology*. 50: 374–379.

Sahgal, A., McKeith, I.G., Galloway, P.H., Tasker, N. and Steckler, T. 1995. Do differences in visuospatial ability between senile dementias of the Alzheimer and Lewy body types reflect differences solely in mnemonic function? *Journal of Clinical and Experimental Neuropsychology*. 17: 35–43.

Saint-Cyr, J.A., Taylor, A.E. and Lang, A.E. 1988. Procedural learning and neostriatal dysfunction in man. *Brain*. 111: 941–959.

Salmon, D.P., Shimamura, A.P., Butters, N. and Smith, S. 1988. Lexical and semantic priming deficits in patients with Alzheimer's disease. *Journal of Clinical and Experimental Neuropsychology*. 10: 477–494.

Shimamura, A.P. and Squire, L.R. 1986. Memory and metamemory: A study of the feeling-of-knowing phenomenon in amnesic patients. *Journal of Experimental Psychology (Learning, Memory and Cognition)*. 12: 452–460.

Shimamura, A.P., Janowsky, J.S. and Squire, L.R. 1990. Memory for the temporal order of events in patients with frontal lobe lesions and amnesic patients. *Neuropsychologia*. 28: 803–813.

Shimamura, A.P., Janowsky, J.S. and Squire, L.R. 1991. What is the role of frontal lobe damage in memory disorders? In *Frontal lobe function and dysfunction*, ed. H.S. Levin, H.M. Eisenberg and A.L. Benton, pp. 173–195. New York: Oxford University Press.

Simon, E., Leach, L., Winocur, G. and Moscovitch, M. 1994. Intact primary memory in mild to moderate Alzheimer's disease: Indices from the California Verbal Learning Test. *Journal of Clinical and Experimental Neuropsychology*. 16: 414–422.

Sinnott, J.D. 1986. Prospective/intentional and incidental everyday memory: Effects of age and passage of time. *Psychology and Aging*. 1: 110–116.

Sohlberg, M.M., White, O., Evans, E. and Mateer, C. 1992a. Background and initial case studies into the effects of prospective memory training. *Brain Injury*. 6: 129–138.

Sohlberg, M.M., White, O., Evans, E. and Mateer, C. 1992b. An investigation of the effects of prospective memory training. *Brain Injury*. 6: 139–154.

Squire, L.R. 1982. Comparisons between forms of amnesia: Some deficits are unique to Korsakoff's syndrome. *Journal of Experimental Psychology (Learning, Memory and Cognition)*. 8: 565–571.

Taylor, A.E. and Saint-Cyr, J.A. 1995. The neuropsychology of Parkinson's disease. *Brain and Cognition*. 28: 281–296.

Taylor, A.E., Saint-Cyr, J.A. and Lang, A.E. 1986. Frontal lobe dysfunction in Parkinson's disease: The cortical focus of neostriatal outflow. *Brain*. 109: 845–883.

Tröster, A.I. and Fields, J.A. 1995. Frontal cognitive function and memory in Parkinson's disease: Toward a distinction between prospective and declarative memory impairments? *Behavioural Neurology*. 8: 59–74.

Van Spaendonck, K.P.M., Berger, H.J.C., Horstink, M.W.I.M., Borm, G.F. and Cools, A.R. 1995. Card sorting performance in Parkinson's disease: A comparison between acquisition and shifting performance. *Journal of Clinical and Experimental Neuropsychology*. 17: 918–925.

Weingartner, H., Grafman, J., Boutelle, W., Kaye, W. and Martin, P.R. 1981. Forms of memory failure. *Science*. 221: 380–382.

West, R.L. 1988. Prospective memory and aging. In *Practical aspects of memory: Current research and issues*, vol. 2, ed. M.M. Gruneberg, P.E. Morris and R.N. Sykes, pp. 119–125. Chichester: Wiley.

Wilkins, A.J. and Baddeley, A.D. 1978. Remembering to recall in everyday life: An approach to absentmindedness. In *Practical aspects of memory: Current research and issues*, vol. 2, ed. M.M. Gruneberg, P.E. Morris and R.N. Sykes, pp. 27–34. Chichester: Wiley.

Wilson, B.A., Cockburn, J. and Baddeley, A.D. 1985. *The Rivermead Behavioural Memory Test*. Bury Saint Edmunds: Thames Valley Test Co.

Wilson, R.S., Como, P.G., Garron, D.C., Klawans, H.L., Barr, A. and Klawans, D. 1987. Memory failure in Huntington's disease. *Journal of Clinical and Experimental Neuropsychology*. 9: 147–154.

Winograd, E. 1988. Some observations on prospective remembering. In *Practical aspects of memory: Current research and issues*, vol. 2, ed. M.M. Gruneberg, P.E. Morris and R.N. Sykes, pp. 348–353. Chichester: Wiley.

10 Remote memory in neurodegenerative disease

ROBERT H. PAUL, JONI R. GRABER,
DAVID C. BOWLBY, JULIE A. TESTA,
MICHAEL J. HARNISH AND
WILLIAM W. BEATTY

INTRODUCTION

Memory is the cognitive domain most vulnerable to brain injury. Accordingly, the research literature on memory impairment in brain damage is vast, but most of it concerns deficits that occur after the time of brain injury (or the presumed onset of degenerative disease), that is, anterograde amnesia. Much less is known about the ability of patients to recollect information acquired prior to the onset of disease, yet the practical consequences of marked impairments in remote memory (i.e. retrograde amnesia) are likely to be more serious for an elderly person with dementia than are equally severe anterograde memory deficits. Specifically, a patient's complete failure to remember any of the items on a grocery list does not meaningfully increase the caregiver's burden, because the patient would not be expected to do the shopping anyway. By contrast, if the dementia patient repeatedly wanders away from home and cannot remember how to return (a failure of remote visuospatial memory), the burden on the caregiver is great and institutionalization of the patient is a likely consequence.

One reason why the study of remote memory has languished is because of theoretical and methodological problems. This chapter reviews the applicability of the theoretical distinction between episodic and semantic memory to remote memory and then the methods used to study remote memory. After highlighting limitations of these methods, the chapter summarizes the findings of studies of remote memory in normal aging, amnesia and neurodegenerative diseases.

THE EPISODIC/SEMANTIC MEMORY DISTINCTION

Tulving (1972) distinguished between two types of memories. 'Semantic' memories were defined as recollections of facts, rules and general knowledge, whereas 'episodic' memories were defined as recollections of personally experienced events anchored to a specific time and place (Chapters 11 and 12). Most tests of autobiographical recall are considered tests of episodic memory as they focus on subjects' memories for personal events or episodes (Baddeley and Wilson 1986). Cermak (1984), however, has raised doubt about the classification of autobiographical memory as 'episodic'. Cermak and O'Connor (1983) described a postencephalitic amnesic patient who was asked to recall episodic memories to cue words (e.g. boat). On this test, the patient was capable of reporting factual information about remote personal events, but was incapable of recalling these events in time and place. Thus, the patient could state that he had sailed in the past, but he could not describe a single episode of sailing. Cermak explained this patient's memory performance by stating that episodic memories devolve into semantic memories over time, i.e. episodic memories lose their orientation to time and place and eventually represent semantic forms of knowledge. If it is true that episodic memories become semantic memories, then tests of remote memory would be biased towards episodic memory for recent time periods and biased towards semantic memory for more distant time periods (Cermak 1984). In addition, tests of autobiographical memory would no longer represent tests of episodic memory but, rather, they would represent tests of both episodic and semantic memories.

While this theory of episodic and semantic memory is

intriguing, its greatest limitation is that the defining parameters of the theory cannot be determined, i.e. determining the time when episodic memories become semantic memories would be difficult if not impossible. Moreover, if subjects are capable of providing very remote episodic memories (specific to time and place), one cannot assume that such memories are simply semantic recollections of the events.

GENERAL METHODS OF STUDYING REMOTE MEMORY

Standardized methods for studying remote memory take one of two approaches. They either present items or questions that tap information that is presumed to be known by most members of a particular age group or they probe for information about the patient's own past personal experiences. The first type of test is easily scored because there are clearly correct answers to each item, but the cause of poor performance is usually unclear, at least for individual patients, because it is impossible to be certain whether the failed items were once known. Tests of autobiographical information focus on knowledge that the patient can be presumed to have once possessed so 'don't know' or extremely vague answers can be interpreted as memory failures. Determining the correctness of complete answers, which is necessary in order to distinguish accurate memories from confabulation, is time-consuming, problematic and sometimes impossible to accomplish.

A particular difficulty common to all tests of remote memory is determining whether subjects learned the test material at the time the events occurred, or if they learned the events at a later date. This distinction is important in order to determine the pattern (i.e. temporal gradient) of remote memory loss for a given subject. If the material was learned or rehearsed after the events had occurred, then test items would not accurately reflect the time periods they were selected to represent. The use of longitudinal studies could resolve this issue by permitting greater control over the acquisition of test material, but the time and cost required for prospective designs are prohibitive. Still, most remote memory tests control this problem by including numerous test items to represent the different time periods. While it remains possible that a subject could have learned a few events from a given decade after they

actually occurred, the possibility that multiple events were learned in the same manner is less probable.

TESTS OF REMOTE MEMORY

The most frequently used measure of memory for public information is the Remote Memory Battery (RMB; Albert et al. 1979). This battery, which has been updated several times, consists of three subtests which require the identification of famous individuals and recollection of public events from the past. On the first test (Famous Faces), individuals are shown photographs of people who became famous at various times and they are asked to name these individuals. The second test consists of a questionnaire which requires recollection of public events from the same time periods tested on the Famous Faces test. The third test is a multiple choice questionnaire pertaining to similar information tested in the first two subtests. Phonemic and semantic cues are provided to patients if they are unable to provide correct answers on the first two tests.

Test items included in the RMB pertain to well-known public information and were selected to represent distinct decades (e.g. the 1920s, 1930s, etc.), but there is no way to be sure that subjects ever knew the information to begin with. The RMB and similar tests are constructed so that normal subjects score about equally well for all decades sampled. This is done to maximize sensitivity to temporal gradients in remote memory loss. Squire et al. (1975) have argued that this procedure can result in artifactual temporal gradients which arise because items from more recent time periods are more difficult; however, because some patient groups (e.g. patients with Huntington's disease (HD)), are equally impaired across decades (Albert et al. 1981), this does not seem to be a serious problem for the original RMB.

The Television Test developed by Squire and Slater (1975) requires identification of the names of television programs that were broadcast for a single season. Programs were selected from the years 1957–1973 using microfilm records of a local newspaper. A significant strength of this test is that recall of the programs is equally difficult for all decades tested as all shows aired for the same length of time (1 year). Because it is not likely that unsuccessful programs will be shown at a later date, the TV test avoids the problem of multiple uncontrolled exposures, which is a serious problem with the RMB and similar measures. The test is inherently flawed because performance is largely dependent on the viewing habits of subjects (Harvey and Crovitz 1979). Thus, failures to accurately identify TV programs could reflect inadequate exposure to the test material rather than indicating true deficits in remote memory. A similar criticism can be made of Brandt's recent 'Oscar' test of remote memory (Brandt and Benedict 1993) which requires identification of the 'Best Picture' (defined by the Academy Awards) from past years.

A third test of remote memory requires the recollection of past Presidents in correct order. Recall failures on this test indicate impaired remote memory because presumably most members of society have been exposed to this information at some point in their lives. Nevertheless, normal controls often make errors, despite the apparent simplicity of the test. For instance, Hamsher and Roberts (1985) tested 250 normal controls' recall of the last six US presidents and only 42% of the subjects performed without error. The President's Test may not detect impairments that are evident on tests like the Famous Faces (Paul et al. 1997), because the number of items is limited and controls do not perform perfectly.

Remote memory for visuospatial memory can be evaluated with the Fargo Map Test (FMT; Beatty 1988) which involves locating geographical features on maps. After providing a residential history, subjects are asked to locate geographical features (e.g. cities and bodies of water) on a map of the United States and on maps of US regions in which the subject has lived or currently resides. As memory for current and previous regions of residence is evaluated, the FMT can be used to establish potential temporal gradients of remote memory loss.

The assessment of autobiographical memories is an alternative means of testing remote memory. A common method of studying autobiographical memories is based on the Crovitz (1970) technique which requires subjects to recall memories in response to cue words. In order to control for confabulation, subjects are tested again with the same cue words after a 24-hour period and are required to reproduce the memories given on the prior day. Memories elicited on the first day are scored using a three-point system based on the specificity of time and place with which the memories were recounted. Responses given on the second day are scored using a three-point scale based on the consistency of information provided compared to that given on day one; a high correlation indicates

verifiable memories, while a low correlation indicates confabulation.

A significant strength of the Crovitz technique is that the cue words require subjects to recall memories in a highly constrained manner. Thus, subjects are not free to recall simply their most salient memories unless they are related to the cue words. By contrast, the Crovitz technique has been criticized because subjects are not required to produce memories from across the lifespan (Kopelman et al. 1989). Thus, if subjects recall a disproportionate number of memories from a time period better preserved than others, their overall performance would be normal. This is an important limitation considering that patients with amnesic syndromes or dementia of the Alzheimer's type typically recall older remote memories better than newer ones.

Beatty et al. (1987) investigated remote autobiographical memories in a patient with severe retrograde amnesia following a hypoxic episode. When given the standard instructions of the Crovitz technique (i.e. to recall memories from any time period), most of the specific memories recalled by the patient were from the first half of his life and his performance was not significantly impaired relative to that of controls. When the subject was asked to recall more recent memories, however, he performed significantly worse than controls, but three of the four specific memories he recalled pertained to events that occurred after the hypoxic incident! These findings clearly indicate that the nature of instructions for the Crovitz test can significantly impact the pattern of performance.

An additional limitation of the Crovitz technique concerns the typical method of controlling confabulation by testing subjects 24 hours later with the same cues. If a subject confabulates on the first day of testing and can reproduce the response on the second day, the consistency of information between both memories would incorrectly rule out confabulation. Alternatively, if a subject has more than one valid memory appropriate for a given cue and produces a different memory to the cue on the second day of testing, the discrepancy between information would indicate confabulation despite the validity of both memories.

In response to the limitations of the Crovitz technique, Kopelman et al. (1989) developed the semi-structured Autobiographical Memory Interview (AMI). The AMI consists of two subtests: the personal semantic schedule and the autobiographical incident schedule, which measure semantic and episodic memory respectively. Both subtests require subjects to recall personal memories from three life periods: childhood, early adulthood and recent adulthood.

Advantages of the AMI include the fact that both semantic and episodic memories are tested and subjects are required to recall memories from their entire lifespan. Thus, the temporal gradient of memory loss can be determined for each subject. Unlike the Crovitz technique, however, the AMI does not restrict the nature of the memories recalled. Therefore, if subjects are capable of recalling a few salient episodic memories for each time period, they will perform normally on this part of the test. Additionally, personal collaterals may not be available for all subjects in order to verify memories, thereby limiting the investigator's ability to identify confabulation. This problem can be serious with older patients who no longer have family members that are capable of recalling information about the subject, especially for information from childhood years.

NORMAL AGING

The notion that remote memory is selectively preserved in the aged has come from the widely accepted observation that the elderly tend to have difficulty remembering recent events but oftentimes recall events of their early lives in accurate and vivid detail. Early research utilizing remote memory questionnaires contradicted this observation by demonstrating significant decrements in performance with increasing age, indicating that remote memory, like other memory functions, is affected by aging (Squire 1974; Wilson et al. 1981). By contrast, more recent studies have concluded that remote memory is not noticeably affected by the aging process (Fozard 1980; Flicker et al. 1993). In part, the ambiguity of these results reflects the large variation in performance of normal individuals on fact-based remote memory tests and the difficulty of constructing test batteries that contain items equally salient for persons of different age groups.

AMNESIA

Although marked retrograde amnesia is usually only observed in patients who also show substantial anterograde amnesia, two lines of evidence make it clear that retrograde amnesia is not simply a function of amnesia severity. First, in two case studies, patients continued to exhibit profound retrograde amnesia after their ability to learn and remember new information had shown substantial recovery (Salmon et al. 1988; Barr et al. 1990). Second, in a study that examined the relationship between amnesics' performance on a version of the RMB and their degree of anterograde amnesia, a significant correlation between anterograde memory test performance and recall of information from the most recent decade was observed, but there were no significant correlations between anterograde amnesia and recall of information from the more distant past (Shimamura and Squire 1986).

Although memory difficulties may accompany damage to many parts of the brain, circumscribed amnesia without other neuropsychological impairment typically follows injury to the basal forebrain, the diencephalon and the medial temporal lobe. Retrograde amnesia following basal forebrain lesions has not received much study, although a temporal gradient of loss has been reported in one study (Gade and Mortensen 1990); retrograde amnesia after diencephalic or medial temporal lobe injury is relatively better studied.

Korsakoff's syndrome has long been considered the prototype of diencephalic amnesia, although it is now recognized that Korsakoff's syndrome commonly also involves cortical atrophy, especially of the frontal lobes and damage to other brain regions (Parkin 1991). In Korsakoff's syndrome patients who recover from the initial Wernicke's phase of the syndrome there is invariably marked atrophy of the mammillary bodies and the dorsal thalamus, especially the dorsomedial thalamic nucleus.

In addition to their anterograde memory deficit, Korsakoff's syndrome patients have severely impaired retrograde memory. This retrograde amnesia is typically temporally graded, with memory for events in the more distant past preserved relative to memory for more recent events. Temporally graded retrograde amnesia has been reported using a variety of assessment techniques, including recall of public events, photographs and voices of famous people and autobiographical knowledge (including, in case PZ, professional knowledge) (Albert et al. 1981; Butters and Cermak 1986; Shimamura and Squire 1986; Butters and Granholm 1987; Parkin 1991).

Reviewing studies of patients with vascular lesions of the diencephalon, Parkin (1991) concludes that *anterograde* amnesia is most common in patients with significant involvement of the mammillothalamic tract and often absent in patients with extensive damage to the dorsomedial thalamic nucleus. The role of the diencephalon in remote memory is not at all clear. Although some patients with vascular lesions of the diencephalon show mild to moderate retrograde amnesia, others do not. For example, Patient N.A., who sustained a stab wound to the brain that destroyed the mamillary bodies bilaterally and the left dorsomedial thalamus (Squire et al. 1989a) exhibits mild retrograde amnesia, but only on the most demanding tests (Cohen and Squire 1981; Parkin 1991).

Amnesia also results from damage to the medial temporal lobes. Perhaps the best known case is H.M., who experienced a severe anterograde memory deficit after bilateral temporal lobe resection for intractable epilepsy. In contrast to Korsakoff's syndrome amnesics, H.M. has only a circumscribed retrograde amnesia, limited to about a 10-year period prior to his surgery (Barr et al. 1990), with good recall for the period prior to that (Kolb and Whishaw 1990).

Another significant cause of amnesia is herpes encephalitis which preferentially damages the limbic system, particularly the medial temporal lobes. Two patients who sustained extensive bilateral lesions of the medial temporal lobes with additional damage to the temporal neocortex have been studied. Both displayed severe anterograde amnesia and a retrograde amnesia for both episodic and semantic knowledge that spanned their entire adult lives (Cermak 1976; Cermak and O'Connor 1983; Warrington and McCarthy 1988; McCarthy and Warrington 1992). When encephalitis causes mainly unilateral temporal lobe damage, circumscribed retrograde amnesia results; qualitatively similarly findings have been described for mainly right (O'Connor et al. 1992) or left-sided lesions (Yoneda et al. 1992).

Circumscribed (i.e. temporally graded) retrograde amnesia also results from bilateral injury to the hippocampi without significant additional neocortical damage as might occur after hypoxia or ischemia. For example, Patient M.R.L., who became amnesic in 1984, exhibited a sharp temporal gradient of retrograde amnesia on the RMB; he was seriously impaired for items from the 1970s and 1980s, but performed normally for items from the 1930s to 1960s. His memories for floor plans of former residencies were intact up to about 1970, but absent thereafter. Finally, M.R.L. showed loss of semantic knowledge of his profession (Beatty et al. 1987). Four other patients

with hippocampal atrophy similar to that of M.R.L. also exhibited temporally graded retrograde amnesia (Squire et al. 1989b).

When the hippocampus is selectively damaged by hypoxia, anterograde amnesia and very slight retrograde amnesia result (Zola-Morgan et al. 1986). Patient R.B. sustained bilateral pyramidal cell loss limited to the CA1 region of the hippocampus, but no other significant damage which might be linked to memory impairment. Patient R.B.'s retrograde amnesia was temporally limited to no more than 3 years based on the TV test, but he performed normally, or even better, than controls on other tests of remote memory.

There is also evidence to suggest that unilateral damage to the left temporal lobe can result in retrograde amnesia. Barr et al. (1990) compared unilateral left and right temporal lobectomy patients to controls on several tests of remote memory: (1) Famous Faces, (2) the Television Test and (3) a remote memory battery which included evaluations of factual, public chronological and autobiographical knowledge. On all three tests the left temporal lobectomy group showed a temporally graded retrograde amnesia compared to the right temporal lobectomy and control groups. The remote memory impairment for both semantic and episodic knowledge was not a result of language impairments.

Limited research with nonhuman primates (Chapter 1) also implicates the temporal lobes in retrograde amnesia. Monkeys with bilateral temporal lobe resections involving the amygdala and part of the hippocampus exhibited extensive retrograde amnesia which was equally severe for all time periods prior to surgery (spanning about 18 months) (Salmon et al. 1989). Thus, the pattern of retrograde amnesia exhibited by these monkeys resembles that shown by patients with extensive bilateral temporal lobe injury which involves the lateral temporal cortices as well as the medial temporal region (e.g. Patient S.S.), yet the combined hippocampus and amygdala (H+A) lesions sustained by the monkeys were designed to approximate the size and location of the tissue resected in patient H.M.! Monkeys with lesions confined to the hippocampus proper exhibit a pattern of temporally graded retrograde amnesia that is similar to that of patients such as M.R.L., with bilateral lesions confined to the hippocampus (Zola-Morgan and Squire 1990).

In summary, most of the available data on retrograde amnesia in subjects with bilateral temporal lobe injury indicate that the extent of retrograde amnesia is proportional to the size of the lesions. Very restricted injury, as in patient R.B., leads to very slight retrograde amnesia. Larger hippocampal lesions, as in patient M.R.L., are associated with temporally graded retrograde amnesia extending back 10–20 years. Still larger bilateral lesions which include the amygdala and portions of the temporal neocortex, as in patient S.S., are accompanied by extensive retrograde amnesia which is not temporally graded. The puzzling exception to these generalizations is patient H.M., the best studied amnesic of all.

CORTICAL DEMENTIA

The study of remote memory deficits in cortical dementia has focused primarily on Alzheimer's disease (AD). In general, remote memory remains relatively intact early in the course of AD. With disease progression, a slight temporal gradient becomes evident and patients demonstrate relatively better memory for information from the distant than recent past (Moss and Albert 1988; Beatty and Salmon 1991). In moderate to severe AD, the temporal gradient disappears and patients show marked retrograde amnesia for all decades of life (Beatty et al. 1988b; Flicker et al. 1993; Butters and Delis 1995). This general pattern of impairment has been demonstrated for memory for famous faces and public events, visuospatial information and autobiographical information. A temporally graded retrograde amnesia has not always been reported for AD patients (Wilson et al. 1981).

Beatty et al. (1988b) found AD patients' cued and uncued recall of famous faces to be severely impaired. Similarly, Sagar et al. (1988) reported AD patients' recall and recognition of news events to be severely impaired. Both of these studies demonstrated a gentle temporal gradient of memory loss in mildly demented patients, characterized by relative preservation of very old memories superimposed on a substantial loss of information from all past decades. More recent work has replicated this pattern of impairment in AD patients when compared to normal elderly controls (Flicker and Ferris 1987; Flicker et al. 1993; Hodges et al. 1993) and to patients with Parkinson's disease (PD; Fozard 1980) or Korsakoff's syndrome (Kopelman 1989).

Geographical knowledge is considered to be a measure of remote memory for visuospatial information and research has shown that AD patients demonstrate marked impairments in this realm (Beatty and Bernstein 1989;

Beatty and Salmon 1991). Furthermore, AD patients are relatively more accurate in locating places on maps of the region where they were born and raised than on maps of the region where they currently reside, thus indicating the same relative sparing of information from the distant past as seen on other remote memory tests (Beatty and Salmon 1991).

A third domain of remote memory that has been examined in AD is autobiographical memory. Normal elderly subjects recall (with or without cues) personal events from specific time periods as well as younger subjects (Howes and Katz 1992) and there is evidence that recall is characterized by a temporal gradient (Sagar et al. 1988). By contrast, AD patients show deficits in remote autobiographical memory regardless of whether recall is cued (Sagar et al. 1984, 1985, 1988; Kopelman 1989; Pillon et al. 1991) or not (Sagar et al. 1985, 1988; Kopelman 1989; Pillon et al. 1991). Kopelman (1989) demonstrated that retrograde amnesia in AD affects not only autobiographical episodic memories, but also personal semantic memories. The memory loss encompasses both the content and date of events (Fozard 1980; Sagar et al. 1988; Dall'Ora et al. 1989); patients give little detail and make chronological mistakes when asked to frame their memory into a given life-period. The loss of *content* of personal events is characterized by a temporal gradient early in the course of dementia, but *dating* of events is markedly poor for all decades and not characterized by a temporal gradient (Sagar et al. 1988; Kopelman 1989).

Two hypotheses have been advanced to account for the observed pattern of remote memory loss in AD. The first hypothesis attributes the deficits in remote memory to faulty retrieval mechanisms, namely a generalized retrieval deficit or a disruption in the organization of retrieval strategies (Kopelman 1992). Support for this theory comes from studies demonstrating that while AD patients have a general deficit in recalling public and autobiographical information, their performance improves with recognition testing (Sagar et al. 1988; Dall'Ora et al. 1989; Kopelman 1989; Finley et al. 1990; Kopelman 1991). Weiskrantz (1985) argues that improved recall of events (that occurred before the onset of dementia) with cuing or recognition indicates an important role for retrieval mechanisms in retrograde amnesia. The notion of a retrieval deficit is also supported by research showing only a weak correlation between retrograde and anterograde amnesia, but significant correlations between scores on remote memory and frontal lobe function tests (Kopelman 1989). It has been suggested that frontal lobe dysfunction, which disrupts retrieval strategies, in conjunction with limbic-diencephalic pathology is the primary cause of the retrograde amnesia seen in AD (Kopelman 1991). The fact that the retrograde amnesia in AD is temporally graded is consistent with the theory that earlier memories are protected from retrieval deficit by virtue of the fact that they are more salient and better rehearsed (Weiskrantz 1985; Sagar 1990). This preservation of older memories may be the result of reminiscence, or of the formation of connections with newly acquired information, which would enhance the retrieval cues available for these older memories (Weiskrantz 1985; Sagar 1990).

An alternative hypothesis for the retrograde amnesia in AD posits that while the deficit in remote memory might involve a retrieval deficit, it is primarily due to a destruction or loss of semantic knowledge (Dall'Ora et al. 1989; Bäckman and Herlitz 1990; Hodges et al. 1993). In theory, recall differs from recognition in that recall requires the integrity of both the stored information and of retrieval processes, while recognition requires primarily intact stored information by minimizing retrieval demands. Thus, studies showing that retrograde amnesia in AD is observed on both recall and recognition tests (Sagar et al. 1985; Flicker and Ferris 1987; Beatty et al. 1988b), suggest that the remote memory impairment in AD involves not only impaired retrieval, but also a breakdown of knowledge (Flicker et al. 1986). Further evidence for this position comes from studies demonstrating that AD patients perform poorly on tests of semantic memory such as visual confrontation naming and category fluency (Flicker and Ferris 1987; Hodges et al. 1992; Beatty et al. 1995) and that naming and remote memory are positively correlated in this population (Flicker and Ferris, 1987; Beatty et al. 1988b). Moreover, on tests such as Famous Faces, AD patients are not only unable to name the pictured individuals, but they are also incapable of producing other descriptive information about these personalities (Hodges et al. 1993). Finally, AD patients do much worse than vascular dementia patients on semantic remote memory measures such as Famous Faces, but the two groups do equally poorly on episodic memory tasks (Ricker et al. 1994). These results further support a degradation in semantic knowledge as being largely responsible for the remote memory deficits seen in AD.

The question of whether the retrograde amnesia in AD reflects impaired retrieval or an additional destruction of semantic memory stores continues to be controversial. Resolution of this issue is of critical importance. If AD patients do indeed have the requisite information available in their memory stores, but are unable to deploy the appropriate strategies to access it, then it might be possible to minimize the impact of remote memory loss by providing patients with appropriate cues.

Little research has been done on remote memory in cortical dementias other than AD. Pick's disease, or dementia of the frontal type, is a rather uncommon cortical dementia, characterized by a clinical presentation similar to AD, but with cellular degeneration and atrophy confined to the frontal and temporal cortex (Cummings 1990). The effect of frontal dementia on remote memory has not been systematically studied, but it is known that interruption of fronto-striatal circuits can lead to a generalized retrieval deficit (Cummings and Benson 1990). Thus, it has been hypothesized that a retrograde amnesia in Pick's disease should have a flat temporal gradient similar to that seen in Huntington's disease. Hodges and Gurd (1994) assessed remote memory for public and autobiographical events in a 67-year-old patient with Pick's disease. At first assessment, early in the disease, remote memory for famous faces and events was relatively spared. In contrast, performance on the Crovitz test for personal remote memory was markedly impaired, as evidenced by difficulties in retrieving time-specific and detailed memories and in dating personal memories. Eighteen months later the patient's performance was severely impaired on all tests of remote memory. As hypothesized, the retrograde amnesia did not have a temporal gradient, which is consistent with the pattern seen in HD, but unlike that seen in AD (Hodges and Gurd 1994).

Another cortical dementia in which remote memory has been examined is corticobasal degeneration, a progressive disorder involving cortical atrophy, concentrated in the posterior frontal and parietal cortices, as well as atrophy of the thalamus, basal ganglia and midbrain (Rebeiz et al. 1968; Gibb et al. 1989; Gibb 1992; Chapter 3). A case study by Beatty et al. (1995) demonstrated marked deficits in a corticobasal degeneration patient on tests of remote memory requiring recall, but normal performance on the same tests requiring recognition. These results provide evidence for a deficit in retrieval, most likely secondary to the frontal pathology present in corticobasal degeneration. The striking contrast between remote memory recognition in corticobasal degeneration and AD might be attributable to the fact that unlike AD, corticobasal degeneration does not affect medial temporal lobe structures. A second possibility is that AD causes more extensive damage to the parietal and lateral temporal cortices than corticobasal degeneration, thus resulting in greater deficits in remote memory (Beatty et al. 1995).

The pathology underlying retrograde amnesia in AD most likely involves the lateral and medial temporal lobe, tertiary parietal areas and entorhinal cortex (Moss and Albert 1988; Kolb and Whishaw 1990), but frontal and parietal pathology might also have a role in retrograde amnesia, at least for certain types of information. It has been demonstrated that bilateral medial temporal lobe damage leads to deficits in remote memory and even more severe deficits are seen with additional involvement of the amygdala and the entorhinal and lateral temporal cortices (Beatty et al. 1987; Squire and Zola-Morgan 1991). Parietal lobe pathology has been implicated as contributing to the deficits in remote memory for geographical knowledge (Beatty and Bernstein 1989; Beatty and Salmon 1991). Frontal lobe dysfunction might play an important role in the inability of AD patients to accurately retrieve and reconstruct autobiographical memories (Dall'Ora et al. 1989; Hodges et al. 1993; Hodges and Gurd 1994). Finally, frontal lobe dysfunction is also thought to be responsible for the presence of the temporal gradient seen in the retrograde amnesia of AD (Kopelman 1991), although the steep temporal gradients seen in the retrograde amnesia of patients with subtotal hippocampal lesions challenge this view.

Remote memory is considered a form of 'crystallized intelligence' that appears to be relatively preserved in normal aging (Fozard 1980; Flicker et al. 1993). Although remote memory is vulnerable to dementia (Flicker et al. 1986), it is noteworthy that of all the mental abilities that are affected by AD, remote memory (especially for personal experiences) appears to be one of the most resistant. Even in the later stages of dementia, some remote memory functions can be measured long after other cognitive functions have reached a floor (Flicker et al. 1993).

SUBCORTICAL DEMENTIA

Albert et al. (1974) introduced the term 'subcortical dementia' to describe the pattern of neuropsychological impairments observed in patients with progressive supra-nuclear palsy. The cognitive and affective changes exhibited by these patients included memory impairment, slowed information processing, abstraction and calculation difficulties and mood disturbance. Subcortical dementia has also been reported in patients with HD (McHugh and Folstein 1975), PD (Albert 1978), multiple sclerosis (Rao 1986) and the AIDS dementia complex (Navia 1986), now called HIV-associated dementia.

Remote memory in subcortical dementia has usually been evaluated with versions of the RMB. Using this test battery, deficits in remote memory have been identified in HD (Albert et al. 1981; Beatty et al.1988b), PD (Freedman et al. 1984; Huber et al. 1986; Sagar et al. 1988) and multiple sclerosis (Beatty et al. 1988a; 1989). In all but one study (Sagar et al. 1988), the magnitude of impairment was equally severe for all decades tested. Venneri et al. (1997) recently confirmed that nondemented PD patients' impairment in retrieving the *contents* of remote events is characterized by a flat temporal gradient, but they found that the loss of ability in *dating* these events was temporally graded (although a similar temporal gradient in the accuracy of dating events was also observed in the control group). The 'flat' temporal gradient characterizing the retrograde amnesia of subcortical dementia is not evident in Korsakoff's syndrome (Albert et al. 1981), mild AD or in patients with bilateral hippocampal lesions and therefore, distinguishes the retrograde amnesia in subcortical dementia from that observed in amnestic syndromes and the most common cortical dementia.

Remote visuospatial memory has not been extensively studied in the subcortical dementias. Mildly demented multiple sclerosis and PD patients showed mild impairments on the FMT. In addition, HD patients showed comparable losses of geographic knowledge for the region in which they were born and raised and for the region of current residence (Beatty 1989). These results generally parallel findings from studies using other remote memory tests; however, the President's Test has not revealed deficits in patients with HD (Caine et al. 1986; Pillon et al. 1991), multiple sclerosis (Caine et al. 1986; Rao et al. 1991), progresive supranuclear palsy (Pillon et al. 1991) or PD (Pillon et al. 1991).

Little information is available about autobiographical memory in subcortical dementias. Paul et al. (1997) recently tested recall of remote autobiographical memories in multiple sclerosis patients using the AMI. Even multiple sclerosis patients who performed normally on the MMSE were significantly impaired in recalling semantic, but not episodic autobiographical memories. Moreover, both old and more recent memories were impaired. Sagar et al. (1988) tested PD patients' remote memory for dates of events using a modified version of the Crovitz (1970) technique. In this test, subjects were required to recall dates of personal memories elicited by 10 word cues. Patients with PD were found to be significantly impaired on this test of autobiographical memory and memories from all decades were similarly impaired.

Only a few studies have investigated the relationship between disease duration and magnitude of remote memory impairment in subcortical dementia. Results from these studies indicate that longer disease duration in HD (Albert et al. 1981) and PD (Huber et al. 1989) is associated with more severe memory deficits. A similar relationship, however, has not been demonstrated in multiple sclerosis (Beatty et al. 1988a; 1989).

Impairments of remote memory in subcortical dementia are believed to result primarily from faulty retrieval processes. This tenet is supported by the observation that patients with subcortical dementia are equally impaired in recalling memories from different time periods and that these patients' performance usually improves with recognition or cueing procedures. As patients are also impaired in recalling information acquired before the onset of their disease, their remote memory dysfunction cannot be attributed to the cumulative effects of impaired anterograde memory. Moreover, a general breakdown in semantic knowledge cannot entirely explain the pattern of remote memory impairments in subcortical dementia because deficits can be demonstrated in patients without naming or other language deficits.

In summary, the integrity of remote memory in subcortical dementia appears to be test-dependent. Patients with subcortical dementia are significantly impaired relative to controls on tests which require identification of famous personalities, recall of public and autobiographical events from the past, but not on the President's Test.

CONCLUSIONS

Despite the methodological difficulties associated with the study of remote memory the overall pattern of results is quite consistent. Patients with subcortical dementias exhibit retrograde amnesia with a flat temporal gradient. The severity of retrograde amnesia is correlated with the degree of global cognitive impairment, but the temporal gradient is the same regardless of overall level of cognitive function. By contrast, in AD a temporally graded retrograde amnesia is evident in the initial stages of the disease when overall cognitive function is only moderately disturbed. As the dementia progresses, the gradient disappears because performance reaches floor, at least on tests like the RMB.

Because HD, PD, progressive supranuclear palsy and multiple sclerosis all disrupt frontostriatal circuits (Domesick 1990), it is tempting to suggest that this pathology underlies the similar patterns of remote memory loss in these diseases. Consistent with this idea is the widespread view that most recall deficits in patients with subcortical diseases or frontal lobe lesions are the result of retrieval difficulties (Shimamura et al. 1991). The striking contrast between recall and recognition of Famous Faces in corticobasal degeneration (Beatty et al., 1995) could lend additional support to this position.

If frontal lobe dysfunction is the source of remote memory deficits in subcortical dementia, then damage to the temporal lobes may be the principal cause of retrograde amnesia in the early stages of AD. Various pathological changes affect the hippocampus and adjacent structures early in the course of AD when temporally graded retrograde amnesia can be demonstrated. Studies of amnesics indicate that when damage is restricted to the hippocampus, temporally graded retrograde amnesia of variable extent occurs. Such studies also indicate that more widespread damage to the temporal lobes is associated with more extensive retrograde amnesia which is not temporally graded. Retrograde amnesia is usually more severe in AD than in amnesia, even when the temporal poles are extensively and bilaterally destroyed. This can probably be attributed to the extensive pathology in prefrontal, parietal and lateral temporal cortices that occurs later in AD but not in temporal lobe amnesia.

Our review of the literature on remote memory revealed some information of relevance to the clinical assessment of retrograde amnesia. The President's Test is brief and widely used, but not particularly sensitive to retrograde amnesia. As tests like the RMB may be too long for use in clinical practice, a standardized test like the AMI may be the best choice for measuring remote memory in the clinical setting. Furthermore, the AMI taps information that the patient once knew and given the low variability in performance by controls, is likely to have high sensitivity.

REFERENCES

Albert, M.L. 1978. Subcortical dementia. In *Alzheimer's disease: Senile dementia and related disorders*, ed. R. Katzman, R.D. Terry and K.L. Bick, pp. 173–180. New York: Raven Press.

Albert, M.L., Feldman, R.G. and Willis, A.L. 1974. The subcortical dementia of progressive supranuclear palsy. *Journal of Neurology, Neurosurgery and Psychiatry*. 37: 121–130.

Albert, M.S., Butters, N. and Brandt, J. 1981. Patterns of remote memory in amnesic and demented patients. *Archives of Neurology*. 38: 495–500.

Albert, M.S., Butters, N. and Levin, J. 1979. Temporal gradients in the retrograde amnesia of patients with alcoholic Korsakoff's disease. *Archives of Neurology*. 36: 211–221.

Bäckman, L. and Herlitz, A. 1990. The relationship between prior knowledge and face recognition memory in normal aging and Alzheimer's disease. *Journal of Gerontology*. 45: 94–100.

Baddeley, A.D. and Wilson, B. 1986. Amnesia, autobiographical memory and confabulation. In *Autobiographical memory*, ed. D. Rubin, pp. 225–252. Cambridge: Cambridge University Press.

Barr, W.B., Goldberg, E., Wasserstein, J. and Novelly, R.A. 1990. Retrograde amnesia following unilateral temporal lobectomy. *Neuropsychologia*. 28: 243–255.

Beatty, W.W. 1988. The Fargo Map Test: A standardized method for assessing remote memory for visuospatial information. *Journal of Clinical Psychology*. 44: 61–67.

Beatty, W.W. 1989. Remote memory for visuospatial information in patients with Huntington's disease. *Psychobiology*. 17: 431–434.

Beatty, W.W. and Bernstein, N. 1989. Geographical knowledge in patients with Alzheimer's disease. *Journal of Geriatric Psychiatry and Neurology*. 2: 76–82.

Beatty, W.W., Goodkin, D.E., Monson, N. and Beatty, P.A. 1989. Cognitive disturbances in patients with relapsing remitting multiple sclerosis. *Archives of Neurology*. 46: 1113–1119.

Beatty, W.W., Goodkin, D.E., Monson, N., Beatty, P.A. and Hertsgaard, D. 1988a. Anterograde and retrograde amnesia in patients with chronic progressive multiple sclerosis. *Archives of Neurology*. 45: 611–619.

Beatty, W.W. and Salmon, D.P. 1991. Remote memory for visuospatial information in patients with Alzheimer's disease. *Journal of Geriatric Psychiatry and Neurology*. 4: 14–17.

Beatty, W.W., Salmon, D.P., Bernstein, N. and Butters, N. 1987. Remote memory in a patient with amnesia due to hypoxia. *Psychological Medicine*.17: 657–665.

Beatty, W.W., Salmon, D.P., Butters, N., Heindel, W.C. and Granholm, E.L. 1988b. Retrograde amnesia in patients with Alzheimer's disease or Huntington's disease. *Neurobiology of Aging*. 9: 181–186.

Beatty, W.W., Scott, J.G., Wilson, D.A. Prince, J.R. and Williamson, D.J. 1995. Memory deficits in a demented patient with probable corticobasal degeneration. *Journal of Geriatric Psychiatry and Neurology*. 8: 132–136.

Brandt, J. and Benedict, R.H.B. 1993. Assessment of retrograde amnesia: Findings with a new public events procedure. *Neuropsychology*. 7: 217–227.

Butters, N. and Cermak, L.S. 1986. A case study of the forgetting of autobiographical knowledge: Implications for the study of retrograde amnesia. In *Autobiographical memory*, ed. D. Rubin, pp. 253–272. Cambridge: Cambridge University Press.

Butters, N., Delis, D. and Lucas, J.A. 1995. Clinical assessment of memory disorders in amnesia and dementia. *Annual Review of Psychology*. 46: 493–523.

Butters, N. and Granholm, E. 1987. The continuity hypothesis: Some conclusions and their implications for the etiology and neuropathology of alcoholic Korsakoff's syndrome. In *Neuropsychology of alcoholism: Implications for diagnosis and treatment*, ed. O.A. Parsons, N. Butters and P.E. Nathan, pp. 176–206. New York: Guilford Press.

Caine, E.D., Bamford, K.A., Schiffer, R.B., Shoulson, I. and Levy, S. 1986. A controlled neuropsychological comparison of Huntington's disease and multiple sclerosis. *Archives of Neurology*. 43: 249–254.

Cermak, L.S. 1976. The encoding capacity of a patient with amnesia due to encephalitis. *Neuropsychologia*. 14: 311–326.

Cermak, L.S. 1984. The episodic-semantic distinction in amnesia. In *Neuropsychology of memory*, ed. L.R. Squire and N. Butters, pp. 55–62. New York: Guilford Press.

Cermak, L.S. and O'Connor, M. 1983. The anterograde and retrograde retrieval ability of a patient with amnesia due to encephalitis. *Neuropsychologia*. 21: 213–224.

Cohen, N.J. and Squire, L.R. 1981. Retrograde amnesia and remote memory impairment. *Neuropsychologia*. 19: 67–76.

Crovitz, H.F. 1970. *Galton's walk: Methods for the analysis of thinking, intelligence and creativity*. New York: Harper and Row.

Cummings, J.L. 1990. Introduction. In *Subcortical dementia*, ed. J.L. Cummings, pp. 3–16. New York: Oxford University Press.

Cummings, J.L. and Benson, D.F. 1990. Subcortical mechanisms and human thought. In *Subcortical dementia*, ed. J.L. Cummings, pp. 251–261. New York: Oxford University Press.

Dall'Ora, P., Della Sala, S. and Spinnler, H. 1989. Autobiographical memory: Its impairment in amnesic syndromes. *Cortex*. 25: 329–336.

Domesick, V.B. 1990. Subcortical anatomy: The circuitry of the striatum. In *Subcortical dementia*, ed. J.L. Cummings, pp. 31–43. New York: Oxford University Press.

Finley, G.E., Sharp, T. and Agramonte, R. 1990. Recall and recognition memory for remotely acquired information in dementia patients. *Journal of Genetic Psychology*. 151: 267–268.

Flicker, C. and Ferris, S.H. 1987. Implications of memory and language dysfunction in the naming deficit of senile dementia. *Brain and Language*. 31: 187–200.

Flicker, C., Ferris, S.H., Crook, T., Bartus, R.T. and Reisberg, B. 1986. Cognitive decline in advanced age: Future directions for the psychometric differentiation of normal and pathological age changes in cognitive function. *Developmental Neuropsychology*. 2: 309–322.

Flicker, C., Ferris, S.H. and Reisberg, B. 1993. A two-year longitudinal study of cognitive function in normal aging and Alzheimer's disease. *Journal of Geriatric Psychiatry and Neurology*. 6: 84–96.

Fozard, J.L. 1980. The time for remembering. In *Aging in the 1980s*, ed. L.W. Poon, pp. 273–287. Washington, D.C.: American Psychological Association.

Freedman, M., Rivoira, P., Butters, N., Sax, D.S. and Feldman, R.G. 1984. Retrograde amnesia in Parkinson's disease. *Canadian Journal of Neurological Science*. 11: 297–301.

Gade, A. and Mortensen, E.L. 1990. Temporal gradient in the remote memory impairment of amnesic patients with lesions in the basal forebrain. *Neuropsychologia*. 28: 985–1001.

Gibb, W.R.G. 1992. Neuropathology of Parkinson's disease and related syndromes. *Neurologic Clinics*. 10: 361–376.

Gibb, W.R.G., Luthert, P.J. and Marsden, C.D. 1989. Corticobasal degeneration. *Brain*. 112: 1171–1192.

Hamsher, K. deS. and Roberts, R.J. 1985. Memory for recent U.S. presidents in patients with cerebral disease. *Journal of Clinical and Experimental Neuropsychology*. 7: 1–13.

Harvey, M.T. and Crovitz, H.F. 1979. Television questionnaire techniques in assessing forgetting in long-term memory. *Cortex*. 15: 609–618.

Hodges, J.R. and Gurd, J.M. 1994. Remote memory and lexical retrieval in a case of frontal Pick's disease. *Archives of Neurology*. 51: 821–827.

Hodges, J.R., Salmon, D.P. and Butters, N. 1992. Semantic memory impairment in Alzheimer's disease: Failure of access or degraded knowledge? *Neuropsychologia*. 30: 301–314.

Hodges, J.R., Salmon, D.P. and Butters, N. 1993. Recognition and naming of famous faces in Alzheimer's disease: A cognitive analysis. *Neuropsychologia*. 31: 775–788.

Howes, J.L. and Katz, A.N. 1992. Remote memory: Recalling autobiographical and public events from across the lifespan. *Canadian Journal of Psychology*. 46: 92–116.

Huber, S.J., Friedenberg, D.L., Shuttleworth, E.C., Paulson, G..W. and Christy, J.A. 1989. Neuropsychological impairments associated with severity of Parkinson's disease. *Journal of Neuropsychiatry and Clinical Neurosciences*. 1: 154–158.

Huber, S.J., Shuttleworth, E.C. and Paulson, G.W. 1986. Dementia in Parkinson's disease. *Archives of Neurology*. 43: 987–990.

Kolb, B. and Whishaw, I.Q. 1990. *Fundamentals of human neuropsychology*, 3rd ed. New York: W.H. Freeman and Company.

Kopelman, M.D. 1989. Remote and autobiographical memory, temporal context memory and frontal atrophy in Korsakoff and Alzheimer patients. *Neuropsychologia*. 27: 437–460.

Kopelman, M.D. 1991. Frontal dysfunction and memory deficits in the alcoholic Korskakoff syndrome and Alzheimer-type dementia. *Brain*. 114: 117–137.

Kopelman, M.D. 1992. Storage, forgetting and retrieval in the anterograde and retrograde amnesia of Alzheimer dementia. In *Memory functioning in dementia*. L. Bäckman ed., pp. 45–71. Amsterdam: Elsevier.

Kopelman, M.D., Wilson, B.A. and Baddeley, A.D. 1989. The Autobiographical Memory Interview: A new assessment of autobiographical and personal semantic memory in amnesic patients. *Journal of Clinical and Experimental Neuropsychology*. 11: 724–744.

McCarthy, R.A. and Warrington, E.K. 1992. Actors but not scripts: The dissociation of people and events in retrograde amnesia. *Neuropsychologia*. 30: 633–644.

McHugh, P.R. and Folstein, M.F. 1975. Psychiatric symptoms of Huntington's chorea: A clinical and phenomenological study. In *Psychiatric aspects of neurological disease*, ed. D.F Benson and D. Blumer, pp. 267–285. New York: Grune and Stratton.

Moss, M.B. and Albert, M.S. 1988. Alzheimer's disease and other dementing disorders. In *Geriatric neuropsychology*, ed. M.S. Albert and M.B. Moss, pp. 146–178. New York: Guilford Press.

Navia, R. 1986. The AIDS dementia complex. I. Clinical features. *Annals of Neurology*, 19: 525–535.

O'Connor, M., Butters, N., Miliotis, P., Eslinger, P. and Cermak, L.S. 1992. The dissociation of anterograde and retrograde amnesia in a patient with herpes encephalitis. *Journal of Clinical and Experimental Neuropsychology*. 14: 159–178.

Parkin, A.J. 1991. Recent advances in the neuropsychology of memory. In *Memory: Neurochemical and abnormal perspectives*, ed. J. Weinman and J. Hunter, pp. 141–162. London: Harwood Academic Publishers.

Paul, R.H., Blanco, C.R., Hames, K.A. and Beatty, W.W. 1997. Autobiographical memory in multiple sclerosis. *Journal of the International Neuropsychological Society*. 3: 246–251.

Pillon, B., Dubois, B., Ploska, A. and Agid, Y. 1991. Severity and specificity of cognitive impairment in Alzheimer's, Huntington's and Parkinson's diseases and progressive supranuclear palsy. *Neurology*. 41: 634–643.

Rao, S.M. 1986. Neuropsychology of multiple sclerosis: A critical review. *Journal of Clinical and Experimental Neuropsychology*. 8: 503–542.

Rao, S.M., Leo, G.J., Bernardin, L. and Unverzagt, F. 1991. Cognitive dysfunction in multiple sclerosis. I. Frequency, patterns and prediction. *Neurology*. 41: 685–691.

Rebeiz, J.J., Kolodny, E.H. and Richardson, E.P. 1968. Corticodentatonigral degeneration with neuronal achromasia. *Archives of Neurology*. 18: 20–33.

Ricker, J.H., Keenan, P.A. and Jacobson, M.W. 1994. Visuoperceptual-spatial ability and visual memory in vascular dementia and dementia of the Alzheimer type. *Neuropsychologia*. 32: 1287–1296.

Sagar, H.J. 1990. Aging and age-related neurological disease: Remote memory. In *Handbook of neuropsychology*, vol. 4, ed. F. Boller and J. Grafman, pp. 311–324. Amsterdam: Elsevier.

Sagar, H.J., Cohen, N.J., Corkin, S. and Growdon, J.H. 1985. Dissociations among processes in remote memory. *Annals of the New York Academy of Sciences*. 444: 533–535.

Sagar, H.J., Cohen, N.J., Sullivan, E.V., Corkin, S. and Growdon, J.H. 1988. Remote memory function in Alzheimer's disease and Parkinson's disease. *Brain*. 111: 185–206.

Sagar, H.J., Corkin, S., Cohen, N.J. and Growdon, J.H. 1984. Remote-memory function in Alzheimer's disease and other neurologic diseases. *Neurology*. 34 (Suppl. 1): 102.

Salmon, D.P., Lasker, B.R., Butters, N. and Beatty, W.W. 1988. Remote memory in a patient with circumscribed amnesia. *Brain and Cognition*. 7: 201–211.

Salmon, D.P., Zola-Morgan, S. and Squire, L.R. 1989. Retrograde amnesia following combined hippocampus-amygdala lesions in monkeys. *Psychobiology*. 15: 37–47.

Shimamura, A.P. and Squire, L.R. 1986. Korsakoff's syndrome: A study of the relation between anterograde amnesia and remote memory impairment. *Behavioral Neuroscience*. 100: 165–170.

Shimamura, A.P., Janowsky, J.S. and Squire, L.R. 1991. What is the role of frontal lobe damage in memory disorders? In *Frontal lobe function and dysfunction*, ed. H.S. Levin, H.M. Eisenberg and A.L. Benton, pp. 173–195. New York: Oxford University Press.

Squire, L. R. 1974. Remote memory as affected by aging. *Neuropsychologia*. 12: 429–435.

Squire, L.R. and Slater, P.C. 1975. Forgetting in very long-term memory as assessed by an improved questionnaire technique. *Journal of Experimental Psychology*. 104: 50–54.

Squire, L.R. and Zola-Morgan, S. 1991. The medial temporal lobe system. *Science*. 253: 1380–1386.

Squire, L.R., Amaral, D.G., Zola-Morgan, S., Kritchevsky, M. and Press, Z.G. 1989a. Description of brain injury in the amnesic patient N.A. based on magnetic resonance imaging. *Experimental Neurology*. 105: 23–35.

Squire, L.R., Chace, P.M. and Slater, P.C. 1975. Assessment of memory for remote events. *Psychological Reports.* 37: 223–234.

Squire, L.R., Haist, F. and Shimamura, A.P. 1989b. The neurology of memory: Quantitative assessment of retrograde amnesia in two groups of amnesics patients. *Journal of Neuroscience.* 9: 828–839.

Tulving, E. 1972. Episodic and semantic memory. In *Organization of memory,* ed. E. Tulving and W. Donaldson, pp. 382–404. New York: Academic Press.

Venneri, A., Nichelli, P., Modonesi, G., Molinari, M.A., Russo, R. and Sardini, C. 1997. Impairment in dating and retrieving remote events in patients with early Parkinson's disease. *Journal of Neurology, Neurosurgery and Psychiatry.* 62: 410–413.

Warrington, E.K. and McCarthy, R.A. 1988. The fractionation of retrograde amnesia. *Brain and Cognition.* 7: 184–200.

Weiskrantz, L. 1985. On issues and theories of the human amnestic syndrome. In *Memory systems of the brain,* ed. N.M. Weinberger, J.L. McGaugh and G. Lynch, pp. 380–418. New York: Guilford Press.

Wilson, R.S., Kaszniak, A.W. and Fox, J.H. 1981. Remote memory in senile dementia. *Cortex.* 17: 41–48.

Yoneda, Y., Yamadori, A., Mori, E. and Yamashita, H. 1992. Isolated prolonged retrograde amnesia. *European Neurology.* 32: 340–342.

Zola-Morgan, S. and Squire, L.R. 1990. The primate hippocampal formation: Evidence for a time-limited role in memory storage. *Science,* 250: 288–290.

Zola-Morgan, S., Squire, L.R. and Amaral, D.G. 1986. Human amnesia and the medial temporal region: Enduring memory impairment following a bilateral lesion limited to field CA1 of the hippocampus. *Journal of Neuroscience.* 6: 2950–2967.

11

Semantic memory in neurodegenerative disease

JOSEPH W. FINK AND
CHRISTOPHER RANDOLPH

INTRODUCTION

Semantic memory is a term for our repository of general knowledge about the world, our representation or 'map' of external reality that invests its referents with meaning. The concept of semantic memory can be traced to Tulving's (1972) bipartite model of long-term memory, in which declarative knowledge could be divided into episodic and semantic memories (Chapters 3 and 12). Whereas episodic memory refers to a system of storing contextually specific episodes or events, semantic memory includes general knowledge about the meaning of concepts, words and objects. According to Tulving (1995), 'semantic memory makes possible the acquisition and retention of factual information in the broadest sense; the structured representation of this information, semantic knowledge, models the world' (p. 841).

The goal of this chapter is to review how semantic memory is affected by various neurodegenerative diseases. We first review evidence that helps elucidate what neurocognitive systems subserve semantic memory. We then examine how semantic memory is affected when these neurocognitive systems are compromised by neurodegenerative disease, with emphasis on Alzheimer's disease (AD) as the prototypical cortical degenerative process. Along the way, we note the inferences that can be drawn about the structure and organization of semantic memory from its disorders in neurodegenerative diseases.

NEURAL SUBSTRATES OF SEMANTIC MEMORY

Before examining what is known about semantic memory in the dementia syndromes that result from neurodegenerative diseases, we will briefly review the neural systems

that seem to be essential to semantic memory. The functional neuroanatomy of semantic memory is complex, but clues to its regional localization and organization come from lesion studies and from functional neuroimaging studies with normals. These areas are covered in more detail elsewhere in this volume (Chapters 3, 5 and 6), but a few main points will be highlighted in order to outline the principal neuroanatomical structures involved in semantic memory.

Lesion studies

Semantic memory is regarded as being relatively resistant to degradation by most forms of acquired brain dysfunction, particularly in the context of diffuse encephalopathic conditions. Indeed, so-called 'hold' measures used to estimate premorbid ability level are probes of semantic memory abilities, including vocabulary, reading recognition and other verbal abilities (Lezak 1995). Nevertheless, there are reports of rare acquired lesions that give rise to a relatively focal impairment of semantic memory. For instance, McKenna and Warrington (1993) compiled a list of 32 cases taken from 25 published case reports in which semantic memory deficits were salient. The etiologies in this case series were largely herpes encephalitis, infarcts and neoplasms. In general, lesion localization was not always clearly-defined in these reports, but all cases had either left hemisphere or bilateral lesions which tended to involve the temporal lobes. McKenna and Warrington (1993) documented many cases of category-specific semantic deficits, in which patients seem to display selective loss of knowledge for specific categories in the presence of preserved knowledge for other categories. The most frequently observed category dissociation is between living things and inanimate objects, though several others have been suggested as well (e.g. concrete/abstract, actions/objects).

In their review of the neuroanatomy underlying acquired semantic memory deficits, Patterson and Hodges (1995) note that the temporal neocortex, particularly the left anterolateral temporal lobe, tends to be implicated as the neuroanatomical common denominator. For example, in cases of herpes encephalitis lesions producing semantic deficits (Warrington and Shallice 1984; Pietrini et al. 1988; Sartori and Job 1988), the common substrate seems to be the temporal neocortex. Similarly, in Bub et al.'s (1988) report of a traumatic brain injury patient with prominent semantic impairments, the predominant site of damage was the left temporal lobe. In a study of temporal lobe epilepsy patients using a verbal fluency paradigm, Tröster et al. (1995b) found that both left and right temporal lobe epilepsy patients exhibited significant semantic impairments relative to normals, with the left temporal lobe epilepsy patients being most impaired.

Patterson and Hodges (1995) also report cases of so-called 'semantic dementia' (which are discussed in more detail later), perhaps a variant of primary progressive aphasia (Weintraub et al. 1990; Weintraub and Mesulam 1993), in which the temporal lobes, particularly the dominant temporal lobe, have been implicated. More specifically, of the few such cases that have come to autopsy, all have exhibited either nonspecific neuronal loss and spongiform changes or Pick's intraneuronal inclusion bodies, concentrated largely in the temporal lobes (Snowden et al. 1992; Patterson and Hodges 1995). The postmortem findings for 'semantic dementia' cases are paralleled by *in vivo* structural (MRI: magnetic resonance imaging) and functional (PET: positron emission tomography and SPECT: single positron emission computed tomography) imaging studies that reveal atrophy and reduced metabolism in the temporal neocortex, predominantly on the left (Hodges et al. 1992; Snowden et al. 1992).

Functional neuroimaging

Recent findings from functional neuroimaging studies with normal subjects complement and refine the localization data from structural lesion studies. Howard et al. (1992) utilized PET techniques to study changes in regional cerebral blood flow associated with word reading and repetition tasks. These investigators argued that their findings were consistent with localization of a semantic lexicon for spoken word recognition in the middle portion of the left superior and middle temporal gyri and a lexicon

for written word recognition in the posterior portion of the left middle temporal gyrus. A drawback of this PET study is that the word reading and repetition tasks it employed did not ensure that subjects were actually engaged in semantic processing of the word stimuli.

Two more recent PET studies have provided further, more elaborate evidence for the importance of the temporal lobes, particularly the left temporal lobe, in the neural networks involved in storage of semantic knowledge. Martin et al. (1995) used PET techniques to measure cerebral blood flow changes in normal subjects in one experiment as they generated words denoting colors and actions typically associated with objects depicted in line drawings. In a second experiment the subjects generated color and action word associations to written names of objects. In both experiments the generation of color word associations selectively activated an area in the ventral temporal lobes just anterior to the region known to be involved in the perception of color. Generation of action word associations activated an area in the left middle temporal gyrus just anterior to the region involved in motion perception. The investigators argued that their findings suggest that object knowledge is organized as a distributed neural system in which the attributes of an object are stored in close proximity to the cortical regions that subserve perception of those attributes.

Martin et al. (1996) used PET to examine the neural correlates associated with naming line drawings of animals and tools. Bilateral activation of the ventral temporal lobes and Broca's area was found during naming of both animals and tools. Moreover, additional brain regions became selectively active as a function of the semantic category (animals versus tools) being processed, i.e. naming of animals also selectively activated the left medial occipital lobe, an 'upstream' area of the occipitofugal stream involved in the earliest stages of visual processing. Naming of tools, by contrast, resulted in the additional activations of a left premotor area known to be activated by imagined hand movements and of a region in the left middle temporal gyrus known to be activated by the generation of action words. Martin et al. (1996) argued that their results 'suggest that semantic representations of objects are stored as a distributed neural network that includes the ventral region of the temporal lobe . . . the location of the other areas recruited as part of this network depends on the intrinsic properties of the object to be identified' (p. 652). Also, their findings are consonant with many of the case reports of patients who exhibit category-specific semantic knowledge deficits, as patients who display specific deficits for naming living things tend to have posterior and ventral lesions, whereas those who display specific deficits for naming man-made objects tend to have more anterior and dorsal lesions (Saffran and Schwartz 1994).

Overall, both the lesion data and functional neuroimaging of healthy volunteers point to a neural model in which semantic knowledge is stored in distributed neural networks with regions in the temporal lobes, particularly the left temporal lobe, at the core. Other cortical areas seem to be recruited into the representational network as a function of the intrinsic properties of the object or concept that is being instantiated. With this conceptual framework as background, we now turn to the neurodegenerative diseases that disrupt these networks of semantic memory.

SEMANTIC MEMORY IMPAIRMENT IN NEURODEGENERATIVE DISEASES

Alzheimer's disease

AD is the most common cortical dementing process (Cummings and Benson 1992) and also by far the greatest focus of work on semantic memory disruption in dementia. Anterograde episodic memory impairment is the virtual sine qua non of AD from very early in the disease course (Flicker et al. 1991; Welsh et al. 1992; Chapter 18). Semantic memory has been somewhat less studied; nonetheless a consensus has emerged from several convergent lines of research that semantic memory is impaired without exception at some point during the AD course. This section will review the converging data that establish and characterize the nature of the semantic memory deficits in AD. Particularly attention will also be given to the chief underlying question that has guided much of the research. Namely, do the observed deficits that AD patients demonstrate on tests of semantic knowledge represent problems in *accessing* semantic knowledge or actual *degradation* of semantic stores?

Numerous methods have been employed to assess the integrity of semantic memory in AD (Nebes 1989). Perhaps the most fruitful and noteworthy paradigms have been studies of naming ability, category fluency, priming and, most recently, multidimensional scaling models of semantic networks.

Naming

Since Alois Alzheimer's first description in 1907 of the disease that now bears his name, a naming disturbance has been recognized as one of the core clinical features of AD (Wilkins and Brody 1969). The anomia tends to be a relatively early manifestation of the disease (Cummings and Benson 1992), it progressively worsens over the disease course (Chertkow and Bub 1990) and is strongly correlated with overall dementia severity (Nebes 1989). In clinical practice, anomia is commonly measured with tests of confrontation naming ability such as the Boston Naming Test (BNT; Kaplan et al. 1983), on which AD patients are impaired (Hodges et al. 1990, 1991). The nature of the anomia in AD has been elucidated by several recent studies. Briefly, Nebes (1989) and others have postulated that the underlying cognitive deficit in AD anomia may derive from three different sources: perceptual misidentification, impaired lexical access and loss of semantic stores. It will be argued that the current evidence strongly points to the degradation of semantic stores as the principal cause for the anomia.

Evidence for naming impairment in AD due to a fundamental semantic disruption rather than visuoperceptual or lexical access problems comes from analyses of naming errors. One line of inquiry has been to characterize the *types* of naming errors made by AD patients. For instance, Martin and Fedio's (1983) classification of naming errors on the BNT found that perceptual errors were quite rare in comparison to language-based errors. In the most comprehensive study to date of naming error patterns, Hodges et al. (1991) compared the naming error patterns of AD patients, Huntington's disease (HD) patients and normal controls on the BNT. They found that, whereas the few errors normals made were predominantly semantic-category (e.g. 'dice' for dominoes) and circumlocutory errors, the AD patients made a significantly greater proportion of semantic-superordinate (e.g. 'vegetable' for asparagus) and semantic-associative errors (e.g. 'blow' for harmonica). The HD group, by contrast, differed from normals only in their increased rate of visually based errors (e.g. 'fountain pen' for asparagus), implying that for these patients the deficit is primarily perceptual. On the other hand, the authors argue that the AD error pattern implies a defect at the level of semantic knowledge, such that specific item knowledge is lost and only more general superordinate category knowledge remains, in keeping with one of Warrington and Shallice's (1984) criteria for a 'semantic storage disorder'. The study also had a longitudinal component whereby 22 of the AD patients were followed for 3 years and retested annually. Their overall naming performance deteriorated over time and their profile of naming errors changed as they became more severely demented, with the proportion of both the semantic-associative errors and visual errors increasing. The authors concluded from these longitudinal findings that semantic degradation progresses with overall disease course and that errors due to perceptual analysis problems only become significant with advancing dementia.

In addition to studies of the *types* of naming errors, stronger evidence for a fundamental semantic memory breakdown in AD comes from studies of the *consistency* of errors, i.e. the demonstration that AD patients lose knowledge pertaining to specific words across multiple probes has been taken as evidence of actual degradation of semantic stores (Huff et al. 1986). By contrast, aphasic patients with lexical access problems evidence inconsistency of the disturbance in naming individual items when tested multiple times or across modalities (Butterworth et al. 1984). In their seminal paper on semantic deficits in AD, Chertkow and Bub (1990) carefully studied the naming errors in a group of AD patients who demonstrated no impairment on measures of visual and verbal perceptual abilities. One of their findings was that the AD patients showed an item-to-item correspondence between naming errors on a picture naming test and loss of name comprehension on a word-to-picture matching test. On follow-up probe questions, the patients showed loss of detailed knowledge for the failed stimuli, but preservation of superordinate knowledge for the items. Moreover, the patients displayed consistency of their anomic responses when retested with the same stimuli one month later. The provision of associative cues (e.g. for lion: 'it is like a tiger') for semantically degraded items resulted in correct naming responses in only 5.4% of the cases. Hence, the marked consistency in loss of knowledge about objects across multiple probes is taken as evidence for a fundamental loss of semantic stores as opposed to an essential problem of access or retrieval.

Hodges and colleagues have developed a semantic test battery that represents the current state of the art for assessing semantic deficits across multiple probes in several modalities (Hodges et al. 1992; Patterson and Hodges 1995). A set of 48 stimulus items (comprised of half animals, half man-made items) is presented to subjects in various combinations of input and output modalities

(i.e. pictures to be named, words to be defined, pictures to be sorted into categories, selecting pictures from a multiple choice array to match a spoken or written word, etc.). In a comparison of AD patients to matched controls, Hodges et al. (1992) essentially replicated Chertkow and Bub's (1990) findings of naming failures for items that were consistently failed across multiple semantic probes. Less frequent exemplars were disproportionately impaired, suggestive of a 'bottom-up' breakdown in the structure of semantic memory. Hence, overall, data from these studies converges to strongly suggest that a breakdown in the integrity of semantic memory in large part accounts for the anomia that is characteristic of AD.

Category fluency

Word-list generation, or verbal fluency, tasks have been widely used for decades to assess lexical retrieval capacities (Milner 1964; Benton 1968; Newcombe 1969). The procedure typically requires the subject to generate as many words as possible in one minute, constrained by a cue provided by the examiner. For letter (or 'phonemic') fluency, the subject is required to produce words that begin with a given letter such as *C* (Benton and Hamsher 1976), whereas for category (or 'semantic') fluency the subject is required to produce exemplars of a given category such as *fruits and vegetables* (Goodglass and Kaplan 1972). Fluency tasks are considered complex and multifactorial, requiring some combination of attention, retrieval strategies, working memory and intact semantic stores (Chertkow and Bub 1990; Hodges et al. 1992; Randolph et al. 1993). Evidence to date indicates that AD patients are disproportionately impaired on category fluency as compared to letter fluency and that this pattern is reflective of a degradation in the semantic stores that are primarily tapped by the category fluency task.

Normal subjects generate more words on average for category fluency as compared to letter fluency; the reverse pattern holds true for AD patients (Monsch et al. 1994). Mildly demented AD patients perform as well as elderly controls on letter fluency, but are impaired on semantic fluency (Butters et al. 1987). In Ober et al.'s (1986) study, for example, mildly demented AD patients generated only half the number of category exemplars produced by normals, their rate of production tended to asymptote more quickly and they produced more inappropriate (i.e. perseverative or noncategory) responses. In a prospective longitudinal study (Baltimore Longitudinal Study of Aging),

Weingartner et al. (1993) found that six subjects who eventually developed AD had generated significantly fewer uncommon category exemplars relative to normal elderly controls two and a half years prior to the presumed onset of the dementia. These six patients had been equivalent to normals on letter fluency. Category fluency is strongly correlated with naming ability (Martin and Fedio 1983; Chertkow and Bub 1990) and it declines steadily as the disease progresses (Nebes 1989).

Although fluency tasks seem to draw upon multiple cognitive functions, recent findings support the notion that category fluency performance is subserved in large part by temporal neocortex, whereas letter fluency is more dependent upon prefrontal systems. It has long been known that brain-injured patients with frontal lesions perform particularly poorly on letter fluency tasks (Milner 1964; Bolter et al. 1983). On the other hand, Newcombe's (1969) study of patients with focal missile wounds found that subjects with left temporal lesions performed most poorly on category fluency. Martin et al. (1994) utilized an interference task paradigm to reveal a double dissociation in normal subjects for letter and category fluency. Subjects performed these two types of fluency tasks alone and while performing two different interference tasks. As hypothesized, letter fluency performance was reduced to a greater extent by concurrent performance of a frontally driven motor sequencing task than by an object decision task known to activate temporal cortex. Category fluency performance was marked by the inverse interference pattern. Although functional neuroimaging studies reviewed by Martin et al. (1994) show both frontal and temporal lobe processes to be involved for both letter and category fluency tasks, the authors conclude that letter fluency seems to be 'more dependent on frontal lobe mediated strategic search than on temporal lobe mediated semantic processes, while the reverse is true for semantic category fluency tasks' (p.1493). Consistent with this conclusion, PET studies of AD patients with salient naming and category fluency deficits have demonstrated relatively selective left temporal hypometabolism (Martin 1990).

What further evidence is there that impaired category fluency in AD is a primary result of degraded semantic memory? Support for this contention comes from several findings. First, AD patients' category fluency performance is not enhanced by provision of retrieval cues. Randolph et al. (1993) compared normals, AD, Huntington's disease

(HD) and Parkinson's disease (PD) patients on two versions of a category fluency test: a standard, 'uncued' version (i.e. *animals* or *items in a supermarket* without further prompts) and a version in which subjects were provided subordinated category cues as retrieval aids during the task (e.g. *animals found on a farm, animals that live in the jungle*, etc.). AD patients did not improve on the cued version, whereas PD and HD patients did improve significantly with the retrieval aids. Also, AD patients' category fluency, but not PD or HD patients', correlated significantly with their naming ability. A second line of support for the degradation hypothesis is the observation that the mean lexical frequency of category words generated by AD patients is significantly higher than that of matched normals (Binetti et al. 1995). Hodges et al. (1992) similarly reported a disproportionate reduction in the production of exemplars from lower order categories. AD patients also have a greater propensity than controls to generate category labels (superordinates) as part of their fluency output (Tröster et al. 1989). Warrington and Shallice (1984) have proposed that disproportionate loss of information about low frequency items represents one of the criteria for a 'semantic storage disorder'. Third, AD patients produce fewer and smaller *clusters* (consisting of contiguous words belonging to the same semantic subcategory; e.g. for animals, clusters would include farm animals, pets, zoo animals, etc.) than normals (Binetti et al. 1995) and PD patients (Troyer et al. 1996). These results would be consistent with a bottom-up breakdown in the availability of subordinate semantic knowledge. Finally, Chertkow and Bub (1990) showed an item-by-item correspondence between category fluency and other probes of semantic knowledge. Items found to be impaired on semantic probes such as confrontation naming virtually never are generated spontaneously on category fluency tests.

In conclusion, findings from studies of category fluency tasks strongly suggest that a fundamental disruption of semantic stores underlies AD patients' impairments on these tests.

Semantic priming

Another of Warrington and Shallice's (1984) originally proposed criteria for a 'semantic storage disorder' is the demonstration of a loss of priming effects. Findings from priming studies with AD patients have been less straightforward than those from naming and fluency paradigms in supporting the semantic degradation hypothesis (Nebes

1989). Priming paradigms are one type of 'implicit' memory measure, in which a subject's response is augmented in some way by prior experience, without necessarily requiring overt recall of that experience (Chapter 12). While certain types of implicit memory place greater demands on retrieval (and perhaps other nonmemory psychological functions; for a discussion, see Randolph et al. 1995), 'on-line' semantic priming places minimal demands on retrieval and attentional processes. This on-line priming involves simply naming, reading, or yes/no decision-making about stimuli as they are presented by computer. Priming is observed when response speed is affected by semantically-related primes that precede the target stimuli. For example, the time taken to read the word 'nurse' is shorter when the preceding word was 'doctor', as opposed to an unrelated word.

Nebes and his colleagues initiated the use of semantic priming paradigms in the investigation of semantic structure in AD. They hypothesized that if semantic systems were disrupted in AD, then these patients should demonstrate diminished priming (Nebes, 1989). The results from a number of studies have demonstrated, however, that AD patients exhibit either preserved or *increased* on-line semantic priming (Chertkow et al. 1989, 1994; Hartman 1991). This finding of 'hyperpriming' relative to matched controls has been interpreted by some as evidence of intact semantic systems in AD patients; however, Martin (1992) argued that hyperpriming would be consistent with degraded representational networks that lose more fine-grained attribute knowledge of objects. Martin suggested that semantically related objects are represented by networks that overlap to a large extent, such that random degradation of unique attribute representations will tend to make representations of semantically related objects even more similar and, in turn, subject to hyperfacilitation by semantically related primes.

In contrast to the majority of the findings from studies of on-line semantic priming with AD patients, Blaxton and Bookheimer (1993) reported *prolongation* of response times in temporal lobe epilepsy patients on stimuli preceded by semantically related primes. This suggests that developmental neuropathology may disrupt semantic network organization, but that neurodegenerative disease, as typified by AD, seems to leave the overarching relational structure of the networks intact.

Semantic 'space': Multidimensional scaling

In one of the newest fronts of inquiry into semantic memory in AD, multidimensional scaling techniques have been used to render spatial models of semantic network structure. Multidimensional scaling refers to a set of multivariate techniques that transform some index of psychological similarity (or 'proximity') between pairs of stimuli into distances between points in a spatial representation that models subjects' schematic organization of the stimuli (Shepard et al. 1972). Thus, multidimensional scaling can be thought of as providing a map that reflects the 'hidden structure' in the data (Kruskal and Wish 1978; p.7) Greater similarity between items is represented by their closeness in geometric space and the geometric axes represent the psychological dimensions along which comparisons are made (Merluzzi 1991).

In the first study to use multidimensional scaling to map the semantic 'space' of AD patients, Chan et al. (1993a) derived proximity data from category fluency (*animals*) data generated by AD and HD patients and normals. Based on the assumption that fluency responses would correspond to automatic spreading activation occurring within the semantic network, the degree of separation between any two given animals in subjects' fluency responses was used as a similarity index for input into multidimensional scaling and follow-up clustering procedures. Chan et al. (1993a) found that the maps of the HD and normal groups were similar, organizing the animal terms along dimensions of domesticity and size, with discrete and interpretable clustering of animal groups. On the other hand, the cognitive map generated from the AD data reflected an anomalous use of the domesticity and size dimensions and follow-up clustering solutions were uninterpretable. These findings were discussed as providing support for the deterioration in AD patients' semantic structure.

In another multidimensional scaling study with AD patients and matched controls, Chan et al. (1993b) used a more direct method for obtaining proximity data than the fluency-based similarity indices used in the first study. Subjects completed a similarity comparison task on all possible triads of 30 animal names to obtain proximity matrices for input into multidimensional scaling analyses. The resultant maps of underlying semantic structure showed that both AD patients and controls used the three dimensions of size, predation and domesticity in their similarity judgments about animals. Closer analysis revealed that AD patients relied most heavily on the relatively concrete perceptual dimension of size, whereas controls relied more on the abstract dimension of domesticity. Additionally, AD patients were less consistent in their use of concepts and showed abnormal clustering of some animals, again suggestive of a breakdown in the structure of semantic knowledge.

Bonilla and Johnson (1995) also used MDS analyses to examine the semantic maps of a small group of AD patients and normals. These investigators employed an unconstrained similarity sort procedure to derive proximity data for the MDS analyses. Their results were consistent with Chan et al.'s (1993b) finding that AD patients make less consistent use of the operative dimensions when categorizing items. Bonilla and Johnson also argued from their results that mildly demented AD patients' organization of semantic knowledge may not be quite as distorted as suggested by Chan and colleagues' studies.

Noteworthy is a longitudinal follow-up to the Chan et al. (1993b) multidimensional scaling study in which Chan et al. (1995) retested 12 of the AD patients and found that an index of semantic network abnormality from initial multidimensional scaling analyses was a strong predictor of subsequent rate of overall decline over the ensuing year. Specifically, using multidimensional scaling data from the initial study, the investigators computed a Similarity Index for each subject, which was a quantitative index of the degree to which a subject's multidimensional scaling map was similar to a standardized normal control map. In multiple regression analysis, the Similarity Index was a highly significant predictor of rate of cognitive decline, as measured by change scores on the Dementia Rating Scale (Mattis 1976) over 1 year. Moreover, in stepwise regression analyses that also included the BNT and letter and category fluency tests, only the Similarity Index was retained as a significant predictor of rate of cognitive decline. The authors suggested that semantic memory dysfunction may serve as a marker for the integrity of association cortices and for their susceptibility to subsequent deterioration. It should be noted, however, that Chan et al.'s (1995) findings were based on only 12 AD cases followed over one year and therefore await replication and extension.

Multidimensional scaling techniques have shown promise for explicating the breakdown in the structure of semantic knowledge in AD patients. Multidimensional scaling offers graphic modeling of semantic organization and preliminary results suggest that it may capture an aspect of semantic structure that has important prognostic value.

'Semantic dementia'

Although AD is the most common cortical neurodegenerative condition that affects semantic memory, there are also reports of focal neurodegenerative processes that degrade semantic networks. As previously discussed, Hodges and colleagues have used the term semantic dementia (originally coined by Snowden et al. 1989) to describe several rare cases of progressive focal atrophy that presented with prominent and circumscribed impairment of semantic memory (Hodges et al. 1992). The core features (Patterson and Hodges 1995) include: (1) impairment of semantic memory manifest in severe anomia, impaired single-word comprehension, reduced category fluency and degraded fund of general knowledge, (2) relative sparing of syntax and phonology, (3) intact perceptual and nonverbal problem-solving abilities, and (4) 'relatively preserved' episodic memory. Semantic dementia is perhaps best understood as a variant of primary progressive aphasia. Early descriptions of primary progressive aphasia (Mesulam 1982) noted non-fluent language output, which is not a feature of Hodges' case series. However, more recent formulations of the syndromal boundaries of primary progresive aphasia (Mesulam and Weintraub 1992; Weintraub and Mesulam 1993) would subsume the constellation of symptoms seen in so-called semantic dementia. Regardless, the focal and progressive changes in semantic memory that are manifest early on in the disease course, as well as the sites and nature of the neuropathology, set this condition apart from the progressive amnestic dementia characteristic of typical AD. The disease process seems to initially strike at the temporal lobe core of the neural networks that subserve semantic memory storage.

Subcortical degenerative dementias

In general, the neurodegenerative diseases that produce so-called subcortical dementias (Cummings and Benson 1992) do not result in prominent disruption of semantic memory stores. From the evidence reviewed thus far regarding the neural substrates of semantic memory, this is not surprising as the principal loci of neuroanatomical changes in subcortical diseases (i.e. white matter, basal ganglia, thalamus, brain stem) do not include the temporal neocortical areas found to be critical for semantic memory. In the following sections we will review the major findings for the status of semantic memory in HD, PD and progressive supranuclear palsy.

Huntington's disease

HD patients may display impaired performance on some standard measures of semantic memory, but on careful analysis these apparent impairments tend to be attributable to initiation and retrieval problems rather than to an actual degradation of semantic knowledge. This pattern is apparent in studies that have used measures of naming ability and verbal fluency. In terms of naming ability, Brown and Marsden's (1988) review of existing studies failed to demonstrate a significant anomia in HD, at least among patients with overall mild to moderate dementia. More recent studies by Hodges and associates show that HD patients do demonstrate some apparent naming impairment. Hodges et al. (1990) matched groups of AD and HD patients on overall dementia and followed them longitudinally for 1 year. These investigators found that the HD patients were mildly impaired on the BNT, but their anomia did not progress as rapidly over 1 year as did the AD patients' anomia. As highlighted previously, in the Hodges et al. (1991) study of naming error patterns among HD and AD patients, the HD patients exhibited a mild anomia on the BNT. Error analysis revealed that the HD patients' anomia was fully attributable to an increased proportion of visually based errors (see also Podoll et al. 1988). Hence, at least among mildly demented HD patients, poor performance on confrontation naming measures appears to stem from the primary visuoperceptual problem HD patients are known to have (Brouwers et al. 1984).

With regard to verbal fluency, HD patients are equally impaired on both letter and category fluency measures, in contrast to AD patients' disproportionate impairment on category fluency (Monsch et al. 1994). Moreover, Hodges et al. (1990) noted that HD patients' letter, but not their category, fluency declined significantly over 1 year (which is the inverse of the pattern observed in AD patients over time). As alluded to already, Randolph et al. (1993) found that, in contrast to AD patients, HD patients' category fluency performance improved significantly with provision of retrieval cues. Hence, it appears that a significant component of the observed fluency deficits in HD patients is attributable to retrieval problems rather than semantic degradation per se.

In Chan et al.'s (1993a) multidimensional scaling study, the HD patients' semantic map for animal terms was highly similar to that of normal controls. That is, in contrast to the AD group, the HD group used the identical dimensions and cluster analysis revealed the same clusters as the normal controls, suggestive of intact semantic organization for mildly demented HD patients. Similarly, the lexical-semantic aspects of language structure such as vocabulary and syntax are generally intact in HD until the disease progresses to the late stages of global dementia (Bayles 1988).

Parkinson's disease

Like HD patients, PD patients are impaired on mechanical aspects of speech and overall output, but lexical-semantic aspects of language such as vocabulary, grammar and syntax tend to be essentially intact (Brown and Marsden 1988; Lezak 1995; for a review, see Bondi and Tröster 1997). Studies of confrontation naming ability among PD patients have been somewhat equivocal overall, with some studies noting a significant anomia and others not (Brown and Marsden 1988). Nonetheless, when PD patients are compared with AD patients carefully matched for age and dementia severity, most studies show that PD patients are less impaired on confrontation naming measures (Bennett et al. 1994). Generally, when naming deficits are present in PD they tend to be mild and have been associated with depressive symptoms (Tröster et al. 1995a). To date there have not been any detailed studies of PD naming error patterns that would help clarify whether the mild anomia sometimes seen in PD is secondary to semantic degradation or, more likely, to other factors such as initiation/retrieval deficits. In two preliminary studies (Fields et al. 1996; Tröster et al. 1996) it was found that patients with PD and dementia, but not PD without dementia, made more naming errors than normal controls. In particular, the PD dementia group tended to make semantic associative errors. The naming impairment of AD is more severe than that of PD when the groups are equated for overall severity of dementia. Although PD dementia and AD groups both make predominantly semantic errors in naming, AD patients make more phonemic errors and 'don't know' responses. Furthermore, the types of semantic errors made by control and PD dementia groups also help distinguish among them. Whereas PD patients tend to make associative semantic errors, normal controls tend to make within-category semantic errors. The naming error pattern in PD dementia suggests that category knowledge is available, but that it is insufficient to generate item names. In AD, in contrast, even category knowledge is often unavailable, consistent with an hypothesized breakdown of semantic memory.

There have likewise been somewhat conflicting findings regarding the nature of the verbal fluency impairments in PD. That is, whereas most studies show that PD patients are impaired on both letter and category fluency relative to normals, there has been more controversy about whether there is a disproportionate impairment of one type of fluency over another (Brown and Marsden 1988; Downes et al. 1993). There is no strong evidence that PD patients are more impaired on either letter or category fluency tasks, as both tasks seem to be negatively affected by retrieval problems. In Randolph et al.'s (1993) study, PD patients exhibited marked facilitation of their category fluency performance when retrieval cues were provided, such that they were able to perform at the same level as normals in the cued condition. Troyer et al. (1996) found that, in contrast to AD patients, PD patients produced clusters of normal size on both category and letter fluency tests; however, the PD patients had fewer *switches* (i.e. number of times patients switch from one cluster to another) than normal controls. These results would be consistent with a fundamental initiation/retrieval problem underlying the verbal fluency deficits in PD, rather than an actual degradation of semantic knowledge. It might be the case, however, that semantic networks are affected once dementia develops in PD, because a recent study shows that patients with PD dementia demonstrate impaired clustering like AD patients (Tröster et al. in press).

Progressive supranuclear palsy

There are very few studies of semantic memory in progressive supranuclear palsy patients. Progressive supranuclear palsy is a subcortical neurodegenerative syndrome first formally recognized in the early 1960s (Richardson et al. 1963), marked by a constellation of supranuclear gaze paresis, pseudobulbar palsy, axial rigidity and dementia (Cummings and Benson 1992). These cardinal neurological features arise from degenerative changes throughout subcortical nuclei that also alter subcortical-cortical connections. There is a relative paucity of literature on the cognitive dysfunction that accompanies progressive supranuclear palsy. Neuropsychological status is difficult to assess reliably secondary to neurological problems (i.e. severe visual disturbance, axial dystonia and dysarthria) and valid evaluation of various cognitive functions can also

be significantly confounded by these patients' marked initiation and set-shifting problems (Lees 1990). Nonetheless, the characteristic clinical features of forgetfulness, bradyphrenia and apathy have made progressive supranuclear palsy a prototypic model of subcortical dementia.

Taken together, the existing studies pertaining to semantic memory function in progressive supranuclear palsy have been difficult to interpret. With regard to naming ability, Pillon et al. (1991) found that progressive supranuclear palsy patients were as impaired as AD patients, whereas Milberg and Albert (1989) found that progressive supranuclear palsy patients had intact naming ability on the BNT compared to AD patients. Pillon et al. (1991) also found that lexical fluency (i.e. a combined index of category and letter fluency) was less impaired in progressive supranuclear palsy patients than in AD and PD patients with overall mild dementia severity. However, lexical fluency was similarly impaired in AD and progressive supranuclear palsy patients with more severe overall dementia. In all studies reviewed by van der Hurk and Hodges (1995), fluency performance was defective for progressive supranuclear palsy patients.

In the most recent and direct study of semantic memory in progressive supranuclear palsy, van der Hurk and Hodges (1995) compared nine progressive supranuclear palsy patients with 13 AD patients carefully matched for demographic variables and overall level of dementia on the Dementia Rating Scale (Mattis 1976). They found relatively spared episodic memory in the progressive supranuclear palsy patients. The investigators hypothesized that AD patients would show disproportionate impairment of semantic memory compared to progressive supranuclear palsy patients. Semantic memory was assessed via confrontation naming performance on the BNT, word comprehension on the Synonym Judgement Test (Franklin et al. 1992) and nonverbal semantic knowledge on the Pyramids and Palm Trees Test (Howard and Patterson 1992). Contrary to their prediction, however, there were no differences between the AD and progressive supranuclear palsy patients on the semantic memory measures, except that the progressive supranuclear palsy patients actually performed worse than the AD patients on the Synonym Judgement Test. Moreover, error pattern analysis for the BNT data did not reveal any differences between the groups. Nonetheless, the authors surmised that the progressive supranuclear palsy patients' apparent problems with semantic memory stemmed from a retrieval deficit secondary to the known frontal systems impairment in progressive supranuclear palsy, rather than from an actual loss of semantic information. Clearly, however, more investigation is necessary to substantiate the nature of the apparent semantic memory problems sometimes seen in progressive supranuclear palsy.

CONCLUSION

For patients with AD, the most common form of neuro-degenerative dementia, anterograde episodic memory impairment is the earliest and most salient feature of the

disease. This deficit robs patients of the ability to lay down new memories from the stream of ongoing events in their lives. In the early stages of the disease, this may be the only deficit that patients must cope with. Language, the ability to reason and stores of knowledge and experience accumulated by these individuals may be largely intact initially. As the disease progresses, however, this repository of information, this substrate for communication, symbolic thought and reason inevitably begins to erode away. This degradation of what is essentially the rich fabric of human experience, woven from both societal and personal history, is arguably the most devastating consequence of the disease.

REFERENCES

Bayles, K.A. 1988. Dementia: The clinical perspective. *Seminars in Speech and Language*. 9: 149–165.

Bennett, D.A., Stebbins, G.T., Gilley, D.W. and Goetz, C.G. 1994. Parkinson's disease. In *Handbook of dementing illnesses*, ed. J.C. Morris, pp. 293–318. New York: Marcel Dekker, Inc.

Benton, A.L. 1968. Differential behavioral effects in frontal lobe disease. *Neuropsychologia*. 5: 53–60.

Benton, A.L. and Hamsher, K. deS. 1976. *Multilingual aphasia examination*. Iowa City: University of Iowa.

Binetti, G., Magni, E., Cappa, S.F., Padovani, A., Bianchetti, A. and Trabucchi, M. 1995. Semantic memory in Alzheimer's disease: An analysis of category fluency. *Journal of Clinical and Experimental Neuro-psychology*. 17: 82–89.

Blaxton, T.A. and Bookheimer, S.Y. 1993. Retrieval inhibition in anomia. *Brain and Language*. 44: 221–237.

Bolter, J.F., Long, C.J. and Wagner, M. 1983. The utility of the Thurstone Word Fluency Test in identifying cortical damage. *Clinical Neuropsy-chology*. 5: 77–82.

Bondi, M.W. and Tröster, A.I. 1997. Parkinson's disease: Neurobehavioral consequences of basal ganglia dysfunction. In *Handbook of neuropsychology and aging*, ed. P.D. Nussbaum, pp. 216–245. New York: Plenum Press.

Bonilla, J.L. and Johnson, M.K. 1995. Semantic space in Alzheimer's disease patients. *Neuropsychology*. 9: 345–353.

Brouwers, P., Cox, C., Martin, A., Chase, T. and Fedio, P. 1984. Differential perceptual-spatial impairment in Huntington's and Alzheimer's dementias. *Archives of Neurology*. 41: 1073–1076.

Brown, R.G. and Marsden, C.D. 1988. 'Subcortical dementia': The neuropsychological evidence. *Neuroscience*. 25: 363–387.

Bub, D., Black, S., Hampson, E. and Kertesz, A. 1988. Semantic encoding of pictures and words: Some neuropsychological observation. *Cognitive Neuropsychology*. 5: 27–66.

Butters, N., Granholm, E., Salmon, D.P., Grant, I. and Wolfe, J. 1987. Episodic and semantic memory: A comparison of amnesic and demented patients. *Journal of Clinical and Experimental Neuropsychology*. 9: 479–497.

Butterworth, B., Howard, D. and McLoughlin, P. 1984. The semantic deficit in aphasia: The relationship between semantic errors in auditory comprehension and picture naming. *Neuropsychologia*. 22: 409–426.

Chan, A.S., Butters, N., Paulsen, J.S., Salmon, D.P., Swenson, M.R. and Maloney, L.T. 1993a. An assessment of the semantic network in patients with Alzheimer's disease. *Journal of Cognitive Neuroscience*. 5: 254–261.

Chan, A.S., Butters, N., Salmon, D.P. and McGuire, K.A. 1993b. Dimensionality and clustering in the semantic network of patients with Alzheimer's disease. *Psychology and Aging*. 8: 411–419.

Chan, A.S., Salmon, D.P., Butters, N. and Johnson, S.A. 1995. Semantic network abnormality predicts rate of cognitive decline in patients with probable Alzheimer's disease. *Journal of the International Neuropsychological Society*. 1: 297–303.

Chertkow, H. and Bub, D. 1990. Semantic memory loss in dementia of the Alzheimer's type: What do various measures measure? *Brain*. 113: 397–417.

Chertkow, H., Bub, D., Bergman, H., Bruemmer, A., Merling, A. and Rothfleiscch, J. 1994. Increased semantic priming in patients with dementia of the Alzheimer's type. *Journal of Clinical and Experimental Neuropsychology*. 16: 608–622.

Chertkow, H., Bub, D. and Seidenberg, M. 1989. Priming and semantic memory loss in Alzheimer's disease. *Brain and Language*. 36: 420–446.

Cummings, J.L. and Benson, D.F. 1992. *Dementia: A clinical approach*, 2nd ed. Boston: Butterworth-Heinemann.

Downes, J.J., Sharp, H.M., Costall, B.M., Sagar, H.J. and Howe, J. 1993. Alternating fluency in Parkinson's disease. *Brain*. 116: 887–902.

Fields, J.A., Paolo, A.M. and Tröster, A.I. 1996. Visual confrontation naming in Parkinson's disease with and without dementia (abstract). *The Clinical Neuropsychologist*. 10: 321–322.

Flicker, C., Ferris, S.H. and Reisberg, B. 1991. Mild cognitive impairment in the elderly: Predictors of dementia. *Neurology*. 41: 1006–1009.

Franklin, S., Turner, J.E. and Ellis, A.W. 1992. *The ADA Comprehension Battery*. University of York: Human Neuropsychology Laboratory.

Goodglass, H. and Kaplan, E. 1972. *Assessment of aphasia and related disorders*. Philadelphia: Lea and Febiger.

Hartman, M. 1991. The use of semantic knowledge in Alzheimer's disease: Evidence for impairments of attention. *Neuropsychologia*. 29: 213–228.

Hodges, J.R., Patterson, K., Oxbury, S. and Funnell, E. 1992. Semantic dementia: Progressive fluent aphasia with temporal lobe atrophy. *Brain*. 115: 1783–1806.

Hodges, J.R., Salmon, D.P. and Butters, N. 1990. Differential impairment of semantic and episodic memory in Alzheimer's and Huntington's diseases: A controlled prospective study. *Journal of Neurology, Neurosurgery and Psychiatry*. 53: 1089–1095.

Hodges, J.R., Salmon, D.P. and Butters, N. 1991. The nature of the naming deficit in Alzheimer's and Huntington's disease. *Brain*. 114: 1547–1558.

Howard, D. and Patterson, K.E. 1992. *The Pyramids and Palm Trees Test*. Bury St. Edmunds, Suffolk, UK: Thames Valley Test Company.

Howard, D., Patterson, K., Wise, R., Brown, W.D., Friston, K., Weiller, C. and Frackowiak, R. 1992. The cortical localization of the lexicons: Positron emission tomography evidence. *Brain*. 115: 1769–1782.

Huff, F.J., Corkin, S. and Growdon, J.H. 1986. Semantic impairment and anomia in Alzheimer's disease. *Brain and Language*. 28: 235–249.

Kaplan, E., Goodglass, H. and Weintraub, S. 1983. *The Boston Naming Test*. Philadelphia: Lea and Febiger.

Kruskal, J.B. and Wish, M. 1978. *Multidimensional scaling*. Beverly Hills, CA: SAGE Publications.

Lees, A.J. 1990. Progressive supranuclear palsy: (Steele–Richardson–Olszewski Syndrome). In *Subcortical dementia*, ed. J. L. Cummings, pp. 123–131. New York: Oxford University Press.

Lezak, M.D. 1995. *Neuropsychological assessment*, 3rd ed. New York: Oxford University Press.

Martin, A. 1990. The neuropsychology of Alzheimer's disease: The case for subgroups. In *Modular deficits in Alzheimer's-type dementia*, ed. M. Schwartz, pp. 143–175. Cambridge, MA: MIT Press.

Martin, A. 1992. Semantic knowledge in patients with Alzheimer's disease: Evidence for degraded representations. In *Memory functioning in dementia*, ed. L. Bäckman, pp. 119–134. Amsterdam: Elsevier.

Martin, A. and Fedio, P. 1983. Word production and comprehension in Alzheimer's disease: The breakdown of semantic knowledge. *Brain and Language*. 19: 124–141.

Martin, A., Haxby, J.V., LaLonde, F.M., Wiggs, C.L. and Ungerleider, L.G. 1995. Discrete cortical regions associated with knowledge of color and knowledge of action. *Science*. 270: 102–105.

Martin, A., Wiggs, LaLonde, F. and Mack, C. 1994. Word retrieval to letter and semantic cues: A double dissociation in normal subjects using interference tasks. *Neuropsychologia*. 32: 1487–1494.

Martin, A., Wiggs, C.L., Ungerleider, L.G. and Haxby, J.V. 1996. Neural correlates of category-specific knowledge. *Nature*. 379: 649–652.

Mattis, S. 1976. Mental status examination for organic mental syndrome in the elderly patient. In *Geriatric psychiatry*, ed. L. Bellak and T.B. Karasu, pp. 77–121. New York: Grune and Stratton.

McKenna, P. and Warrington, E.K. 1993. The neuropsychology of semantic memory. In *Handbook of neuropsychology*, vol. 8, ed. F. Boller and J. Grafman, pp. 193–213. Amsterdam: Elsevier.

Merluzzi, T.V. 1991. Representation of information about self and other: A multidimensional scaling analysis. In *Person schemas and maladaptive interpersonal patterns*, ed. M.J. Horowitz, pp. 155–166. Chicago: University of Chicago Press.

Mesulam, M.M. 1982. Slowly progressive aphasia without generalized dementia. *Annals of Neurology*. 11: 592–598.

Mesulam, M.M. and Weintraub, S. 1992. Spectrum of primary progressive aphasia. *Baillière's Clinical Neurology*. 1: 583–609.

Milberg, W. and Albert, M. 1989. Cognitive differences between patients with progressive supranuclear palsy and Alzheimer's disease. *Journal of Clinical and Experimental Neuropsychology*. 11: 605–614.

Milner, B. 1964. Some effects of frontal lobotomy in man. In *The frontal granular cortex and behavior*, ed. J.M. Warren and U. Aker, pp. 313–334. New York: McGraw-Hill.

Monsch, A.U., Bondi, M.W., Butters, N., Paulsen, J.S., Salmon, D.P., Brugger, P. and Swenson, M.R. 1994. A comparison of category and letter fluency in Alzheimer's disease and Huntington's disease. *Neuropsychology*. 8: 25–30.

Nebes, R.D. 1989. Semantic memory in Alzheimer's disease. *Psychological Bulletin*. 106: 377–394.

Newcombe, F. 1969. *Missile wounds of the brain*. London: Oxford University Press.

Ober, B.A., Dronkers, N.F., Koss, E., Delis, D.C. and Friedland, R.P. 1986. Retrieval from semantic memory in Alzheimer-type dementia. *Journal of Clinical and Experimental Neuropsychology*. 8: 75–92.

Patterson, K. and Hodges, J.R. 1995. Disorders of semantic memory. In *Handbook of memory disorders*, ed. A.D. Baddeley, B.A. Wilson and F.N. Watts, pp. 167–186. New York: Wiley.

Pietrini, V., Nertempi, P., Vaglia, A., Revello, M.G., Pinna, V. and Ferro-Milone, F. 1988. Recovery from herpes simplex encephalitis: Selective impairment of specific semantic categories with neuroradiological correlation. *Journal of Neurology, Neurosurgery and Psychiatry*. 51: 1284–1293.

Pillon, B., Dubois, B., Ploska, A. and Agid, Y. 1991. Severity and specificity of cognitive impairment in Alzheimer's, Huntington's and Parkinson's diseases and progressive supranuclear palsy. *Neurology*. 41: 634–643.

Podoll, K., Caspary, P., Lange, H.W. and Noth, J. 1988. Störungen der Objektbenennung bei Chorea Huntington. *Zeitschrift für Experimentelle und Angewandte Psychologie*. 35: 242–258.

Randolph, C., Braun, A.R., Goldberg, T.E. and Chase, T.N. 1993. Semantic fluency in Alzheimer's, Parkinson's and Huntington's disease: Dissociation of storage and retrieval failures. *Neuropsychology*. 7: 82–88.

Randolph, C., Tierney, M. and Chase, T.N. 1995. Implicit memory in Alzheimer's disease. *Journal of Clinical and Experimental Neuropsychology*. 17: 343–351.

Richardson, J.C., Steele, J. and Olszewski, J. 1963. Supranuclear ophthalmoplegia, pseudobulbar palsy, nuchal dystonia and dementia. *Transcripts of the American Neurological Association*. 88: 25–27.

Saffran, E.M. and Schwartz, M.F. 1994. Of cabbages and things: Semantic memory from a neuropsychological perspective – a tutorial review. In *Attention and performance*, vol. 15, ed. C. Umilta and M. Moscovitch, pp. 507–536. Cambridge, MA: MIT Press.

Sartori, G. and Job, R. 1988. The oyster with four legs: A neuropsychological study on the interaction of visual and semantic information. *Cognitive Neuropsychology*. 4: 105–132.

Shepard, R.N. Romney, A.K. and Nerlove, S.B. 1972. *Multidimensional scaling: Theory and application in the behavioral sciences, Vol. I*. New York: Seminar Press.

Snowden, J.S., Goulding, P.J. and Neary, D. 1989. Semantic dementia: A form of circumscribed cerebral atrophy. *Behavioural Neurology*. 2: 167–182.

Snowden, J.S., Neary, D., Mann, D.M.A., Goulding, P.J. and Testa, H.J. 1992. Progressive language disorder due to lobar atrophy. *Annals of Neurology*. 31: 174–183.

Tröster, A.I., Fields, J.A., Paolo, A.M., Pahwa, R. and Koller, W.C. 1996. Visual confrontation naming in Alzheimer's disease and Parkinson's disease with dementia (abstract). *Neurology*. 46 (Suppl.): A292-A293.

Tröster, A.I., Fields, J.A., Testa, J.A., Paul, R.H., Blanco, C.R. Hames, K.A., Salmon, D.P. and Beatty, W.W. In press. Cortical and subcortical influences on clustering and switching in the performance of verbal fluency tasks. *Neuropsychologia*.

Tröster, A.I., Salmon, D.P., McCullough, D. and Butters, N. 1989. A comparison of the category fluency deficits associated with Alzheimer's and Huntington's disease. *Brain and Language*. 37: 500–513.

Tröster, A.I., Stalp, L.D., Paolo, A.M., Fields, J.A. and Koller, W.C. 1995a. Neuropsychological impairment in Parkinson's disease with and without depression. *Archives of Neurology*. 52: 1164–1169.

Tröster, A.I., Warmflash, V., Osorio, I., Paolo, A.M., Alexander, L.J. and Barr, W.B. 1995b. The roles of semantic networks and search efficiency in verbal fluency performance in intractable temporal lobe epilepsy. *Epilepsy Research*. 21: 19–26.

Troyer, A.K., Moscovitch, M. and Winocur, G. 1996, February. *Clustering and switching on verbal fluency tests: Evidence from healthy controls and patients with Alzheimer's and Parkinson's disease*. Paper presented at the Annual Meeting of the International Neuropsychological Society, February 14–17, 1996; Chicago, IL.

Tulving, E. 1972. Episodic and semantic memory. In *Organization of memory*, ed. E. Tulving and W. Donaldson, pp. 381–403. New York: Academic Press.

Tulving, E. 1995. Organization of memory: Quo vadis? In *The cognitive neurosciences*, ed. M.S. Gazzaniga, pp. 839–847. Cambridge, MA: MIT Press.

Van der Hurk, P.R. and Hodges, J.R. 1995. Episodic and semantic memory in Alzheimer's disease and progressive supranuclear palsy: A comparative study. *Journal of Clinical and Experimental Neuropsychology*. 17: 459–471.

Warrington, E.K. and Shallice, T. 1984. Category specific semantic impairments. *Brain*. 107: 829–854.

Weingartner, H.J., Kawas, C., Rawlings, R. and Shapiro, M. 1993. Changes in semantic memory in early stage Alzheimer's disease patients. *The Gerontologist*. 33: 637–643.

Weintraub, S. and Mesulam, M. 1993. Four neuropsychological profiles in dementia. In *Handbook of neuropsychology*, vol. 8, ed. F. Boller and J. Grafman, pp. 253–282. Amsterdam: Elsevier.

Weintraub, S., Rubin, N. and Mesulam, M. 1990. Primary progressive aphasia: Longitudinal course, neuropsychological profile and language features. *Archives of Neurology*. 47: 1329–1335.

Welsh, K.A., Butters, N., Hughes, J.P., Mohs, R.C. and Heyman, A. 1992. Detection and staging of dementia in Alzheimer's disease. *Archives of Neurology*. 49: 448–452.

Wilkins, R.H. and Brody, I.A. 1969. Alzheimer's disease. *Archives of Neurology*. 21: 109–110.

12 Nondeclarative memory in neurodegenerative disease

DAVID P. SALMON, TARA T. LINEWEAVER
AND WILLIAM C. HEINDEL

INTRODUCTION

A number of recently conceived models of memory draw a distinction between relatively independent memory systems that differ from one another in the type of information stored and in the processes acting upon that information (Squire 1987; Tulving and Schacter 1990). One memory system dichotomy that has generated considerable theoretical and empirical interest is the distinction between declarative (or explicit) and nondeclarative (or implicit or procedural) forms of memory (Cohen and Squire 1980; Squire 1987). Declarative memory refers to knowledge of episodes and facts that can be consciously recalled and related (i.e. declared) by the rememberer. It has been characterized as 'knowing that' and includes such things as memory for the words on a recently presented list and knowledge that a cat is an animal. Nondeclarative memory, in contrast, is described as 'knowing how' and pertains to an unconscious form of remembering that is expressed only through the performance of the specific operations comprising a particular task. The use of nondeclarative memory is indicated by the performance of a newly acquired motor, perceptual or cognitive skill, for example, and by the unconscious facilitation in processing a stimulus that occurs following its previous presentation (i.e. priming).

The distinction that has been drawn between declarative and nondeclarative memory is based not only on conceptual grounds but also on the dissociation of these two forms of memory in patients with circumscribed amnesia arising from damage to medial temporal lobe or midline diencephalic brain structures. Despite severe deficits in declarative memory, amnesic patients demonstrate normal lexical and semantic priming (Warrington and Weiskrantz 1968, 1970; Gardner et al. 1973; Graf et al. 1984; Shimamura and Squire 1984; Cermak et al. 1985;

Shimamura 1986) and a preserved ability to learn and retain a variety of motor, perceptual and cognitive skills (e.g. Corkin 1968; Cermak et al. 1973; Brooks and Baddeley 1976; Cohen and Squire 1980; for a review, see Squire 1987). The preservation of nondeclarative memory in patients with circumscribed amnesia indicates that this form of memory does not rely on the same medial temporal and diencephalic brain structures that are thought to mediate declarative memory and suggests that declarative and nondeclarative memory are neurobiologically as well as conceptually distinct.

While studies of patients with circumscribed amnesia provide abundant evidence that the medial temporal and diencephalic brain regions that mediate declarative memory are not necessary for nondeclarative memory, they provide little information about the neurological bases of nondeclarative memory. Nondeclarative memory encompasses a wide variety of learning and memory abilities and it is unlikely that a single set of brain structures underlies all of its forms. Rather, each form of nondeclarative memory may be mediated by those brain structures that are directly involved in the initial processing and performance of a particular task (Cohen and Squire 1980). As a result of this diversity, the neurobiological basis of nondeclarative memory cannot be fully explored within a single patient group, but must be examined through the careful investigation of patients with neurodegenerative diseases that affect a variety of brain regions beyond those involved in circumscribed amnesia. In this way, one can determine if unique patterns of preserved and impaired nondeclarative memory abilities are associated with particular sites of brain pathology.

The present chapter will describe some of the recent research on nondeclarative memory in patients with neurodegenerative disorders and will discuss the implications of this research for our understanding of the neurobiological bases of this form of memory. This research has primarily focused on dementing disorders that have relatively diffuse cortical or subcortical neuropathological abnormalities. The majority of studies have centered on patients with Alzheimer's disease (AD), a progressive neurodegenerative disorder characterized by neuron and synapse loss and the presence of neuritic plaques and neurofibrillary tangles, primarily in the hippocampus and entorhinal cortex and in the association cortices of the temporal, parietal and frontal lobes (Brun 1983; Terry and Katzman 1983; Chapter 3). AD is also characterized by a pronounced reduction of cortical acetylcholine due to damage to the nucleus basalis of Meynert and in many cases by a reduction of cortical norepinephrine due to damage to the nucleus locus coeruleus. The nondeclarative memory performance of patients with dementia of AD is often compared and contrasted to that of patients with Huntington's disease (HD), a genetically transmitted disorder which results in the gradual deterioration of the basal ganglia (Bruyn et al. 1979), or Parkinson's disease (PD), a disease producing extensive cell loss and other neuropathological abnormalities (e.g. Lewy bodies) in the substantia nigra, the primary source of dopaminergic projection to the basal ganglia and neocortex. The first part of the chapter will focus on priming in patients with various neurodegenerative diseases, while the second part will examine the ability of these patients to learn and retain motor, perceptual and cognitive skills.

PRIMING

During the past decade a number of studies have examined priming in patients with various neurodegenerative disorders. These studies have most commonly employed a repetition paradigm in which a stimulus is presented and after some interval (ranging from fractions of a second to minutes or hours) the original stimulus, or some degraded form of the original stimulus, is presented again. The initial presentation of the stimulus is assumed to produce some activation that facilitates its subsequent processing. This facilitation is reflected by faster processing of the stimulus on its second presentation or by an enhanced ability to identify the stimulus in its degraded form.

An associative paradigm has also been used to examine priming in patients with neurodegenerative diseases. Associative priming refers to a procedure in which a stimulus is presented and after some interval a second, lexically- or semantically-related stimulus is presented. The presentation of the first stimulus is assumed to activate the second stimulus through their lexical or semantic association (e.g. through spreading activation within the semantic network) and this activation facilitates the processing of the second stimulus in some subsequent task (e.g. deciding whether it is a word or nonword).

A theoretical distinction has been made by some investigators between perceptual (or data-driven) and conceptual priming (Roediger and Blaxton 1987; Blaxton 1989). Perceptual priming involves processes that operate at the level of the visual or auditory form of a target stimulus and is not affected by the particular meaning or content of the stimulus. It can, however, be influenced by manipulations of the stimulus' surface features (e.g. changes in modality or type face). Conceptual priming, in contrast, does involve processes that operate at the level of the meaning or content of a target stimulus and is influenced by manipulations of the depth of conceptual analysis of the stimulus. Repetition priming may have both a perceptual and conceptual component, depending on the nature of the stimulus material and the initial processing task. Associative priming, however, is always conceptually based because it relies on activation of a stimulus through its associations rather than through its direct presentation (as in repetition priming).

Gabrieli and colleagues have recently suggested that the distinction between perceptual and conceptual priming may have a neurological as well as a psychological basis (Fleischman et al. 1995; Gabrieli et al. 1995). These investigators propose that evidence from priming studies in patients with neurodegenerative diseases (reviewed below) indicates that conceptual and perceptual priming can be dissociated in patients with different sites of brain pathology. It is important to point out, however, that tasks used to assess priming in patients with neurodegenerative diseases often do not exclusively engage either conceptual or perceptual processes. Rather, both types of processing may contribute to normal priming performance, with the relative contribution of each depending on the specific features of the task. Priming effects in normal individuals and amnesic patients on the widely-used word-stem completion task (see below), for example, have been shown to be greater following elaborative processing of a semantic, rather than a physical, feature of the stimulus during study (indicating a conceptual processing component), as well as when the stimulus is presented in the same modality, rather than in different modalities, at study and test (indicating a perceptual processing component) (Carlesimo 1994). With this caveat in mind, the effects of various neurodegenerative diseases on conceptual and perceptual priming will be discussed in turn.

Conceptual priming

Two of the first studies to examine priming in patients with neurodegenerative diseases (Shimamura et al. 1987; Salmon et al. 1988) compared the performance of patients with AD to those of HD patients, patients with circumscribed amnesia associated with alcoholic Korsakoff's syndrome and normal control subjects, on a word–stem completion task previously used by Graf et al. (1984). In this task, subjects were first exposed to a list of 10 target words (e.g. MOTEL, ABSTAIN) and asked to rate each word in terms of its 'likability'. Following two presentations and ratings of the entire list, the subjects were shown three-letter stems (e.g. MOT, ABS) of words that were and were not on the presentation list and asked to complete the stems with the 'first word that comes to mind'. Half of the stems could be completed with previously presented words, while the other half were used to assess baseline guessing rates. Other lists of words were used to assess the subjects' ability at free recall and recognition.

Although all three patient groups were severely and equally impaired on free recall and recognition of presented words, the groups differed with regard to their ability to prime. The stem-completion priming of the alcoholic Korsakoff's and HD patients was comparable to that of the normal control subjects. The patients with AD, in contrast, exhibited impaired priming relative to both normal control subjects and the other two patient groups. This deficit in the stem–completion priming performance of AD patients was subsequently replicated in numerous studies (Heindel et al. 1989; Keane et al. 1991; Randolph 1991; Bondi et al. 1993; Perani et al. 1993; but see Deweer et al. 1994; Huberman et al. 1994).

Salmon and colleagues (Salmon et al. 1988) also compared the priming performance of AD, HD and normal control subjects on an associative (i.e. semantic) priming test which employed a paired-associate procedure. In this task, subjects were first asked to judge the degree of relatedness of categorically or functionally related word pairs (e.g. BIRD-ROBIN, NEEDLE-THREAD) and later to 'free-associate' to the first words of the previously presented pairs and to words that were not presented as part of the paired-associates. The results with this priming task showed that AD patients were significantly less likely to produce the second word of the semantically-related pair than were the other two subject groups. In fact, the priming score for the AD patients did not differ from baseline guessing rates.

A similar free-association procedure was used by Brandt et al. (1988) to assess verbal priming in AD patients. These investigators first read a list of 10 stimulus words to AD and normal control subjects. After a short delay, an unrelated free-association task was administered in which the subject was asked to say a word in response to a probe word read by the experimenter. For half of the probe words, a previously presented stimulus word was the third most common associate according to normative data. The other half of the probe words were not associated with any of the 10 stimulus words. Priming of the stimulus words was demonstrated in the normal control subjects by their increased tendency to produce the previously presented stimulus words as the primary associate in the free-association task. Patients with AD also showed a slightly increased tendency to produce the previously presented words, but this priming was impaired relative to that of the normal control subjects.

The studies described above were among the first to demonstrate significant deficiencies in long-term priming in any neurologically impaired patient group and suggest that priming may be mediated by neural substrates that are selectively disrupted in AD. Since AD patients and not HD or amnesic patients, have marked pathology in temporal, parietal and frontal association cortices (Brun 1983; Terry and Katzman 1983), impaired priming may be the result of damage to those neocortical association areas which are presumed to store the representations of semantic memory. According to this view, cortical damage in AD patients may result in a breakdown in the organization of semantic knowledge that is necessary to support priming, i.e. the hierarchical associative network underlying semantic knowledge may have deteriorated sufficiently in the AD patients to greatly limit the capacity of available cues to activate traces of previously presented stimuli. For example, the cue 'bird' may not evoke an unconscious activation of the categorical associate 'robin' on the semantic priming task because the association between the two words has been greatly weakened. Similarly, the representation of the concept MOTEL may be degraded to such an extent that it cannot be activated by its prior presentation in the stem-completion task to a level that facilitates its subsequent identification in a degraded form.

This interpretation of the priming deficit exhibited by patients with AD is consistent with their known semantic memory impairment (for reviews, see Salmon and Chan 1994; Chapter 11) and receives additional support from several recent studies that examined semantic memory through the use of semantically-based event-related potentials. In one of these studies, Iragui et al. (1996) compared the N400 component of the event-related potentials of patients with AD with those of young and elderly normal control subjects. The N400 component is elicited as an individual reads or listens to meaningful material and is sensitive to semantic and associative relationships among lexical items (Kutas and Hillyard 1980, 1983, 1984). It is thought to be a reliable index of semantic processes because the N400 amplitude is typically larger when a subject hears or sees a word that is incongruous with the semantic context that preceded it (provided by a word or sentence; e.g. The bird ate the *nail*) than when the word matches its context (e.g. The hammer hit the *nail*). Iragui and colleagues found that the N400 component of the event-related potentials produced by AD patients was abnormal in that it occurred later and was broader and of lower amplitude than that of either control group.

In a related study, Schwartz et al. (1996) found similar abnormalities in the N400 component of AD patients who were performing a task in which they first heard a category name and were then shown a related or an unrelated target item. The AD patients also produced abnormal reaction time data when they were required to press a key to indicate whether or not the target item was a member of the category; however, these data indicated greater than normal priming (i.e. hyperpriming) in the AD patients. The results of this study, in conjunction with those of Iragui et al. (1996), indicate that AD patients are impaired in their ability to analyse and integrate semantic information and suggest that this impairment may be related to their semantic or conceptual priming deficits.

In contrast to the studies presented above, several recent studies fail to support the notion that the priming deficit of AD patients is related to a breakdown in the organization of semantic memory. These studies demonstrate that, under certain conditions, AD patients can exhibit normal performance on semantic or conceptual priming tasks. One such study, for example, examined verbal priming in AD patients using a homophone spelling bias task (Fennema-Notestine et al. 1994). In the initial phase of this study, it was determined that across two test sessions normal control subjects, AD patients and amnesic patients all spontaneously shifted their preferred spelling on approximately 30% of homophonic words. With this baseline rate of shifting in mind, subjects were asked to spell a series of homophonic words (to establish the initial spelling preference) and then to spell these words again a few minutes later after they had been biased against their preference by presenting the homophone within a semantic context. For example, if a subject's preferred spelling had initially been *son*, he or she was asked in the second phase to spell this word immediately after having heard *moon* and *stars*. Conversely, if their preferred spelling had been *sun*, they were biased with *father* and *daughter* in the second phase. After the biasing trials, all subject groups tended to shift to their nonpreferred spelling on approximately 60% of the homophonic words. This doubling of the shift to nonpreferred spelling by the biasing presentation suggests that the semantic relationship between the biasing and target words was intact enough in the AD patients to activate the nonpreferred spelling to a normal level.

Additional evidence of intact semantic or conceptual priming in patients with AD has been provided by studies which employed the stem-completion priming paradigm, but ensured that subjects fully processed the target words at a semantic level during the initial orienting phase of the task (Grosse et al. 1990; Partridge et al. 1990). These studies demonstrated that when patients with AD were required to attend to the semantic aspects of the target stimulus, they exhibited priming that was equivalent to that of normal control subjects. Unfortunately, however, the interpretation of the results of these studies is complicated by several methodological issues. For example, AD subjects who were unable to perform the semantic encoding task were eliminated from the Partridge et al. study and these may have been the very subjects with semantic memory deterioration who would have exhibited impaired priming on the stem-completion task. In addition, the semantic orienting task used by Grosse et al. resulted in considerably less priming in normal control subjects than usually observed in other studies that have used the stem-completion procedure. Finally, neither of these studies directly compared the 'likability judgement' and 'semantic processing' orienting tasks, so alternative explanations (e.g. subject differences) for the differences in Grosse et al.'s and Partridge et al.'s results and those of Shimamura et al. (1987) and Salmon et al. (1988) cannot be ruled out.

It should also be noted that the results of these studies do not necessarily indicate that semantic memory is completely intact in patients with AD. As Fennema-Notestine et al. (1994) point out, there are likely to be degrees of semantic degradation in patients with AD and priming tasks differ in the demands they place on semantic memory. A patient with partial deterioration of semantic memory may perform normally on a conceptual priming task that places few demands on semantic memory, but be impaired on a task with greater semantic memory demands. In addition, enriching the semantic context in which a target stimulus is presented may allow a patient with a partially degraded semantic memory to achieve a level of activation necessary for normal priming (Grosse et al. 1990).

Other studies that demonstrate normal semantic or conceptual priming in patients with AD (for a review, see Nebes 1989) suggest that previous findings of impaired priming may be related to a deficiency in controlled, effortful retrieval processes, rather than to semantic memory deterioration. According to this view, semantic knowledge is intact in patients with AD, but can only be accessed in a normal fashion through automatic retrieval processes. Thus, priming tasks that engage 'automatic' cognitive processes such as naming or pronunciation, or that measure priming over extremely short time intervals (e.g. less than 400 msec) that preclude the use of controlled processes such as expectancy or semantic matching, should be performed normally by patients with AD.

Support for this hypothesis was provided in a study by Nebes et al. (1984) that examined the difference in naming latencies of AD patients and normal control subjects for target words that were preceded (by approximately 500 msec) either by a semantically related word (primed trials) or by an unrelated word (unprimed trials). Both the AD patients and normal control subjects had a slight and equivalent facilitation in naming (or pronunciation) latency when a word was preceded by a semantic associate (i.e. semantic priming). Based on these data, Nebes et al. concluded that priming and semantic memory are normal in AD patients when they are assessed with techniques which rely solely upon automatic information processing.

A number of subsequent studies have examined priming and semantic memory in patients with AD using naming (i.e. reading or pronunciation) and lexical decision tasks that are thought to involve automatic processes. Ober et al. (1991), for example, examined priming in AD patients with a naming procedure similar to the one used by Nebes et al. (1984) and with a lexical decision procedure (both with 250 msec interstimulus intervals). In the lexical decision task, a series of letter strings is presented visually and the subject is asked to indicate, as quickly as possible, whether or not each string represents a real word. Pairs of prime and target words (e.g. SPINACH, LETTUCE) are embedded in the series and priming is reflected by the facilitation of the subject's reaction time in making the word/nonword decision when a target item is preceded by a related prime relative to when it is preceded by an unrelated prime. Ober and colleagues observed no significant differences in the magnitude of priming exhibited by the AD patients and elderly normal control subjects on either type of task; however, these results are difficult to interpret because either the AD patients or the normal control subjects failed to prime significantly above baseline performance in a number of the many semantic conditions that were included in this study. Therefore, the priming tasks used in this study may have lacked the sensitivity to consistently measure semantic priming effects.

Albert and Milberg (1989), like Ober et al. (1991) found no significant difference in the magnitude of priming exhibited by AD patients and elderly normal control subjects in a lexical decision task with a 500 msec interstimulus interval. When these investigators calculated a proportional priming score to correct for the generally slower reaction times of the AD patients (i.e. unprimed minus primed reaction times divided by baseline reaction time), they found that the patients exhibited significantly less priming than the normal control subjects which suggests that they had difficulty with the semantic processing required by this task. Similarly, Ober and Shenaut (1988) observed no significant priming in AD patients on a lexical decision task (with a 1000 msec interstimulus interval) in which target words were primed by semantically related words.

Several additional studies that employed lexical decision or naming (i.e. reading) tasks have revealed abnormal priming in AD patients, even though these tasks are thought to minimize the use of controlled, effortful access of semantic memory. For example, Glosser and Friedman

(1991), using a threshold oral reading task, found that AD patients were impaired on a short-term priming task when the prime and target words were semantically related (e.g. *sheep-goat*), but not when they were only lexically related (e.g. *cottage-cheese*). In a number of other studies using a lexical decision or naming procedure, abnormal priming in AD patients was reflected by significantly *greater* than normal associative semantic priming (i.e. hyperpriming; Chertkow et al. 1989; Nebes et al. 1989; Balota and Duchek 1991; Hartman, 1991; Chenery et al. 1994; Chertkow et al. 1994).

Although this latter abnormality is difficult to interpret, Martin (1992) has suggested that these hyperpriming effects in AD patients may be the direct result of underspecified, overgeneralized semantic representations created by the loss of item-specific attributes. In this view, AD patients are not able to distinguish between items that are closely related in semantic memory (e.g. ROBIN and FINCH) because their knowledge of detailed attributes (e.g. respective size and colorings of the birds) no longer exists. Thus, activating one representation in the semantic memory of a AD patient serves to activate to the same degree all other representations with which it has become generalized. For example, the activation of ROBIN may activate FINCH to the same extent as the overgeneralized representation essentially imposes the same meaning on both items. Once this overgeneralization has occurred, associative priming (e.g. ROBIN-FINCH) virtually becomes repetition priming (e.g. ROBIN-ROBIN) for the AD patient. As repetition priming effects are almost always larger than associative priming effects, AD patients exhibit greater than normal priming (i.e. hyperpriming).

Taken together, the results of the studies reviewed above suggest that, under most conditions, the conceptual priming of patients with AD is abnormal. This abnormality may be manifested as a priming deficit on stem-completion and free-association priming tasks, or may be revealed as hypopriming or hyperpriming on short-term priming tasks that use naming or lexical decision procedures. The abnormal priming exhibited by patients with AD stands in contrast to the normal priming produced by patients with circumscribed amnesia or other degenerative neurological disorders such as HD. This dissociation suggests that the conceptual priming abnormalities of the AD patients are not due to the general effects of impaired declarative memory or dementia that these patients share

with the amnesic and HD patients. Rather, some evidence suggests that it may be related to the deterioration of semantic memory that is unique to patients with AD. The mechanisms that underlie the conceptual priming deficit of AD patients remain unknown, however, and other factors such as deficient effortful retrieval processes or a general decline in the ability to activate representations (see Salmon and Heindel 1992) may be involved.

Perceptual priming

Studies of repetition priming in patients with AD have almost exclusively demonstrated normal performance when procedures are utilized that allow priming to occur at a perceptual level. Normal repetition priming effects have been observed with AD patients on lexical decision tasks (Ober and Shenaut 1988), on simple reading tasks (Balota and Duchek 1991), on reading tasks using geometrically transformed script (Moscovitch et al. 1986; Grober et al. 1992; Deweer et al. 1993) and on tasks which require the identification of briefly presented words that have been encountered previously in an unrelated reading task (Keane et al. 1991; but see Ostergaard 1994). In the study by Keane and colleagues (1991), normal perceptual repetition priming was evident even though the patients were impaired on a stem-completion priming task that was similar to the one employed by Shimamura et al. (1987). Ostergaard (1994), in contrast, observed impaired priming in AD patients on a task requiring the identification of briefly presented words and suggested that the priming of the control subjects in the Keane et al. (1991) study may have been attenuated by a ceiling effect in their baseline performance.

Normal perceptual repetition priming effects were also observed in AD patients in several studies that examined real-time cognitive processing with event-related potentials (Friedman et al. 1992; Rugg et al. 1994). In studies by Friedman et al. (1992) and Rugg et al. (1994), a continuous list of words was presented and the subject was required to respond with a keypress to any animal names that appeared in the list. Repetition priming was examined in nontarget (i.e. nonanimal) words that were repeated after lags of either one or six intervening items (Rugg et al. 1994) or that averaged 14 intervening items (Friedman et al. 1992). Repetition priming was revealed by a greater positivity within a set of complex event-related potentials components for repeated items than for unrepeated items. There were no significant differences in repetition priming between the AD patients and normal control subjects in either study.

The preservation of perceptual priming in patients with AD suggests that this form of priming involves processing within brain regions different from those that are damaged by AD. Consistent with this suggestion, Gabrieli, Fleischman and their colleagues (Fleischman et al. 1995; Gabrieli et al. 1995) have recently presented evidence that perceptual priming may be mediated by a putative visual memory mechanism (similar to the presemantic Perceptual Representation System proposed by Tulving and Schacter, 1990) in the right occipital cortex, a brain area not prominently affected by AD. These investigators examined explicit memory and perceptual identification priming in a patient (M.S.) with a left homonymous hemianopsia due to a right hemisphere temporal lobectomy performed as treatment for pharmacologically intractable epilepsy. Despite normal performance on a visually-based explicit recognition memory test, patient M.S. was impaired on a perceptual identification priming test.

Preserved perceptual priming in AD patients may also have important implications for the variability in their performance across studies of verbal priming. As mentioned previously, several investigators (e.g. Tulving and Schacter 1990; Keane et al. 1991; Carlesimo 1994) have suggested that most verbal priming tasks involve both a semantic (i.e. conceptual) and a presemantic perceptual processing component, but that the relative contribution of each component varies across tasks. As the demands of priming tasks become more heavily weighted towards perceptual processing, the performance of patients with AD may approach normal. Thus, AD patients may exhibit normal priming on a perceptual identification task that can be performed solely on the basis of perceptual processes, some residual (albeit, less than normal) priming on a stem-completion priming task that invokes both conceptual and perceptual processes and almost no priming on a paired-associate priming task that precludes the use of perceptual processes and is solely dependent on conceptual processes.

SKILL LEARNING

A number of recent studies have examined the neurobiological bases of motor, perceptual and cognitive skill learning in patients with various neurodegenerative diseases.

The results of these studies suggest that the corticostriatal system (i.e. reciprocal connections between the neocortex and the basal ganglia via the thalamus), the cerebellum and the primary motor and sensory cortices may all play important roles in at least some forms of nondeclarative learning and memory. The basal ganglia have been implicated in the acquisition of motor, perceptual and cognitive skills (Saint-Cyr et al. 1988; Butters et al. 1994). In addition, the cerebellum appears to have an integral role in motor skill learning (Sanes et al. 1990) and in light of recent speculation about the role of the cerebellum in nonmotor cognitive processes (Daum et al. 1993; Leiner et al. 1993), this structure may also contribute to the acquisition of perceptual and cognitive skills. Finally, the motor and sensory cortical regions involved in performing a particular skill may also be modified during the development of skilled behavior (Seitz et al. 1990; Grafton et al. 1992).

Motor skill learning

In order to explore the neurological correlates of motor skill learning, Heindel et al. (1988) compared the ability of AD, HD and amnesic patients to learn the motor skills underlying performance of a pursuit rotor task. In this task, subjects were required to maintain contact between a hand-held stylus and a rotating metallic disk. The amount of time the stylus was kept in contact with the disk on each 20-second trial was measured across blocks of trials. To ensure that any observed group differences in skill acquisition could not be attributable to ceiling or floor effects, the initial levels of performance among the groups was equated by manipulating the difficulty (i.e. speed of rotation of the disk) of the task.

The results of the study showed that AD and amnesic patients demonstrated rapid and extensive motor learning across trials and that this learning was equivalent to that of normal control subjects. The preserved motor skill learning exhibited by the AD and amnesic patients was consistent with previous reports (Corkin 1968; Eslinger and Damasio 1986) and indicates that this form of nondeclarative memory is not dependent on the medial temporal lobe structures damaged in both of these disorders, nor on the temporal, parietal or frontal association cortices affected by AD. This result has been replicated in a number of subsequent studies (Heindel et al. 1989; Bondi et al. 1993) and has been generalized to the ability to learn the visuomotor skills necessary to trace a pattern seen in a mirror-reversed view (Gabrieli et al. 1993; Rouleau et al. unpublished results).

In contrast to the AD and amnesic patients, HD patients were impaired in learning the motor skills underlying pursuit rotor task performance. This motor learning deficit suggests that this form of nondeclarative memory may be mediated by the corticostriatal system that is severely compromised in HD (Bruyn et al. 1979). Heindel and colleagues (1988) postulated that the neostriatal damage suffered by HD patients may lead to a deficiency in developing the motor programs that are necessary to perform the pursuit rotor task. In learning a motor skill, appropriate movements comprising the target skill must be combined in a correct temporal sequence (i.e. a motor program). In the early stages, an elementary closed-loop negative feedback system is employed in which new motor commands are generated in direct response to visually perceived errors. As motor programs are acquired and modified through practice, a sequence of movements can be organized in advance of their performance (rather than simply responding to errors) and smooth, coordinated motor performance ensues. If, as suspected, the neostriatal damage in the HD patients precludes their developing motor programs, these patients may demonstrate some improvement in the early stages of motor skill acquisition by relying upon their error-correction mode of performance. Their inability to generate new motor programs would prevent them from adopting the more effective predictive mode of performance utilized by AD patients, amnesics and normal control subjects.

Although Heindel et al. (1988) found no significant relationship between the severity of HD patients' primary motor dysfunction and their ability to learn the pursuit rotor task, some concern about this potential confound remained. To address this concern, Heindel et al. (1991) examined the sensitivity of HD and AD patients to classical adaptation-level effects observed in a weight judgement task (Benzig and Squire 1989). Like learning the pursuit rotor task, the manifestation of adaptation effects in the weight judgement task may rely on the development of motor programs; however, the weight judgement task is much less reliant than the pursuit rotor task on overt movement. In this task, AD and HD subjects were first exposed to either a relatively heavy (heavy bias) or a relatively light (light bias) set of weights and were later asked to rate the heaviness of a standard set of 10 weights using a nine-point scale. Patients with AD, like normal control

subjects, perceived the standard set of weights as heavier following the light bias trials and lighter following the heavy bias trials, despite their poor explicit memory for the initial biasing session. In contrast, the weight judgements of the HD group were not significantly influenced by prior exposure to relatively heavy or light weights.

The results with the weight biasing task are of particular interest since the perceptual biasing may involve the modification of programmed movement parameters. A number of studies (for a review, see Jones 1986) have demonstrated that the perception of weight is normally mediated by centrally generated motor commands rather than by peripheral sensory information. The sensation of heaviness is then influenced by discrepancies between the intended, or programmed, force and the actual force needed to lift an object. Prior exposure to relatively heavy or light weights (i.e. the biasing trials) may result in an increase or decrease in the amount of force programmed for lifting weights, which would then lead to an illusory decrease or increase in the perceived heaviness of the standard set of weights. Thus, the impaired weight biasing performance of the HD patients, like their skill learning deficits shown with the pursuit rotor task, may be due to a motor programming deficit resulting from neostriatal dysfunction.

In a related study, Paulsen et al. (1993) compared the performance of AD and HD patients on a perceptual adaptation task involving laterally displaced vision. In this task, subjects were required to point to a target while wearing distorting prisms that shifted the perceived location of objects 20 degrees to the right or left. Quantitative indices of pointing accuracy were obtained under several conditions. First, baseline performance was assessed without prisms or visual feedback regarding accuracy. Second, preadaptation performance was assessed with prisms and without visual feedback. Third, a series of 30 adaptation trials were carried out with prisms and visual feedback. Fourth, postadaptation performance was assessed with prisms and without visual feedback. Finally, aftereffects were assessed without prisms or visual feedback.

The results of this study demonstrated that AD patients exhibited normal adaptation to the prisms after visual feedback and normal negative aftereffects when the prisms were removed. In contrast, HD patients failed to exhibit normal adaptation or negative aftereffects on this task. As adaptation to such lateral spatial distortion is thought to be mediated by the modification of central motor programs through visual feedback regarding the accuracy of intended movements, these results are consistent with the motor skill learning deficits exhibited by HD patients on the pursuit rotor and biasing of weight judgement tasks.

A number of additional studies provide evidence for the critical role of the basal ganglia in the acquisition and retention of motor skills. Nondemented patients who had recovered from hemiparesis following basal ganglia strokes were impaired in learning to skillfully produce a specific triangular movement with their previously affected hand (Platz et al. 1994). In addition, a subgroup of patients in the clinically asymptomatic stages of human immuno-deficiency virus (HIV) infection (Martin et al. 1993) and rhesus monkeys infected with the simian immuno-deficiency virus (SIV) (Rausch et al. 1994), demonstrated impaired learning on the pursuit rotor task and in both cases this deficiency was significantly related to increased levels of quinolinic acid, an excitotoxic N-methyl-D-aspartate (NMDA) agonist that may be particularly detrimental to the NMDA receptor-rich basal ganglia. Finally, schizophrenic patients with tardive dyskinesia exhibited poorer learning on the pursuit rotor task than patients without tardive dyskinesia and poor learning of the motor skill was correlated with caudate nucleus abnormalities revealed by magnetic resonance imaging (MRI) (Granholm et al. 1993).

Recent evidence from studies examining the performance of patients with neurodegenerative diseases on a serial reaction time task (Nissen and Bullemer 1987) suggests that a primary role of the basal ganglia in the acquisition of skilled motor behavior may involve sequencing of motor acts (Aldridge et al. 1993; Pellis et al. 1993; Willingham and Koroshetz 1993). The serial reaction time task is a four-choice procedure in which a subject must respond as quickly as possible to the illumination of one of four lights, each located immediately above a corresponding response key. During the first four blocks of trials, the stimuli are presented in a particular 10-item sequence that is repeated 10 times in each block. The stimuli are presented in a new random sequence during the fifth block of trials. Learning is indicated by a reduction in response latency over the first four blocks of trials as the subject benefits from the sequence repetition. An increase in response time is anticipated on the fifth block of trials (i.e. the new random sequence) if the initial response time

decline is due to learning of the stimulus sequence rather than to learning nonspecific aspects of the task.

In studies comparing the performances of AD and normal control subjects on the serial reaction time task (Knopman and Nissen 1987; Grafman et al. 1990), patients with AD had generally slower response times than normal control subjects, but demonstrated the same rate of decline in response latency over the blocks of trials that contained a repeating sequence and a normal increase in response latency when a random sequence was presented (but see Ferraro et al. 1993). This performance was similar to that of amnesic patients (Nissen and Bullemer 1987) and indicates that these patients learn and retain the sequence despite an inability to recall it explicitly.

In contrast to the AD patients' normal learning on this task, Knopman and Nissen (1991) found that HD patients demonstrated significantly less decline in response latency than normal control subjects over the repeating sequence trials and showed less increase in response latency than controls during the block of trials in which a new random stimulus sequence was presented. Willingham and Koroshetz (1993) observed a similar nondeclarative learning impairment on the serial reaction time task in HD patients and other investigators have noted a mild, but significant, deficit in patients with PD (Ferraro et al. 1993; Pascual-Leone et al. 1993).

Learning on the serial reaction time task may not be solely a function of the basal ganglia, but may also involve the cerebellum. Pascual-Leone and colleagues (1993) found that patients with cerebellar degeneration (i.e. olivo-pontocerebellar or cerebellar-cortical atrophy) failed to show improvement in reaction time across the repeating-sequence trials of the serial reaction time task. In addition, these patients were unable to acquire declarative knowledge of the repeating sequence even when they were given specific instructions regarding the possibility of a repeating sequence and the stimuli only had to be viewed across trials without a motor response. These results led Pascual-Leone et al. to conclude that the cerebellum may be performing an operation common to a number of tasks: specifically, the indexing and ordering of events in the time domain. Such a deficit would lead to poor declarative or nondeclarative learning on the serial reaction time task since the stimuli must be kept in a temporary memory buffer in their proper temporal sequence in order for the repeating sequence to be learned. This explanation would also account for the previously demonstrated inability of patients with cerebellar degeneration to effectively plan a series of actions to solve a problem (Grafman et al. 1992).

Changes in the motor cortex may also play a prominent role in the initial acquisition of new motor skills. Using maps of cortical motor potentials evoked by focal transcranial magnetic stimulation, Pascual-Leone et al. (1994) found that as normal individuals learned a repetitive motor sequence in a serial reaction time task, progressively larger maps of cortical outputs to the muscles involved in the task were generated. When subjects eventually developed declarative knowledge of the entire motor sequence, the cortical maps returned to baseline levels. These results suggest that sustained cortical modulation is important for initially learning a new motor sequence, but as the sequence is instantiated as a unitary motor plan, the contribution of the motor cortex is attenuated and other brain structures (e.g. the basal ganglia) assume greater importance in performing the task. A similar initial involvement of primary motor (M1), premotor, sensorimotor and somatosensory cortex in motor skill learning has been reported from studies using positron emission tomography (PET) in humans (Jenkins et al. 1994; Kawashima et al. 1994; Schlaug et al. 1994) and from lesion studies with non-human primates (Pavlides et al. 1993).

Taken together, these studies of motor skill learning in patients with neurodegenerative diseases suggest that this form of nondeclarative learning and memory involves processes that are mediated by the motor cortex, the cerebellum and the basal ganglia. One framework might suggest that sustained cortical processing is important for the initial performance and acquisition of the motor movements, while the cerebellum is important for the timing and indexing of events that allows the motor movements to be initially ordered into a sequence. The sequence of movements may then be processed and stored in the basal ganglia where, with repetition and practice, it becomes consolidated as a central motor program that underlies skilled motor behavior.

This putative sequence receives some support from a recent PET study (Kawashima et al. 1994) that demonstrated increased activation in the prefrontal, premotor and parietal association cortices and the cerebellum when normal individuals were learning a new motor sequencing task relative to when they were performing a prelearned sequencing task. The basal ganglia, in contrast, were equally activated in both motor performance conditions.

These results suggest that the cerebellum and motor cortex may be involved in developing motor automaticity, whereas the basal ganglia are involved in both the learning of new motor patterns and the retrieval of old patterns.

Perceptual and cognitive skill learning

Although the basal ganglia are primarily thought of as structures involved in skilled motor performance, they have also been implicated in the acquisition and maintenance of cognitive and perceptual skills. Patients with HD, for example, have been found to be impaired in acquiring the visuoperceptual skill of reading mirror-reversed text (Martone et al. 1984) or the cognitive skills necessary to efficiently solve a complex problem solving task, the Tower of Hanoi puzzle (Butters et al. 1985). Bondi and colleagues (Bondi and Kaszniak 1991; Bondi et al. 1993) found that PD patients showed marginally less facilitation than control subjects in identifying new fragmented pictures following a prior training session. These perceptual and cognitive skill deficits appear to be somewhat specific to patients with basal ganglia damage as they are not apparent in patients with AD (Deweer et al. 1993, 1994; Perani et al. 1993; Huberman et al. 1994) or circumscribed amnesia (for review, see Squire 1987).

A recent study examined the ability of PD patients and patients with circumscribed amnesia to acquire the cognitive skill necessary to perform a probabilistic classification task (Knowlton et al. 1996). In this task, subjects were required to classify stimulus patterns as being associated with one of two outcomes which occurred equally often. The stimulus patterns were composed of four stimuli which were each independently and probabilistically related to the two outcomes (i.e. correctly predicted one of the outcomes 25, 43, 57 or 75% of the time). The probabilistic structure of the task discouraged attempts to learn the relationship between the stimuli and outcomes using declarative memory, but allowed nondeclarative learning of these relationships to take place.

The results of this study showed that amnesic patients were able to learn the probabilistic relationship as well as normal control subjects, despite impaired declarative memory for the training episode. Non-demented PD patients, in contrast, recalled the training episode normally, but were impaired in learning the probabilistic relationship between the stimuli and outcomes. This double dissociation of declarative and nondeclarative memory between PD and amnesic patients indicates that this form of cognitive skill learning is not mediated by the medial temporal lobe structures damaged in the amnesic patients. Rather, the basal ganglia structures that are dysfunctional in patients with PD appear to be critical for normal cognitive skill learning.

It should be noted that perceptual and cognitive skill learning deficits have not been observed in all studies of patients with basal ganglia dysfunction. Appollonio et al. (1994), for example, found normal perceptual skill learning in PD patients using a fragmented picture task. Normal acquisition of a mirror-reading skill by both demented and nondemented PD patients has also been reported (Huberman et al. 1994). These conflicting results indicate the need for further investigation of this aspect of nondeclarative memory in patients with neurodegenerative diseases.

In contrast to the deficient motor skill learning exhibited by patients with cerebellar degeneration and despite the growing awareness of the potential role of the cerebellum in nonmotor cognitive processes (Leiner et al. 1993; Canavan et al. 1994; Middleton and Strick 1994), two recent studies failed to demonstrate a decrement in perceptual or cognitive skill learning in these patients. In the first study, Appollonio et al. (1993) found that patients with cerebellar degeneration were equivalent to normal control subjects in terms of perceptual learning on a picture fragment completion task (it should be noted, however, that little or no skill learning was demonstrated by either group in this study). In a second study, Daum et al. (1993) observed no difference between patients with cerebellar degeneration and normal control subjects in their rates of learning the perceptual skill of reading mirror-reversed text or the cognitive skills necessary to efficiently solve the Tower of Hanoi puzzle. Although suggestive, these negative results must be interpreted with caution until confirmed by further research examining a variety of perceptual and cognitive skills in patients with varying degrees of cerebellar damage.

Just as plasticity in the motor and somatosensory cortices may contribute to the learning of new motor skills, perceptual learning may be mediated by changes in the cortical regions that are involved in basic perception. Recent studies have shown, for example, that large and consistent improvements in visual and auditory discrimination occur with practice and psychophysical evidence suggests that this perceptual skill learning is likely to result from improved neuronal sensitivity in the visual and auditory cortices due to synaptic plasticity (Karni and Sagi 1991, 1993; Ahissar and Hochstein 1993; Edeline and Weinberger 1993; Karni et al. 1994; Sakurai 1994; Zohary et al. 1994).

SUMMARY AND CONCLUSIONS

The studies of nondeclarative memory in patients with neurodegenerative diseases reviewed in this chapter indicate that a dissociation exists between AD and HD patients in their patterns of impaired and preserved nondeclarative memory abilities. Patients with AD are impaired on some tests of verbal priming that are performed normally by HD patients, while HD patients are impaired on many skill learning tasks that are easily mastered by patients with AD. This apparent dissociation was verified in a study that directly compared the performance of amnesic, AD, HD and PD patients on the pursuit rotor skill learning task and the stem-completion priming task (Heindel et al. 1989). Although amnesics performed normally on both tasks, a double dissociation was observed between AD and HD patients. The AD patients were severely impaired on verbal priming but showed normal acquisition of the pursuit rotor skill, while the HD patients showed the opposite pattern of spared and impaired abilities. The performance of the PD patients was dependent upon whether they were demented or not. Demented PD patients were impaired on both memory tasks, whereas the nondemented PD patients were intact on both.

The double dissociation of priming and motor skill learning in AD and HD patients provides important information about the neurological substrates of nondeclarative memory. The HD patients' impairment on the pursuit rotor task is consistent with the proposed association between the acquisition of motor skills and the neostriatum and is complemented by studies demonstrating the role of the cerebellum and primary motor cortex in this form of nondeclarative memory. In contrast, the verbal priming deficit exhibited by patients with AD (and their deficit in semantic memory in general) may be attributable to the neocortical and basal forebrain damage that occurs in this disease. Thus, these results demonstrate that nondeclarative memory is not subserved by a single brain system and are consistent with the notion that this form of memory is mediated by those brain structures that are directly engaged in processing information during learning of a given task (Squire 1987). Patients with HD who have damage to the basal ganglia structures that are involved in processing motor information have difficulty in learning and retaining new motor skills. Similarly, patients with AD who have damage in neocortical regions that are thought to process semantic information are impaired on some verbal priming tasks.

ACKNOWLEDGMENTS

The preparation of this manuscript was supported in part by funds from NIA grants AG–05131 and AG–12963 and NIMH grant MH–48819.

REFERENCES

Ahissar, M. and Hochstein, S. 1993. Attentional control of early perceptual learning. *Proceedings of the National Academy of Science.* 90: 5718–5722.

Albert, M. and Milberg, W. 1989. Semantic processing in patients with Alzheimer's disease. *Brain and Language.* 37: 163–171.

Aldridge, J.W., Berridge, K.C., Herman, M. and Zimmer, L. 1993. Neuronal coding of serial order: Syntax of grooming in the neostriatum. *Psychological Science.* 4: 391–395.

Appollonio, I., Grafman, J., Clark, K., Nichelli, P., Zeffiro, T. and Hallett, M. 1994. Implicit and explicit memory in patients with Parkinson's disease with and without dementia. *Archives of Neurology.* 51: 359–367.

Appollonio, I.M., Grafman, J., Schwartz, V., Massaquoi, S. and Hallett, M. 1993. Memory in patients with cerebellar degeneration. *Neurology.* 43: 1536–1544.

Balota, D. A. and Duchek, J. M. 1991. Semantic priming effects, lexical repetition effects and contextual disambiguation effects in healthy aged individuals and individuals with senile dementia of the Alzheimer's type. *Brain and Language.* 40: 181–201.

Benzig, W.C. and Squire, L.R. 1989. Preserved learning and memory in amnesia: Intact adaptation-level effects and learning of stereoscopic depth. *Behavioral Neuroscience.* 103: 538–547.

Blaxton, T.A. 1989. Investigating dissociations among memory measures: Support for a transfer-appropriate processing framework. *Journal of Experimental Psychology (Learning, Memory and Cognition).* 15: 657–668.

Bondi, M.W. and Kaszniak, A.W. 1991. Implicit and explicit memory in Alzheimer's disease and Parkinson's disease. *Journal of Clinical and Experimental Neuropsychology.* 13: 339–358.

Bondi, M.W., Kaszniak, A.W., Bayles, K.A. and Vance, K.T. 1993. Contributions of frontal system dysfunction to memory and perceptual abilities in Parkinson's disease. *Neuropsychology.* 7: 89–102.

Brandt, J., Spencer, M., McSorley, P. and Folstein, M.F. 1988. Semantic activation and implicit memory in Alzheimer disease. *Alzheimer Disease and Associated Disorders.* 2: 112–119.

Brooks, D.N. and Baddeley, A.D. 1976. What can amnesic patients learn? *Neuropsychologia.* 14: 111–122.

Brun, A. 1983. An overview of light and electron microscopic changes. In *Alzheimer's disease*, ed. B. Reisberg, pp. 37–47. New York: The Free Press.

Bruyn, G.W., Bots, G. and Dom, R. 1979. Huntington's chorea: Current neuropathological status. In *Advances in neurology,* vol. 23: *Huntington's disease*, ed. T. Chase, N. Wexler and A. Barbeau, pp. 83–94. New York: Raven Press.

Butters, N., Salmon, D.P. and Heindel, W.C. 1994. Specificity of the memory deficits associated with basal ganglia dysfunction. *Revue Neurologique.* 150: 580–587.

Butters, N., Wolfe, J., Martone, M., Granholm, E. and Cermak, L.S. 1985. Memory disorders associated with Huntington's disease: Verbal recall, verbal recognition and procedural memory. *Neuropsychologia.* 6: 729–744.

Canavan, A.G.M., Sprengelmeyer, R., Diener, H.C. and Homberg, V. 1994. Conditional associative learning is impaired in cerebellar disease in humans. *Behavioral Neurosciences.* 108: 475–485.

Carlesimo, G.A. 1994. Perceptual and conceptual priming in amnesic and alcoholic patients. *Neuropsychologia.* 32: 903–921.

Cermak, L.S., Lewis, R., Butters, N. and Goodglass, H. 1973. Role of verbal mediation in performance of motor tasks by Korsakoff patients. *Perceptual and Motor Skills.* 37: 259–262.

Cermak, L.S., Talbot, N., Chandler, K. and Wolbarst, L.R. 1985. The perceptual priming phenomenon in amnesia. *Neuropsychologia.* 23: 615–622.

Chenery, H. J., Ingram, J. C. L. and Murdoch, B. E. 1994. The effect of repeated prime-target presentation in manipulating attention-induced priming in persons with dementia of the Alzheimer's type. *Brain and Cognition.* 25: 108–127.

Chertkow, H., Bub, D., Bergman, H., Bruemmer, A., Merling, A. and Rothfleisch, J. 1994. Increased semantic priming in patients with dementia of the Alzheimer's type. *Journal of Clinical and Experimental Neuropsychology*. 16: 608–622.

Chertkow, H., Bub, D. and Seidenberg, M. 1989. Priming and semantic memory loss in Alzheimer's disease. *Brain and Language*. 36: 420–446.

Cohen, N. and Squire, L.R. 1980. Preserved learning and retention of pattern analyzing skills in amnesia: Dissociation of knowing how and knowing that. *Science*. 210: 207–210.

Corkin, S. 1968. Acquisition of motor skill after bilateral medial temporal lobe excision. *Neuropsychologia*. 6: 255–265.

Daum, I., Ackerman, H., Schugens, M.M., Reimold, C., Dichgans, J. and Birbaumer, N. 1993. The cerebellum and cognitive functions in humans. *Behavioral Neuroscience*. 107: 411–419.

Deweer, B., Ergis, A.M., Fossati, P., Pillon, B., Boller, F., Agid, Y. and Dubois, B. 1994. Explicit memory, procedural learning and lexical priming in Alzheimer's disease. *Cortex*. 30: 113–126.

Deweer, B., Pillon, B., Michon, A. and Dubois, B. 1993. Mirror reading in Alzheimer's disease: Normal skill learning and acquisition of item-specific information. *Journal of Clinical and Experimental Neuropsychology*. 15: 789–804.

Edeline, J.M. and Weinberger, N.M. 1993. Receptive field plasticity in the auditory cortex during frequency discrimination training: Selective retuning independent of task difficulty. *Behavioral Neuroscience*. 107: 82–103.

Eslinger, P.J. and Damasio, A.R. 1986. Preserved motor learning in Alzheimer's disease: Implications for anatomy and behavior. *Journal of Neuroscience*. 6: 3006–3009.

Fennema-Notestine, C., Butters, N., Heindel, W.C. and Salmon, D.P. 1994. Semantic homophone priming in patients with dementia of the Alzheimer type. *Neuropsychology*. 8: 579–587.

Ferraro, F.R., Balota, D.A. and Connor, L.T. 1993. Implicit memory and the formation of new associations in nondemented Parkinson's disease individuals and individuals with senile dementia of the Alzheimer type: A serial reaction time (SRT) investigation. *Brain and Cognition*. 21: 163–180.

Fleischman, D.A., Gabrieli, J.D.E., Reminger, S., Rinaldi, J., Morrell, F. and Wilson, R. 1995. Conceptual priming in perceptual identification for patients with Alzheimer's disease and a patient with right occipital lobectomy. *Neuropsychology*. 9: 187–197.

Friedman, D., Hamberger, M., Stern, Y. and Marder, K. 1992. Event-related potentials (ERPs) during repetition priming in Alzheimer's patients and young and older controls. *Journal of Clinical and Experimental Neuropsychology*. 14: 448–462.

Gabrieli, J.D.E., Corkin, S., Mickel, S.F. and Growdon, J.H. 1993. Intact acquisition and long-term retention of mirror-tracing skill in Alzheimer's disease and global amnesia. *Behavioral Neuroscience*. 107: 899–910.

Gabrieli, J.D.E., Fleischman, D.A., Keane, M.M., Reminger, S.L. and Morrell, F. 1995. Double dissociation between memory systems underlying explicit and implicit memory in the human brain. *Psychological Science*. 6: 76–82.

Gardner, H., Boller, F., Moreines, J. and Butters, N. 1973. Retrieving information from Korsakoff patients: Effects of categorical cues and reference to the task. *Cortex*. 9: 165–175.

Glosser, G,. and Friedman, R.B. 1991. Lexical but not semantic priming in Alzheimer's disease. *Psychology and Aging*. 6: 522–527.

Graf, P., Squire, L. and Mandler, G. 1984. The information that amnesic patients do not forget. *Journal of Experimental Psychology [Human Learning and Memory]*. 10: 164–178.

Grafman, J., Litvan, I., Massaquoi, S., Stewart, M., Sirigu, A. and Hallett, M. 1992. Cognitive planning deficit in patients with cerebellar degeneration. *Neurology*. 42: 1493–1496.

Grafman, J., Weingartner, H., Newhouse, P.A., Thompson, K., Lalonde, F., Litvan, I., Molchan, S. and Sunderland, T. 1990. Implicit learning in patients with Alzheimer's disease. *Pharmacopsychiatry*. 23: 94–101.

Grafton, S.T., Mazziotta, J.C., Presty, S., Friston, K.J., Frackowiak, R.S.J. and Phelps, M.E. 1992. Functional anatomy of human procedural learning determined with regional cerebral blood flow and PET. *Journal of Neuroscience*. 12: 2542–2548.

Granholm, E., Bartzokis, G., Asarnow, R.F. and Marder, S.R. 1993. Preliminary associations between motor procedural learning, basal ganglia T2 relaxation times and tardive dyskinesia in schizophrenia. *Psychiatry Research: Neuroimaging*. 50: 33–44.

Grober, E., Ausubel, R., Sliwinski, M. and Gordon, B. 1992. Skill learning and repetition priming in Alzheimer's disease. *Neuropsychologia*. 30: 849–858.

Grosse, D.A., Wilson, R.S. and Fox, J.H. 1990. Preserved word-stem-completion priming of semantically encoded information in Alzheimer's disease. *Psychology and Aging*. 5: 304–306.

Hartman, M. 1991. The use of semantic knowledge in Alzheimer's disease: evidence for impairments of attention. *Neuropsychologia*. 29: 213–228.

Heindel, W., Butters, N. and Salmon, D. 1988. Impaired learning of a motor skill in patients with Huntington's disease. *Behavioral Neuroscience*. 102: 141–147.

Heindel, W., Salmon, D. and Butters, N. 1991. The biasing of weight judgments in Alzheimer's and Huntington's disease: A priming or programming phenomenon? *Journal of Clinical and Experimental Neuropsychology*. 13: 189–203.

Heindel, W., Salmon, D., Shults, C., Walicke, P. and Butters, N. 1989. Neuropsychological evidence for multiple implicit memory systems: A comparison of Alzheimer's, Huntington's and Parkinson's disease patients. *Journal of Neuroscience*. 9: 582–587.

Huberman, M., Moscovitch, M. and Freedman, M. 1994. Comparison of patients with Alzheimer's and Parkinson's disease on different explicit and implicit tests of memory. *Neuropsychiatry, Neuropsychology and Behavioral Neurology*. 7: 185–193.

Iragui, V., Kutas, M. and Salmon, D.P. 1996. Event-related brain potentials during semantic categorization in normal aging and senile dementia of the Alzheimer's type. *Electro-encephalography and Clinical Neurophysiology* 4: 1–15.

Jenkins, I.H., Brooks, D.J., Nixon, P.D., Frackowiak, R.S.J. and Passingham, R.E. 1994. Motor sequence learning: A study with positron emission tomography. *Journal of Neuroscience*. 14: 3775–3790.

Jones, L.A. 1986. Perception of force and weight: Theory and research. *Psychological Bulletin*. 100: 29–42.

Karni, A. and Sagi, D. 1991. Where practice makes perfect in texture discrimination: Evidence for a primary visual cortex plasticity. *Proceedings of the National Academy of Sciences*. 88: 4966–4970.

Karni, A. and Sagi, D. 1993. The time course of learning a visual skill. *Nature*. 365: 250–252.

Karni, A., Tanne, D., Rubenstein, B.S., Askenasy, J.M. and Sagi, D. 1994. Dependence on REM sleep of overnight improvement of a perceptual skill. *Science*. 265: 679–682.

Kawashima, R., Roland, P.E. and O'Sullivan, B.T. 1994. Fields in human motor areas involved in preparation for reaching, actual reaching and visuomotor learning: A positron emission tomography study. *Journal of Neuroscience*. 14: 3462–3474.

Keane, M.M., Gabrieli, J.D.E., Fennema, A.C., Growdon, J.H. and Corkin, S. 1991. Evidence for a dissociation between perceptual and conceptual priming in Alzheimer's disease. *Behavioral Neuroscience*. 105: 326–342.

Knopman, D.S. and Nissen, M.J. 1987. Implicit learning in patients with probable Alzheimer's disease. *Neurology*. 37: 784–788.

Knopman, D.S. and Nissen, M.J. 1991. Procedural learning is impaired in Huntington's disease: Evidence from the serial reaction time test. *Neuropsychologia*. 29: 245–254.

Knowlton, B.J., Mangels, J.A. and Squire, L.R. 1996. A neostriatal habit learning system in humans. *Science*, 273: 1399–1402.

Kutas, M. and Hillyard, S.A. 1980. Reading senseless sentences: Brain potentials reflect semantic incongruity. *Science*. 207: 203–205.

Kutas, M. and Hillyard, S.A. 1983. Event related brain potentials to grammatical errors and semantic anomalies. *Memory and Cognition*. 11: 539–550.

Kutas, M. and Hillyard, S.A. 1984. Brain potentials during reading reflect work expectancy and semantic association. *Nature*. 307: 161–163.

Leiner, H.C., Leiner, A.L. and Dow, R.S. 1993. Cognitive and language functions of the human cerebellum. *Trends in Neurosciences*. 16: 444–447.

Martin, A. 1992. Degraded knowledge representations in patients with Alzheimer's disease: Implications for models of semantic and repetition priming. In *Neuropsychology of memory*, 2nd ed., ed. L. R. Squire and N. Butters, pp. 220–232. New York: Guilford Press.

Martin, A., Heyes, M.P., Salazar, A.M., Law, W.A. and Williams, J. 1993. Impaired motor-skill learning, slowed reaction time and elevated cerebrospinal-fluid quinolinic acid in a subgroup of HIV-infected individuals. *Neuropsychology*. 7: 149–157.

Martone, M., Butters, N., Payne, M., Becker, J. and Sax, D. 1984. Dissociations between skill learning and verbal recognition in amnesia and dementia. *Archives of Neurology*. 41: 965–970.

Middleton, F.A. and Strick, P.L. 1994. Anatomical evidence for cerebellar and basal ganglia involvement in higher cognitive function. *Science*. 266: 458–461.

Moscovitch, M., Winocur, G. and McLachlan, D. 1986. Memory as assessed by recognition and reading time in normal and memory-impaired people with Alzheimer's disease and other neurological disorders. *Journal of Experimental Psychology (General)*. 115: 331–347.

Nebes, R. 1989. Semantic memory in Alzheimer's disease. *Psychological Bulletin*. 106: 377–394.

Nebes, R. D., Brady, C. B. and Huff, F. J. 1989. Automatic and attentional mechanisms of semantic priming in Alzheimer's disease. *Journal of Clinical and Experimental Neuropsychology*. 11: 219–230.

Nebes, R., Martin, D. and Horn, L. 1984. Sparing of semantic memory in Alzheimer's disease. *Journal of Abnormal Psychology*. 93: 321–330.

Nissen, M.J. and Bullemer, P. 1987. Attentional requirements of learning: Evidence from performance measures. *Cognitive Psychology*. 19: 1–32.

Ober, B. A. and Shenaut, G. K. 1988. Lexical decision and priming in Alzheimer's disease. *Neuropsychologia*. 26: 273–286.

Ober, B. A., Shenaut, G. K., Jagust, W. J. and Stillman, R. C. 1991. Automatic semantic priming with various category relations in Alzheimer's disease and normal aging. *Psychology and Aging*. 6: 647–660.

Ostergaard, A.L. 1994. Dissociations between word priming effects in normal subjects and patients with memory disorders: Multiple memory systems or retrieval? *Quarterly Journal of Experimental Psychology*. 47A: 331–364.

Partridge, F., Knight, R. and Feehan, M. 1990. Direct and indirect memory performance in patients with senile dementia. *Psychological Medicine*. 20: 111–118.

Pascual-Leone, A., Grafman, J., Clark, K., Stewart, M., Massaquoi, S., Lou, J. and Hallett, M. 1993. Procedural learning in Parkinson's disease and cerebellar degeneration. *Annals of Neurology*. 34: 594–602.

Pascual-Leone, A., Grafman, J. and Hallett, M. 1994. Modulation of cortical motor output maps during development of implicit and explicit knowledge. *Science*. 263: 1287–1289.

Paulsen, J.S., Butters, N., Salmon, D.P., Heindel, W.C. and Swenson, M.R. 1993. Prism adaptation in Alzheimer's and Huntington's disease. *Neuropsychology*. 7: 73–81.

Pavlides, C., Miyashita, E. and Asanuma, H. 1993. Projection from the sensory to the motor cortex is important in learning motor skills in monkeys. *Journal of Neurophysiology*. 70: 733–741.

Pellis, S.M., Castenada, E., McKenna, M.M., Tran-Nguyen, L.T.L. and Whishaw, I.Q. 1993. The role of the striatum in organizing sequences of play fighting in neonatally dopamine-depleted rats. *Neuroscience Letters*. 158: 13–15.

Perani, D., Bressi, S., Cappa, S.F., Vallar, G., Alberoni, M., Grassi, F., Caltagirone, C., Cipolotti, L., Franceschi, M., Lenzi, G.L. and Fazio, F. 1993. Evidence of multiple memory systems in the human brain. *Brain*. 116: 903–919.

Platz, T., Denzler, P., Kaden, B. and Mauritz, K.H. 1994. Motor learning after recovery from hemiparesis. *Neuropsychologia*. 32: 1209–1223.

Randolph, C. 1991. Implicit, explicit and semantic memory functions in Alzheimer's disease and Huntington's disease. *Journal of Clinical and Experimental Neuropsychology*. 13: 479–494.

Rausch, D.M., Heyes, M.P., Murray, E.A., Lendvay, J., Sharer, L.R., Ward, J.M., Rehm, S., Nohr, D., Weihe, E. and Eiden, L.E. 1994. Cytopathologic and neurochemical correlates of progression to motor/cognitive impairment in SIV-infected rhesus monkeys. *Journal of Neuropathology and Experimental Neurology*. 53: 165–175.

Roediger, H.L. and Blaxton, T.A. 1987. Effects of varying modality, surface features and retention interval on priming in word fragment completion. *Memory and Cognition*. 15: 379–388.

Rugg, M. D., Pearl, S., Walker, P., Roberts, R. C. and Holdstock, J. S. 1994. Word repetition effects in event-related potentials in healthy young and old subjects and in patients with Alzheimer-type dementia. *Neuropsychologia*. 32: 381–398.

Saint-Cyr, J.A., Taylor, A.E. and Lang, A.E. 1988. Procedural learning and neostriatal dysfunction in man. *Brain*. 111: 941–959.

Sakurai, Y. 1994. Involvement of auditory cortical and hippocampal neurons in auditory working memory and reference memory in the rat. *Journal of Neuroscience*. 14: 2606–2623.

Salmon, D.P. and Chan, A.S. 1994. Semantic memory deficits associated with Alzheimer's disease. In *Neuropsychological explorations of memory and cognition: Essays in honor of Nelson Butters*, ed. L.S. Cermak, pp. 61–76. New York: Plenum Press.

Salmon, D.P. and Heindel, W.C. 1992. Impaired priming in Alzheimer's disease: Neuropsychological implications. In *Neuropsychology of memory*, 2nd ed., ed. L.R. Squire and N. Butters, pp. 179–187. New York: Guilford Press.

Salmon, D., Shimamura, A., Butters, N. and Smith, S. 1988. Lexical and semantic priming deficits in patients with Alzheimer's disease. *Journal of Clinical and Experimental Neuropsychology*. 10: 477–494.

Sanes, J.N., Dimitrov, B. and Hallett, M. 1990. Motor learning in patients with cerebellar dysfunction. *Brain*. 113: 103–120.

Schlaug, G., Knorr, U. and Seitz, R.J. 1994. Inter-subject variability of cerebral activations in acquiring a motor skill: A study with positron emission tomography. *Experimental Brain Research*. 98: 523–534.

Schwartz, T. J., Kutas, M., Butters, N., Paulsen, J. S. and Salmon, D. P. 1996. Electrophysiological insights into the nature of the semantic deficit in Alzheimer's disease. *Neuropsychologia*. 34: 827–841.

Seitz, R.J., Roland, P.E., Bohm, C., Greitz, T. and Stone-Elander, S. 1990. Motor learning in man: A positron emission tomographic study. *Neuroreport*. 1: 17–20.

Shimamura, A.P. 1986. Priming effects in amnesia: Evidence for a dissociable memory function. *Quarterly Journal of Experimental Psychology*. 38A: 619–644.

Shimamura, A.P. and Squire, L.R. 1984. Paired-associate learning and priming effects in amnesia: A neuropsychological study. *Journal of Experimental Psychology (General)*. 113: 556–570.

Shimamura, A.P., Salmon, D.P., Squire, L.R. and Butters, N. 1987. Memory dysfunction and word priming in dementia and amnesia. *Behavioral Neurosciences*. 101: 347–351.

Squire, L.R. 1987. *Memory and brain*. New York: Oxford University Press.

Terry, R.D. and Katzman, R. 1983. Senile dementia of the Alzheimer type. *Annals of Neurology*. 14: 497–506.

Tulving, E. and Schacter, D. 1990. Priming and human memory systems. *Science*. 247: 301–306.

Warrington, E.K. and Weiskrantz, L. 1968. New method of testing long-term retention with special reference to amnesic patients. *Nature*. 217: 972–974.

Warrington, E.K. and Weiskrantz, L. 1970. Amnesic syndrome: Consolidation or retrieval? *Nature*. 228: 628–630.

Willingham, D.B. and Koroshetz, W.J. 1993. Evidence for dissociable motor skills in Huntington's disease patients. *Psychobiology*. 21: 173–182.

Zohary, E., Celebrini, S., Britten, K.H. and Newsome, W.T. 1994. Neuronal plasticity that underlies improvement in perceptual performance. *Science*. 263: 1289–1292.

13

Memory in neurodegenerative disease: what has been learned about the organization of memory?

ANDREW R. MAYES

INTRODUCTION

It is very widely believed that memories are stored where the remembered information is represented in the brain (Ungerleider 1995). Thus, distinct kinds of information will be stored in different brain regions. There is certainly evidence that most, if not all, regions of the brain show the kinds of plastic change at synapses that could underlie long-term memory (McGaugh et al. 1995). Whether the intraneuronal and organizational extraneuronal storage processes for two kinds of memory are qualitatively dissimilar cannot be determined at present, but this may be more likely if the brain regions involved have radically different cytoarchitectures (as may be the case, for example, with the cerebellum and the neocortex). Whether the encoding and retrieval of information depends on different regions from those involved in storage is also hard to determine in a principled way at present, but, for example, is likely to be the case when encoding and/or retrieval are nonroutine and require the planning of mental operations, as is often the case with episodic and semantic memory.

Structural damage to different brain regions disrupts memory for distinct kinds of information. I have suggested five broad groups of memory disorders caused by brain damage (Mayes 1988). First, there are disorders of short-term or working memory, which are selective for specific kinds of information such as phonological sequences and which are caused by parietal and possibly by frontal lobe lesions. Second, there are disorders of previously well-established semantic memory, which are caused by association neocortex lesions, particularly those affecting the temporal association neocortex. Third, there are the memory disorders resulting from damage to the prefrontal association cortex, which may all be caused by distur-

bances to the executive processes believed to be mediated primarily by this brain region. Fourth, there is the amnesic syndrome, which affects recall and recognition of fact and episode information and is caused mainly by lesions to the medial temporal lobe and midline diencephalic regions. These first four groups of memory disorders are all of aware memory, variously called declarative or explicit memory. Fifth, there is a much more heterogeneous group of disorders of those kinds of memory often referred to as procedural, nondeclarative or implicit memory. These forms of unaware memory may be for conditioning or motor, perceptual and cognitive skills, forms of which are disrupted by cerebellar and basal ganglia lesions, respectively. They also include priming or information-specific implicit memory (ISIM), perceptual forms of which some recent evidence suggests can be damaged by posterior cortical lesions (Keane et al. 1995).

The differences between the different kinds of disorder of the fifth type seem to be so great that they may differ more from each other than they do from the other four groups of memory disorders. Even with the other four groups of organic memory disorders it is currently unclear whether they have been correctly characterized. Two illustrations may clarify this point. First, it is uncertain whether working memory deficits do not also affect long-term memory, but theoretically important to know. With phonological short-term memory disorder, however, it has been shown that long-term memory is only normal for spoken verbal material which can be rapidly recoded semantically. If this is made impossible by requiring memory for spoken words in an incomprehensible foreign language, then long-term as well as short-term memory is devastated (Vallar and Papagno 1995). Second, although semantic memory disorders dissociate from amnesia, it will be argued later in this chapter that this does not mean that semantic memory depends primarily on the association cortex whereas episodic memory depends primarily on medial temporal lobe and diencephalic limbic structures. Rather, it will be argued that very long-term storage of both facts and episodes depends on association cortex whereas shorter-term storage of this information depends on the limbic system.

Since the late 1980s, it has become possible to extend our knowledge about the location of particular kinds of memory by using neuroimaging procedures whilst scanned subjects perform selected encoding and retrieval procedures, the activations of which can be compared with those of appropriately selected baseline conditions. In general, these neuroimaging procedures have produced results consistent with the implications of the lesion reported in literature. Both the lesion and the neuroimaging literatures on memory suggest that dementing patients, like those with unchanging brain lesions, should show memory deficits that can be predicted from the location of their lesions.

As the chapter indicates, this suggestion is well supported. Thus, dementia of the Alzheimer type, in which damage to the posterior neocortical association cortex is particularly prominent fairly early in the disease, is associated with impaired performance on working memory tests, certain kinds of information-specific implicit memory or priming deficit, amnesia and semantic memory deficits. It is not associated with impairments in skill acquisition and memory, however, which is to be expected because these seem to be more susceptible to the basal ganglia damage suffered by patients with Huntington's disease (HD), who do have impaired skill memory. In contrast to patients with Alzheimer's disease (AD), those with HD perform normally on priming tasks which involve semantic information (as well as perceptual priming tasks) and do not show deficits on semantic memory tasks except when performance is disrupted by visually based errors or depends on active search processes during retrieval. HD disrupts frontal lobe function both indirectly because of the frontal lobe projections of the caudate nucleus and because of frontal lobe degeneration that occurs later in the disease. This frontal lobe dysfunction probably disrupts strategic retrieval that may be important in recalling both semantic and episodic information (at which HD patients are also impaired). It also disrupts the kinds of executive operations important for working memory and patients with HD are impaired at working memory as well.

WORKING MEMORY AND NEURODEGENERATIVE DISEASE

The question immediately raised is whether working memory is impaired in AD and HD for the same or different reasons. In Chapter 8, Owen and his colleagues suggest a way in which this kind of question may be answered. They use evidence both from lesion and neuroimaging studies to identify regions of the frontal association cortex that mediate different executive or short-term memory holding operations. Evidence from both sources suggests that the ventrolateral frontal cortex mediates the organization of response sequences that map directly on to sequences held in short-term memory, whereas the dorsolateral frontal cortex plays a more active role in manipulating and monitoring information held in short-term memory. Both these frontal regions, however, work as part of a larger system that includes reciprocally connected posterior neocortical structures. There is indeed good evidence that lesions in posterior association cortex disrupt short-term memory for auditory and visual verbal information and for visuospatial information, more than do frontal association cortex lesions (McCarthy and Warrington 1990).

Owen and his colleagues have compared working memory in several kinds of dementia using two tasks. One of these tasks (tapping) is a computerized version of Corsi's block tapping procedure (Milner 1971), performance on which requires relatively passive copying of the order of tapping of spatial locations and so is presumably mainly dependent on short-term storage. There is evidence that performance on this task depends on the ventrolateral, but not dorsolateral frontal cortex. The second task (strategic) is a computerized equivalent of a radial maze working memory task that requires subjects to reorganize and change the information they are holding in short-term storage. Performance on this task should depend on both short-term storage and executive functions. Indeed, Owen and his colleagues have found that performance on a similar task to this second one involves both dorsolateral and ventrolateral frontal cortex. The second task allows a measure of the effectiveness of the search strategy used as well as of short-term memory storage. Use of the tasks illuminates two broad features of dementia. First, as different dementias progress, performance deteriorates on new tasks in a fairly regular fashion. For example, Parkinson's disease (PD) patients in the early disease stage were only impaired at the tapping task whereas later they were impaired at both tasks. Consistent with this, Owen and his colleagues cite evidence that it is the caudate regions projecting to the dorsolateral frontal cortex that show the earliest and greatest dopamine loss in PD patients. Second, dementing patients in whom the illness disrupted the functioning of the frontal lobes tended to show problems with both of the tasks. Interestingly, patients with HD, who showed a similar order of breakdown on the two tasks as did PD patients, were more impaired on both tasks than AD patients who were matched for degree of dementia.

These observations on working memory warrant some comments. Depending on how stored information needs to be manipulated, performance on working memory tasks requires a neural system that holds the information in short-term storage and other neural systems that mediate the executive processes needed. Short-term storage may well depend on the continuance of the neural activity involved in the initial representation and so will inevitably be in the representing brain region, which will certainly include the posterior association cortex. The precise region will vary depending on the exact information being held in short-term memory. Although most researchers seem to believe that the prefrontal association cortex primarily mediates different executive processes, there is a growing body of opinion that it is concerned with short-term storage with different kinds of information being stored in distinct frontal cortex regions (Goldman-Rakic 1990). There are four possibilities: (1) the frontal cortex mediates different executive processes, (2) the frontal cortex mediates short-term storage for different kinds of information, (3) it does both these things, (4) it does neither of these things. Damage to a short-term memory holding system is likely to have a disruptive effect on planning ability and, as Owen and his colleagues argue, damage to executive function may well disturb short-term memory performance. Nevertheless, they seem to be arguing for the view that frontal cortex mediates both short-term storage and executive processes.

For example, there was evidence of a deficit in strategy use on the strategy task in patients with HD and progressive supranuclear palsy, suggesting that performance on this task in these patients may have been bad at least in part because of impaired executive processes. A similar argument has been made by Sahgal et al. (1995), who compared a group of patients with mild Lewy body dementia

with a group of equivalently demented AD patients on the same tapping and strategy working memory tasks. The Lewy body dementia patients were only more impaired than the AD patients on the strategy task and on this task they also showed more problems with strategic planning. This accords with evidence that Lewy body dementia particularly affects the frontal association cortex. In contrast, in patients with multiple system atrophy, there was no evidence for impaired strategy use, which suggests that their deficit on the strategy task was caused by an impaired ability to hold visuospatial information for short periods of time. The pattern of working memory deficits in dementia is, therefore, compatible with the proposal that the frontal lobes are involved in mediating both short-term storage and executive functions with the precise effects of lesions depending on the location of damage within the frontal association neocortex.

As already indicated, however, there is evidence that posterior cortex lesions impair several kinds of short-term memory more severely than do frontal cortex lesions. Both posterior cortex connectivity and this evidence strongly suggest that this broad region contains neural systems mediating short-term storage operations. It is, therefore, surprising that patients with AD, who fairly early in their illness suffer atrophy of the parieto-temporal cortex, were found to be less impaired than HD patients, matched for dementia, on Owen and colleagues' two spatial working memory tasks. Although it might be argued that, relatively speaking, short-term memory for visuospatial information depends more on frontal cortex mechanisms than does short-term memory for phonology, Baddeley (1986) has nevertheless suggested that the primary deficit in AD patients' short-term memory impairment in phonology is with the central executive component of working memory because patients are: (1) impaired at dual task performance, (2) have intact articulatory loops and (3) at least in the mild stage of the disease, show a relatively intact recency effect. This raises two issues. First, do AD patients, early in the disease, have problems with short-term storage operations of the kind that might result from posterior cortex atrophy and, if not, why not? Second, do AD patients, early in the disease, show executive function deficits other than with dual task performance and, if so, what lesions are responsible for these deficits? Little can currently be said about the first issue and the second is hard to test. For example, P. Broks et al. (personal communication) have shown that patients with mild AD were impaired at some tests of executive function, including the Tower of London test, two verbal fluency tests and the Stroop test, but preserved at others, including the Luria tests and tests of auditory sustained attention and cognitive estimation. It is hard to know from the pattern of results whether the deficits seen were caused by an impairment in one or more executive processes or by a deficit in the basic processes (perhaps mediated by posterior association cortex) on which these executive processes operate. A deficit in the basic processes would impair task performance and might also cause an overload and breakdown of otherwise unimpaired executive processes. If so, the pattern as well as the severity of impairment might well be indistinguishable from that caused by a selective failure of executive processes.

Future work needs to identify the cortical regions involved in the short-term storage of different kinds of information and of the regions that mediate the executive processes that may be involved in manipulating this stored information. Only then will it be possible to specify the location of the lesions and the functional deficits that disrupt AD patients' performance on working memory and executive tasks. Future work also needs to sort out three further problems. The first is the kinds of long-term memory tasks that are impaired in patients with dementia affecting basal ganglia–frontal cortex systems. One would expect deficits on tasks that depend on executive mediation (Mayes 1988) such as free recall of organizable materials, prospective memory, source memory and temporal memory (as in questions like 'when was Sadat assassinated'?), but which tasks are disrupted should depend on the specific executive processes affected. Second, if there is impairment on other long-term memory tasks, this may indicate that some of these dementias involve disruption to more posterior cortical systems' functioning as well, in the way that Owen and his colleagues suggest. This must be resolved. Third, if there are short-term storage deficits caused by a dementia, then long-term memory for the same information, however tested, should be impaired for the same information unless it is possible to recode the information into a code for which storage is unaffected. Thus, patients with any of the above kinds of dementia should have long-term recognition memory deficits for the appropriate kinds of visuospatial information. This is supported by the work of Baddeley et al. (1988) who found that patient P.V. with her impairment in phonological short-term memory was unable to learn spoken Russian words that she could not understand.

PROSPECTIVE MEMORY AND FRONTAL CORTEX FUNCTION

It is widely believed that prospective memory, or remembering to remember, depends on executive functions mediated by the frontal cortex as well as on episodic memory and will, therefore, be disrupted in dementing conditions that affect the frontal association cortex. Knight convincingly supports this interpretation by pointing out that very often remembering to remember must take place under dual task conditions, performance on which, Baddeley (1986) and others have argued, depends on specific executive processes and is mediated by the frontal cortex. As Knight indicates, however, success at prospective memory must depend on several processes, particularly including the ability to recall things and intentions from the past, i.e. aspects of episodic memory. It has now been shown by several workers that prospective memory declines with age at least when conditions are made difficult as is more likely to apply when the remembering to remember is cued by a time-based cue rather than an event-based cue. This is consistent with the view that failure at prospective memory results from a difficulty with initiating retrieval when a cue is presented rather than because the significance of the cue has simply been forgotten. Initiation of retrieval, particularly under dual task conditions, requires executive processes and it is known that aging is especially associated with atrophy in the frontal association cortex. Although elderly people do have deficits in episodic memory as well, it is likely that their prospective memory failures are most often caused by an executive processing inadequacy because they can remember a cue's significance when directly challenged after showing a failure of prospective memory.

The only kind of dementia for which prospective memory has been assessed is AD, which has been shown to be very sensitive to deficits in this kind of memory. Given that AD might cause a deficit for several reasons, it is interesting that Knight notes that prospective memory remained impaired in the study of Huppert and Beardsall (1993) even when retrospective memory scores were covaried. This suggests that at least one cause of the prospective memory deficit in AD could be an executive processing problem, perhaps related to dual task performance. This would be consistent with evidence that working memory is impaired in AD mainly because of the impairment of executive processing. If so, there are three possible explanations of why executive processing should be impaired early in AD: (1) AD leads to disruptive structural loss in the frontal cortex earlier than is generally supposed; (2) Although damage early in the disease is mainly confined to posterior association cortex, the frontal cortex becomes functionally disturbed and performs sub-optimally because of direct links between it and the damaged posterior regions. There is some evidence against both these possibilities in that AD patients, early in the course of the disease, show hypometabolism in the posterior association cortex, but usually not in the frontal region (Chawluk et al. 1990) except perhaps in cases with a familial history of AD (D. Neary, personal communication); and (3) Certain executive functions and, consequently, the forms of memory that depend on them, are mediated by posterior as well as frontal association cortex. Some evidence of this in relation to prospective memory was found in a recent study in which prospective memory was examined in normal control subjects and patient groups with either frontal cortex or posterior cortex lesions (Mayes and Daum 1997). We found that both groups of patients were impaired at a prospective memory task even when we were able to show that they retained what it was that they had been asked to remember at the end of the session. Although they could do this, both patient groups were impaired at remembering to respond to the event-related cues during the session, which suggests that their failure on the prospective memory task was caused by a deficit in certain executive processes. In support of this possibility, both groups of patients were equally impaired on several tests of executive functions.

Deficits in prospective memory particularly affect the ability to cope in daily life so it is surprising that it has been so little examined in dementing patients. This is likely to be rapidly remedied, however, as there is now considerable interest in this form of memory (Brandimonte et al. 1996). Future work should use the methodological control mentioned above in which subjects are asked after they have failed on the prospective memory component of a task whether they remember what they should have done to what cue. It is only when failure occurs in the presence of accurate episodic memory that one can be fairly confident of executive processes being implicated. The nature of these processes and the brain regions that mediate them need to be more fully specified, but one would probably predict that those dementias which particularly affect the frontal association cortices should show prospective memory failure at an early stage. In general, early in their development 'frontal' dementias should affect several forms of memory including prospective memory, working memory, recall of organizable materials, temporal memory, source memory and metamemory, which have all been shown to be disrupted by frontal cortex lesions (Mayes 1988). It remains possible that different 'frontal' dementias will be found to disrupt these forms of memory differentially because the dementias affect somewhat different frontal regions and the forms of memory depend on executive processes mediated by distinct frontal (and possibly posterior) cortical regions.

REMOTE EPISODIC MEMORY IN DEMENTIA

In Chapter 10, Paul and his colleagues focus on the impairments shown by dementing patients in memory for facts and episodes first experienced in the remote past before illness should have seriously affected brain function. They consider tests both of remote memory for public information involving famous events and people and of autobiographical materials. Relative to what is usually counted as semantic memory, none of the material in such tests has been heavily rehearsed. Nevertheless, strictly speaking, knowledge of who Clement Attlee was or what happened at Mount St. Helens, depends on semantic memory although there is nothing to prevent the rememberer drawing on memory of past episodes that they have experienced to aid retrieval of the critical facts.

Paul and his colleagues compare the remote memory deficits of AD patients with those of patients with dementing conditions which affect the frontal lobes (or the fronto-striatal system) more dramatically in their relatively early stages. These dementias include HD, PD, progressive supranuclear palsy, the AIDS dementia complex (now called human immunodeficiency virus (HIV)-associated dementia) and Pick's disease when it primarily affects the frontal lobes. Whereas early in its course, AD causes a remote memory deficit with relative sparing of older memories, this is not so with the dementias which primarily affect the frontal lobes or the fronto-striatal system as they produce a remote memory deficit without a temporal gradient that becomes more severe as the dementia advances. In AD also, the temporal gradient is eventually lost, but it is not clear whether this is not simply caused by a floor effect.

It is suggested that remote memory may be impaired either because storage has been disrupted or because active retrieval search processes have been disturbed. Any dementia which disturbs the functioning of the frontal association cortex could damage the executive processes that underlie the effective use of strategic search processes. The purpose of such processes is to find and encode cues that will automatically reactivate a target memory representation when the initially encoded cues fail to do this as is usually the case. How would one know that poor memory results from this kind of problem rather than the loss or partial loss of the target information from memory itself? Paul and his colleagues argue that one relevant criterion is whether remote memory deficits are reduced when tested by recognition compared to free recall. This is based on the view that strategic retrieval is not needed for recognition or that it is at least less important than it is with free recall. As already indicated, patients with frontal cortex damage do indeed seem to be markedly more impaired at free recall than they are at recognition although this does not prove that the problem is one of strategic retrieval. There is some evidence that this is also the case with dementias that primarily affect the frontal lobe system although this needs to be much more systematically tested.

Although it is very likely true that free recall depends much more than does recognition on strategic retrieval search processes, there is another difference between the two which means that free recall may be more impaired than recognition even when there is no active search process deficit. Free recall and recognition are typically of items in remote memory tests, so free recall can require that more complex associative information has to be retrieved than with recognition. This is because free recall works by retrieving links between items and the contexts in which they appeared whereas there is evidence that recognition does not need to retrieve these links. If there is a problem with storing complex associative information relative to simpler associations and item information, then recall will be more impaired than recognition. This is exactly what Aggleton and Shaw (1996) have claimed is true of amnesics who have sustained selective damage to the hippocampus or other structures in the hippocampal circuit of Papez. If these patients have an impaired ability to consolidate complex associations into long-term memory, then they should be impaired at recognition when it taps complex associations rather than single items. This can be tested by devising foils that comprise studied items that have been recombined into different associations than those they were in during study. Patients with dementias that primarily attack frontal cortex functioning should not show disrupted performance on these kinds of recognition test of remote memory to any greater extent than they do on standard recognition tests if their problem is genuinely one of strategic retrieval.

They should also show deficits on executive function tests that depend minimally on memory and performance on some of these tests should correlate with their degree of impairment for recall of remote memories. Paul and his colleagues do not reject the possibility that part of the problem of AD patients with remote memory may arise because of a deficit in executive processes underlying active retrieval search. This is possible, but is subject to the comments that have already been made about AD and deficits in working and prospective memory. Paul and his colleagues also consider the view that the primary cause of the AD deficit in remote memory is the loss of semantic knowledge suffered by this patient group. Their main support for this view seems to be that semantic memory is impaired in AD and that the remote memory deficit is one of storage rather than access because it affects recognition as well as free recall. If the view is correct, however, it should be possible to show that: (1) there is breakdown in the storage of semantic information for reasons independent of any impairment in recognition memory, (2) this impairment disrupts the ability to retrieve episodic information that somehow relies on the semantic information, memory for which has been impaired, and (3) this mechanism can explain why, early in the disease's course, more remote episodic memories are less impaired.

These things have not yet been done, but as will be discussed in the next section, evidence from semantic dementia suggests that semantic memory loss per se may have a relatively insignificant effect on episodic memory. It seems more likely that AD in its early stages disrupts remote episodic memory for the same reasons that disruption occurs in medial temporal lobe amnesia. Although the reasons for this are not fully understood, it is clear that amnesics' remote memory loss is not primarily caused by a loss of semantic knowledge. It is also probable that the loss is not primarily caused by a failure of strategic search operations at retrieval. Amnesics show an impairment in remote memory for both facts and events despite the preservation of their memory for overlearnt semantic information, perhaps because key aspects of the relevant kinds of information are initially stored in the damaged medial temporal lobe structures.

According to Alvarez and Squire (1994), the hippocampus is initially critical for fact and event memory but, with the passage of time, responsibility is gradually passed to the posterior association neocortex. If they are correct, then, in the early stages of AD, when damage is typically greatest in the region of the medial temporal lobes, there will be a deficit in memory for both facts and events which still depend on the medial temporal lobe region for their storage. Older memories should not be affected if the responsibility for their storage has been passed to the association neocortex so this view has no problem explaining a temporal gradient. Relatively early in their disease, however, patients with AD suffer degeneration in their posterior temporal cortices. The damage they suffer is likely to cause some degradation in the storage of older fact and event memories which no longer rely on the medial temporal lobe structures that are damaged in some amnesics. This damage, which may affect episodic memory and both heavily rehearsed and less rehearsed semantic memory equally, when combined with the damage to the medial temporal lobe area, should produce a very extended temporal gradient in which the remotest memories are still impaired, but less so than more recent memories.

Remote memory impairment fairly early in AD may, therefore, be caused by: (1) failures of strategic search during retrieval that are caused by damage to the frontal lobes or a larger circuit that includes frontal and posterior associations cortices, and (2) storage degradation caused by medial temporal lobe and posterior association cortex damage. The relative contribution of each of these functional deficits may be hard to determine as is considered in the next section, which also indicates why loss of semantic knowledge per se is unlikely to be a major factor underlying the remote memory deficit for episodes and facts that have not been greatly overlearnt.

SEMANTIC MEMORY AND DEMENTIA

Fink and Randolph (Chapter 11) review the relevant lesion and neuroimaging literature and conclude that available evidence suggests that well established semantic memory is stored in a neural network at the core of which probably lies the temporal lobe (particularly the left side). Interestingly, a recent neuroimaging study has provided evidence that there is a distributed neural system that probably stores associative and visual semantic information related both to words and pictures, which includes the junction between parietal and temporal cortices and between fusiform and inferior temporal cortex on the left, the left middle temporal cortex and the left inferior frontal gyrus (Vandenberghe et al. 1996). This study, therefore, suggests that the parietal and frontal cortices, as well as parts of the temporal association cortex, may be involved in storing semantic information. Although Fink and Randolph suggest that the involvement of other cortical areas may relate to the specific kinds of semantic information that are being stored, it is not clear that their suggestion explains the results of Vandenberghe and his colleagues because the critical parietal and frontal regions were activated indiscriminately during the retrieval of both associative and visual semantic information. If, as Fink and Randolph argue, representations are stored close to where they are represented in perception, the inferior frontal gyrus might be expected to be involved in storing functional information about inanimate objects like hammers as this region may represent the kinds of action likely to be performed with a hammer. The results of Vandenberghe and his colleagues suggest that the inferior frontal gyrus stores perceptual as well as functional information.

Fink and Randolph review the evidence concerning semantic memory breakdown in different kinds of dementia using the principle that if there is structural deterioration within the neocortical region where semantic information is probably stored, then there will be a deficit in semantic storage. Dementia might not otherwise be expected to cause a deficit in semantic memory unless performance on the tests used is strongly dependent on strategic search processes during retrieval. AD patients, who clearly suffer deterioration in critical posterior association neocortex structures early in the course of the disease, have been shown to have semantic memory deficits as do patients with semantic dementia, who show focal atrophy in the inferolateral temporal cortex (usually bilaterally or on the left side). Dementing patients with deterioration that affects the frontal or fronto–striatal system may show deficits on semantic memory tests. Indeed, patients with progressive supranuclear palsy dementia may show more severe deficits than equivalently demented AD patients.

Fink and Randolph consider the evidence that these deficits arise because of a breakdown in the organization of strategic search processes or from other factors unrelated to semantic information storage disturbances. For example, there is evidence that the naming deficits shown by early HD patients are associated with visually based errors, which suggests that their poor confrontation naming stems from their known visuoperceptual problems. Similarly, the impaired category fluency performance of PD patients is markedly improved by cueing, which implies that search processes may be impaired in this patient group.

One would expect that damage within the neocortical regions that Vandenberghe et al.'s (1996) neuroimaging study indicates to be activated by retrieving semantic information about words and pictures should produce an impairment in semantic memory storage rather than access. In other words, one should expect that patients with AD and semantic dementia should have deficits in semantic memory storage whereas patients with dementias affecting the frontal or striato-frontal circuits should show semantic memory access problems unless the dementia has affected the left inferior frontal region.

Shallice (1988) has proposed five criteria for distinguishing between storage and access failure. Storage deficits should (1) cause items to be consistently retrieved or not retrieved across time, (2) cause ISIM or priming to be impaired for information no longer stored, (3) cause superordinate information to be preserved relative to subordinate features, (4) cause memory for less frequently rehearsed information to be more impaired than memory for more frequently rehearsed information and (5) cause the allowance of greater search time not to decrease the size of the deficit. As I have argued before (Mayes 1988), if these criteria are appropriate, then they should follow from a well-supported theoretical account of storage and retrieval, but this is not the case. One should, therefore, treat cautiously any claims based upon them.

Perhaps the least contentious of the five criteria are the first two, although even with these criteria care should be applied. If storage of particular information is only partially disrupted by a lesion, then it seems quite feasible that retrieval should be inconsistent across time depending on the exact state of the brain and the quality of the cues actually encoded. Nevertheless, it might be argued that it is hard to imagine a kind of retrieval deficit that would produce a consistent pattern of performance across time. An argument to the contrary might run along the follow-

ing lines: If accessing a still stored memory is impaired, the problem is most likely to be caused by a deficit in the executive processes that underlie active search, which is the process of identifying cues that when encoded will automatically activate a representation of the target information. Encoding of information is almost certain to be idiosyncratic with the result that active search for appropriate cues for some memories is likely to be very easy whereas the search for appropriate cues for other memories may be very hard. If this is so, subjects might regularly achieve the simple searches despite a deficient active search mechanism and regularly fail on the hard searches because the search mechanism is impaired. It is, therefore, not enough to merely assert that storage deficits cause consistent patterns of success or failure across time whereas access deficits cause inconsistent patterns. In particular, there needs to be a convincing demonstration that retrieval success across time is very inconsistent on an item-by-item basis when there is direct evidence for an access problem specifically related to the ability to actively search for cues. Such a deficit is most likely to be found in patients with frontal association cortex lesions. If there are other kinds of access process that can break down, these processes need to be convincingly distinguished from storage processes and a theoretical reason given for why deficits in the processes lead to inconsistent patterns of memory performance across time.

As Fink and Randolph point out, there is good evidence that AD patients show a consistent pattern of retrieval success or failure for specific semantic information across time and the same is probably true of semantic dementia patients. Use of Hodges' semantic memory test battery also shows that AD and semantic dementia patients show consistent success or failure on semantic tasks with verbal and pictorial stimuli. This supports the Vandenberghe et al. (1996) notion of a common semantic storage system for pictorial and word inputs. The application of multidimensional scaling techniques to produce spatial models of semantic structure is also finding evidence that the organization of semantic information is subtly deranged in AD patients.

This subtle derangement may be relevant to what has been found with AD patients' ability to show information-specific implicit memory for semantic information. If storage of such information has been completely destroyed, then subjects should be unable to show either aware (explicit) or unaware (implicit) memory for the longer stored information provided one accepts the reasonable assumption that information is stored only once and in one system of neurons. If, however, the store is only partially damaged, then whether information-specific implicit memory is impaired will very much depend on one's theoretical assumptions. This can be illustrated by an example. If the organization of semantic memory is subtly deranged, then concepts that were previously distinguishable in terms of their detailed features may become harder or impossible to discriminate. This will impair explicit semantic memory for the concepts, but may even improve performance on certain semantic priming tasks as has sometimes been reported in AD patients (Chertkow et al. 1994). Improvement may occur because semantic priming is weaker than repetition priming and the effect of semantic related concepts becoming more similar to each other is to make the first kind of priming more like the second. If information-specific implicit memory tasks can be made to depend on retrieving more complex semantic information, which closely matches that retrieved by explicit memory, then deficits are more likely to be seen in AD and semantic dementia patients.

In the first section, it was suggested that very long-term storage of both facts and events probably depends on association neocortex structures whereas shorter term storage depends more on the medial temporal lobe structures, such as the hippocampus, which are damaged in organic amnesia. Ironically, some of the best evidence for this view has emerged from study of patients with *semantic* dementia. These patients, who typically have bilateral or predominantly left-sided atrophy of the inferolateral temporal cortex, were originally regarded as having deficits in semantic memory in the face of relative preservation of most of their other cognitive abilities. They may have relatively good preservation of their memory for recent personal episodes, particularly if these episodes do not relate to semantic knowledge which the patient has lost. Interestingly, the patients do not usually seem to be more than mildly impaired at remembering episodes involving semantic knowledge that they have lost (for a discussion, see Graham and Hodges 1997), although this issue needs much more extensive investigation before the degree of preservation can be confidently characterized.

In contrast to patients with semantic dementia, patients with medial temporal lobe amnesia were often regarded as having a problem with episodic memory. This view of

amnesia cannot be correct, however, because amnesics are very impaired at learning about new facts as well as about new episodes. As has already been stated, Alvarez and Squire (1994) have advanced a view of medial temporal lobe amnesia in which the hippocampus initially stores information critical for the reactivation of fact and event memories that are represented in the neocortex. With time and presumably rehearsal of these memories, they eventually cease to depend on the hippocampus and are stored instead by connections between the representing regions in the association neocortex. As patients with semantic dementia have damage to a cortical region likely to be involved in very long-term storage of facts and episodes, but show relatively little damage to the medial temporal lobe system that, according to Alvarez and Squire, mediates the shorter term storage of facts and episodes, they should show severe and approximately equal deficits in memory for facts and episodes that have been in memory for a long time. Exactly this has been shown by Graham and Hodges (1997). Relative to AD patients, they found that semantic dementia patients have a very severe memory deficit for personal episodes that were experienced many years previously although their ability to acquire new episodes is much less affected. One semantic dementia patient, given the Galton–Crovitz test, showed relatively preserved recall of personal episodes experienced in the last 5 years, but not from further in the past. His recall from the past one and one-half years seemed to be the most detailed and normal. If these findings are correct, then semantic dementia is not really semantic at all, but a dementia that primarily affects memory storage of facts and personally experienced episodes that have been in the memory sufficiently long for storage to have been transferred to the association neocortex.

The above findings are important and clearly need to be replicated. They also raise three issues. The first issue concerns the view that young fact and episode memories depend on the hippocampus whereas older memories of these kinds depend on the kinds of association neocortex regions identified by the neuroimaging study of Vandenberghe et al. (1996). Underlying the view is the concept that complex memories involve components that are represented in several neocortical regions and that originally the components are bound together at the level of the hippocampus, but that with time and rehearsal, they are eventually bound together at neocortical level.

McClelland et al. (1995) argued that the neocortical system uses an interleaved learning strategy where the contents of remembered episodes can be compared with the contents of current episodes so as to extract common features. This sounds like a system for acquiring particular kinds of semantic memory slowly, but it seems that it also allows episodic memories to become dependent on the neocortex because McClelland and Goddard (1996) talk about childhood episodic memories no longer being hippocampally dependent in old people. It remains to be shown conclusively that this is true and that the neocortex stores old personally experienced episodes in much the same way that it stores facts even if these facts have been abstracted from many episodes.

The second issue relates to the ability of patients with semantic dementia to learn new episodes relatively normally. If memory for these episodes initially depends on the hippocampus somehow reactivating representations of components of the episodes in the distributed regions of the neocortex, it is not clear how even young episodic memories can be relatively normal in semantic dementia patients. The reason is, of course, that some of the cortical representing regions will be damaged in this dementia because this is the reason why similar episodes, experienced in the remote past, are not stored effectively. The model needs to be developed to explain how younger episodic memories can be preserved when similar older episodic memories are impaired. One possible reason is that the links between different cortical regions that are hypothesized to underlie old memories may be more susceptible to cortical damage than are the links between the hippocampus and the cortical regions that are hypothesized to underlie young memories.

The third issue is a puzzle about why semantic dementia patients are so little impaired at remembering episodes that seem to depend on semantic information that they have no longer. There is very good evidence that recall and recognition in normal people is quite strongly affected by whether or not they encode new inputs semantically (Craik and Tulving 1975). One would, therefore, expect patients who cannot engage in such semantic processing to show episodic memory deficits. Clearly, more research needs to be done on the new learning abilities of semantic dementia patients to resolve this tension convincingly.

NONDECLARATIVE MEMORY IN DEMENTIA

Nondeclarative or implicit forms of memory are heterogeneous and hence mediated by different brain structures. It is, therefore, likely that information-specific implicit memory for perceptual and semantic information will be particularly disrupted by dementias, such as AD and semantic dementia, that affect the posterior association cortices (and the left inferior frontal gyrus according to Vandenberghe et al. 1996). Skill memory will be particularly disrupted by dementias, like HD, which affect the basal ganglia and motoric classical conditioning will be particularly disrupted by dementias that affect the cerebellum. The data that Salmon and his colleagues review basically confirms these likelihoods with respect to the brain regions that mediate information-specific implicit memory, skill memory and motoric conditioning.

Not only is motoric classical conditioning of the eye blink reflex impaired after cerebellar lesions in animals (Thompson 1991), but subsequent work showed this to be true in humans as well (Lye et al. 1988). It was not, therefore, surprising to find that this form of conditioning was not only impaired in patients with olivopontocerebellar atrophy, but also in patients with idiopathic cerebellar ataxia who had selective cerebellar cortical atrophy (Daum et al. 1993a). Interestingly, Daum and her colleagues found that although patients with selective cerebellar atrophy were impaired at the learning of motoric classical conditioning, they acquired autonomic conditioned responses normally as they did slow cortical potentials so that both these responses occurred between the tone conditioned stimulus and the airpuff unconditioned stimulus. Daum and her colleagues argued that the motoric conditioning deficit could not have resulted from the timing disturbances, known to be produced by cerebellar lesions, as the patients' deficient rate of conditioned response production remained even when slow conditioned responses were included. Their results were also consistent with the possibility that autonomic (or fear) conditioning is not mediated by the cerebellum, but in other brain regions (such as the amygdala). If this is so, then classical conditioning of different kinds of responses must be mediated by different brain regions and classical conditioning of autonomic responses might be impaired in AD, although patients with AD should show preserved classical conditioning of motor responses.

Salmon and his colleagues argue that both lesion and neuroimaging evidence suggests that the basal ganglia constitute the storage region for skills, particularly motor skills. In keeping with this, there is good evidence that HD disrupts motor skill acquisition whereas patients with AD develop and retain motor skills normally. Perceptual and cognitive skill acquisition has been less examined, although HD patients have been shown to be worse at learning to read mirror-reversed words (Martone et al. 1984) and at learning to solve the Tower of Hanoi puzzle (Butters et al. 1985). Although the cerebellum may be involved in motor skill acquisition, Daum et al.'s (1993b) results indicate that, when degeneration is confined to the cerebellum, learning to read mirror-reversed text or to solve the Tower of Hanoi puzzle is not impaired.

There is some direct evidence that information-specific implicit memory depends on storage processes in the neocortical regions likely to be involved in representing the information that is being remembered. For example, Keane et al. (1995) found that a patient with damage focused primarily on the right posterior neocortex was impaired at certain visual perceptual repetition priming tasks, but performed normally on semantic priming tasks and on recognition of visually presented words. This suggests that patients in the relatively early stages of AD should have preserved information-specific implicit memory for visual items, which are represented in fairly posterior visual association areas that are unaffected until late in the disease's progression. In contrast, AD patients, early in the course of the disease, should be impaired at information-specific implicit memory for semantic information as this is likely to be represented in more anterior association cortex, particularly the regions identified by Vandenberghe et al.'s (1996) neuroimaging study, which are usually affected early in AD. The evidence that Salmon and his colleagues review is consistent with the view that perceptual priming is preserved in AD. They also conclude on the balance of the evidence that AD leads to abnormal priming of semantic information. In contrast, HD patients show preserved priming on for both perceptual and conceptual information despite their explicit memory deficits for facts and episodes, which is consistent with their illness only minimally affecting posterior association neocortex.

Several comments are warranted about the evidence. First, it needs to be proved that the semantic hyperpriming, that some researchers have observed, with short-term naming or lexical procedures is caused by a degradation of the semantic store causing associative priming to become more like repetition priming. Second, if priming is preserved because the representing neocortical region is relatively unaffected by the dementing process, then information-specific implicit memory should also be preserved for priming of novel information of the same kind. This possibility remains to be systematically tested although Postle et al. (1996) have reported that AD patients showed priming of a form of novel pattern priming. The authors argued that the patterns should be represented in the peristriate cortex, which should be relatively preserved in AD patients. Third, comparison of AD patients' and normal subjects' performances on most repetition priming tasks is not straightforward as baseline performance is usually markedly inferior in patients. Ideally, some attempt should be made to manipulate normal subjects' performance so that their baseline levels correspond to those of AD patients in order to see whether their perceptual priming performance still remains matched to that of the patients.

A fourth comment relates to stem completion priming at which AD patients have sometimes been found to be normal and sometimes impaired. Keane et al. (1991) as well as others believe that this form of priming involves unaware memory for both perceptual and semantic features. The key point to note about stem completion priming is that not all studies have reported an impairment in AD and those that do typically find some priming rather than none at all (for a review, see Downes et al. 1996). Salmon and his colleagues argue that the patients only show normal stem completion priming when they are required to attend to the semantic features of the words. In contrast, Downes et al., who analysed 21 studies, 11 of which found stem completion priming deficits in AD patients, argued that the key requirement for obtaining preserved priming was that subjects should read aloud the target words during study. The presence or absence of this encoding requirement correctly classified 85% of the studies analysed whereas semantic encoding was found to be similar in studies finding deficits and studies finding preserved priming. To test whether the conclusion of their analysis was correct, these researchers compared the effects of two encoding conditions on stem completion performance in a group of AD patients. In one condition, subjects made a pleasantness judgement and, in the other, they read the words aloud. In the pleasantness judgement condition, the patients were impaired whereas, in the word reading condition, they showed preserved priming. Broadly similar results were found in a recent study by Fleischman et al. (1997) in which AD patients showed normal stem completion priming not only when they read words at study, but also when they said them after generating them from definitions. As stem completion priming was greater following the nonsemantic encoding condition it is difficult to see how this form of priming depends appreciably on semantic memory.

Contrary to the view that stem completion priming is partially a semantic task, Downes and his colleagues argued that, unlike other visual priming tasks, it is phonologically driven because it depends on derived phonology in the lexical selection process. Support for this argument derives from the demonstration that both normal subjects and AD patients show an indirect form of stem completion priming, called cohort priming, when they read words aloud at study. Cohort priming is the increased likelihood that, for nontarget completions, there is overlap with the initial stem phonology of target words. When words were not spoken aloud at study, then AD patients were markedly impaired at cohort as well as stem completion priming. Even though AD patients probably suffer an impairment in lexical semantics, this does not explain why getting patients to articulate target words generally produces normal levels of stem completion whereas not doing so produces a stem completion priming deficit. Patients with AD do have phonological processing deficits (Biassou et al. 1995), but the precise nature of the phonological processing deficit that sometimes causes problems with this kind of priming still needs to be characterized.

CONCLUSIONS

As was indicated in the Introduction to this chapter, memory is primarily mediated by the brain regions that represent the stored information so that dementing conditions cause breakdowns in those forms of memory where the stored information is represented in brain regions that are affected by the illness. As the deficits are progressive, the impairments should worsen as the dementia advances.

There is one qualification to this summary statement and one research implication that should be drawn from it. The qualification is that, at least for explicit memory for episodes and facts, a region other than the storage site seems to be involved in memory performance such that damage to this region will impair episodic and semantic memory. This is the frontal region, which is probably the critical brain area concerned with active search without which access to stored facts and episodes would be a great deal worse. One would, therefore, predict that those dementias that affect the frontal association neocortex are likely to disrupt active search processes, depending on which frontal regions are affected. In order to pursue research on this issue, it will be necessary to develop good measures of the effectiveness of active search and to relate these to precisely which frontal regions are not working properly as ascertained by neuroimaging studies.

The research implication is that it is critically important to analyse memory tasks correctly, not only with respect to what underlying processes (such as active search) performance depends upon, but also what kinds of information are being retrieved. This is not as obvious as it may seem as the example of stem completion priming in the last section should make plain. The importance of being correct is obvious if memories are stored where the stored information is represented during encoding. It should also be emphasized that although we have reasonable knowledge of where different kinds of information are represented, this knowledge is still far from precise and needs to be improved by future lesion and neuroimaging studies. For example, how good is the evidence that motor skills are stored only in basal ganglia structures and, even if this is true, exactly which basal ganglia structures are involved?

Despite the above caveat, it can be said with some confidence that if a dementing patient has a clear deficit in a particular kind of memory, this generally gives a good indication of the location of the brain structures that the dementing process is affecting. Future work will increase the precision of this knowledge and will be able to check it more precisely through the use of functional as well as structural neuroimaging methods.

REFERENCES

Aggleton, J.P. and Shaw, C. 1996. Amnesia and recognition memory: A re-analysis of psychometric data. *Neuropsychologia*. 34: 51–62.

Alvarez, R. and Squire, L.R. 1994. Memory consolidation and the medial temporal lobe: A simple network model. *Proceedings of the National Academy of Sciences (USA)*. 91: 7041–7045.

Baddeley, A. 1986. *Working memory*. Oxford: Clarendon Press.

Baddeley, A.D., Papagno, C. and Vallar, G. 1988. When long-term learning depends on short-term storage. *Journal of Memory and Language*. 27: 586–595.

Biassou, N., Grossman, M., Onishi, K., Mickanin, J., Hughes, E., Robinson, K.M. and D'Esposito, M. 1995. Phonological processing deficits in Alzheimer's disease. *Neurology*. 45: 2165–2169.

Brandimonte, M., Einstein, G.O. and McDaniel, M.A. 1996. *Prospective memory: Theory and applications*. Mahwah, NJ: Lawrence Erlbaum Associates.

Butters, N., Wolfe, J., Martone, M., Granholm, E. and Cermak, L.S. 1985. Memory disorders associated with Huntington's disease: Verbal recall, verbal recognition and procedural memory. *Neuropsychologia*. 6: 729–744.

Chawluk, J.B., Grossman, M., Calcano-Perez, J.A., Alavi, A., Hurtig, H.I. and Reivich, M. 1990. Positron emission tomographic studies of cerebral metabolism in Alzheimer's disease. In *Modular deficits in Alzheimer-type dementia*, ed. M.F. Schwartz, pp. 101–141. Cambridge: MIT Press.

Chertkow, H., Bub, D., Bergman, H., Bruemmer, A., Merling, A. and Rothfleisch, J. 1994. Increased semantic priming in patients with dementia of the Alzheimer's type. *Journal of Clinical and Experimental Neuropsychology*. 16: 608–622.

Craik, F.I.M. and Tulving, E. 1975. Depth of processing and the retention of words in episodic memory. *Journal of Experimental Psychology (General)*. 104: 268–294.

Daum, I., Ackerman, H., Schugens, M.M., Reimold, C., Dichgans, J. and Birnbaumer, N. 1993b. The cerebellum and cognitive functions in humans. *Behavioral Neuroscience*. 107: 411–419.

Daum, I., Schugens, M.M., Ackerman, H., Lutzerberger, W., Dichgans, J. and Birnbaumer, N. 1993a. Classical conditioning after cerebellar lesions in humans. *Behavioral Neuroscience*. 107: 748–756.

Downes, J.J., Davis, E.J., De Mornay Davies, P., Perfect, T.J., Wilson, K., Mayes, A.R. and Sagar, H.J. 1996. Stem-completion priming in Alzheimer's disease: The importance of target word articulation. *Neuropsychologia*. 34: 63–75.

Fleischman, D.A., Gabrielli, J.D.E., Rinaldi, J.A., Reminger, S.L., Grinnell, E.R., Lange, K.L. and Shapiro, R. 1997. Word-stem completion priming for perceptually and conceptually encoded words in patients with Alzheimer's disease. *Neuropsychologia*. 35: 25–35.

Goldman-Rakic, P.S. 1990. Cellular and circuit basis of working memory in prefrontal cortex of nonhuman primates. In *Progress in Brain Research*, vol. 85, ed. H.B.M. Uylings, C.G. Van Eden, J.P.C. De Bruin, M.A. Corner and M.G.P. Feenstra, pp. 325–336. Amsterdam: Elsevier Science Publishers (Biomedical Division).

Graham, K.S. and Hodges, J.R. 1997. Differentiating the roles of the hippocampal system and the neocortex in long-term memory storage. *Neuropsychology*. 11: 77–89.

Huppert, F.A. and Beardsall, L. 1993. Prospective memory impairment as an early indicator of dementia. *Journal of Clinical and Experimental Neuropsychology*. 15: 805–821.

Keane, M.M., Gabrieli, J.D.E., Fennema, A.C., Growdon, J.H. and Corkin, S. 1991. Evidence for a dissociation between perceptual and conceptual priming in Alzheimer's disease. *Behavioral Neuroscience*. 105: 326–342.

Keane, M.M., Gabrieli, J.D.E., Mapstone, H.C., Johnston, K.A. and Corkin, S. 1995. Double dissociation of memory capacities after bilateral occipital-lobe or medial temporal-lobe lesions. *Brain*. 118: 1129–1148.

Lye, R.H., O'Boyle, D.J., Ramsden, R.T. and Schady, W. 1988. Effects of a unilateral cerebellar lesion on the acquisition of eyeblink conditioning in man. *Journal of Physiology*. 403: 58.

Martone, M, Butters, N., Payne, M., Becker, J. and Sax, D. 1984. Dissociations between skill learning and verbal recognition in amnesia and dementia. *Archives of Neurology*. 41: 965–970.

Mayes, A.R. 1988. *Human organic memory disorders*. Cambridge: Cambridge University Press.

Mayes, A.R. and Daum, I. 1997. How specific are the memory and other cognitive deficits caused by frontal lobe lesions? In *Methodology of frontal and executive function*, ed. P. Rabbitt. Hove, UK: Lawrence Erlbaum Associates.

McCarthy, R.A. and Warrington, E.K. 1990. *Cognitive neuropsychology*. London: Academic Press.

McClelland, J.L. and Goddard, N.H. 1996. Considerations arising from a complementary learning systems perspective on hippocampus and neocortex. *Hippocampus*. 6: 654–665.

McClelland, J.L., McNaughton, B.L. and O'Reilly, R.C. 1995. Why there are complementary learning systems in the hippocampus and neocortex: Insights from the successes and failures of connectionist models of learning and memory. *Psychological Review*. 102: 419–457.

McGaugh, J.L., Bermudez-Rattoni, F. and Prado-Alcala, R.A. 1995. *Plasticity in the central nervous system: Learning and memory*. Mahwah, NJ: Lawrence Erlbaum Associates.

Milner, B. 1971. Interhemispheric differences in the localization of psychological processes in man. *British Medical Bulletin*. 27: 272–277.

Postle, B.R., Corkin, S. and Growdon, J.H. 1996. Intact implicit memory for novel patterns in Alzheimer's disease. *Learning and Memory*. 3: 305–312.

Sahgal, A., McKeith, I.G., Galloway, P.H., Tasker, N. and Steckler, T. 1995. Do differences in visuospatial ability between senile dementias of the Alzheimer and Lewy body types reflect differences solely in mnemonic function? *Journal of Clinical and Experimental Neuropsychology*. 17: 35–43.

Shallice, T. 1988. *From neuropsychology to mental structure*. Cambridge: Cambridge University Press.

Thompson, R.F. 1991. Are memory traces localized or distributed? *Neuropsychologia*. 29: 571–582.

Ungerleider, L.G. 1995. Functional brain imaging studies of cortical mechanisms of memory. *Science*. 270: 769–775.

Vallar, G. and Papagno, C. 1995. Neuropsychological impairments of short-term memory. In *Handbook of memory disorders*, ed. A.D. Baddeley, B. Wilson and F.N. Watts, pp. 135–166. Chichester: Wiley and Sons.

Vandenberghe, R., Price, C., Wise, R., Josephs, O. and Frackowiak, R.S.J. 1996. Functional anatomy of a common semantic system for words and pictures. *Nature*. 383: 254–256.

PART III

Clinical perspectives

14 Biological and psychosocial risk factors for dementia and memory loss

DIANE M. JACOBS AND PETER SCHOFIELD

INTRODUCTION

The process of identifying risk factors for dementia is a long one, that typically begins with an astute clinician who observes that a given factor or agent seems to be associated with a specific disorder. These initial observations often are followed by case-control studies, in which patients with the disease of interest are compared with healthy control subjects to determine whether or not the suspected risk factors are more frequent among those with the disease than those without. While clinical observations and case-control studies provide important clues about potential risk factors, limitations inherent in these methods (e.g. selection bias) restrict conclusions about risk factors that can be drawn from them. Large-scale, population- or community-based epidemiological investigations can control for some of the limitations associated with clinical research and can more definitively assess potential risk factors.

In recent years, there have been a number of community-based epidemiological studies of dementia and associated risk factors. In this chapter, we review studies of the incidence and prevalence of dementia associated with various disorders. Prevalence represents the total number of cases of a disease in a defined population at a given time; incidence represents the number of people in a defined population who *develop* a disease in a given time period. The prevalence of a disease in a population is the function of both the incidence rate and the duration of the disease. As a result, incidence and prevalence rates do not necessarily go hand in hand: a disease with low incidence but long duration may have high prevalence, while a disease with high incidence but short duration could have low prevalence; therefore, incidence, but not prevalence, can provide a direct measure of the risk or probability of developing a disease – in this case, dementia.

We describe biological and psychosocial risk factors for dementia and memory loss associated with Alzheimer's (AD), Parkinson's (PD) and Huntington's disease (HD), vascular dementia and AIDS. Memory loss and dementia are, of course, the defining features of AD. For the other diseases, our discussion focuses on risk factors associated with dementia among patients with these conditions rather than on risk factors for the disorders, as these have been described elsewhere. Although not a ubiquitous feature, the risk of dementia in patients with PD is far greater than that among age-matched controls (Rajput et al. 1987; Mayeux et al. 1990; Marder et al. 1993). Dementia is an inevitable feature of HD; however, the onset and course of cognitive impairment do vary from patient to patient and this heterogeneity is in part a function of biological and psychosocial risk. Patients with a history of stroke are at significantly greater risk for dementia than their stroke-free peers (Tatemichi et al. 1993). Stroke characteristics associated with increased dementia risk include left-side or bilateral infarcts, recurrent stroke and the presence of white matter lesions; medical risk factors for vascular dementia among patients with stroke include hypertension, history of myocardial infarction and diabetes mellitus (Skoog 1994). In addition, psychosocial factors mediate risk of dementia associated with cerebrovascular disease and stroke. Similarly, while medical factors are strongly associated with risk for AIDS-associated dementia (e.g. low hemoglobin and body mass index, more constitutional symptoms prior to AIDS diagnosis) (McArthur et al. 1993), psychosocial factors also mediate dementia risk.

EMPIRICAL FINDINGS

Age

Age is a major risk factor for all types of dementia and advancing age is the single most important risk factor for

AD. The prevalence of AD rises exponentially with age, doubling approximately every 5 years, at least up to age 90 years (Jorm 1990). Approximately 2% of the population between ages 65 and 69 years is affected, with prevalence estimates rising to over 20% of individuals age 85–90 years. Age-specific incidence rates, which are less affected by survivor bias than prevalence rates, also appear to increase exponentially. For example, the incidence of AD rose steeply in the Bronx Aging Study from 1.3 per 100 per year in 75–79 year-olds to 3.5 per 100 per year in 80–84-year-olds and 6.0 per 100 per year among subjects 85 years and older (Aronson et al. 1991). Although this exponential rise in incidence with advancing age is remarkably consistent across studies, specific incidence rates vary widely, in part due to differences across studies in the criteria used to diagnose incident cases. Prevalence and incidence data on individuals over age 90 years are not sufficient to determine whether the exponential trends continue. Some investigators have suggested that the incidence may begin to level off in the very old (Mortimer et al. 1981).

Among patients with PD, later age at onset of motor manifestations is associated with a significantly increased risk of dementia (Lieberman et al. 1979; Mayeux et al. 1992; Stern et al. 1993; Marder et al. 1995). From a population-based registry of PD, Mayeux et al. (1992) estimated that the prevalence of PD with dementia increased with age from zero for patients younger than 50 to 787.1 per 100 000 for those aged 80 years and older. In a prospective cohort study, Stern et al. (1993) found that PD patients over 70 years of age had nearly three times the risk of incident dementia compared to PD patients less than 70 years.

The association between age and dementia in HD is the inverse of the other dementias: the juvenile onset form is associated with severe and rapidly progressive dementia, whereas cognitive dysfunction is relatively mild and slowly progressive in patients with onset of motor symptoms after age 50 years (Bird 1978). The dementia associated with midlife onset of HD, the most frequent presentation, is intermediate between the juvenile and late onset in terms of severity and rapidity of course.

In addition to being a risk factor for stroke, age is a risk factor for dementia among stroke patients (Tatemichi et al. 1992a, 1993). Tatemichi et al. (1993) examined 251 patients 3 months after the onset of acute ischemic stroke. Dementia was present in 26.3% of patients. Age significantly increased the risk of dementia, even after controlling for other demographic and stroke-related factors.

Compared with patients aged 60–69 years, stroke patients over 80 years of age had a sixfold increased risk of vascular dementia and a 14-fold increased risk of mixed dementia (i.e. coincident AD and vascular dementia); patients aged 70–79 years had a twofold increased risk of vascular dementia and a threefold increased risk of mixed dementia.

There is some evidence that increasing age is a risk factor for dementia associated with human immunodeficiency virus (HIV–1) Associated Dementia Complex. McArthur et al. (1993) found that the risk of dementia among AIDS patients in the Multicenter AIDS Cohort Study was higher among patients who were older at AIDS onset. Comparisons of HIV-seropositive (symptomatic and asymptomatic) and seronegative control subjects in the Multicenter AIDS Cohort Study, however, yielded no significant interaction between age and serostatus (van Gorp et al. 1994). In an investigation of AIDS cases reported to the Centers for Disease Control, the prevalence of HIV encephalopathy among patients with AIDS was highest among the very young and the very old: HIV encephalopathy was present in 13% of AIDS patients less that 15 years old; in AIDS patients more than 15 years old, the proportion with HIV encephalopathy progressively increased with age from 6% in persons 15–34 years old to 19% in individuals over age 75 years (Janssen et al. 1992). This study did not, however, include formal measures of cognitive function. Further investigation is needed to definitively determine whether or not increasing age is associated with greater risk for dementia in HIV–1 infection and AIDS.

Education

There have been numerous investigations of educational attainment as a risk factor for dementia in AD. Several population-based investigations of the prevalence of AD have reported higher rates of AD among individuals with fewer years of education (Sulkava et al. 1985; Zhang et al. 1990; Korczyn et al. 1991). The results of recent incidence studies, however, have been conflicting. In a community-based cohort in North Manhattan, New York, subjects with less that 8 years of education were at significantly greater risk for incident AD during the 4 years of follow-up than subjects with 8 or more years of education (Stern et al. 1994). In contrast, the incidence of AD in the Framingham Study (Cobb et al. 1995) and Mayo Clinic Rochester Epidemiology Project (Beard et al. 1992) was not affected by educational attainment. Differences between these studies in the range of education in the populations studied and in the methods used to assess cognition and diagnose dementia, may have contributed to their disparate results.

Education generally has not been associated with risk of dementia among patients with PD (Jacobs et al. 1995; Marder et al. 1995), although borderline associations have been reported (Salganik and Korczyn 1990). In their prospective cohort study of community-dwelling patients with PD, Marder et al. (1995) found that while level of education did not contribute significantly to the prediction of incident dementia, subjects who developed dementia during the 3.5 year follow-up period had an average of two fewer years of formal education than subjects who remained nondemented.

Low educational attainment has been associated with significantly increased risk of vascular dementia (Gorelick et al. 1992; Tatemichi et al. 1992a, 1993; Mortel et al. 1995). In a case-control study of dementia following stroke, education was significantly and independently associated with dementia, even after controlling for age, race and stroke risk factors (Tatemichi et al. 1993). Relative to patients who had completed some education beyond high school, patients who had less that 9 years of schooling had a fourfold increased risk of dementia and those completing between nine and 12 years of schooling had over a twofold increased risk.

Data from the Multicenter AIDS Cohort study suggest that education is not a significant, independent risk factor for dementia among patients with AIDS (McArthur et al. 1993), although low education was associated with increased risk for cognitive abnormalities in asymptomatic HIV-1 infected subjects (Satz et al. 1993). The prevalence of cognitive abnormality in seropositive subjects with 12 or fewer years of education was 38%, compared to less than 17% in the other education-serostatus groups.

In summary, many studies suggest that educational attainment is inversely associated with dementia risk, i.e. low educational attainment is a risk factor for dementia. One methodological concern of studies investigating the influence of education on dementia is the potential for detection bias: poorly educated individuals are less accomplished at test taking and are therefore more likely to perform poorly on the kinds of cognitive tests that are used to diagnose dementia. Detection bias is particularly a problem for prevalence studies because the effects of pre-

morbid cognitive functioning and disease status cannot be disentangled. Incidence studies address the problem somewhat because, by definition, incident cases must score in the normal range at the baseline study visit and only subsequently score in the demented range. Nevertheless, the possibility remains that because persons with limited education generally obtain lower scores on formal measures of cognition, they are closer to 'failing' the cognitive evaluation at any study visit.

Occupation

Occupational attainment is a significant predictor of incident AD, independent of its association with education; individuals with low educational and low occupational attainment, however, have a further increased risk of AD (Stern et al. 1994). Stern et al. (1994) followed a cohort of nondemented elders for 1–4 years. At the initial visit, each subject's primary occupation was classified according to the US census categories. Based upon these categories, subjects were grouped into low (unskilled/semiskilled, skilled trade or craft and clerical/office worker) and high (manager business/government and professional/technical) occupational levels. Subjects with lower occupational attainment were at more than twice the risk of incident AD. The increased risk for subjects with low educational and occupational attainment approached threefold.

Several studies have shown that occupational attainment may influence dementia following stroke (Tatemichi et al. 1993; Mortel et al. 1995). Tatemichi et al. (1993) reported a higher percentage of unskilled laborers in the group of subjects with dementia following stroke compared to stroke patients without dementia. Occupation, however, was not a significant independent correlate of dementia when other demographic and clinical characteristics were included in the predictor model.

Gender

The relationship between gender and risk for AD is unclear. Several prevalence studies have found a higher rate of AD among women (Sulkava et al. 1985; Rocca et al. 1990; Zhang et al. 1990). There is also evidence, however, that men with AD may be at disproportionate risk for death compared to female cases and that the apparently higher prevalence of AD among women may simply reflect this differential mortality (Perls et al. 1993; Corder et al. 1995). Incidence studies of AD avoid the potential problem of differential mortality and most – but not all – incidence studies of AD have found no difference in the risk of AD by gender (Letenneur et al. 1994; Paykel et al. 1994; Schoenberg et al. 1987; Katzman et al. 1989; Li et al. 1991). Aronson et al. (1991) reported higher incidence rates of dementia in women up to the age of 84 years, after which the incidence was slightly higher in men.

PD is more prevalent in men than in women (Mayeux et al. 1992), but gender generally has not been associated with an increased risk for dementia or cognitive impairment among PD patients (Ebmeier et al. 1990; Jacobs et al. 1995; Marder et al. 1995).

Risk factors for vascular dementia generally are the same as those for stroke (Skoog 1994). Therefore, sex differences in risk for vascular dementia largely reflect group differences in stroke risk factors. Population-based prevalence studies generally have found that vascular dementia is more common in men (Sulkava et al. 1985; Hasegawa et al. 1986; Rocca et al. 1990, 1991); however, there are some indications that this difference diminishes with increasing age and that there may be a female preponderance in the oldest age groups (Molsa et al. 1982; Aronson et al. 1990; Rocca et al. 1991; Skoog et al. 1993). Nevertheless, among stroke patients, gender does not appear to be associated with dementia risk (Tatemichi et al. 1992a, 1993).

Ethnicity

Limited data are available on race or ethnicity as potential risk factors for dementia and memory loss. Community-based incidence studies of AD and dementia in the USA, western Europe, Japan and China have yielded similar age-specific incidence rates up to age 75 years, after which there is considerable divergence (van Duijn 1996). This divergence in results may in part be due to differences between studies in terms of diagnostic criteria, competing mortality and comorbidity. There is some suggestion that the etiology of dementia may vary cross-nationally, with AD being the most common cause of dementia in Caucasian populations from the USA and Europe and vascular dementia predominating in Asian populations (Jorm 1991). Several biracial investigations in the USA have reported a higher prevalence of dementia in African-Americans than in white people (Schoenberg et al. 1985; Heyman et al. 1991); it may be that the higher prevalence of dementia in African-Americans was associated with an increased risk of vascular dementia due to the higher prevalence of hypertension and stroke in this group. In

their cohort of stroke patients, Tatemichi et al. (1993) did find a significantly increased risk of vascular dementia in African-American and Hispanic patients as compared to white subjects.

Family history of dementia and genetic risk factors

There have been major advances in our understanding of the genetics of AD in the past 5 years (Chapter 18). It is now clear that AD is a genetically heterogeneous condition: genes on four different chromosomes have been implicated in familial AD (St.George-Hyslop et al. 1987, 1992; Pericak-Vance et al. 1991; Levy-Lahad et al. 1995). In recent years, there have been numerous reports of an association between the apolipoprotein E (APOE) gene on chromosome 19 and AD. The three common alleles of APOE, designated APOE $\varepsilon2$, $\varepsilon3$ and $\varepsilon4$, occur in approximately 7%, 78% and 14% of chromosomes, respectively, although these estimates vary according to the ethnic/racial background and age of the population (Strittmatter and Roses 1995). Strittmatter et al. (1993) showed an association between APOE $\varepsilon4$ and late onset familial AD. A subsequent report showed that there was also a strong association between sporadic late onset AD and APOE $\varepsilon4$ (Saunders et al. 1993). A gene dose effect of APOE $\varepsilon4$ has been shown, such that homozygotes are at risk of AD at an earlier age (Corder et al. 1993). The presence of APOE $\varepsilon2$, by contrast, has been shown to be protective for AD in some studies using prevalent cases; however, others have found increased risk of AD with APOE $\varepsilon2$ and reduced survival of AD subjects with APOE $\varepsilon2$, suggesting that survival bias may account for these findings (van Duijn et al. 1995). The process by which APOE affects disease expression in AD is unknown; however, evidence of isoform-specific associations of APOE with neurofibrillary tangles and senile plaques, the pathological hallmarks of AD, suggest two potential mechanisms. Specifically, APOE $\varepsilon4$ is associated with increased amyloid beta-peptide deposition in senile plaques (Schmechel et al. 1993) and with an increased rate of formation of neurofibrillary tangles (Strittmatter et al. 1994).

Numerous reports have supported the association between APOE $\varepsilon4$ and the increased risk of AD; however, the predictive value of APOE genotyping as a screening test is limited: about one-half of AD patients do not have the $\varepsilon4$ allele and many APOE $\varepsilon4$ carriers do not develop dementia (Myers et al. 1996). Further, the association of

APOE ε4 and dementia is not specific for AD. APOE ε4 has been associated with an increased risk of non-AD dementias as well, including vascular dementia (Frisoni et al. 1994; Isoe et al. 1996; Myers et al. 1996) and diffuse Lewy body disease (Arai et al. 1994; Benjamin et al. 1994; Pickering-Brown et al. 1994). APOE genotype does not, however, appear to be associated with dementia in PD, suggesting that the biological basis for dementia in PD and AD differ (Benjamin et al. 1994; Marder et al. 1994; Koller et al. 1995).

A family history of dementia is associated with an increased risk of dementia among patients with PD (Marder et al. 1990) and familial aggregation of AD and PD has been reported (Hofman et al. 1989). Marder et al. (1990) administered a structured risk-factor interview to surrogates of 17 demented PD patients and 54 nondemented patients. Family history of PD was not associated with an increased risk of dementia; however, PD patients with a family history of dementia had an over sixfold increased risk of dementia. A family history of dementia was present in 30% of the demented group and 5.6% of the nondemented group. Significant family history was most often reported among siblings. At present it is unclear whether the familial clustering of AD and PD reflects a shared genetic influence or common environmental exposures. Recent evidence of an association of CYP2D6B, a genetic mutation associated with increased risk of PD (Smith et al. 1992), to the Lewy body variant of AD (Saitoh et al. 1995) and synaptic pathology in AD (Chen et al. 1995) support a common genetic origin of these disorders. The CYP2D6 gene encodes an enzyme, debrisoquine 4-hydroxylase, that is involved in detoxifying environmental toxins and the mutant B allele is associated with reduced levels of the active enzyme in brain. These findings suggest that both genetic and environmental factors are involved in the etiology of these diseases.

The rate of cognitive decline in HD has been associated with the length of the trinucleotide (CAG) repeat expansion in the gene IT–15 on chromosome 4. Brandt et al. (1996) reported that although patients with long versus short repeat lengths did not differ in disease severity at baseline, over a 2-year follow-up period patients with longer repeat lengths experienced significantly greater neurological and cognitive decline. There is a strong inverse correlation between repeat length and age at onset of HD (Ranen et al. 1995; Brandt et al. 1996); this association elucidates the inverse association of age with demen-

tia in HD, described earlier. Juvenile onset HD and genetic anticipation (i.e. earlier disease onset in successive generations within a pedigree) are associated with paternal transmission of the disease gene (Telenius et al. 1993; Ranen et al. 1995).

A family history of dementia has not been associated with an increased risk for dementia among patients with cerebrovascular disease. Although genetic background clearly influences risk factors for cerebrovascular disease and stroke, an independent genetic risk for vascular dementia has not been identified.

Head injury

Evidence of head injury as a risk factor for dementia comes primarily from investigations of AD. The first systematic attempt to determine if a significant association existed between head injury and AD was a case-control study by Mortimer et al. (1983). In that study, a history of head injury with loss of consciousness was nearly five times more common in AD cases than in hospital and community controls. There have been numerous subsequent studies which have examined the association between history of head injury and AD. A collaborative re-analysis of case-control studies found a significant association of head injury with AD, particularly if the trauma occurred within the 10 years preceding dementia onset (Mortimer et al. 1991). One limitation of case-control studies, however, is the potential for recall bias (i.e. the possibility that cases/informants are more likely to recall past exposures that might be relevant or explanatory for the disease of interest than controls because they are more motivated to identify a reason for the disease). Recall bias might therefore lead to an apparent association between the exposure of interest (e.g. head injury) and the disease when no such association really exists. It is notable that two cohort studies, in which recall bias is not a potential problem, failed to find an association between AD and head injury (Katzman et al. 1989; Williams et al. 1991). One recent study suggests that the association between head injury and AD may be modified by APOE genotype: head trauma was associated with an increased risk of AD only in carriers of the APOEε4 allele (Mayeux et al. 1995).

Depression

Although the effects of depression on memory in neurodegenerative disease are discussed in Chapter 19, it is worth noting here that depression has been identified as a risk factor for dementia. Epidemiological evidence from case-control studies suggests that a history of medically treated depression is more common in AD patients than in healthy control subjects (Heyman et al. 1984; Kokmen et al. 1991). A recent prospective, longitudinal investigation found that nondemented elders with depressed mood were nearly three times more likely to become demented over 2.5 years of follow-up (Devanand et al. 1996). Similarly, depression is associated with an approximately threefold increased risk of incident dementia associated with PD (Starkstein et al. 1992; Stern et al. 1993; Marder et al. 1995). Depression may be an early manifestation of dementia in AD and PD, or it may increase susceptibility for dementia through another mechanism. Depression is common in HD, occurring at some time in nearly 40% of patients (Caine and Shoulson 1983), but the influence of depression on the onset or course of dementia in HD is unknown. Depression also is common after stroke (Robinson and Starkstein 1990); however, there does not appear to be a causal link between depression and dementia in stroke patients (Tatemichi et al. 1992b).

IMPLICATIONS

In this chapter we have briefly reviewed the evidence implicating certain patient characteristics (age, education, occupational attainment), biological variables (genetics) and exogenous factors (head injury) as risk factors for dementia. The clinical syndrome of dementia reflects dysfunction of the neural substrates for memory and cognition and may arise in the course of many different diseases. We have considered just a few neurodegenerative diseases, albeit the most common. It is notable, however, that age and education appear as risk factors for dementia associated with most of these diseases, despite profound differences in their underlying pathology. Why might this be so?

Dementia severity has been shown to correlate with the extent of pathological brain changes (Terry et al. 1991), but clinicopathological studies have also clearly indicated that modest amounts of brain pathology are compatible with normal cognition (Tomlinson et al. 1968), which suggests that a threshold of damage must be exceeded before cognitive impairment and dementia arise. These observations have led to the concept of 'brain reserve capacity' implying a structural or functional buffer which mini-

mizes the cognitive consequences of relatively circumscribed brain damage. The concept of brain reserve is useful when considering the roles of aging and perhaps education, as dementia risk factors.

Studies of the aging brain have yielded somewhat conflicting results, but there is general agreement that certain involutional brain changes are a constant. Reduction in brain size (Davis and Wright 1977), reduction in large neurons (Terry et al. 1987) and some loss of synaptic density (Masliah et al. 1993) are typical brain changes which may commence as early as in the fifth decade of life. In the elderly, therefore, brain damage caused by neurological diseases is superimposed upon age-related brain changes which, by lowering cerebral reserve, increase the likely cognitive consequences of an added burden of pathology.

Some authors have suggested that education may increase brain reserve (Katzman 1993). Results from animal investigations of environmental influences on brain morphology have been cited in support of this contention. Studies have demonstrated that trophic brain changes (e.g. increases in cortical mantle thickness, size and branching of synapses, ratio of neuroglia to neurons and volume of dendritic neuropil) occur in rats raised in an 'enriched environment' in which adequate nutrition is supplemented by an 'interesting and stimulating environment' (e.g. Diamond 1988). Similar structural brain changes might be promoted in humans by appropriately stimulating and challenging environments. In fact, autopsy studies of humans who were free of cognitive impairment prior to death indicated an inverse correlation between dendritic complexity and age (Jacobs and Scheibel 1993) and a direct correlation between dendritic complexity and educational attainment (Jacobs et al. 1993).

Support for the brain reserve theory also comes from a number of clinical studies. Although not a study of dementia, a report by Gronwall and Wrightson (1975) is particularly illustrative. These investigators studied cognitive recovery after concussive head injury and found that young adults who had previously sustained a concussion recovered cognitive function more slowly than did control subjects following their first head injury. They concluded, 'concussion produces some persisting change which increases the damage caused by further concussion . . . the most probable explanation of the cumulation of the effects of concussion is that each event destroys neurons, diminishing the reserve available and making the loss evident under the stress of further injury' (Gronwall and Wrightson, 1975). A similar mechanism of summating pathology has been proposed to explain why head injury may be a risk factor for AD: subclinical brain damage due to trauma might lower the reserve causing subsequent, entirely unrelated, AD to become symptomatic earlier in its course.

Of more direct relevance to the issue of cerebral reserve, education and dementia was a brain imaging study of AD patients reported by Stern et al. (1992). These investigators examined the association between education and an index of AD pathology, namely regional cerebral blood flow in the parietal lobe. They found an inverse correlation between years of education and parietal perfusion, suggesting more advanced AD pathology in patients with more years of education, despite comparable clinical severity. In other words, at a given level of clinical impairment, well-educated patients had more pathology than did less educated patients. In a subsequent study, a similar relationship was found between occupational experience and AD pathology: patients whose occupations were associated with higher interpersonal skills and physical demands had less relative perfusion in the parietal region (i.e. greater pathology), even after controlling for age, severity of dementia and education (Stern et al. 1995).

In summary, the fact that psychosocial factors, such as age and education, influence risk for dementia, regardless of the specific underlying disease, suggests that they are important modifiers of the response to the disease process: the brain reserve theory offers an intuitively appealing interpretation for this empirical finding. Other interpretations are clearly possible, however. One concern, discussed in some detail earlier, is that all dementia studies, irrespective of the specific target disease, are subject to educational biases in case detection. This is a methodological issue that has been addressed extensively elsewhere. In the case of AD, the only condition we reviewed in which dementia is the defining characteristic of the disease, low educational attainment might be a proxy for lifestyle or environmental factors more directly implicated in disease causation. Epidemiological studies continue to address these issues.

ACKNOWLEDGMENTS

Support was provided by Federal Grants AG07232, AG08702 and AG07370 and by the Charles S. Robertson Memorial Gift for Alzheimer's Disease Research from the Banbury Fund.

REFERENCES

Arai, H., Higuchi, S., Muramatsu, T., Iwatsubo, T., Sasaki, H. and Trojanowski, J.Q. 1994. Apolipoprotein E gene in diffuse Lewy body disease with or without co-existing Alzheimer's disease. *Lancet*. 344: 1307.

Aronson, M.K., Ooi, W.L., Geva, D.L., Masur, D., Blau, A. and Frishman, W. 1991. Age-dependent incidence, prevalence and mortality in the old old. *Archives of Internal Medicine*. 151: 989–992.

Aronson, M.K., Ooi, W.L., Morgenstern, H., Hafner, A., Masur, D., Crystal, H., Frishman, W.H., Fisher, D. and Katzman, R. 1990. Women, myocardial infarction and dementia in the very old. *Neurology*. 40: 1102–1106.

Beard, C.M., Kokmen, E., Offord, K. and Kurland, L.T. 1992. Lack of association between Alzheimer's disease and education, occupation, marital status or living arrangement. *Neurology*. 42: 2063–2068.

Benjamin, R., Leake, A., Edwardson, J.A., McKeith, I.G., Ince, P.G., Perry, R.H. and Morris, C.M. 1994. Apolipoprotein E genes in Lewy body and Parkinson's disease. *Lancet*. 343: 1565.

Bird, E.D. 1978. The brain in Huntington's chorea. *Psychological Medicine*. 8: 357–360.

Brandt, J., Bylsma, F.W., Gross, R., Stine, O.C., Ranen, N. and Ross, C.A. 1996. Trinucleotide repeat length and clinical progression in Huntington's disease. *Neurology*. 46: 527–531.

Caine, E. and Shoulson, I. 1983. Psychiatric syndromes in Huntington's disease. *American Journal of Psychiatry*. 140: 728–733.

Chen, X., Xia, Y., Alford, M., DeTeresa, R., Hansen, L., Klauber, M.R., Katzman, R., Thal, L., Masliah, E. and Saitoh, T. 1995. The CYP2D6B allele is associated with a milder synaptic pathology in Alzheimer's disease. *Annals of Neurology*. 38: 653–658.

Cobb, J.L., Wolf, P.A., Au, R., White, R. and D'Agostino, R.B. 1995. The effect of education on the incidence of dementia and Alzheimer's disease in the Framingham Study. *Neurology*. 45: 1707–1712.

Corder, E.H., Saunders, A.M., Strittmatter, W.J., Schmechel, D.E., Gaskell Jr., P.C., Rimmler, J.B., Locke, P.A., Conneally, P.M., Schmader, K.E., Tanzi, R.E., Gusella, J.F., Small, G.W., Roses, A.D., Pericak-Vance, M.A. and Haines, J.L. 1995. Apolipoprotein E, survival in Alzheimer's disease patients and the competing risks of death and Alzheimer's disease. *Neurology*. 45: 1323–1328.

Corder, E.H., Saunders, A.M., Strittmatter, W.J., Schmechel, D.E., Gaskell, P.C., Small, G.W., Roses, A.D., Haines, J.L. and Pericak-Vance, M.A. 1993. Gene dose of Apolipo-protein E type 4 allele and the risk of Alzheimer's disease in late onset families. *Science*. 261: 921–923.

Davis, P.J.M. and Wright, E.A. 1977. A new method for measuring cranial cavity volume and its application to the assessment of cerebral atrophy at autopsy. *Neuropathology and Applied Neurobiology*. 3: 341–358.

Devanand, D.P., Sano, M., Tang, M-X., Taylor, S., Gurland, B., Wilder, D., Stern, Y. and Mayeux, R. 1996. Depressed mood and the incidence of Alzheimer's disease in the community elderly. *Archives of General Psychiatry*. 53: 175–182.

Diamond, M.C. 1988. *Enriching heredity: The impact of the environment on the anatomy of the brain*. New York: The Free Press.

Ebmeier, K.P., Calder, S.A., Crawford, J.R., Stewart, L., Besson, J.A.O. and Mutch, W.J. 1990. Clinical features predicting dementia in idiopathic Parkinson's disease: A follow-up study. *Neurology*. 40: 1222–1224.

Frisoni, G.B., Calabresi, L., Geroldi, C., Bianchetti, A., D'Acquarica, A.L., Govoni, S., Sirtori, C.R., Trabucchi, M. and Franceschini, G. 1994. Apolipoprotein E epsilon 4 allele in Alzheimer's disease and vascular dementia. *Dementia*. 5: 240–242.

Gorelick, P.B., Chatterjee, A., Patel, D., Flowerdew, F., Dollear, W., Taber, J. and Harris, Y. 1992. Cranial computed tomographic observations in multi-infarct dementia: A controlled study. *Stroke*. 23: 804–811.

Gronwall, D. and Wrightson, P. 1975. Cumulative effect of concussion. *Lancet*. 2: 995–997.

Hasegawa, K., Homma, A. and Imai, Y. 1986. An epidemiology study of age-related dementia in the community. *International Journal of Geriatric Psychiatry*. 1: 45–55.

Heyman, A., Fillenbaum, G., Prosnitz, B., Raiford, K., Burchett, B. and Clark, C. 1991. Estimated prevalence of dementia among elderly black and white community residents. *Archives of Neurology* 48: 594–598.

Heyman, A., Wilkinson, W.E., Stafford, J.A., Helms, M.J., Sigmon, A.H. and Weinberg, T. 1984. Alzheimer's disease: A study of epidemiological aspects. *Annals of Neurology* 15: 335–341.

Hofman, A., Shulte, W., Tanja, R., van Duijn, C., Haaxma, R., Lameris, A., Otten, V. and Saan, R. 1989. History of dementia and Parkinson's disease in 1st degree relatives of patients with Alzheimer's disease. *Neurology*. 39: 1589–1592.

Isoe, K., Urakami, K., Saato, K. and Takahashi, K. 1996. Apolipoprotein E in patients with dementia of the Alzheimer type and vascular dementia. *Acta Neurologica Scandinavica*. 93: 133–137.

Jacobs, B., Schall, M. and Scheibel, A.B. 1993. A quantitative dendritic analysis of Wernicke's area in humans. II. Gender, hemispheric and environ-mental factors. *Journal of Comparative Neurology*. 327: 97–111.

Jacobs, B. and Scheibel, A.B. 1993. A quantitative dendritic analysis of Wernicke's area in humans. I. Lifespan changes. *Journal of Comparative Neurology*. 327: 83–96.

Jacobs, D.M., Marder, K., Cote, L.J., Sano, M., Stern, Y. and Mayeux, R. 1995. Neuropsychological charac-teristics of preclinical dementia in Parkinson's disease. *Neurology*. 45: 1691–1696.

Janssen, R.S., Nwanyanwu, O.C., Selik, R.M. and Stehr-Green, J.K. 1992. Epidemiology of human immuno-deficiency virus encephalopathy in the United States. *Neurology*. 42: 1472–1476.

Jorm, A.F. 1990. *The epidemiology of Alzheimer's disease and related disorders*. London: Chapman and Hall.

Jorm, A.F. 1991. Cross-national comparison of the occurrence of Alzheimer's disease and vascular dementia. *European Archives of Psychiatry and Clinical Neuroscience*. 240: 218–222.

Katzman, R. 1993. Education and the prevalence of dementia and Alzheimer's disease. *Neurology.* 43: 13–20.

Katzman, R., Aronson, M., Fuld, P., Kawas, C., Brown, T., Morgenstern, H., Frishman, W., Gidez, L., Eder, H. and Ooi, W.L. 1989. Development of dementing illnesses in an 80-year-old volunteer cohort. *Annals of Neurology.* 25: 317–324.

Kokmen, E., Beard, C.M., Chandra, V., Offord, K.P. and Schoenberg, B.S. 1991. Clinical risk factors for Alzheimer's disease: A population based case-control study. *Neurology.* 41: 1393–1397.

Koller, W.C., Glatt, S.L., Hubble, J.P., Paolo, A., Tröster, A.I., Handler, M.S., Horvat, R.T., Martin, C., Schmidt, K., Karst, A., Wijsman, E.M., Yu, C.-E. and Schellenberg, G.D. 1995. Apolipoprotein E genotypes in Parkinson's disease with and without dementia. *Annals of Neurology.* 37: 342–345.

Korczyn, A.D., Kahana, E. and Galper, Y. 1991. Epidemiology of dementia in Ashkelon, Israel (abstract). *Neuroepidemiology.* 10: 100.

Letenneur, L., Commenges, D., Dartigues, J.F. and Barberger-Gateau, P. 1994. Incidence of dementia and Alzheimer's disease in elderly community residents of south-western France. *International Journal of Epidemiology.* 23: 1256–1261.

Levy-Lahad, E., Wijsman, E.M., Nemens, E. Anderson, L., Goddard, K.A.B., Weber, J.L., Bird, T.D. and Schellenberg, G.D. 1995. A familial Alzheimer's disease locus on Chromosome 1. *Science.* 269: 970–973.

Li, G., Shen, Y.C., Chen, C.H., Zhau, Y.W., Li, S.R. and Lu, M. 1991. A three-year follow-up study of age-related dementia in an urban area of Beijing. *Acta Psychiatrica Scandinavica.* 83: 99–104.

Lieberman, A., Dziatolowski, M., Kupersmith, M., Serby, M., Goodgold, A., Korein, J. and Goldstein, M. 1979. Dementia in Parkinson disease. *Annals of Neurology.* 6: 355–359.

Marder, K., Flood, P., Cote, L. and Mayeux, R. 1990. A pilot study of risk factors for dementia in Parkinson's disease. *Movement Disorders.* 5: 156–161.

Marder, K., Maestre, G., Cote, L., Mejia, H., Alfaro, B., Halim, A., Tang, M., Tycko, B. and Mayeux, R. 1994. The apolipoprotein epsilon 4 allele in Parkinson's disease with and without dementia. *Neurology.* 44: 1330–1331.

Marder, K., Tang, M.-X., Cote, L.J., Stern, Y. and Mayeux, R. 1993. Predictors of dementia in community-dwelling elderly patients with Parkinson's disease. *Neurology.* 43: S115.

Marder, K., Tang, M.-X., Cote, L., Stern, Y. and Mayeux, R. 1995. The frequency and associated risk factors for dementia in patients with Parkinson's disease. *Archives of Neurology.* 52: 695–701.

Masliah, E., Mallory, M., Hansen, L., DeTeresa, R. and Terry, R.D. 1993. Quantitative synaptic alterations in the human neocortex during normal aging. *Neurology.* 43: 192–197.

Mayeux, R., Chen, J., Mirabello, E., Marder, K., Bell, K., Dooneief, G., Cote, L. and Stern, Y. 1990. An estimate of the incidence of dementia in idiopathic Parkinson's disease. *Neurology.* 40: 1513–1517.

Mayeux, R., Denaro, J., Hemenegildo, N., Marder, K., Tang, M.X., Cote, L.J. and Stern, Y. 1992. A population-based investigation of Parkinson's disease with and without dementia: Relationship to age and gender. *Archives of Neurology.* 49: 492–497.

Mayeux, R., Ottman, R., Maestre, G., Ngai, C., Tang, M.-X., Ginsberg, H., Chun, M., Tycko, B. and Shelanski, M. 1995. Synergistic effects of traumatic head injury and apolipo-protein-ε4 in patients with Alzheimer's disease. *Neurology.* 45: 555–557.

McArthur, J.C., Hoover, D.R., Bacellar, H., Miller, E.N., Cohen, B.A., Becker, J.T., Graham, N.M.H., McArthur, J.H., Selnes, O.A., Jacobson, L.P., Visscher, B.R., Concha, M. and Saah, A. for the Multicenter AIDS Cohort Study. 1993. Dementia in AIDS patients: Incidence and risk factors. *Neurology.* 43: 2245–2252.

Molsa, P., Marttila, R. and Rinne, U. 1982. Epidemiology of dementia in a Finnish population. *Acta Neurologica Scandinavica.* 65: 541–552.

Mortel, K.F., Meyer, J.S., Herod, B. and Thornby, J. 1995. Education and occupation as risk factors for dementia of the Alzheimer and ischemic vascular types. *Dementia.* 6: 55–62.

Mortimer, J.A., French, L.R., Hutton, J.T., Schuman, L.M., Christians, B. and Boatman, R.A. 1983. Reported head trauma in an epidemiologic study of Alzheimer's disease. *Neurology.* 33 (Suppl. 2): 85.

Mortimer, J.A., Schuman, L.M. and French, L.R. 1981. Epidemiology of dementing illness. In *The epidemiology of dementia*, ed. J.A. Mortimer and L.M. Schuman, pp. 3–23. New York: Oxford University Press.

Mortimer, J.A., van Duijn, C.M., Chandra, V., Fratiglioni, I., Graves, A.B., Heyman, A., Jorm, A.F., Kokmen, E., Kondo, K., Rocca, W.A., Shalat, S.L., Soininen, H. and Hofman, A. for the Eurodem Risk Factors Research Group. 1991. Head trauma as a risk factor for Alzheimer's disease: A collaborative re-analysis of case-control studies. *International Journal of Epidemiology*. 20: S28-S35.

Myers, R.H., Schaefer, E.J., Wilson, P.W.F., D'Agostino, R., Ordovas, J.M., Espino, A., Au, R., White, R.F., Knoefel, J.E., Cobb, J.L., McNulty, K.A., Beiser, A. and Wolf, P.A. 1996. Apolipoprotein E ε4 association with dementia in a population-based study: The Framingham Study. *Neurology*. 46: 673–677.

Paykel, E.S., Brayne, C., Huppert, F.A., Gill, C., Barkley, C., Gehlhaar, E., Beardsall, L., Girling, D.M., Pollitt, P. and O'Connor, D. 1994. Incidence of dementia in a population older than 75 years in the United Kingdom. *Archives of General Psychiatry*. 54: 325–332.

Pericak-Vance, M.A., Bebout, J.L., Gaskell Jr, P.C., Yamaoka, L.H., Hung, W.-Y., Alberts, M.J., Walker, A.P., Bartlett, R.J., Haynes, C.A., Welsh, K.A., Earl, N.L., Heyman, A., Clark, C.M. and Roses, A.D. 1991. Linkage studies in familial Alzheimer disease: Evidence for chromosome 19 linkage. *American Journal of Human Genetics*. 48: 1034–1050.

Perls, T.T., Morris, J.N., Ooi, W.L. and Lipsitz, L.A. 1993. The relationship between age, gender and cognitive performance in the very old: The effect of selective survival. *Journal of the American Geriatric Society*. 41: 1193–1201.

Pickering-Brown, S.M., Mann, D.M.A., Bourke, J.P., Roberts, D.A., Balderson, D., Burns, A., Byrne, J. and Owen, F. 1994. Apolipoprotein ε4 and Alzheimer's disease pathology in Lewy body disease and in other B-amyloid-forming diseases. *Lancet*. 343: 1155.

Rajput, A.H., Offord, K.P., Beard, C.M. and Kurland, L.T. 1987. A case-control study of smoking habits, dementia and other illnesses in idiopathic Parkinson's disease. *Neurology*. 37: 226–232.

Ranen, N.G., Stine, O.C., Abbott, M.H., Sherr, M., Codori, A.M., Franz, M.L., Chao, N.I., Chung, A.S., Pleasant, N., Callahan, C., Kasch, L.M., Ghaffari, M., Chase, G.A., Kazazian, H.H., Brandt, J., Folstein, S.E. and Ross, C.A. 1995. Anticipation and instability of IT–15 CAGn repeats in parent-offspring pairs with Huntington disease. *American Journal of Human Genetics*. 57: 593–602.

Robinson, R.G. and Starkstein, S.E. 1990. Current research in affective disorders following stroke. *Journal of Neuropsychiatry and Clinical Neuroscience*. 2: 1–14.

Rocca, W.A., Bonaiuto, S., Lippi, A., Luciani, P., Turtu, F., Cavarzeran, F. and Amaducci, L. 1990. Prevalence of clinically diagnosed Alzheimer's disease and other dementing disorders: A door-to-door survey in Appignano, Macerata Province, Italy. *Neurology*. 40: 626–631.

Rocca, W.A., Hofman, A., Brayne, C., Breteler, M.M, Clarke, M., Copeland, J.R., Dartigues, J.F., Engedal, K., Hagnell, O., Heeren, T.J., Jonker, C., Lindesay, J., Lobo, A., Mann, A., Molsa, P.K., Morgan, K., O'Connor, D.W., da Silva Droux, A., Sulkava, R. and Kay, D.W. 1991. The prevalence of vascular dementia in Europe: Facts and fragments from 1980–1990 studies. *Annals of Neurology*. 30: 817–824.

Saitoh, T., Xia, Y., Chen, X., Masliah, E., Galasko, D., Shults, C., Thal, L.J., Hansen, L.A. and Katzman, R. 1995. The CPY2D6B mutant allele is overrepresented in the Lewy body variant of Alzheimer's disease. *Annals of Neurology*. 37: 110–112.

Salganik, I. and Korczyn, A. 1990. Risk factors for dementia in Parkinson's disease. In *Parkinson's disease: Anatomy, pathology and therapy*, ed. M.B. Streifler, A.D. Korczyn, E. Melamed and M.B.H. Youdim, pp. 343–347. New York: Raven Press.

Satz, P., Morgenstern, H., Miller, E.N., Selnes, O.A., McArthur, J.C., Cohen, B.A., Wesch, J., Becker, J.T., Jacobson, L., D'Elia, L.F., van Gorp, W. and Visscher, B. 1993. Low education as a possible risk factor for cognitive abnormalities in HIV–1: Findings from the Multicenter AIDS Cohort Study MACS. *Journal of Acquired Immune Deficiency Syndromes*. 6: 503–511.

Saunders, A.M., Strittmatter, W.J., Schmechel, D., St.George-Hyslop, P.H., Pericak-Vance, M.A., Joo, S.H., Rosi, B.L., Gusella, J.F., Crapper-MacLachlan, D.R., Alberts, M.J., Hulette, C., Crain, B., Goldgaber, D. and Roses, A.D. 1993. Association of apolipoprotein E allele ε4 with late-onset familial and sporadic Alzheimer's disease. *Neurology*. 43: 1467–1472.

Schmechel, D.E., Saunders, A.M., Strittmatter, W.J., Crain, B.J., Hulette, C.M., Joo, S.H., Pericak-Vance, M.A., Goldgaber, D. and Roses, A.D. 1993. Increased amyloid beta-peptide deposition in cerebral cortex as a consequence of apolipoprotein E genotype in late-onset Alzheimer disease. *Proceedings of the National Academy of Sciences*. 90: 9649–9653.

Schoenberg, B.S. Anderson, D.W. and Haeren, A.F. 1985. Severe dementia: Prevalence and clinical features in a biracial US population. *Archives of Neurology*. 42: 740–743.

Schoenberg, B.S., Kokmen, E. and Okazaki, H. 1987. Alzheimer's disease and other dementing illnesses in a defined United States population: incidence rates and clinical features. *Annals of Neurology*. 22: 724–729.

Skoog, I. 1994. Risk factors for vascular dementia: A review. *Dementia*. 5: 137–144.

Skoog, I., Nilsson, L., Palmertz, B. Andreasson, L.A. and Svanborg, A. 1993. A population-based study of dementia in 85-year-olds. *New England Journal of Medicine*. 328: 153–158.

Smith, C.A.D., Gough, A.C., Leigh, P.N., Summers, B.A., Harding, A.E., Maraganore, D.M., Sturman, S.G., Schapira, A.H.V., Williams, A.C., Spurr, N.K. and Wolf, C.R. 1992. Debrisoquine hydroxylase gene polymorphism and susceptibility to Parkinson's disease. *Lancet*. 339: 1375–1377.

St.George-Hyslop, P.H., Tanzi, R.E., Polinsky, R.J., Haines, J.L., Nee, J., Watkins, P.C., Myers, R.H., Feldman, R.G., Pollen, D., Drachman, D., Growdon, J., Bruni, A., Foncin, J-F., Salmon, D., Frommelt, P., Amaducci, L., Sorbi, S., Piacentini, S., Stewart, G.D., Hobbs, W.J., Conneally, P.M. and Gusella, J.F. 1987. The genetic defect causing familial Alzheimer's disease maps on chromosome 21. *Science*. 235: 885–890.

St.George-Hyslop, P., Haines, J., Rogaev, E., Mortilla, M., Vaula, G., Pericak-Vance, M., Foncin, J-F., Montesi, M., Bruni, A., Sorbi, S., Rainero, I., Pinessi, L., Pollen, D., Polinski, R., Nee, L., Kennedy, J., Macciardi, F., Rogaeva, E., Liang, Y., Alexandrova, N., Lukiw, W., Schlumpf, K., Tanzi, R., Tsuda, T., Farrer, L., Cantu, J-M., Duara, R., Amaducci, L., Bergamini, L., Gusella, J., Roses, A. and Crapper McLachlan, D. 1992. Genetic evidence for a novel Alzheimer's disease locus on chromosome 14. *Nature Genetics*. 2: 330–334.

Starkstein, S.E., Mayberg, H.S., Leiguarda, R., Preziosi, T.J. and Robinson, R.G. 1992. A prospective longitudinal study of depression, cognitive decline and physical impairments in patients with Parkinson's disease. *Journal of Neurology, Neurosurgery and Psychiatry*. 55: 377–382.

Stern, Y., Alexander, G.E., Prohovnik, I. and Mayeux, R. 1992. Inverse relationship between education and parietotemporal perfusion deficit in Alzheimer's disease. *Annals of Neurology*. 32: 371–375.

Stern, Y., Alexander, G.E., Prohovnik, I., Stricks, L., Link, B., Lennon, M.C. and Mayeux, R. 1995. Relationship between lifetime occupation and parietal flow: Implications for a reserve against Alzheimer's disease pathology. *Neurology*. 45: 55–60.

Stern, Y., Gurland, B., Tatemichi, T.K., Tang, M.X., Wilder, D. and Mayeux, R. 1994. Influence of education and occupation on the incidence of Alzheimer's disease. *Journal of the American Medical Association*. 271: 1004–1010.

Stern, Y., Marder, K., Tang, M.X. and Mayeux, R. 1993. Antecedent clinical features associated with dementia in Parkinson's disease. *Neurology*. 43: 1690–1692.

Strittmatter, W.J. and Roses, A.D. 1995. Apolipoprotein E and Alzheimer disease. *Proceedings of the National Academy of Sciences*. 92: 4725–4727.

Strittmatter, W.J., Saunders, A.M., Goedert, M., Weisgraber, K.H., Dong, L.M., Jakes, R., Huang, D.Y., Pericak-Vance, M., Schmechel, D. and Roses, A.D. 1994. Isoform-specific interactions of apolipoprotein E with microtubule-associated protein tau: Implications for Alzheimer's disease. *Proceedings of the National Academy of Sciences*. 91: 11183–11186.

Strittmatter, W.J., Saunders, A.M., Schmechel, D., Pericak-Vance, M., Enghild, J. and Salvesen, G.S. 1993. Apolipoprotein E: High avidity binding to β-amyloid and increased frequency of type 4 allele in late onset familial Alzheimer disease. *Proceedings of the National Academy of Sciences*. 90: 1977–1981.

Sulkava, R., Wikstrom, J., Aromaa, A., Raitasalo, R., Lahtinen, V., Lahtela, K. and Palo, J. 1985. Prevalence of severe dementia in Finland. *Neurology*. 35: 1025–1029.

Tatemichi, T.K., Desmond, D.W., Mayeux, R., Paik, M., Stern, Y., Sano, M., Remien, R.H., Williams, J.B., Mohr, J.P., Hauser, W.A. and Figueroa, M. 1992a. Dementia after stroke: baseline frequency, risks and clinical features in a hospitalized cohort. *Neurology*. 42: 1185–1193.

Tatemichi, T.K., Desmond, D.W., Paik, M., Figueroa, M., Gropen, T.I., Stern, Y., Sano, M., Remien, R., Williams, J.B., Mohr, J.P. and Mayeux, R. 1993. Clinical determinants of dementia related to stroke. *Annals of Neurology*. 33: 568–575.

Tatemichi, T.K., Rosenstein, B., Remien, R.H., Williams, J.B.W., Desmond, D.W., Sano, M., Stern, Y. and Mayeux, R. 1992b. Depression and intellectual impairment after stroke: Causally linked? *Annals of Neurology*. 32: 267.

Telenius, H., Kremer, H.P., Theilmann, J., Andrew, S.E., Almqvist, E., Anvret, M., Greenberg, C., Greenberg, J., Lucotte, G., Squitieri, F., Starr, E., Goldberg, Y.P. and Hayden, M.R. 1993. Molecular analysis of juvenile Huntington disease: The major influence on CAGn repeat length is the sex of the affected parent. *Human Molecular Genetics*. 2: 1535–1540.

Terry, R.D., DeTeresa, R. and Hansen, L.A. 1987. Neocortical cell counts in normal human adult aging. *Annals of Neurology*. 21: 530–539.

Terry, R.D., Masliah, E., Salmon, D.P., Butters, N., DeTeresa, R., Hill, R., Hansen, L.A. and Katzman, R. 1991. Physical basis of cognitive alterations in Alzheimer's disease: Synapse loss is the major correlate of cognitive impairment. *Annals of Neurology*. 30: 572–580.

Tomlinson, B.E., Blessed, G. and Roth, M. 1968. Observations on the brains of non-demented old people. *Journal of the Neurological Sciences*. 7: 331–356.

Van Duijn, C.M. 1996. Epidemiology of the dementias: Recent developments and new approaches. *Journal of Neurology Neurosurgery and Psychiatry*. 60: 478–488.

Van Duijn, C.M., de Knijff, P., Wehnert, A., De Voecht, J., Bronzova, J.B., Havekes, L.M., Hofman, A. and Van Broeckhoven, C. 1995. The apolipoprotein E ε2 allele is associated with an increased risk of early-onset Alzheimer's disease and a reduced survival. *Annals of Neurology*. 37: 605–610.

Van Gorp, W.G., Miller, E.N., Marcotte, T.D., Dixon, W., Paz, D., Selnes, O., Wesch, J., Becker, J.T., Hinkin, C.H., Mitrushina, M., Satz, P., Weisman, J.D., Buckingham, S.L. and Stenquist, P.K. 1994. The relationship between age and cognitive impairment in HIV–1 infection: Findings from the Multicenter AIDS Cohort Study and a clinical cohort. *Neurology*. 44: 929–935.

Williams, D.B., Annegers, J.F., Kokmen, E., O'Brien, P.C. and Kurland, L.T. 1991. Brain injury and neurologic sequelae: A cohort study of dementia, parkinsonism and amyotrophic lateral sclerosis. *Neurology*. 41: 1554–1557.

Zhang, M., Katzman, R., Salmon, D., Jin, H., Cai, G., Wang, Z., Qu, G., Grant, I., Yu, E., Levy, P., Klauber, M.R. and Liu, W.T. 1990. The prevalence of dementia and Alzheimer's disease in Shanghai, China: Impact of age, gender and education. *Annals of Neurology*. 27: 428–437.

15

Cross-cultural issues in the neuropsychological assessment of neurodegenerative disease

ANDREAS U. MONSCH, KIRSTEN I. TAYLOR
AND MARK W. BONDI

INTRODUCTION

As we approach the year 2000, research has increasingly become an international venture. Modern technology offers clinicians and researchers the possibility of communicating and comparing the results of their investigations almost immediately through globally-linked telecommunication networks. This development, which will undoubtedly increase in the coming decades, will not only provide new and exciting opportunities but will also raise new questions about the comparability and generalizability of research findings across international borders.

The purpose of this chapter is to discuss conceptual and methodological issues involved in cross-cultural research pertaining to neurodegenerative diseases. The chapter focuses on dementia and the cross-cultural issues related to its diagnosis. As neuropsychological assessment is a critical part of the diagnostic process, we address the utilization of dementia screening instruments in a cross-cultural context. As similar issues arise in investigations comparing neuropsychological functioning in different ethnic groups (Olmedo 1981), cross-ethnic studies are also addressed.

METHODOLOGICAL AND CONCEPTUAL ISSUES

Cross-cultural research in neurodegenerative diseases has primarily been carried out in an attempt to compare prevalence rates of these diseases to discover possible risk and/or protective factors (i.e. genetic and environmental) (Katzman 1987; Chang et al. 1993). In a literature review of 47 prevalence studies on dementia from Asia, Europe,

North America and South Africa, Jorm et al. (1987) identified age as a consistent risk factor for dementia. A relationship between age and prevalence rate was found across all studies, with the prevalence rate doubling approximately every 5 years after the age of 60 years. Sixteen of the 47 studies had data appropriate for an analysis of the relative frequency of dementia of the Alzheimer type and multi-infarct dementia. Upon reviewing these studies, Jorm et al. (1987) found that the prevalence of multi-infarct dementia was significantly higher than that of Alzheimer's disease (AD) among Japanese and Russian populations. In contrast, among Scandinavian and British populations there was an excess of AD over multi-infarct dementia cases. Finnish and US populations, however, exhibited no differences in the prevalence rates of multi-infarct dementia and AD. Overall, there was a tendency for AD to be more prevalent among females than males, whereas multi-infarct dementia was more common among males.

The major hindrances to cross-cultural comparisons of dementia prevalence rates, and hence the search for possible risk and/or protective factors, have been the use of inconsistent diagnostic criteria and practices and a lack of reliable and valid neuropsychological screening and assessment instruments (Katzman 1987). Furthermore, the confounding variables encountered in studies carried out within one culture (e.g. age, language, education, understanding of mental health and illness, family and social networks, alcohol use, ecological demands, genetic differences, etc.) are magnified when two groups from different cultures are compared (Favazza and Oman 1978; Ardila 1995). These latter difficulties have led Ardila to point out: 'We barely have dealt with individual differences in neuropsychological performance; and our understanding of cultural differences is, to be optimistic, very insufficient'

(Ardila 1995, p. 143). The two largest challenges facing cross-cultural research on neurodegenerative diseases, then, are the implementation of standardized diagnostic strategies within the cultures under investigation and the development and validation of culturally appropriate neuropsychological instruments which possess adequate normative data (Westermeyer 1985; Katzman 1987; Fuld et al. 1988).

In the past, many cross-cultural studies have simply implemented in one culture (A) tests which were developed, standardized and validated in another culture (B). Frequently, test scores obtained by members of culture A were then interpreted with respect to the normative data gathered in culture B. This approach gives rise to the obvious criticism: How can one assume that the norms or behaviors of culture B are valid for culture A? Cross-cultural studies are, by definition, empirical investigations which compare groups who have had different experiences that have led to predictable and significant differences in behavior (Brislin 1976). This dilemma involves one of the most important methodological distinctions in cross-cultural research: the emic-etic distinction. Emic analyses focus on one single culture and attempt to derive valid principles that describe indigenous psychological phenomena. Etic analyses, on the other hand, are concerned with universal, generalizable principles that account for all human behavior and fulfill comparative goals (Berry 1989).

An emic approach appears, at first glance, to have many characteristics well-suited for cross-cultural neuropsychological comparisons. Construct validity is preserved and many of the confounds inherent in cross-cultural research are resolved because native investigators independently decide on the most culturally relevant means to measure a neuropsychological construct. A dilemma might arise, however, when investigators from different cultures attempt to compare their results. Inherent differences in the relative function, use and importance of the neuropsychological construct under investigation lead by definition to different assessment instruments and items – investigators would thus be attempting to compare the incomparable (Brislin 1976; Favazza and Oman 1978). On the other hand, if investigators independently conclude that identical test items best reflect the construct under investigation in each culture, then one could assume that the construct measured by these items is similar for both cultures. These etic items would then be appropriate for use in quantitative, cross-cultural comparisons once normative data had been collected within each culture. The question in cross-cultural research is therefore not whether the approach is emic or etic, but to what extent it is emic and to what extent it is etic (Brislin 1976; Westermeyer 1985).

A combined emic-etic approach, the so-called imposed-etic methodology, is often adopted in different cultures for the neuropsychological assessment of neurodegenerative diseases. This approach is exemplified by the utilization of internationally accepted diagnostic criteria in different cultures (Westermeyer 1985). The DSM-IV (American Psychiatric Association 1994) or the ICD–10 (World Health Organization 1992) diagnostic criteria for dementia, then, can be likened to etic constructs; the criteria are assumed to be universally valid and sufficient to define the presence of dementia in all human subjects. For example, DSM-IV criteria for dementia require the presence of multiple cognitive deficits, including memory impairment and at least one of the following: aphasia, apraxia, agnosia or a disturbance in executive functioning (Chapter 3; Chapter 18). In addition, these cognitive deficits are required to 'cause significant impairment in social or occupational functioning and must represent a significant decline from a previous level of functioning' (American Psychiatric Association 1994, p. 86). These deficits may manifest themselves in different behaviors across cultures, necessitating an emic approach to their assessment. Each culture must independently determine how to assess memory, language, gnosis, praxis and executive functioning in a culturally meaningful way and decide whether results of the emic-driven assessment fit the etic diagnostic criteria.

Cross-cultural comparisons of the neuropsychological performances of individuals identified as demented require culturally appropriate instruments. The most common approach to developing such instruments has been to literally translate and culturally adapt tests from another culture (for a neuropsychologically relevant example, see Tollman and Msengana 1990). Van de Vijver and Hambleton (1996) point out three major sources of bias that must be taken into consideration in translating test instruments: (1) construct bias, i.e. will the test be measuring the same neuropsychological principle (construct) in both cultures? (2) item bias, i.e. is the literal translation of the individual items adequate? and (3) administration bias, i.e. are the administration procedures comparable?

The Chinese version of the Mini Mental State Examination (CMMS; Katzman et al. 1988) offers a good example of construct preservation during cultural adaptation. In the American MMSE (Folstein et al. 1975), subjects are asked to write a sentence. This item measures the ability to form and express an understandable statement in the form of writing. As many Chinese have never learned to write, however, the item 'Write a sentence' had to be culturally adapted to 'Say a sentence' (Salmon et al. 1989). Although writing and speaking are clearly distinctly different cognitive processes, the superordinate construct had been preserved.

Attempts to reduce item bias have included back-translation. With this method, an instrument is constructed in one language, a bilingual translates it into the target language and finally another, independent bilingual translates the test back into the original language. The two versions of the test are compared to judge the quality of the translation. Additional quality can be added to the back-translation by a cultural adaptation of test items with the help of bilingual speakers. This might include a change in the phrasing of test items to most closely reflect their original meaning in the target culture, or the choice of new items or words based on target culture frequency norms (Brislin 1976; Van de Vijver and Hambleton 1996). For example, the American MMSE item 'Repeat the phrase "No ifs ands, or buts"' was culturally adapted into '44 stone lions', an alliterative phrase in Chinese, for the CMMS (Salmon et al. 1989).

Sources of administration bias include different physical testing situations, communication problems between the examiner and examinee and culturally influenced strategies of dealing with frustration, anxiety and embarrassment over poor performance (Van de Vijver and Hambleton 1996). Avoiding these types of biases necessitates the active collaboration of professionals from each culture involved in the study (Ardila 1995).

FINDINGS FROM CROSS-CULTURAL AND CROSS-ETHNIC STUDIES

Cross-cultural studies

One of the largest cross-cultural studies on the neuropsychological assessment of dementia has been the Shanghai survey of dementia, a two-phase dementia prevalence survey carried out by investigators from the Shanghai Mental Health Center in collaboration with

investigators from the University of California at San Diego's (UCSD) Alzheimer's Disease Research Center (ADRC) (Salmon et al. 1989; Zhang et al. 1990; Hill et al. 1993).

Phase I of the Shanghai survey of dementia involved the screening of more than 5000 residents of the Jing-An district of Shanghai aged 55 years or older with the CMMS and a home interview. Education-corrected CMMS cut-off scores were calculated from this sample. Subjects who fell below an education-adjusted CMMS cut-off score ($N=510$) and a 5% sample from the cohort who scored above the cut-off score ($N=241$) entered the second phase of the study (total $N=751$) (Zhang et al. 1990).

Phase II was composed of extensive diagnostic and clinical examinations including medical, psychiatric, neurological, neuropsychological and functional assessments. The neuropsychological evaluation consisted of the Chinese version of the Blessed Information Memory Concentration Test, the Hasegawa Dementia Scale, the Object Memory Evaluation, Verbal Fluency, Digit Span and WISC-R Block Design. Education-corrected cut-off scores were calculated for all neuropsychological instruments and were used in subsequent analyses. The functional assessment consisted of Chinese versions of the Pfeffer Outpatient Disability Scale (POD), Activities of Daily Living (ADL), Instrumental Activities of Daily Living (IADL) and a short set of history questions. The diagnosis of dementia was made by three independent clinicians employing the criteria outlined in DSM-III. Two thirds of all patients with dementia fulfilled the diagnostic criteria for AD (McKhann et al. 1984; Zhang et al. 1990; Hill et al. 1993).

The prevalence of AD in the Shanghai dementia survey was much higher and the proportion of AD to multi-infarct dementia cases much lower than in previously published studies from China and Japan (Jorm et al. 1987). These differences may be attributed to two factors. First, the Shanghai survey utilized a comprehensive battery of tests, including diagnostic, neuropsychological and functional assessments and a large subject pool. A much more sensitive investigation into the prevalence and causes of dementia was therefore possible. For example, the outcome on the functional assessments, the brief history, IADL and POD, but not the ADL, were significant predictors of dementia (Hill et al. 1993) and were employed for the diagnosis. Second, the researchers identified education (or the lack thereof) as the major confounding variable in neuropsychological test results and were able to statistically control for this bias by calculating education-corrected cut-off scores. For example, extensive analyses of the CMMS revealed that the appropriate cutoff score for Chinese individuals with no formal education was 17/30. In contrast, individuals with at least 6 years of education required use of a cut-off score of 20/30 and those with more than 6 years of education required use of a cut-off score of 24/30 (Zhang et al. 1990).

One of the most significant findings from the Shanghai survey was that elderly subjects with no education and with 6 or fewer years of education were significantly more likely to be clinically diagnosed as demented compared with those individuals possessing 6 or more years of education. This finding does not appear to be an artifact as all neuropsychological examination scores had been statistically corrected for education. Instead, it seems that no or low education is an independent risk factor for dementia and that real differences in the prevalence rates of dementia are observed among groups with different levels of formal education (Hill et al. 1993). An association between low educational attainment and an increased risk for dementia has also been reported in North American studies (e.g. Stern et al. 1994; Cobb et al. 1995), supporting the Shanghai survey findings. Zhang et al. (1990) offer a possible explanation for this phenomenon: no formal education may be associated with early deprivation, thereby lowering brain reserve and allowing dementia symptoms to appear at an earlier stage during disease progression (Chapter 14).

Salmon et al. (1989) compared the MMSE scores in a cross-cultural study of China, Finland and the USA. The CMMS scores were obtained for 1601 Chinese subjects from the Shanghai survey who had at least some formal education. The Finnish participants were 525 randomly selected elderly individuals from the city of Kuopio who were administered a literal translation of the MMSE. Ninety elderly volunteers from the UCSD ADRC were matched to the Finnish and Chinese samples with respect to their distribution of MMSE scores. All subjects were between the ages of 65 and 74 years.

Although the overall performances on the respective MMSEs were nearly identical in the Chinese, Finnish and American groups, an item analysis revealed different patterns of performance on the individual test items. Most notably, the Chinese subjects performed better on an item

requiring object recall, but more poorly on items requiring reading of a sentence and copying of two intersecting pentagons than did the Finnish and American subjects. With respect to the latter finding, it is important to note that more than half of the Chinese participants had been educated with Si-Shu, an informal mode of literacy training devoted to the study of classics, calligraphy, literary works and history, but with no systematic training in science and mathematics. Thus, although these individuals had a comparable amount of education, they may have been relatively disadvantaged when asked to copy a complex geometric figure. The better performance of the Chinese subjects on the recall item remains unexplained and further research is necessary to determine if this is indeed a culturally specific characteristic (Salmon et al. 1989).

Fuld et al. (1988) administered the Object-Memory Evaluation (OME) to an elderly American sample and a culturally adapted OME to a Japanese sample (both aged 70–89 years) in order to investigate cross-cultural differences in memory and language performances and to evaluate the utility of the OME in detecting these differences. The American sample was screened for dementia with the Fuld adaptation of the Blessed 'Mental Test' (Fuld 1978) and the Japanese sample was screened with the Hasegawa Mental Status Test (Hasegawa et al. 1974). A detailed comparison of these tests was not undertaken because of the use of different screening measures. Comparison of OME performances, however, revealed interesting results. The very old (ages 80–89 years) Japanese subjects performed better than the very old American subjects on recall and retrieval of OME items. With respect to language, as measured by a verbal fluency task requiring oral generation of first names for 1 minute, the very old Japanese subjects performed worse than any of the American subjects or the old (ages 70–79 years) Japanese subjects. Although the memory performances of the Asian and American subjects were similar to those reported by Salmon et al. (1989), Fuld et al.'s findings must be interpreted with caution for several reasons. First, the Blessed 'Mental Test' may have been easier than the Hasegawa Mental Status Test, thereby allowing patients already in the very early stages of a dementing illness into the American sample. Second, the cultural adaptation of the OME into Japanese necessitated the selection of a set of objects different from that used in the American OME version. Although a separate group of American patients performed similarly on both versions, it remains unknown whether a separate group of Japanese subjects would also perform similarly. Furthermore, comparisons were not reported for either the delayed recall measure of the OME or the verbal fluency distractor trials. Despite these shortcomings, Fuld et al.'s (1988) investigation represents a valuable attempt to compare the results from memory and language evaluations across two cultures.

Cross-ethnic studies

As a whole, the results from cross-ethnic dementia prevalence studies remain inconclusive. For example, Fillenbaum et al. (1990) compared the performance of 83 black and 81 white community residents (aged 65 years and older, cognitively impaired and nonimpaired) on six dementia screening instruments. They found that scores on these measures correlated with race and education: black people and less well-educated individuals performed more poorly on the tests than did white people and more educated individuals. The impact of education did not vary as a function of ethnicity. Stern et al. (1992), using the results from a neuropsychological paradigm as the criterion for dementia, found differences in the dementia classification rates of self-identified non-Hispanic white ($N=158$), non-Hispanic black ($N=123$) and Hispanic ($N=141$) ethnic groups. All neuropsychological test scores, however, were significantly correlated with education. Once the influence of education on the assessment instruments had been statistically controlled, there no longer were any differences in the prevalence rates of dementia among the ethnic groups. Clearly, more cross-ethnic investigations are needed to elucidate the possible impact of ethnicity on neuropsychological test performance and consequently, ethnic differences in dementia prevalence rates. As memory impairment, by definition, is required to be demonstrated before dementia can be diagnosed, a necessary first step in stimulating further cross-ethnic research is the development of appropriate memory measures. At least with regard to Spanish-speaking groups in the USA, recent efforts have been directed at the development of ethnically appropriate memory measures (Ardila et al. 1994; Harris et al. 1995; Jacobs et al. 1997).

CONCLUSIONS

Cross-cultural research on the neuropsychological assessment of dementia poses a number of conceptual and methodological difficulties that have only recently begun to be addressed. In designing a neuropsychological instrument for cross-cultural or -ethnic use, the construct, item and administration biases must be considered. Furthermore, it is imperative that test scores be interpreted relative to normative data obtained within the cultures of interest and that all cross-cultural comparisons be made relative to appropriate normative data. Differences in either the amount or type of education between two cultures might independently influence performance on even well-developed neuropsychological assessment instruments. These confounds must be adequately documented and controlled for before a comparative study of two cultural or ethnic groups can be considered reliable or valid. The possibility remains, however, that the magnitude of differences between two very distant cultures may affect respective neuropsychological test performances to such a degree that a cross-cultural comparison becomes meaningless; it would represent an attempt to compare the incomparable.

Future cross-cultural research on neurodegenerative diseases will need to include clinico-pathological, clinico-chemical and genetic components if neuropsychological test scores and diagnostic criteria are to be independently validated. Such studies will have the power to substantiate or repudiate what have been considered naturally occurring differences in dementia prevalence rates across cultures. They will aid in the detection of risk and/or protective factors, thus improving our understanding of the etiologies of neurodegenerative diseases.

ACKNOWLEDGMENTS

Preparation of this chapter was supported in part by a grant from the La Roche Foundation (AUM), by NIH grant AG12674 (MWB) and by funds from the Medical Research Service of the Department of Veterans Affairs (MWB).

REFERENCES

American Psychiatric Association. 1994. *Diagnostic and statistical manual of mental disorders*, 4th ed. Washington DC: Author.

Ardila, A. 1995. Directions of research in cross-cultural neuropsychology. *Journal of Clinical and Experimental Neuropsychology*. 17: 143–150.

Ardila, A., Roselli, M. and Puente, A.E. 1994. *Neuropsychological evaluation of the Spanish speaker*. New York: Plenum Press.

Berry, J.W. 1989. Imposed etics-emics-derived etics: The operationalization of a compelling idea. *International Journal of Psychology*. 24: 721–735.

Brislin, R.W. 1976. Comparative research methodology: Cross-cultural studies. *International Journal of Psychology*. 11: 215–229.

Chang, L., Miller, B.L. and Lin, K.-M. 1993. Clinical epidemiologic studies of dementias: Cross-ethnic perspectives. In *Psychopharmacology and psychobiology of ethnicity. Progress in psychiatry*, vol. 39, ed. K.-M. Lin, R.E. Poland and G. Nagasaki, pp. 223–252. Washington DC: American Psychiatric Press.

Cobb, J.L., Wolf, P.A., Au, R., White, R. and D'Agostino, R.B. 1995. The effect of education on the incidence of dementia and Alzheimer's disease in the Framingham Study. *Neurology*. 45: 1707–1712.

Favazza, A.R. and Oman, M. 1978. Overview: Foundations of cultural psychiatry. *American Journal of Psychiatry*. 135: 293–303.

Fillenbaum, G., Heyman, A., Williams, K., Prosnitz, B. and Burchett, B. 1990. Sensitivity and specificity of standardized screens of cognitive impairment and dementia among elderly black and white community residents. *Journal of Clinical Epidemiology*. 43: 651–660.

Folstein, M.F., Folstein, S.E. and McHugh, P.R. 1975. 'Mini Mental State': A practical method for grading the cognitive state of patients for the clinician. *Journal of Psychiatry Research*. 12: 189–198.

Fuld, P.A. 1978. Psychological testing in the differential diagnosis of the dementias. In *Alzheimer's disease: Senile dementia and related disorders. Aging*, vol. 7, ed. R. Katzman, R.D. Terry and K.L. Bick, pp. 185–193. New York: Raven Press.

Fuld, P.A., Muramoto, O., Blau, A., Westbrook, L. and Katzman, R. 1988. Cross-cultural and multi-ethnic dementia evaluation by mental status and memory testing. *Cortex*. 24: 511–519.

Harris, J.G., Cullum, C.M. and Puente, A.E. 1995. Effects of bilingualism on verbal learning and memory in Hispanic adults. *Journal of the International Neuropsychological Society*. 1: 10–16.

Hasegawa, K., Inoue, K. and Moriya, K. 1974. An investigation of dementia rating scale for the elderly. *Seishinigaku*. 16: 965–969.

Hill, L.R., Klauber, M.R., Salmon, D.P., Yu, E.S.H., Liu, W.T., Zhang, M. and Katzman, R. 1993. Functional status, education and the diagnosis of dementia in the Shanghai survey. *Neurology*. 43: 138–145.

Jacobs, D.M., Winston, T.D. and Polanco, C.L. 1997. Assessment of verbal memory in Spanish-speaking elders: Development of two frequency-matched list learning tests. *Journal of Clinical and Experimental Neuropsychology*. 19: 119–125.

Jorm, A.F., Korten, A.E. and Henderson, A.S. 1987. The prevalence of dementia: A quantitative integration of the literature. *Acta Psychiatrica Scandinavica*. 76: 465–479.

Katzman, R. 1987. Alzheimer's disease: Advances and opportunities. *Journal of the American Geriatrics Society*. 35: 69–73.

Katzman, R., Zhang, M., Qu, O.-Y., Wang, Z., Liu, W.T., Yu, E., Wong, S.-C., Salmon, D.P. and Grant, I. 1988. A Chinese version of the Mini-Mental State Examination: Impact of illiteracy in a Shanghai dementia survey. *Journal of Clinical Epidemiology*. 41: 971–978.

McKhann, G., Drachman, D., Folstein, M., Katzman, R., Price, D. and Stadlan, E.M. 1984. Clinical diagnosis of Alzheimer's disease: Report of the NINCDS-ADRDA work group under the auspices of Department of Health and Human Services task force on Alzheimer's disease. *Neurology*. 34: 939–944.

Olmedo, E.L. 1981. Testing linguistic minorities. *American Psychologist*. 36: 1078–1085.

Salmon, D.P., Riekkinen, P.J., Katzman, R., Zhang, M., Jin, H. and Yu, E. 1989. Cross-cultural studies of dementia: A comparison of Mini-Mental State Examination performance in Finland and China. *Archives of Neurology*. 46: 769–772.

Stern, Y., Andrews, H., Pittman, J., Sano, M., Tatemichi, T., Lantigua, R. and Mayeux, R. 1992. Diagnosis of dementia in a heterogeneous population: Development of a neuro-psychological paradigm-based diagnosis of dementia and quantified correction for the effects of education. *Archives of Neurology*. 49: 453–460.

Stern, Y., Gurland, B., Tatemichi, T.K., Tang, M.X., Wilder, D. and Mayeux, R. 1994. Influence of education and occupation on the incidence of Alzheimer's disease. *Journal of the American Medical Association*. 271: 1004–1010.

Tollman, S.G. and Msengana, N.B. 1990. Neuropsychological assessment: Problems in evaluating the higher mental functioning of Zulu-speaking people using traditional western techniques. *South African Journal of Psychology*. 20: 20–24.

Van de Vijver, F. and Hambleton, R.K. 1996. Translating tests: Some practical guidelines. *European Psychologist*. 1: 89–99.

Westermeyer, J. 1985. Psychiatric diagnosis across cultural boundaries. *American Journal of Psychiatry*. 142: 798–805.

World Health Organization. 1992. *Tenth Revision of the International Classification of Diseases, Chapter V (f): Mental and Behavioural Disorders. Clinical Descriptions and Diagnostic Guidelines*. Geneva, Switzerland: Author.

Zhang, M., Katzman, R., Salmon, D., Jin, H., Cai, G., Wang, Z., Qu, G., Grant, I., Yu, E., Levy, P., Klauber, M. and Liu, W.T. 1990. The prevalence of dementia and Alzheimer's disease in Shanghai, China: Impact of age, gender and education. *Annals of Neurology*. 27: 428–437.

16

Psychometric issues in the clinical assessment of memory in aging and neurodegenerative disease

ANTHONY M. PAOLO

INTRODUCTION

The psychometric issues pertaining to the assessment of memory in elderly persons concern the reliability, validity and normative data available for memory tests. This chapter first discusses patient factors that influence the reliability and validity of memory evaluations and then describes the psychometric properties of memory assessment devices commonly used with the elderly. Methods for estimating premorbid memory abilities and detecting possible changes in memory functions are briefly presented.

It is known that older individuals are more likely than the general population to experience visual and auditory deficits and to be more susceptible to fatigue that may impede the evaluation process. To reduce fatigue, frequent breaks should be taken, testing may need to be conducted over several days and/or abbreviated versions of memory tests may need to be considered. Sensory deficits associated with advancing age also need to be considered.

SENSORY–PERCEPTUAL FACTORS INFLUENCING MEMORY EVALUATIONS

Visual functions

Visual efficiency tends to decline with advancing age. It has been estimated that 91% of the severely visually impaired are over the age of 45 years and that 68% of the severely visually impaired are 65 years of age and older (Shindell 1989). Although it is good practice to have examinees who wear glasses bring them to the testing session, wearing glasses does not necessarily ensure adequate visual acuity. It is essential that the examiner determine whether each client's vision is sufficient to allow for valid test administration. For instance, elderly subjects who successfully

read material printed in elite type (i.e. 12 characters per inch) have no difficulty with the visual requirements of the Picture Completion and Picture Arrangement subtests of the Wechsler Adult Intelligence Scale (Storandt and Futterman 1982). It is suggested that such a procedure would likely generalize to most of the commonly used memory tests. Nevertheless, it is also a good idea to have a magnifying glass or large print versions of test materials available during the assessment. If significant visual impairment is present, administration and interpretation of verbal memory tests should be given priority.

The relationship between cognitive status and acquired visual impairment in the elderly is largely unknown. It is possible that visual deterioration is related to changes in central nervous system structures that also impact mental integrity. Snyder et al. (1976) demonstrated that elderly persons with visual deficiencies (i.e. acuity less than 20/70) performed more poorly on a verbal mental status questionnaire than did persons with visual acuity better than 20/70.

Auditory functions

Hearing impairment is common among the elderly, with prevalence estimates ranging from 30 to 60% (Mader 1984). The type of hearing loss most common in the elderly makes it difficult for them to distinguish speech sounds from background noise, especially as the background noise increases (Milne 1977). As such, examiners should inquire about hearing aids that the examinee may use and ascertain that the examinee uses those devices during testing. Examiners should also inquire about results of audiological examinations and be familiar with the symptoms of hearing loss. Hearing loss should be suspected when the examinee: (1) has a history of tinnitus or ear infections, (2) makes responses suggesting that sounds were heard but not understood (e.g. mistakes *drapes* for *grapes*, etc.), (3) is socially withdrawn, (4) frequently asks that instructions be repeated, (5) has loud speech, (6) reports that she has trouble understanding speech in a group situation, (7) is reported to turn the television and radio up loud, and (8) watches the speaker's mouth intently (Vernon 1989).

In cases where significant hearing loss is documented or suspected, the examiner can ask the client to repeat a few complex sentences (e.g. 'Each fight readied the boxer for the championship bout') prior to initiating the test session. If repetition is accurate, the examiner can be reasonably confident that hearing proficiency is sufficient for testing. Conversely, an inability to accurately repeat sentences should prompt further evaluation for hearing loss, aphasia and problems with attention and memory. For clients whose only difficulty appears to be diminished hearing acuity, administration of nonverbal or figural memory tests should be given priority.

The specific relationship between hearing impairment and cognitive decline in the elderly remains unknown. Several studies have found an association between hearing and cognitive impairment (Granick et al. 1976; Ohta et al. 1981; Peters et al. 1988; Hertzog and Schear 1989; Uhlmann et al. 1989), while others have not (Herbst and Humphrey, 1980; Jones et al. 1984; Vesterager et al. 1988). A recent longitudinal investigation suggests that hearing and cognitive impairments are unrelated in healthy elderly, but that they are related in demented elderly (Gennis et al. 1991). For individuals with dementing disorders, it is possible that pathological changes in neurological structures contribute to both hearing loss and cognitive impairment (Grimes et al. 1985).

Language functions

Elderly persons referred for memory evaluation may display age-related communication problems; therefore, it is important for clinicians to distinguish the language changes of normal aging from those associated with diseases of the brain. Normal language functions for persons 70 years of age and older include a fluent speech pattern (above 100 words per minute) with numerous adjectives, adverbs and complicated syntax (Albert 1981; Obler and Albert 1984, 1985). They tend to be redundant, repetitive and include commentary on what they are saying. There is also frequent personalization and use of judgmental words (e.g. *unfortunately*). If a client displays problems with verbal productivity, reduced phrase length, articulation

difficulty, grammatical errors or paraphasias, these observations may reflect an organically based language disorder that may hinder valid memory testing and require further investigation.

MEMORY ASSESSMENT BATTERIES

It is beyond the scope of this chapter to provide a detailed description of every available memory test (for test descriptions, see Lezak 1995). Rather, this section will focus on the reliability, validity and normative data of memory tests commonly used with elderly persons. Memory instruments without psychometric data relevant to the elderly are not reviewed. Table 16.1 summarizes the available normative and psychometric information for each test.

Wechsler Memory Scales (WMS/WMS-R/WMS-III)

Normative data

The original WMS (Wechsler 1945) has a long clinical history, but since the revised editions (WMS-R; Wechsler 1987; WMS-III; Wechsler 1997) are superior in many ways (D'Elia et al. 1989; Chelune et al. 1990; Bowden and Bell 1992), this section will focus on them. There are two elderly normative samples for the WMS-R. The original normative sample provided in the manual (Wechsler 1987) extends to persons 74 years of age and the Mayo's Older American Normative Studies (MOANS; Ivnik et al. 1992b) sample provides normative information for persons 56–94 years old.

For elderly persons, the original normative sample is divided into age ranges of 55 to 64 ($N=54$), 65 to 69 ($N=55$) and 70 to 74 years ($N=50$), with approximately equal numbers of males and females in each age group. The sample was designed to be representative of the USA population according to the 1980 US Census in terms of age, race, education and geographical region. All age groups also had an average IQ, based on either the full WAIS-R or a four-subtest short form.

The recently published MOANS (Ivnik et al. 1992a,b) elderly sample is comprised of 441 normal volunteers selected to be representative of elderly in Olmstead County, Minnesota. The majority are Caucasian (99%) and most have at least a high school education (88%). Normative tables were developed using overlapping,

Table 16.1. *Summary of normative and psychometric data*

Test	Normative sample size	Age range	Education range	Adequacy of Psychometric data	
				Test–retest stability[a]	Validity[b]
Wechsler Memory Scale-Revised:					
Manual	316	16–74	0–13+	*Good* – Summary Indexes, Logical Memory I and II, Digit and Visual Span, Visual Reproduction II *Fair* – Visual Paired Assoc. I and II, Verbal Paired Assoc I, Visual Reproduction *Poor* – Verbal Paired Assoc II	Good
Ivnik et al. 1992a	441	56–94	0–18+	Not provided	Not provided
Giuliano et al. 1994	113	55–98	<11	Not provided	Not provided
Wechsler Memory Scale-III					
Technical Manual (Weschler 1997)	1250	16–89	0–16+	*Good* – Logical Memory, Verbal Paired Associates I, Auditory Immediate and Delayed, Immediate General, and Working memory *Fair* – All other primary subtest and index scores	Preliminary data is good
Rivermead Behavioural Memory Test:					
Test manual	118	16–69	Not provided	Good	Preliminary data is good
Cockburn and Smith 1989	119	70–94	9.5[c]		
Memory Assessment Scale:					
Manual	843	18–70+	0–13+	Summary indexes – good, Most subtests – good, except Verbal and Visual Span, List Recall, and Immediate Visual Recognition which have fair stability	Preliminary data is good
California Verbal Learning Test:					
Manual	273	17–80	13.83 ± 2.7[c]	61% of the scores have poor stability over a 1 year period	Good
Paolo et al. (1997)	212	53–94	8–20	Not provided	Not provided
Rey Auditory Verbal Learning Test:					
see Table 16.2 for norms	—	—	—	Poor to fair	Good
Selective Reminding Test:					
Ruff et al. 1988	392	16–70	0–16+	Fair	Good
Masur et al. 1989	360	75–85	0–12+	*Good* – Sum Recall, Long term retrieval, Consistent retrieval *Fair* – Short term retrieval, Consistent long term storage *Poor* – Intrusions	Not provided
Schmidt et al. 1992	420	20–79	0–16+	Not provided	Not provided

Table 16.1. (*cont.*)

Test	Normative sample size	Age range	Education range	Adequacy of Psychometric data	
				Test–retest stability[a]	Validity[b]
Fuld Object Memory Test:					
Giuliano et al. 1994	133	55–98	<11	Not provided	Good
Fuld et al. 1990	474	75–85	0–12+	Not provided	Not provided
Benton Visual Retention Test:					
Manual	185	60–89	13.5[c]	Not provided	Good
Robertson-Tchabo et al. 1989	1643	20–89	Not provided	Not provided	Not provided
Youngjohn et al. 1993	1128	17–84	12–25	Poor (Youngjohn et al. 1992a)	Not provided
Rey Complex Figure:					
Meyers and Meyers 1995a	601	18–89	Not provided	Fair to good	Preliminary data is adequate
Meyers and Meyers 1995a; Census matched	394	18–89	13.9±2.5[c]	Fair to good	Same as above
Spreen and Strauss 1991	37	50–85	13.2[c]	Poor	Adequate
Berry and Carpenter 1992	60	68±8.5	15±3.1[c]	Not provided	Not provided
Boone et al. 1993	91	45–83	14.5±2.5[c]	Not provided	Not provided
Continuous Visual Memory Test:					
Manual	310	18–91	13.9[c]	*Good* – Total Score and d-Prime *Fair* – Delayed Recognition	Questionable for the elderly

Notes:

[a] Good is: 0.80, fair: 0.60–0.79, poor: 0.59 or below.

[b] Validity judgments are based on research concerning the test's ability to distinguish normal persons from those with memory impairment in general.

[c] Average age or education, rather than range. Number following is the standard deviation, if provided.

mid-point age ranges. Such a procedure maximizes sample size and provides the broadest possible normative base for each midpoint age. The sample sizes range from 53 subjects for persons 83 years and older (midpoint age=88), to 178 subjects for persons 68–78 years old (midpoint age=73). The MOANS norms extend the clinical usefulness of the WMS-R to the very old, but they may not be appropriate for persons with limited formal education and for nonwhites.

To address the lack of normative information for elderly persons with lower levels of education (i.e. less than 11 years), Giuliano et al. (1994) collected data on 133 non-demented, community-dwelling volunteers from rural counties in central Virginia. The sample consisted of 105 females and 28 males, of whom 69 are African-Americans and 64 are Caucasians. Means for age and education are

76.5 years (SD=7.9) and 6.7 years (SD=2.1), respectively. Means and standard deviations by age and education are provided for the immediate and delayed recall trials of the Logical Memory and Visual Reproduction subtests. The sample size per group is small with the largest cell containing only 15 subjects. As the cell sizes are small and the sample it is not representative of elderly persons in general, caution must be used when interpreting scores from this sample. Nevertheless, this study is an important step in the process of providing more adequate normative data for elderly persons.

Psychometric properties

The internal consistency reliabilities of the WMS-R subtests for elderly persons range from 0.27 for Figural Memory to 0.92 for Digit Span. Only the Digit Span subtest meets the recommended minimum cut-off of 0.80 (Anastasi 1988; Sattler 1988) for tests used in clinical decision making. The summary Index scores, except the Visual Memory Index ($r=0.69$), all meet this minimum criterion for ages 65 and older. Test-retest stability for the summary indexes over 4–6 weeks for persons 70–74 years old was adequate and ranged from 0.80 to 0.93; however, for subtests, test-retest stability for this oldest group was adequate ($r=0.80$ or above) for only six out of 17 subtests. As the time interval between testings increases, the stability coefficients will likely decrease. Ivnik et al. (1995) reported test-retest coefficients for WMS-R summary indexes that were 10–20 points lower than those in the WMS-R manual for elderly persons retested after an average of 3.7 years. From a clinical standpoint, low stability means that relatively large differences are needed in order to conclude that a change in score on retest is beyond measurement error and thus, reflects an actual alteration in memory performance (Atkinson 1991; Mittenberg et al. 1991).

Numerous factor analytical studies of the WMS-R have been conducted, with most supporting an attention/concentration factor and a general memory component (Wechsler 1987; Bornstein and Chelune 1988; Roid et al. 1988). A recent confirmatory factor analysis using the WMS-R standardization sample found support for three factors consisting of attention/concentration, immediate memory and delayed memory (Burton et al. 1993). A factor analysis across three different age groups from a clinical sample revealed a tendency for visual memory tests to load on a verbal factor with increasing age (Bornstein and Chelune 1989), which suggests that older individuals may rely more on verbal strategies in the recall of 'nonverbal' or spatial material. Overall, there is good support for an attention-concentration factor and a memory factor, but evidence for separate verbal and visual memory factors in normal persons is tenuous.

Many studies support the validity of the WMS-R subtests and indexes in the detection of memory impairment. WMS-R subtests and indexes differentiate normal persons from individuals with AD, Huntington's disease (HD), Parkinson's disease (PD), alcoholic Korsakoff's syndrome and multiple sclerosis (Butters et al. 1988; Fischer 1988; Tröster et al. 1995). The subtests have also been found useful in distinguishing among memory impairments associated with different neurodegenerative diseases (Chapter 18). Butters et al. (1988) reported that the WMS-R is not only useful in differentiating demented patients from amnesics, but that savings scores (i.e. percent retained

on delayed recall) for the Logical Memory and Visual Reproduction subtests distinguish AD from HD subjects. Tröster et al. (1993) evaluated Logical Memory and Visual Reproduction savings scores among AD and HD patients with mild and moderate degrees of dementia. Not only did each patient group perform more poorly than their respective control group, but the moderately demented subjects were significantly impaired relative to the mildly demented group, which suggests that the savings scores are sensitive to the progression of memory impairment.

While the WMS-R is a vast improvement over the original WMS, it has several psychometric weaknesses. The original normative sample is small. Although the MOANS sample is larger, it is not representative of elderly persons in general. The reliability for most subtests is poor, yielding large errors of measurement, which suggests that the WMS-R provides only an approximate estimate of overall memory functions (Elwood 1991). The latter observation also suggests that confidence intervals be used when conveying results from the WMS-R. Finally, the multidimensional structure of the WMS-R Index scores is not adequately supported. (*See also* Psychological Corporation 1997; and Weschler 1997 for a substantial revision of WMS-R.)

Rivermead Behavioural Memory Test (RBMT)

The RBMT (Wilson et al. 1985, 1991) was developed to detect impairment of everyday memory functions. Tasks include remembering a name, an appointment and a newspaper article; finding a hidden object; recognizing faces and remembering a route. RBMT norms are based on 118 subjects from 16 to 69 years of age. Elderly norms (Cockburn and Smith 1989) consist of 119 community-dwelling persons ranging from 70 to 94 years of age with an average educational level of 9.5 years. Inter-rater reliability is excellent with 100% agreement and parallel-form reliability is adequate for the complete form (all *r*s more than 0.82). Test-retest stability for the complete form is good ($r=0.85$), but the retest interval was not reported (Wilson et al. 1989). The RBMT has adequate validity in distinguishing normal persons from those with cerebral dysfunction (Wilson et al. 1989) and in detecting mild and moderate dementia (Huppert and Beardsall 1993).

Memory Assessment Scales (MAS)

The MAS (Williams 1991) is an individually administered battery of tasks developed to assess three areas of memory: (1) attention, concentration and short-term memory;

(2) learning and immediate memory; and (3) delayed recall. Normative data for elderly persons is limited. The normative sample described in the manual consists of 190 persons between 60–69 years of age and 156 persons aged 70 years or older. Age and education adjusted norms as well as census corrected norms are included in the manual.

Psychometric properties

No test-retest information for elderly persons is available. Nevertheless, the manual reports generally good stability coefficients that range from 0.70 to 0.95 for subtests and from 0.85 to 0.86 for summary scales, for 30 subjects (mean age=42 years) retested after 6 months.

Unfortunately, little research with the MAS has been conducted on elderly persons. Preliminary data reported in the manual suggest that the MAS subtests and summary scores are sensitive to closed head injury, stroke, and AD. For instance, persons with left hemisphere lesions performed worse than patients with right hemisphere lesions on verbal memory tests, while patients with right hemisphere lesions performed worse on visual memory tasks. Persons with AD scored at least one standard deviation below the average of normal persons on every summary score and they tended to score lower than those with closed head injury or stroke. Although these preliminary studies are encouraging, additional research is needed prior to the routine use of the MAS with elderly persons.

INDIVIDUAL MEMORY TESTS

California Verbal Learning Test (CVLT)

The CVLT (Delis et al. 1987) quantifies numerous components of verbal learning and memory, including different learning strategies, processes and errors that subjects may display. Many of these indices allow quantification of memory constructs derived from cognitive neuroscience. For example, how subjects organize material that they are learning provides information concerning their encoding strategies. The CVLT provides measures of learning strategies through the semantic- and serial-clustering scores. Semantic clustering is an active and efficient learning/encoding strategy so that semantic clustering scores indicate the extent to which a subject has identified the categories represented within the word list, has learned to associate the category name with the instances on the list and can retrieve the category names during recall. Serial clustering is less effective for recalling words than is seman-

tic clustering and the serial clustering score reveals the extent to which an examinee recalled the words in the order in which they were presented. With the semantic- and serial-clustering scores, the CVLT can document not only the presence of a memory problem, but also identify the deficient learning strategy that may contribute to poor performance. In addition, the CVLT assesses free recall, cued recall and recognition, allowing for inferences about the presence of encoding, storage and/or retrieval deficits.

Psychometric properties.

The CVLT normative sample consists of 104 males and 169 females ranging in age from 17 to 80 years. Means for age and education are 58.93 years (SD=15.35) and 13.83 years (SD=2.70), respectively. Information regarding the racial composition of the standardization sample is not provided. Normative data are provided for seven age groups separately for males and females, but no information concerning the sample size of these groups is provided. Paolo et al. (1997) recently extended the CVLT norms using 212 healthy elderly persons ranging from 53 to 94 years of age (M=70.58 years; SD=6.98). Average education was relatively high with an average of 14.92 years (SD=2.56). Ninety-eight percent of the sample is Caucasian and 93% are right-handed. The normative information is provided through overlapping cell tables that maximizes sample size and clinical utility of the information. In addition, norms are presented for additional CVLT measures, including rate of forgetting (percentage retained) and the proportions of intrusion and perseverative errors to words recalled. Other normative data has been published but these are for younger persons with average ages of 38.8 years (Otto et al. 1994) and 29.1 years (Wiens et al. 1994). Internal consistency reliability ranges from 0.70 to 0.92 and test-retest stability for 21 normal adults retested 1 year later ranges from 0.12 to 0.79.

The construct validity of the multiple indexes assessed by the CVLT has been generally supported through factor analytical studies (Delis et al. 1988; Wiens et al. 1994). Clinical investigations have demonstrated the validity of the CVLT in identifying verbal learning and memory deficits in persons with AD, HD and PD (Kramer et al. 1989; Delis et al. 1991a; Bondi et al. 1994; Buytenhuijs et al. 1994; Köhler 1994), multiple sclerosis (Kessler et al. 1992) and human immunodeficiency virus (HIV) infection (Peavy et al. 1994).

The quantification of numerous verbal learning and memory processes and the provision of good validity

Table 16.2. *Summary of Rey Auditory Verbal Learning Test normative samples*[a]

Sample	Gender	Age group (years)	N	Average		Recognition Test
				Age	Education	
Bleecker et al. 1988	Male	50–59	20	55	13	50-word list
		60–69	23	65	13	No delay
		70–79	18	74	15	
		80–89	11	83	18	
	Female	50–59	22	55	14	
		60–69	29	65	14	
		70–79	29	74	15	
		80–89	13	84	15	
Geffen et al. 1990	Male	50–59	11	56	12	50-word list
		60–69	10	66	10	20 min delay
		70+	10	77	12	
	Female	59–59	9	58	12	
		60–69	12	63	10	
		70+	10	74	11	
Mitrushina et al. 1991	N/A	57–65	28	63	14	Story
		66–70	45	68	14	10 min delay
		71–75	57	73	15	
		76–85	26	79	13	
Savage and Gouvier 1992	Male	50–59	9	N/A	≥12	Story
		60–69	9	N/A	≥12	30 min delay
		70–76	10	N/A	≥12	
	Female	50–59	10	N/A	≥12	
		60–69	10	N/A	≥12	
		70–76	9	N/A	≥12	
MOANS[b] Ivnik et al. 1992b	N/A	56–66	143	61	N/A	30-word list
		59–69	168	64	N/A	30 min delay
		62–72	182	67	N/A	
		65–75	194	70	N/A	
		68–78	214	73	N/A	
		71–81	203	76	N/A	
		74–84	196	79	N/A	
		77–87	168	82	N/A	
		80–90	131	85	N/A	
		83+	98	88	N/A	

Notes:

N/A: not available.

[a] Only age groups for elderly persons are summarized. Some of the studies have normative data for younger persons not presented in this table.

[b] For the MOANS norms, the age provided is actually the midpoint age for the corresponding age group.

information, are major strengths of the CVLT. In addition, an alternate form of CVLT, which should be useful in retest situations, has been developed (Delis et al. 1991b); however, the reliability of many scores is below that suggested for tests used in clinical decision making and additional, demographically representative normative data would improve the clinical utility of this promising test.

Rey Auditory Verbal Learning Test (RAVLT)

The RAVLT (Rey 1964) is a brief, easily administered measure of verbal learning and memory similar to the CVLT. The RAVLT provides measures of registration, verbal learning, overall verbal memory functioning, immediate and delayed recall and recognition. Several RAVLT norms are available for elderly persons and characteristics of these normative samples are summarized in Table 16.2. Generally, the normative samples consist of well-educated Caucasians. The test scores provided for each sample, and the method of test administration, differ slightly across the studies. For instance, the recognition trial may be a 30-item word list, a 50-item word list or in story format. Delayed recall intervals range from none to 30 minutes. Selection of RAVLT norms must therefore consider the demographic characteristics of the patient and the test administration method employed. A recently published manual (Schmidt 1996) is helpful in this regard as it characterizes the various normative samples and also provides compilations of normative data for a variety of alternative test forms.

Test-retest stability for the RAVLT in elderly persons has been reported across three separate testing periods. Mitrushina and Satz (1991) reported stability coefficients ranging from 0.41 to 0.79 for different RAVLT scores over a 1-year interval. All stability coefficients are below the minimum suggested criterion of 0.80 for tests used in clinical decision making. The validity of the RAVLT in detecting memory impairment has been demonstrated in persons with AD (Bigler et al. 1989; Mitrushina et al. 1994; Tierney et al. 1994), PD (Tierney et al. 1994), AIDS (Ryan et al. 1992; Mitrushina et al. 1994) and closed head injury (Bigler et al. 1989). The pattern of performance among AD and PD patients reveals that persons with AD evidence problems with all aspects of memory (i.e. encoding, storage and retrieval), while persons with PD demonstrate a retrieval deficit. The latter is suggested by relatively poor free recall, but adequate scores on recognition.

Selective Reminding Test (SRT)

The SRT (Buschke 1973; Buschke and Fuld 1974) is a free recall test in which the patient is asked to learn and remember a list of 10–15 common nouns; after each recall attempt, the person is reminded only of the items that they did not recall. Ruff et al. (1988) provide age- (16–70 years old) and education- (12 or less, 13–15, and 16 or more years) corrected norms for a 12-item list presented for 12 trials. The total sample consisted of 392 normal, healthy subjects with groups ranging from 30 to 36 persons with approximately equal numbers of men and women in each group; 95% of the sample was Caucasian. Women tended to perform better than men and scores tended to be higher for well-educated and younger persons. Test-retest reliability for 141 subjects (based on alternate forms administered 6 months apart) ranged from 0.66 to 0.73. Youngjohn et al. (1992a) assessed the stability of a computerized version of the SRT over a 21-day interval in 115 normal persons (mean age=49 years) and reported test-retest coefficients of 0.64 to 0.74.

Masur et al. (1989) provided normative information for 360 healthy elderly ranging in age from 75 to 85 years old (M=80 years; SD=3). Sixty-two percent of this sample was female and 92% was Caucasian. Delayed recall was tested after a 5-minute period of interference that consisted of a category verbal fluency task. This delay period differs from the 1-hour delay employed by Ruff et al. (1988). Test-retest stability over a 2-hour interval ranged from 0.42 to 0.92 in a sample of 16 persons with AD. Schmidt et al. (1992) presented normative data for 420 subjects, aged 20–79 years, for a 15-item, 5-trial version of the SRT. Approximately equal numbers of males and females were included in six 10-year age groups, except for persons 70–79 years old, where females outnumbered males (45 versus 25). No information concerning the sample's racial composition or the delay interval was presented.

Masur et al. (1989) found the SRT to have sensitivity of 80% and specificity of 95% in persons with AD relative to healthy elderly. In addition, Masur et al. (1990) reported that the *sum of recall* and *delayed recall* scores were the most useful in predicting the development of dementia, demonstrating specificity of 86% and 88%, respectively and sensitivities of 47% and 46%, respectively. The low sensitivities suggest that persons who may develop dementia can still perform adequately on the SRT a year or two before the cognitive loss becomes clinically apparent.

Paulsen et al. (1995) utilized a 10-item, 6-trial version of the SRT and reported good discrimination between normal subjects and persons with AD or HD. The SRT was not useful for differentiating AD from HD. Hart et al. (1987) reported that *total recall*, *storage* and *recognition* scores from the SRT were useful for distinguishing mild AD from patients with depression.

The SRT, although a useful memory test, may be difficult or frustrating for some older persons. The development of SRT short forms (Smith et al. 1995) may minimize this disadvantage. Parallel forms are also available for repeat testing (Hannay and Levin 1985; Ruff et al. 1988; Masur et al. 1989; Deptula et al. 1990). Given the many available versions of the SRT, clinicians must be careful to select normative data appropriate to the test version they are using.

Fuld Object Memory Evaluation (FOME)

The FOME (Fuld 1981) was developed specifically for persons 70 years and older and to be useful with nursing home and community residents. Patients are asked to remember 10 common objects that they identify tactually and visually prior to the first recall trial. Five recall trials are administered, separated by 30 or 60 seconds of distraction. Selective reminding is provided at the end of each recall trial. Normative data provided in the FOME manual consists of small groups of persons 70–79 years and 80–89 years old (Fuld 1981). Giuliano et al. (1994) present additional norms for elderly persons with low education levels. The FOME has been found useful for differentiating both dementia and depression from healthy aging (La Rue et al. 1986). A short form of the FOME, using one immediate recall trial and a 10-minute delay and recognition trial, has been normed on 474 persons, 75–85 years old (Fuld et al. 1990). This sample is two-thirds female and predominantly Caucasian. The short form has utility comparable to the SRT in predicting the development of dementia over a span of 1–2 years (Fuld et al. 1990).

Benton Visual Retention Test (BVRT)

The BVRT (Sivan 1992) evaluates visual memory, visual perception and visuo-constructive abilities. There are three, roughly equivalent, alternate forms, each comprised of 10 unique designs and four different administration methods. The most common administration consists of having the subject view each design for 10 seconds and then immediately reproduce it from memory. The normative

data for elderly provided in the manual consists of means and standard deviations for persons 60–89 years of age, with sample sizes ranging from eight to 62 subjects. Robertson-Tchabo and Arenberg (1989) provide normative information for number of errors (i.e. means, standard deviations and frequency distributions) by gender and education for ages 20–89 years. Sample sizes for the elderly age groups range from 9 to 123 subjects. More recently, Youngjohn et al. (1993) presented age- and education-corrected normative information for 464 males and 664 females (mean age=59 years) that were well-educated (mean of 16 years).

Inter-rater reliability for the *number correct* and *number of errors* scores is high with coefficients of at least 0.94. Test-retest reliability coefficients over a 21-day interval for a young (mean age=49 years) and well-educated (mean education=16 years) sample of 115 persons were 0.53 for *number of errors* and 0.57 for *number correct*. These stability coefficients are poor considering the short retest interval. The BVRT is reported to be valid for the detection of memory impairment associated with dementia (Eslinger et al. 1985; Youngjohn et al. 1992b).

Rey Complex Figure (RCF)

The RCF (Rey 1941) was designed to assess visuospatial constructional ability and visual memory. Administration involves having the subject copy the complex figure, then without prior warning, reproduce it from memory. Some investigators give both immediate and delayed recall trials, others only delayed recall trials. The delayed recall intervals range from 3 to 45 minutes. Normative data provided in the manual (Meyers and Meyers 1995a) is based on 601 persons, 18–89 years of age. No information is provided concerning the sample's educational, racial or gender characteristics. The sample sizes for elderly age groups range from 15 (ages 80–89 years) to 49 (ages 70–74 years). A smaller sample of 394 subjects was used to provide US Census age-matched normative data. The average education for this Census age-matched group was 13.91 (SD=2.48). The administration method utilized for this normative sample consists of four separate tasks: (1) Copy, (2) recall following a 3-minute delay, (3) recall after 30 minutes and (4) recognition. The normative sample described in the manual is clearly the largest, but other normative information has been presented. Spreen and Strauss (1991) provide means and standard deviations for 13 persons 60–69 years old and 10 persons 70 years and older. Berry and Carpenter (1992) provide data for four small groups of well-educated persons, with an average age of 68 years, for four different delayed recall intervals (i.e. 15, 30, 45 and 60 minutes). Boone et al. (1993) provide means and standard deviations separately for three age groups (45–59, 60–69 and 70–83 years) and by WAIS-R Full Scale IQ. Their sample consists of 34 men and 57 women with an average education of 15 years; 78% were Caucasian.

Unfortunately, there are numerous administration and scoring methods for the RCF (Stern et al. 1994; Meyers and Meyers 1995b; Berry and Carpenter 1992; Duley et al. 1993; Hamby et al. 1993), making comparisons across studies and choice of the appropriate normative data difficult. The recent publication of the updated manual (Meyers and Meyers, 1995a) may permit greater standardization of administration and scoring procedures.

Psychometric properties

The inter-rater reliability across the different scoring methods is generally high and typically greater than 0.90. Test-retest stability for a small group ($n=12$) of young persons (mean age = 33.9 years) over a 6-month interval is generally adequate, ranging from 0.76 to 0.89. Temporal stability over a 1 year period for older adults (mean age 65 years) was below the 0.80 criterion, ranging from 0.18 for copy to 0.59 for a 30 minute delayed recall (Berry et al. 1991).

Although the RCF has been found useful in detecting visual-constructional and visual-memory impairment in persons with head injury, psychiatric disturbance and PD (Grossman et al. 1993; Meyers and Meyers 1995a), the poor temporal stability for elderly persons and the fact that many normal and high functioning older persons find the task difficult (Van Gorp et al. 1990; La Rue 1992), suggests that the RCF be used cautiously with older adults.

Continuous Visual Memory Test (CVMT)

The CVMT (Trahan and Larrabee 1988) consists of three tasks: (1) an 'acquisition' task which tests recognition memory by requiring subjects to discriminate 'new' versus 'old' (repeated) complex visual designs, (2) a 30-minute delayed recognition task that requires the subject to recognize the 'old' stimuli from perceptually similar distractors and (3) a visual discrimination task which serves to distinguish visual memory problems from visual discrimina-

tion deficits. The standardization sample consists of 310 normal, healthy adults ranging from 18 to 91 years of age. Most of the subjects (72%) were 49 years of age or younger.

There is little test reliability and validity information for elderly persons. Test-retest stability coefficients based on 12 persons retested after seven days ranged from 0.76 to 0.85. Although the coefficients are adequate, the sample size and retest interval are completely inadequate for a test used in clinical decision making. As an age-related decline in CVMT scores has been reported (Trahan et al. 1990), the adequacy of the normative data for persons 60 years and older has been questioned (Hall et al. 1995). In a preliminary study of healthy normal elderly, Hall et al. (1996) found that 7–63% of persons 60 years and older actually scored within the impaired range using the age-corrected cut-off scores provided in the CVMT manual. These authors suggested that the CVMT may not be an appropriate measure of nonverbal memory in older adults. The latter conclusion, in conjunction with the inadequate stability data, suggests that the CVMT performance of elderly persons be interpreted conservatively.

DETECTING CHANGES IN MEMORY FUNCTIONS

The ideal method for detecting change, or more specifically deterioration in memory functions, is to compare an individual's current and premorbid test scores. Unfortunately, premorbid test data are rarely available and alternative methods are required to *estimate* premorbid memory function. One such method uses current scores from neuropsychological tests relatively resistant to brain dysfunction, alone or in combination with patient demographic data, to statistically estimate premorbid functioning. For example, Schlosser and Ivison (1989) developed regression equations (using word reading ability and age as predictors) to estimate premorbid scores on the Australian version of the Wechsler Memory Scale (Ivison 1977). Unfortunately, this method has not been cross-validated and alternative, objective methods for estimating premorbid memory functions have not been published.

Although premorbid memory test results are rarely available, it is quite common to have repeat memory evaluation data available for patients with known or suspected dementia. Several methods are available for determining if the observed changes in two test scores are meaningful. Statistical methods include the use of the standard errors of measurement and prediction (Lord and Novik 1968), the reliable change index based on the standard error of the difference between two scores (Jacobson and Truax 1991; Chelune et al. 1993), or hierarchical linear modeling (HLM; Bryk and Raudenbush 1992). A clinical method for deciding whether a test score change is meaningful depends on 'the rarity' with which test-retest differences of a given magnitude occur in normal samples (Matarazzo and Herman 1984).

The HLM method is relatively new and has demonstrated usefulness in the detection of improvement over time; however, it cannot be recommended for the detection of possible memory decline until it is further developed and refined (Speer and Greenbaum 1995). The other statistical methods are based on the standard error of measurement and provide a way of determining whether a score obtained on retest represents a change (i.e. gain or loss) not attributable to measurement error. Atkinson (1991) and Mittenberg et al. (1991) provide tables, based on the standard error of measurement for the WMS-R standardization sample, that can be used to determine if a given WMS-R score represents a meaningful change from one obtained earlier.

Most memory test manuals do not contain tables that provide cut-off scores for what constitutes an 'abnormal' (i.e. unusual) difference between scores, but most test manuals do provide standard error of measurement statistics or reliability coefficients and standard deviations from which the standard error can be computed. As such, clinicians can compute the appropriate standard error of measurement for most memory test scores and these can be used as a rough guide in detecting meaningful change upon repeat testing.

CONCLUSIONS

This chapter discussed the visual, auditory and language changes associated with aging that may influence the reliability and validity of memory assessment and suggested brief screening methods that can be used to assess whether such changes may significantly impact the evaluation of memory. The chapter then summarized the reliability, validity and normative data for commonly used memory tests. Most of the memory tests discussed have adequate validity in detecting memory impairments in elderly persons. At this time the RCF and CVMT should be used with caution in elderly persons pending further investigation of their reliability and validity in the elderly population. The test-retest stability of most of the memory tests falls below the recommended minimum cut-off for tests used in clinical decision making, which suggests that relatively large test-retest differences are needed in order to conclude that a significant change in memory functions has occurred over time. As repeated assessments are commonly used to evaluate memory deterioration due to disease, good test-retest normative data are sorely needed. None of the memory tests reviewed, however, provides adequate information in this regard. Current methods available for assisting clinicians in detecting significant change on retesting were briefly discussed.

The normative data available for elderly persons are generally poor for many of the most commonly used memory tests. The recent co-development of the WAIS-III and WMS-III, and the MOANS project are notable exceptions. It is hoped that these projects represent the future of norm devleopment in that they clearly demonstrate the importance of adequate normative information for elderly persons. More representative elderly normative data is still needed for many commonly used memory assessment devices.

REFERENCES

Albert, M.L. 1981. Changes in language with aging. *Seminars in Neurology.* 1: 43–46.

Anastasi, A. 1988. *Psychological testing,* 6th ed. New York: Macmillan.

Atkinson, L. 1991. Three standard errors of measurement and the Wechsler Memory Scale – Revised. *Psychological Assessment.* 3: 136–138.

Berry, D.T.R. and Carpenter, G.S. 1992. Effect of four different delay periods on recall of the Rey-Osterrieth Complex Figure by older persons. *Clinical Neuropsychologist.* 6: 80–84.

Berry, D.T.R., Allen, R.S. and Schmitt, F.A. 1991. Rey-Osterrieth Complex Figure: Psychometric characteristics in a geriatric sample. *Clinical Neuropsychologist*. 5: 143–153.

Bigler, E.D., Rosa, L., Schultz, F., Hall, S. and Harris, J. 1989. Rey-Auditory Verbal Learning and Rey-Osterrieth Complex Figure Design performance in Alzheimer's disease and closed head injury. *Journal of Clinical Psychology*. 24: 277–280.

Bleecker, M.L., Bolla-Wilson, K., Agnew, J. and Meyers, D.A. 1988. Age-related sex differences in verbal memory. *Journal of Clinical Psychology*. 44: 403–411.

Bondi, M.W., Monsch, A.U., Galasko, D., Butters, N., Salmon, D.P. and Delis, D.C. 1994. Preclinical cognitive markers of dementia of the Alzheimer's type. *Neuropsychology*. 8: 374–384.

Boone, K.B., Lesser, I.M., Hill-Gutierrez, E., Berman, N.G. and D'Elia, L.F. 1993. Rey-Osterrieth Complex Figure performance in healthy, older adults: Relationship to age, education and IQ. *Clinical Neuropsychologist*. 7: 22–28.

Bornstein, R.A. and Chelune, G.J. 1988. Factor structure of the Wechsler Memory Scale – Revised. *Clinical Neuropsychologist*. 2: 107–115.

Bornstein, R.A. and Chelune, G.J. 1989. Factor structure of the Wechsler Memory Scale – Revised in relation to age and educational level. *Archives of Clinical Neuropsychology*. 4: 15–24.

Bowden S.C. and Bell, R.C. 1992. Relative usefulness of the WMS and WMS-R: A comment on D'Elia et al. (1989). *Journal of Clinical and Experimental Neuropsychology*. 14: 340–346.

Bryk, A.S. and Raudenbush, S.W. 1992. *Hierarchical linear models: Applications and data analysis methods*. Newbury Park, CA: Sage.

Burton, D.B., Mittenberg, W. and Burton, C.A. 1993. Confirmatory factor analysis of the Wechsler Memory Scale – Revised standardization sample. *Archives of Clinical Neuropsychology*. 8: 467–475.

Buschke, H. 1973. Selective reminding for analysis of memory and learning. *Journal of Verbal Learning and Verbal Behavior*. 12: 543–550.

Buschke, H. and Fuld, P.A. 1974. Evaluating storage, retention and retrieval in disordered memory and learning. *Neurology*. 24: 1019–1025.

Butters, N., Salmon, D.P., Cullum, C.M., Cairns, P., Tröster, A.I., Jacobs, D., Moss, M. and Cermak, L.S. 1988. Differentiation of amnesic and demented patients with the Wechsler Memory Scale – Revised. *Clinical Neuropsychologist*. 2: 133–148.

Buytenhuijs, E.L., Berger, H.J., Van Spaendonck, K.P., Horstink, M.W., Borm, G.F. and Cools, A.R. 1994. Memory and learning strategies in patients with Parkinson's disease. *Neuropsychologia*. 32: 335–342.

Chelune, G.J., Bornstein, R.A. and Prifitera, A. 1990. The Wechsler Memory Scale – Revised: Current status and applications. In *Advances in psychological assessment*, vol. 7, ed. P. McReynolds, J.C. Rosen and G.J. Chelune, pp. 65–99. New York: Plenum Press.

Chelune, G.J., Naugle, R.I., Lüders, H., Sedlak, J. and Awad, I.A. 1993. Individual change after epilepsy surgery: Practice effects and base-rate information. *Neuropsychology*. 7: 41–52.

Cockburn, J. and Smith, P.T. 1989. *Rivermead Behavioural Memory Test (Suppl. 3): Elderly people*. Reading: Thames Valley Test Company.

D'Elia, L., Satz, P. and Schretlen, D. 1989. Wechsler Memory Scale: A critical appraisal of the normative studies. *Journal of Clinical and Experimental Neuropsychology*. 11: 551–568.

Delis, D.C., Freeland, J., Kramer, J.H. and Kaplan, E. 1988. Integrating clinical assessment with cognitive neuroscience: Construct validation of the California Verbal Learning Test. *Journal of Consulting and Clinical Psychology*. 56: 123–130.

Delis, D. C., Kramer, J.H., Kaplan, E. and Ober, B.A. 1987. *The California Verbal Learning Test*. New York: The Psychological Corporation.

Delis, D.C., Massman, P.J., Butters, N., Salmon, D.P., Cermak, L.S. and Kramer, J.H. 1991a. Profiles of demented and amnesic patients on the California Verbal Learning Test: Implications for the assessment of memory disorders. *Psychological Assessment*. 3: 19–26.

Delis, D.C., Massman, P.J., Kaplan, E., McKee, R., Kramer, J.H. and Gettman, D. 1991b. Alternate form of the California Verbal Learning Test: Development and reliability. *Clinical Neuropsychologist*. 5: 154–162.

Deptula, D., Singh, R. and Goldsmith, S. 1990. Equivalence of five forms of the Selective Reminding Test in young and elderly subjects. *Psychological Reports*. 67: 1287–1295.

Duley, J.F., Wilkins, J.W., Hamby, S.L., Hopkins, D.G., Burwell, R.D. and Barry, N.S. 1993. Explicit scoring criteria for the Rey-Osterrieth and Taylor complex figures. *Clinical Neuropsychologist*. 7: 29–38.

Elwood, R.W. 1991. The Wechsler Memory Scale – Revised: Psychometric characteristics and clinical application. *Neuropsychology Review*. 2: 179–201.

Eslinger, P.J., Damasio, A.R., Benton, A.L. and VanAllen, M. 1985. Neuropsychologic detection of abnormal mental decline in older persons. *Journal of the American Medical Association*. 253: 670–674.

Fischer, J.S. 1988. Using the Wechsler Memory Scale – Revised to detect and characterize memory deficits in multiple sclerosis. *Clinical Neuropsychologist*. 2: 149–172.

Fuld, P.A. 1981. *The Fuld Object-Memory Evaluation*. Chicago: Stoelting Instrument.

Fuld, P.A., Masur, D.M., Blau, A.D., Crystal, H. and Aronson, M.K. 1990. Object-Memory evaluation for prospective detection of dementia in normal functioning elderly: Predictive and normative data. *Journal of Clinical and Experimental Neuropsychology*. 12: 520–528.

Geffen, G., Moar, K.J., O'Hanlon, A.P., Clark, C.R. and Geffen, L.B., 1990. Performance measures of 16- to 86-year-old males and females on the Auditory Verbal Learning Test. *Clinical Neuropsychologist*. 4: 45–63.

Gennis, V., Garry, P.J., Haaland, K.Y., Yeo, R.A. and Goodwin, J.S. 1991. Hearing and cognition in the elderly: New findings and a review of the literature. *Archives of Internal Medicine*. 151: 2259–2264.

Giuliano, A.J., McLain, C.A. and Marcopulos, B.A. 1994. Memory assessment in low education rural elderly (abstract). *Journal of the International Neuropsychological Society*. 1: 166.

Granick S., Kleban, M.H. and Weiss, A.D. 1976. Relationship between hearing loss and cognition in normally hearing aged persons. *Journal of Gerontology*. 31: 434–440.

Grimes, A.M., Grady, C.L., Foster, N.L., Sunderland, T. and Patronas, M.J. 1985. Central auditory function in Alzheimer's disease. *Neurology*. 35: 352–358.

Grossman, M., Carvell, S., Peltzer, L., Stern, M.B., Gollomp, S. and Hurtig, H.I. 1993. Visual constructional impairments in Parkinson's disease. *Neuropsychology*. 7: 536–547.

Hall, S., Pinkston, S.L., Szalda-Petree, A.C. and Coronis, A.R. 1996. The performance of healthy older adults on the Continuous Visual Memory Test and the Visual-Motor Integration Test: Preliminary findings. *Journal of Clinical Psychology*. 52: 449–454.

Hamby, S.L., Wilkins, J.W. and Barry, N.S. 1993. Organizational quality on the Rey-Osterrieth and Taylor Complex Figure Tests: A new scoring system. *Psychological Assessment*. 5: 27–33.

Hannay, H.J. and Levin, H.S. 1985. Selective Reminding Test: An examination of the equivalence of four forms. *Journal of Clinical and Experimental Neuropsychology*. 7: 251–263.

Hart, R.P., Kwentus, J.A., Hamer, R.M. and Taylor, J.R. 1987. Selective reminding procedure in depression and dementia. *Psychology and Aging*. 2: 111–115.

Herbst, K.G. and Humphrey, C. 1980. Hearing impairment and mental state in the elderly living at home. *British Medical Journal*. 281: 903–905

Hertzog, C. and Schear, J. M. 1989. Psychometric considerations in testing the older person. In *Testing older adults: A reference guide for geropsychological assessments*, ed. T. Hunt and C.J. Lindley, pp. 24–50. Austin, Texas: Pro-Ed.

Huppert, F.A. and Beardsall, L. 1993. Prospective memory impairment as an early indicator of dementia. *Journal of Clinical and Experimental Neuropsychology*. 15: 805–821.

Ivison, D. 1977. The Wechsler Memory Scale: Preliminary findings toward an Australian standardization. *Australian Psychologist*. 12: 303–312.

Ivnik, R.J., Malec, J.F., Smith, G.E., Tangalos, E.G., Petersen, R.C., Kokmen, E. and Kurland, L.T. 1992a. Mayo's Older American Normative Studies: WMS-R norms for ages 56 to 94. *The Clinical Neuropsychologist*. 6 (Suppl.): 49–82.

Ivnik, R.J., Malec, J.F., Smith, G.E., Tangalos, E.G., Petersen, R.C., Kokmen, E. and Kurland, L.T. 1992b. Mayo's Older American Normative Studies: Updated AVLT norms for ages 56 to 97. *The Clinical Neuropsychologist*. 6 (Suppl.): 83–104.

Ivnik, R.J., Smith, G.E., Malec, J.F., Petersen, R.C. and Tangalos, E.G. 1995. Long-term stability and intercorrelations of cognitive abilities in older persons. *Psychological Assessment*. 7: 155–161.

Jacobson, N.S. and Truax, P. 1991. Clinical significance: A statistical approach to defining meaningful change in psychotherapy research. *Journal of Consulting and Clinical Psychology*. 59: 12–19.

Jones, D.A., Victor, C.R. and Vetter, N.J. 1984. Hearing difficulty and its psychological implications for the elderly. *Journal of Epidemiology and Community Health*. 38: 75–78.

Kessler, H.R., Cohen, R.A., Lauer, K. and Kausch, D.F. 1992. The relationship between disability and memory dysfunction in multiple sclerosis. *International Journal of Neuroscience*. 62: 17–24.

Köhler, S. 1994. Quantitative characterization of verbal learning deficits in patients with Alzheimer's disease. *Journal of Clinical and Experimental Neuropsychology*. 16: 749–753.

Kramer, J.H., Levin, B.E., Brandt, J. and Delis, D.C. 1989. Differentiation of Alzheimer's, Huntington's and Parkinson's disease patients on the basis of verbal learning characteristics. *Neuropsychology*. 3: 111–120.

La Rue, A. 1992. *Aging and neuropsychological assessment*. New York: Plenum Press.

La Rue, A., D'Elia, L.F., Clark, E.O., Spar, J.E. and Jarvik, L.F. 1986. Clinical tests of memory in dementia, depression and healthy aging. *Psychology and Aging*. 1: 69–77.

Lezak, M.D. 1995. *Neuropsychological assessment*, 3rd ed. New York: Oxford University Press.

Lord, F.M. and Novik, M.R. 1968. *Statistical theories of mental test scores*. Reading , MA: Addison-Wesley.

Mader, S. 1984. Hearing Impairment in elderly persons. *Journal of the American Geriatrics Society*. 32: 548–553.

Masur, D.M., Fuld, P.A., Blau, A.D., Crystal, H. and Aronson, M.K. 1990. Predicting development of dementia in the elderly with the Selective Remind-ing Test. *Journal of Clinical and Experimental Neuropsychology*. 12: 529–538.

Masur, D.M., Fuld, P.A., Blau, A.D., Thal, L.J., Levin, H.S. and Aronson, M.K. 1989. Distinguishing normal and demented elderly with the Selective Reminding Test. *Journal of Clinical and Experimental Neuropsychology*. 11: 615–630.

Matarazzo, J.D. and Herman, D.O. 1984. Base rate data for the WAIS-R: Test-retest stability and VIQ-PIQ differences. *Journal of Clinical Neuropsychology*. 6: 351–366.

Meyers, J.E. and Meyers, K.R. 1995a. *Rey Complex Figure Test and Recognition Trial: Professional manual*. Odessa, FL: Psychological Assessment Resources.

Meyers, J.E. and Meyers, K.R. 1995b. Rey Complex Figure Test under four different administration procedures. *The Clinical Neuropsychologist*. 9: 63–67.

Milne, J.S. 1977. A longitudinal study of hearing loss in older people. *British Journal of Audiology*. 11: 7–14.

Mitrushina, M. and Satz, P. 1991. Effect of repeated administration of a neuropsychological battery in the elderly. *Journal of Clinical Psychology*. 47: 790–801.

Mitrushina, M., Satz, P., Chervinsky, A. and D'Elia, L. 1991. Performance of four age groups of normal elderly on the Rey Auditory-Verbal Learning Test. *Journal of Clinical Psychology*. 47: 351- 357.

Mitrushina, M., Satz, P., Drebing, C., Van Gorp, W., Mathews, A., Harker, J. and Chervinsky, A. 1994. The differential pattern of memory deficit in normal aging and dementias of different etiology. *Journal of Clinical Psychology*. 50: 246–252.

Mittenberg, W., Thompson, G.B. and Schwartz, J.A. 1991. Abnormal and reliable differences among Wechsler Memory Scale – Revised subtests. *Psychological Assessment*. 3: 492–495.

Obler, L.K. and Albert, M.L. 1984. Language in aging. In *Clinical neurology of aging*, ed. M.L. Albert, pp. 245–253. New York: Oxford University Press.

Obler, L.K. and Albert, M.L. 1985. Language skills across adulthood. In *Handbook of the psychology of aging*, 2nd ed., ed. J.E. Birren and K.W. Schaie, pp. 463–473. New York: Van Nostrand Reinhold Company.

Ohta, R.J., Carlin, M.F. and Harmon, B.M. 1981. Auditory acuity and performance on the Mental Status Questionnaire in the elderly. *Journal of the American Geriatrics Society*. 32: 476–478.

Otto, M.W., Bruder, G.E., Fava, M., Delis, D.C., Quitkin, F.M. and Rosenbaum, J.F. 1994. Norms for depressed patients for the California Verbal Learning Test: Associations with depression severity and self-report of cognitive difficulties. *Archives of Clinical Neuropsychology*. 9: 81–88.

Paolo, A.M., Tröster, A.I. and Ryan, J.J. 1997. California Verbal Learning Test: Normative data for the elderly. *Journal of Clinical and Experimental Neuropsychology*. 19: 220–234.

Paulsen, J.S., Salmon, D.P., Monsch, A.U., Butters, N., Swenson, M.R. and Bondi, M.W. 1995. Discrimination of cortical from subcortical dementias on the basis of memory and problem-solving tests. *Journal of Clinical Psychology*. 51: 48–58.

Peavy, G., Jacobs, D., Salmon, D., Butters, N., Delis, D., Taylor, M., Massman, P., Stout, J., Heindel, W., Kirson, D., Atkinson, J., Chandler, J., Grant, I. and the HNRC Group. 1994. Verbal memory performance of patients with human immunodeficiency virus infection: Evidence of subcortical dysfunction. *Journal of Clinical and Experimental Neuropsychology*. 16: 508–523.

Peters, C.A., Potter, J.F. and Scholer, S.G. 1988. Hearing impairment as a predictor of cognitive decline in dementia. *Journal of the American Geriatrics Society*. 36: 981–986.

Psychological Corporation. 1997. *WAIS-III/WMS-III Technical Manual*. San Antonio: The Psychological Corporation.

Rey, A. 1941. L'examen psychologique dans les cas d'encéphalopathie traumatique. *Archives de Psychologie*. 28: 286–340.

Rey, A. 1964. *L'examen clinique en psychologie*. Paris: Presses Universitaires de France.

Robertson-Tchabo, E.A. and Arenberg, D. 1989. Assessment of memory in older adults. In *Testing older adults: A reference guide for geropsychological assessments*, ed. T. Hunt and C. Lindley, pp. 200–231. Austin, TX: Pro-Ed.

Roid, G.H., Prifitera, A. and Ledbetter, M. 1988. Confirmatory analysis of the factor structure of the Wechsler Memory Scale – Revised. *The Clinical Neuropsychologist*. 2: 116–120.

Ruff, R.M., Light, R.H. and Quayhagen, M. 1988. Selective Reminding Tests: A normative study of verbal learning in adults. *Journal of Clinical and Experimental Neuropsychology*. 11: 539–550.

Ryan, J.J., Paolo, A.M. and Skrade, M. 1992. Rey Auditory Verbal Learning Test performance of a federal corrections sample with Acquired Immunodeficiency Syndrome. *International Journal of Neuroscience*. 64: 177–181.

Sattler, J.M. 1988. *Assessment of children*, 3rd ed. San Diego: Author.

Savage, R.M. and Gouvier, W.D. 1992. Rey Auditory-Verbal Learning Test: The effects of age and gender and norms for delayed recall and story recognition trials. *Archives of Clinical Neuropsychology*. 7: 407–414.

Schmidt, J.P, Tombaugh, T.N. and Faulkner, P. 1992. Free-recall, cued-recall and recognition procedures with three verbal memory tests: Normative data from age 20 to 79. *The Clinical Neuropsychologist*. 6: 185–200.

Schmidt, M. 1996. *Rey Auditory and Verbal Learning Test: A handbook*. Los Angeles: Western Psychological Services.

Schlosser, D. and Ivison, D. 1989. Assessing memory deterioration with the Wechsler Memory Scale, the National Adult Reading Test and the Schonell Graded Word Reading Test. *Journal of Clinical and Experimental Neuropsychology*. 11: 785–792.

Shindell, S. 1989. Assessing the visually impaired older adult. In *Testing older adults: A reference guide for geropsychological assessments*, ed.T. Hunt and C.J. Lindley, pp.135–149. Austin, TX: Pro-Ed.

Sivan, A.B. 1992. *Benton Visual Retention Test*, 5th ed. San Antonio: The Psychological Corporation.

Smith, R.L., Goode, K.T., La Marche, J.A. and Boll, T.J. 1995. Selective Reminding Test short form administration: A comparison of two through twelve trials. *Psychological Assessment*. 7: 177–182.

Snyder, L.H., Pyrek, J. and Smith, K.C. 1976. Vision and mental function of the elderly. *Gerontologist*. 16: 491–495.

Speer, D.C. and Greenbaum, P.E. 1995. Five methods for computing significant individual client change and improvement rates: Support for an individual growth curve approach. *Journal of Consulting and Clinical Psychology*. 63: 1044–1048.

Spreen, O. and Strauss, E. 1991. *A compendium of neuropsychological tests*. New York: Oxford University Press.

Stern, R.A, Singer, E.A., Duke, L.M., Singer, N.G., Morey, C.E., Daughtrey, E.W. and Kaplan, E. 1994. The Boston qualitative scoring system for the Rey-Osterrieth Complex Figure: Description and interrater reliability. *The Clinical Neuropsychologist*. 8: 309–322.

Storandt, M. and Futterman, A. 1982. Stimulus size and performance on two subtests of the Wechsler Adult Intelligence Scale by younger and older adults. *Journal of Gerontology*. 37: 602–603.

Tierney, M.C., Nores, A., Snow, W.G., Fisher, R.H., Zorzitto, M.L. and Reid, D.W. 1994. Use of the Rey Auditory Verbal Learning Test in differentiating normal aging from Alzheimer's and Parkinson's dementia. *Psychological Assessment*. 6: 129–134.

Trahan, D.E. and Larrabee, G.J. 1988. *Continuous Visual Memory Test: Professional manual*. Odessa, FL: Psychological Assessment Resources.

Trahan, D.E., Larrabee, G.J. and Quintana, J.W. 1990. Visual recognition memory in normal adults and patients with unilateral vascular lesions. *Journal of Clinical and Experimental Neuropsychology*. 12: 857–872.

Tröster, A.I., Butters, N., Salmon, D.P., Cullum, C.M., Jacobs, D., Brandt, J. and White, R.F. 1993. The diagnostic utility of savings scores: Differentiating Alzheimer's and Huntington's diseases with the Logical Memory and Visual Reproduction tests. *Journal of Clinical and Experimental Neuropsychology*. 15: 773–788.

Tröster, A.I., Stalp, L.D., Paolo, A.M., Fields, J.A. and Koller, W.C. 1995. Neuropsychological impairment in Parkinson's disease with and without depression. *Archives of Neurology*. 52: 1164–1169.

Uhlmann, R.F., Larson, E.B., Rees, T.S., Koepsell, T.D. and Duckert, L.G., 1989. Relationship of hearing impairment to dementia and cognitive dysfunction in older adults. *Journal of the American Medical Association*. 261: 1916–1919.

Van Gorp, W.G., Satz, P. and Mitrushina, M. 1990. Neuropsychological processes associated with normal aging. *Developmental Neuropsychology*. 6: 279–290.

Vernon, M. 1989. Assessment of persons with hearing disabilities. In *Testing older adults: A reference guide for geropsychological assessments*, ed. T. Hunt and C.J. Lindley, pp. 150–162. Austin, Texas: Pro-Ed.

Vesterager, V., Salomon, G. and Jagd, M. 1988. Age-related hearing difficulties. II. Psychological and sociological consequences of hearing problems: A controlled study. *Audiology*. 27: 179–192.

Wechsler, D.A. 1945. A standardized memory scale for clinical use. *Journal of Psychology*. 19: 87–95.

Wechsler, D. 1987. *Manual for the Wechsler Memory Scale – Revised*. San Antonio: The Psychological Corporation.

Wechsler, D. 1997. *The Wechsler Memory Scale – Third Edition*. San Antonio: The Psychological Coroporation.

Wiens, A.N., Tindall, A.G. and Crossen, J.R. 1994. California Verbal Learning Test: A normative data study. *The Clinical Neuropsychologist*. 8: 75–90.

Williams, J. M. 1991. *MAS: Memory Assessment Scales professional manual*. Odessa, FL: Psychological Assessment Resources.

Wilson, B.A., Cockburn, J. and Baddeley, A.D. 1991. *The Rivermead Behavioral Memory Test*, 2nd ed. Titchfield: Thames Valley Test Company.

Wilson, B.A., Cockburn, J. and Baddeley, A.D. 1985. *The Rivermead Behavioural Memory Test*. Titchfield: Thames Valley Test Company.

Wilson, B., Cockburn, J., Baddeley, A. and Hiorns, R. 1989. The development and validation of a test battery for detecting and monitoring everyday memory problems. *Journal of Clinical and Experimental Neuropsychology*. 11: 855–870.

Youngjohn, J.R., Larrabee, G.J. and Crook, T.H. 1992a. Test-retest reliability of computerized, everyday memory measures and traditional memory measures. *Clinical Neuropsychologist*. 6: 276–286.

Youngjohn, J.R., Larrabee, G.J. and Crook, T.H. 1992b. Discriminating age-associated memory impairment from Alzheimer's disease. *Psychological Assessment*. 4: 54–59.

Youngjohn, J.R., Larrabee, G.J. and Crook, T.H. 1993. New adult age- and education-correction norms for the Benton Visual Retention Test. *Clinical Neuropsychologist*. 7: 155–160.

17

The role of memory assessment in the preclinical detection of dementia

MARK W. BONDI AND ANDREAS U. MONSCH

INTRODUCTION

As the baby boom generation approaches retirement age and average life expectancy continues to rise, dementia will become an increasingly prevalent syndrome (Manton 1990; Myers 1990; Chapter 14). For example, estimates in the USA project that Alzheimer's disease (AD) will increase from its current level of approximately 4 million to more than 14 million affected individuals over the next 50 years (Khachaturian et al. 1994). Thus, neuropsychological research on dementia has increasingly focused on identifying the pattern, progression and neuropathological correlates of the cognitive deficits associated with various dementing disorders (La Rue 1992; Poon et al. 1992). These efforts have led to an increased understanding of the particular neuropsychological deficits that occur in the early stages of dementia. Furthermore, investigators have recently begun to identify cognitive changes that appear to presage the development of dementia. These recent advances in research on the neuropsychological detection of preclinical dementia, and their potential clinical implications, will be discussed in the present chapter.

PRECLINICAL DETECTION OF ALZHEIMER'S DISEASE

To date, the available epidemiological and biological evidence suggest a view of AD as a chronic disease, and the emerging picture is that of a long preclinical period of neuropathological changes prior to the appearance of the full dementia syndrome (for a discussion, see Katzman and Kawas 1994). Many of the recent attempts to identify cognitive markers of incipient AD are also consistent with the view of AD as a chronic disease.

Much like cancer or heart disease, an individual is predisposed by genetic factors, traumatic events or other un-

known factors towards entering a malignant phase which, in the case of AD, is characterized by intracellular events that lead to neuritic degeneration, the formation of neurofibrillary tangles and neuron and synapse loss (Katzman and Kawas 1994) (Figure 17.1). Over a period of time, the neural degeneration gradually reaches a level that initiates the clinical symptoms of the dementia syndrome. This framework for understanding the development of AD suggests that cognitive deficits associated with the disease also appear gradually and might be identified before the degree of neural degeneration reaches a level necessary to produce clinically diagnosable dementia (i.e. when both cognitive and functional impairments are evident, as required by both DSM and the NINCDS-ADRDA criteria).

Memory decline in early Alzheimer's disease

Although AD involves significant impairments in attention, 'executive' functions, language and visuospatial and constructional abilities, failure of recent memory is usually the most prominent feature during the early stages of the disease (Chapters 12 and 18). Accordingly, much of the neuropsychological research concerning early detection of AD has focused on learning and memory. Numerous studies have shown that measures of the ability to learn new information and retain it over time are quite sensitive in differentiating between mildly demented patients with clinically diagnosed AD and normal older adults (Storandt et al. 1984; Eslinger et al. 1985; Kaszniak et al. 1986; Bayles and Kaszniak 1987; Delis et al. 1991; Welsh et al. 1991; Petersen et al. 1994).

For example, Welsh et al. (1991) found that a delayed free recall measure on a verbal memory task was highly effective (i.e. had 90% accuracy) in distinguishing between very mildly demented patients with AD (all with MMSE scores above 24 out of 30) and elderly normal control subjects and that this measure was significantly more effective than measures of learning, confrontation naming, verbal

Figure 17.1. Chronic disease model of Alzheimer's disease. Adapted from Katzman and Kawas (1994), with permission of Raven Press.

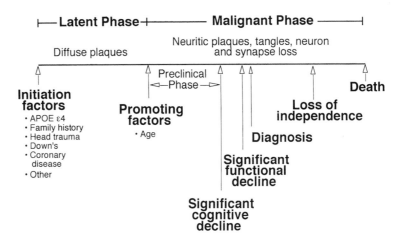

Chronic Disease Model of Alzheimer's Disease

fluency and constructional ability. Similar results have been obtained in other studies (Knopman and Ryberg 1989; Flicker et al. 1991; Morris et al. 1991; Petersen et al. 1994) and in one case (Morris et al. 1991) the effectiveness of memory measures for detecting early AD was confirmed by histopathological verification of AD at autopsy.

Although measures of learning and retention are the most effective neuropsychological indices for differentiating between mildly demented and normal elderly individuals, measures of language, 'executive' functions and constructional abilities also have some diagnostic value (Salmon et al. in press). For example, Monsch et al. (1992) compared the performances of mildly demented patients with probable AD and normal elderly control subjects on several types of verbal fluency tasks and found that the semantic category fluency task had greater than 90% sensitivity and specificity for the diagnosis of dementia. Similarly high sensitivity (94%) and specificity (87%) for the diagnosis of dementia was demonstrated for the number of categories achieved on a modified version of the Wisconsin Card Sorting Task in a study that compared the performances of mildly demented probable AD patients to normal elderly subjects (Bondi et al. 1993).

Nevertheless, the primacy and prominence of memory impairment in AD is consistent with evidence suggesting that neuropathological changes in the hippocampus and entorhinal cortex are the first and most severe to occur in the disease (Hyman et al. 1984; Braak and Braak 1991).

There is now considerable evidence from both human and animal studies that these brain structures are critical for the acquisition and retention of new information (for a review, see Squire et al. 1993). It is also possible that early involvement of these structures in AD may lead to decrements in learning and memory during a preclinical phase of AD (Katzman 1994) in which subtle cognitive changes are evident before gradual neural degeneration has spread and reached a level sufficient to produce the full clinical manifestation of the dementia syndrome.

Utility of cognitive measures in predicting the development of dementia

Although the precise length of a preclinical phase of AD is not known and may vary considerably among affected individuals, a growing body of evidence demonstrates that subtle cognitive impairments can be detected several years or more prior to the clinical diagnosis of dementia (La Rue and Jarvik 1987; Katzman et al. 1989; Fuld et al. 1990; Bondi et al. 1994, 1995; Masur et al. 1994; Linn et al. 1995). Some of the earliest evidence for this possibility was provided by La Rue and Jarvik (1980; 1987), who longitudinally studied aging twins. These investigators found that poor performance by nondemented subjects on three subtests of the Wechsler Adult Intelligence Scale (WAIS; Vocabulary, Similarities and Digit Symbol) was associated with the development of dementia some 20 years later.

The studies of La Rue and Jarvik have important

theoretical significance, because they were the first to explore the possibility of detecting cognitive decline in individuals who would eventually develop dementia years later. Building upon these initial findings, Katzman and colleagues (1989) undertook a longitudinal investigation from the Bronx Aging Study in which 434 community-dwelling older adults were evaluated for dementia over a 5-year period. When enrolled in the study, all subjects were ambulatory, nondemented, functionally independent and between the ages of 75 and 85 years. The results demonstrated that the 59% of the cohort who made zero to two errors (out of 33 possible errors) on the Information-Memory-Concentration test (IMC; Blessed et al. 1968) during the initial evaluation had a less than 0.6% per year chance of developing probable or possible AD, whereas the 16% of the cohort with five to eight errors on this test (but who were not clinically demented) developed probable or possible AD at a rate of over 12% per year. Thus, difficulty on this brief cognitive screening measure predated the subsequent clinical diagnosis of AD by 2–5 years. It should also be noted that more than 90% of those who scored over five errors on the IMC test at the initial evaluation made errors in all or part of the 5-point memory phrase questions.

Tröster et al. (1994) recently investigated the utility of another cognitive screening test, the Dementia Rating Scale (DRS; Mattis 1976), in predicting the development of dementia among a group of individuals judged to be at risk for AD on the basis of subclinical memory impairment. Of the 30 subjects originally assigned to this group at the initial evaluation, four subjects were subsequently diagnosed with AD at the 4–6-year follow-up evaluation. The remaining 26 subjects remained free of dementia at follow-up; 21 were deemed healthy and five remained at risk by virtue of their subclinical memory impairment. Of the five DRS subscales, the Memory subscale predicted with considerable accuracy (93% at a cut-off score of 20/25) which subjects with subclinical memory impairment would develop AD 4–6 years later. Neither the DRS Total score nor any of the other subscales were useful in this regard. Thus, although the results of Tröster et al. (1994) and Katzman et al. (1989) demonstrate the potential utility of cognitive screening measures in the preclinical detection of AD, an item-wise inspection of both the DRS and the IMC test revealed that their sensitivity was primarily due to the memory-related items in each case.

Another study by Snowdon et al. (1996) demonstrated that linguistic ability, and not memory, in early life was a potent marker of poor cognitive function and AD in late life. In an intriguing and unique design, the handwritten autobiographies of 93 sisters who were participants of the Nun Study (Snowdon et al. 1989) were retrieved from the convent's archives and analysed for idea density (i.e. the average number of ideas expressed per 10 words) and grammatical complexity (i.e. an 8-point scale ranging from simple one-clause sentences to complex sentences with multiple forms of embedding and subordination). The sisters wrote their autobiographies, which were 200–300 words in length and limited to a single sheet of paper, at an average age of 22 years and had their cognitive function assessed an average of 58 years later, when they were 75–87 years old. Least squares regression analysis indicated that cognitive function, as indexed by the MMSE score, was associated with idea density, grammatical complexity and years of education. Forty-five per cent of the variance in MMSE score was explained by this model. Idea density (37%) and grammatical complexity (20%), however, had the strongest independent associations with MMSE score (years of education accounted for 13% of the variance).

Jacobs et al. (1995) also found that poor word-finding and verbal abstract reasoning abilities, in addition to immediate memory, were associated with the later diagnosis of AD. Using Cox regression analyses, they examined the associations between baseline neuropsychological test scores and the subsequent development of AD. Controlling for the effects of age, education, sex and language of test administration, the results demonstrated that baseline scores on the Boston Naming Test, immediate recall on the Buschke Selective Reminding Test and the Similarities subtest of the WAIS-R were significantly and independently associated with the later diagnosis of AD.

Thus, the findings of Jacobs et al. (1995) and Snowdon et al. (1996) support a relationship between language and linguistic abilities and poor cognitive function and AD in late life. These data also appear to be among the first to corroborate the initial findings of La Rue and Jarvik (1987) that nonmemory measures (i.e. WAIS Vocabulary, Similarities and Digit Symbol) are potentially associated with the development of dementia some years later, as prior studies suggest that idea density is associated with vocabulary skill and general knowledge (for a discussion, see Snowdon et al. 1996).

Memory measures in the preclinical detection of Alzheimer's disease

Although a growing body of evidence demonstrates that subtle cognitive decline can be detected in individuals a number of years prior to their meeting established criteria for a clinical diagnosis of AD (La Rue and Jarvik 1980, 1987; Bayles and Kaszniak 1987; Katzman et al. 1989; Fuld et al. 1990; Masur et al. 1990, 1994; La Rue et al. 1992; Bondi et al. 1994, 1995; Linn et al. 1995; Snowdon et al. 1996), the majority of these recent studies indicate that measures of learning and memory are particularly effective in this regard (Fuld et al. 1990; Masur et al. 1990, 1994; Bondi et al. 1994, 1995; Linn et al. 1995; Zonderman et al. 1995). Fuld and colleagues (Fuld et al. 1990; Masur et al. 1990), for example, demonstrated that poor performance on measures of recall from the Fuld Object Memory Test (Fuld 1977) or the Selective Reminding Test (Buschke and Fuld 1974) correctly predicted the subsequent development of AD within the next 5 years (Chapter 16). In an extensive follow-up to these studies, Masur and colleagues (1994) found that a logistic regression model of performance on four neuropsychological measures (a delayed recall measure from the Selective Reminding Test, a recall measure from the Fuld Object Memory Test, the Digit Symbol Substitution subtest from the Wechsler Adult Intelligence Scale and a measure of verbal fluency) was moderately effective in identifying individuals who later developed AD (32/64; 50%) and provided excellent specificity for identifying individuals who remained free of dementia (238/253; 94%) over a subsequent 11-year period.

A similar result was obtained in a large epidemiological study examining initial neuropsychological test performance of over 1000 nondemented elderly individuals who were followed over the subsequent 13 years (Linn et al. 1995). Fifty-five individuals developed AD during the study and development of the disorder was accurately predicted by their initial performance on a delayed recall measure from the Logical Memory subtest of the Wechsler Memory Scale and on the Digit Span subtest from the WAIS. Interestingly, subjects who later developed AD initially performed worse on the delayed recall measure, but better on the Digit Span subtest, than those who remained nondemented. It is also interesting to note that recall and digit span measures predicted subsequent development of dementia even when the initial neuropsychological evaluation preceded clinical onset of dementia by 7 years or more.

Preclinical detection of Alzheimer's disease in 'at risk' individuals

Another approach to examining potential decrements in learning and memory during a preclinical phase of AD has been to compare the performance of nondemented older adults who have an increased risk for developing the disease due to a positive family history or the presence of the epsilon 4 allele of the apolipoprotein E gene (ApoE-ε4) to that of individuals who do not have these risk factors (La Rue et al. 1992; Smalley et al. 1992; Bondi et al. 1994, 1995; Hom et al. 1994; Chapters 14 and 18). This approach assumes that nondemented elderly individuals with the risk factor for AD are more likely to be in the preclinical phase of the disease than those who do not have the risk factor and therefore are likely to perform worse on sensitive neuropsychological tests.

In one study using this approach, Hom et al. (1994) demonstrated that a group of 20 nondemented elderly individuals with a positive family history (FH+) of AD performed significantly worse than 20 age- and education-matched nondemented individuals with a negative family history (FH−) of AD on tests of verbal intelligence and verbal learning and memory. This difference occurred despite the fact that the average performances of both groups on these tests were within normal limits. In a similar study, Bondi et al. (1994) longitudinally assessed nondemented FH+ and FH− individuals with quantitative and qualitative indices derived from the California Verbal Learning Test (CVLT; Delis et al. 1987). Although the groups were carefully matched in terms of demographic variables and performance on standardized mental status examinations, the FH+ subjects recalled significantly fewer items during learning and delayed recall, produced more intrusion errors and demonstrated a greater recency effect than the FH− individuals. In addition, five of the nondemented subjects in this study performed on the CVLT in a manner qualitatively similar to that of a group of mildly impaired AD patients and were subsequently diagnosed with AD 1–2 years following their initial evaluation.

With the identification of a common and specific genetic risk factor for AD, the ApoE-ε4 allele, several recent studies have focused on episodic memory changes in nondemented elderly subjects who possess this risk factor. In one study, Reed et al. (1994) found that nondemented elderly male individuals with the ε4 allele exhib-

Figure 17.2. California Verbal
Learning Test raw scores of
nondemented older adults with the
apolipoprotein ε4 allele (*n* = 17)
compared to those lacking an ε4
allele (*n* = 35). Adapted from Bondi
et al. (1995), with permission of the
American Academy of Neurology.

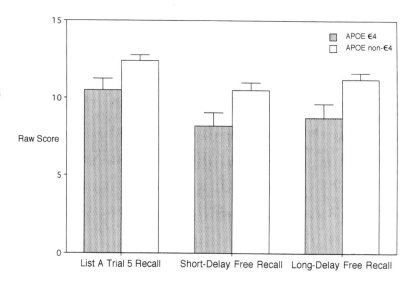

ited poorer mean performance on a test of visual memory than their dizygotic twin who did not have the ε4 allele. Bondi et al. (1995) demonstrated that the verbal learning and memory performance of nondemented subjects with the ApoE-ε4 allele was qualitatively (though not quantitatively) similar to that of early stage patients with AD. Furthermore, nondemented subjects with the ApoE-ε4 allele recalled fewer items during the learning trials and over delay intervals and utilized a less effective organizational strategy for learning than carefully matched nondemented subjects without the ApoE-ε4 allele (see Figure 17.2). Follow-up examinations revealed that six of 14 subjects with the ε4 allele subsequently developed either probable or possible AD or questionable AD (i.e. cognitive decline without evidence of significant functional impairment), whereas none of 26 subjects without an ε4 allele demonstrated any cognitive decline.

Tierney and colleagues (1996a,b) have also utilized information about an individual's ApoE genotype to determine whether such knowledge improves the prediction of which memory-impaired subjects will eventually develop AD. One hundred and seven subjects with memory impairment, but not dementia, were referred to the study from community physicians and were prospectively followed over a 2-year period. Twenty-nine subjects developed AD during this period and 78 did not develop dementia. Tierney et al. found that ApoE genotype, although a statistically significant predictor, was a reliable

prognostic indicator only when memory test performance was included in the predictive model. They suggest that ApoE genotyping in isolation is not likely to be useful as a prognostic indicator of AD.

The 29 subjects who developed AD during this period also performed significantly below that of the 78 who did not progress to AD at entry into the study (i.e. at a time point when neither group was considered to be demented). For example, the two groups were sufficiently different at entry on cognitive screening measures, as shown by the significant differences between the two groups on both the MMSE (Folstein et al. 1975) and the Dementia Rating Scale (Mattis 1976). Given these large differences at entry, it is not surprising that other sensitive neuropsychological measures, particularly delayed recall, also showed significant differences at entry and perhaps why ApoE genotype was not particularly predictive of progression. In other words, the liberal cut off scores of the MMSE (24 or more) and DRS (123 or more) used by Tierney et al. may have resulted in the inclusion of very mildly demented individuals into the study, thereby diluting any potential utility of ApoE genotype to predict progression beyond that already accounted for by memory impairment.

Petersen and colleagues (Petersen et al. 1995, 1996; Smith et al. 1996), however, came to different conclusions from those of Tierney et al. in a longitudinal study of patients with mild cognitive impairment but who did not meet criteria for dementia (i.e. Clinical Dementia Rating=

0.5). This group of mild cognitive impairment patients were at risk for dementia by virtue of having a significant memory impairment. Over the course of several years of follow-up, these subjects' mild cognitive impairment evolved to dementia at a rate of approximately 15% per year. The presence of an ApoE ε4 allele was the best predictor of subsequent development of dementia in these individuals. Thus, Petersen et al. (1995, 1996) indicate that ApoE is an important risk factor for AD and, in patients with a mild cognitive impairment, ApoE may be quite useful in predicting who is likely to progress to dementia.

Hyman et al. (1996), in a much larger study of 1899 individuals 65 years and older, provided some similar, though less compelling, findings of the importance of ApoE genotype in predicting progression to dementia. Although analyses demonstrated a significant effect of ApoE-ε4 allele in predicting performance on a delayed recall task over a 4–7-year period, the magnitude of this effect was fairly modest, with an odds ratio for developing impairment of approximately 1.37 (95% confidence interval: 1.007–1.850). Thus, many individuals reach old age without cognitive impairment despite inheritance of one or two ApoE-ε4 alleles. Hyman et al. (1996) conclude by suggesting that ApoE genotyping alone will have limited utility as a diagnostic or prognostic indicator of cognitive decline in older adults. Unfortunately, no formal diagnoses were made over the 4–7-year period and thus conclusions about the diagnostic utility of ApoE are more limited in this study.

It should also be noted that recent evidence suggests that ApoE-ε4 associated risk for AD is age dependent and that the risk related to the ε4 allele appears to wane with increasing age (Rebeck et al. 1994; Petersen et al. 1996). For individuals older than 75 years of age who carry an ApoE ε4 allele, the attributable risk of developing AD is considerably lower than for subjects ages 60–74 years. Regardless of age or ApoE genotype, however, investigators have demonstrated that recall measures remain a strong preclinical predictor of AD in cohorts of individuals older than 75 years of age (Katzman et al. 1989; Fuld et al. 1990; Masur et al. 1994). Thus, irrespective of the ApoE genotype of a very elderly individual, neuropsychological indices such as delayed recall may provide sensitive markers of preclinical AD. The importance of memory assessment is also highlighted by the finding that ApoE genotyping lacks the sensitivity and specificity to be used alone in diagnosing AD (Mayeux et al. 1998).

Neuroimaging procedures in the preclinical detection of Alzheimer's disease

Building upon the findings from neuropsychological studies of individuals at risk for AD, a number of preliminary imaging studies have also recently examined subjects in the early stages of AD or at risk for developing dementia through the use of structural (i.e. magnetic resonance or MRI) or functional (i.e. positron emission tomography or PET) imaging procedures (Haxby et al. 1986, 1988; Soininen et al. 1994, 1995; Small et al. 1995; Reiman et al. 1996). Haxby et al. (1986, 1988), for example, measured cerebral metabolism with PET in AD patients and found differing patterns of decreased metabolism in the association cortex. The individual patterns of decreased metabolism correlated with neuropsychological test scores purported to reflect information processing in particular brain regions. The decreased neocortical metabolism was found even in patients in the earliest stages of dementia, in whom neuropsychological testing revealed little or no deficits other than amnesia. This finding suggests that functional neuroimaging may provide evidence of metabolic alterations very early in the course of AD (Chapters 6 and 7). Haxby et al. (1986, 1988) also suggest that neocortical metabolic abnormalities can be observed with PET before associated impairments of neocortically mediated visuospatial and language functions are demonstrable.

With respect to functional metabolic activity in subjects at risk for AD, Small et al. (1995) performed PET scans and ApoE genotyping on a group of older adults with a positive family history for AD and mild memory complaints (but normal cognitive performance). Despite equivalent MMSE scores (means of 28.8 versus 29.3 points), parietal lobe metabolism was significantly lower in the at-risk subjects with an ApoE-ε4 allele than in those without an ε4 allele. Similarly, Reiman et al. (1996) compared the PET scans of 11 cognitively-normal, middle-aged ε4/ε4 homozygotes and 22 non-ε4 control subjects. Results revealed that the ε4 homozygotes had reduced glucose metabolism in brain regions similar to those showing reductions in AD. Reiman et al. concluded that these findings provide preclinical evidence that the presence of the ε4 allele is a risk factor for AD.

In structural volumetric studies of AD, Soininen et al. (1995) demonstrated that nondemented older adults homozygous for the ε4 allele may have minor damage to their hippocampal formation. This finding is concordant with their previous finding (Soininen et al. 1994) that subjects fulfilling criteria for age-associated memory impairment demonstrated less volumetric asymmetry between right and left hippocampal formations than matched control subjects without memory disturbance.

PRECLINICAL DETECTION OF HUNTINGTON'S DISEASE

Since the advent of DNA markers for Huntington's disease (HD) (Gusella et al. 1983) and the recent discovery of the gene responsible for HD (i.e. the trinucleotide repeat (CAG) on chromosome 4; Huntington's Disease Collaborative Research Group 1993), investigators have examined the potential neuropsychological detection and characterization of the preclinical period of HD prior to the onset of motor impairments.

Jason et al. (1988) were among the first to explore pre-symptomatic neuropsychological changes in seven individuals at high risk for HD based on DNA and linkage analysis. In this study, five of the seven high risk individuals demonstrated impairments on tests of visuospatial and frontal system functioning. The authors suggest that clear neuropsychological impairment may be present in HD even when overt signs and symptoms are not expected for a number of years. Diamond et al. (1992) also found evidence of presymptomatic cognitive decline in persons at risk for HD. Probable HD gene carriers were inferior to probable noncarriers on several individual tests of learning and memory. Diamond et al. (1992) concluded, based on these preliminary findings, that cognitive decline may be present prior to identifiable motor impairments in HD.

Other teams of investigators (Strauss and Brandt 1990; Rothlind et al. 1993; Giordini et al. 1995), however, have not supported these early findings of cognitive impairment in individuals at genetic risk for HD. Strauss and Brandt (1990), for example, found no differences between 12 probable HD gene carriers and 15 noncarriers on an extensive battery of neuropsychological tests. In addition, Rothlind et al. (1993) found no significant differences in young, asymptomatic adults at very high genetic risk for HD on tests of verbal learning and memory and on tests of oculomotor functioning. In a longitudinal design, Giordini et al. (1995) also did not find evidence of neuropsychological impairment in eight subjects at risk for HD on three separate assessments over a 4-year span. This latter study was one of the first to include both linkage analysis (G8 probe)

and examination of the trinucleotide repeats on most of the subjects.

In all of these prior studies, sample sizes were quite small and power was extremely limited, especially in those studies which failed to demonstrate any differences between high and low risk subjects (i.e. insufficient power to reject a null hypothesis when it is false). In a large study that overcame these limitations, Foroud and colleagues (1995) were among the first to examine the HD gene and its relative contribution to neuropsychological functioning in 394 HD gene carriers and noncarriers. In this study Foroud et al. quantified the number of trinucleotide triplet repeats on chromosome 4. One allele of 40 or more triplet repeats was considered to be disease-producing and individuals with this genetic mutation were designated as gene carriers. Individuals with 31 or fewer triplet repeats were considered to be in the normal range and classified as noncarriers. Subjects in the border region of 32–39 triplet repeats were considered uninformative and excluded from analysis because of uncertainty surrounding the development of HD within this range of triplet repeats. Thus, of the 394 individuals genotyped, 120 were HD gene carriers and 260 were considered noncarriers.

The results showed that the Digit Symbol and Picture Arrangement subtests of the WAIS-R were significantly lower in the HD gene carrier group, even after the scores from all gene carriers with any positive findings on their neurological motor examination were removed. Results also demonstrated statistically significant negative correlations between the number of CAG repeats and cognitive performance on the Vocabulary and Digit Symbol subtests of the WAIS-R in the asymptomatic HD gene carriers. The authors suggest that cognitive changes occur very early in the course of HD and that the degree of cognitive deficit is proportional to the number of CAG repeats in the HD allele. Future large-scale studies of this kind, with more sensitive neuropsychological indices of frontal system functioning, visuospatial processing and recall and recognition memory, may reveal other manifestations of the cognitive changes that precede the motor impairments of HD.

CONCLUSIONS

It is clear from the results of studies reviewed in this chapter that decrements in learning and memory are particularly evident in the early stages of dementia and are likely to presage the development of the full dementia syndrome. A growing number of investigations provide converging evidence that a preclinical phase of detectable cognitive decline, and structural or metabolic changes, can precede the clinical diagnosis of dementia by several years. Furthermore, many of these studies suggest that the detection of preclinical AD may be enhanced, but not supplanted, if risk factors such as a positive family history or the presence of the ApoE-ε4 allele are considered in conjunction with cognitive and imaging findings. It should be emphasized, however, that the combination of various risk factors can only provide for an estimate of an individual's risk of eventually developing AD. Therefore, regardless of an individual's age, ApoE genotype or family history for AD, sensitive neuropsychological and perhaps brain metabolic measures, appear to provide some of the most salient markers of preclinical AD.

Beyond a 5- to 10-year period prior to the onset of dementia, however, perhaps other measures of cognitive ability (e.g. vocabulary skill or linguistic ability) may be better predictors of the development of dementia later in life because they may represent markers of neurocognitive development and brain reserve capacity established early in life (La Rue and Jarvik 1987; Snowdon et al. 1996; Chapter 14). Reduced reserve capacity may then make individuals more vulnerable later in life to the consequences of the neuropathological cascade of AD. Alternatively, as Snowdon et al. (1996) suggest, perhaps low linguistic ability may actually be a direct early expression of subtle neuropathological changes in early life that precede the neuritic plaques and neurofibrillary tangles of AD in late life. For example, one autopsy study of individuals aged 20–100 years showed that the neurofibrillary tangles and neuropil threads found in AD developed over approximately five decades (Ohm et al. 1995). Thus, it is unclear whether there are direct but subtle neuropathological changes in individuals destined to develop AD that are detected by sensitive

cognitive tests (e.g. linguistic ability in early life) or, instead, reduced reserve capacity to make one more vulnerable later in life to the consequences of the shorter term cascade of neuropathological changes in AD. In the latter case, then, measures of learning and memory would appear to provide greater sensitivity because the hippocampus and entorhinal cortex would be the earliest and most severely affected sites of neuropathology. Regardless of the mechanism (i.e. reduced reserve capacity versus direct early expression of AD-related neuropathology), the studies reviewed in this chapter attest to the notion that cognitive decline can be detected a number of years prior to the full clinical manifestation of the dementia syndrome.

Finally, La Rue and Markee (1995) rightly caution that it is important to note that the predictive utility of many of the test findings in the studies outlined above is modest (e.g. positive predictive value=68% in the study by Masur et al. 1994) and that the range of time over which prediction has been demonstrated is typically short (1–3 years). Additional long-term studies are needed before conclusions can be drawn about the predictive validity of cognitive tests vis-à-vis new-onset dementia (La Rue and Markee 1995). Although considerable progress has been made, additional studies are necessary to enhance our ability to clinically detect dementia in its earliest stages when neuroprotective agents designed to impede the progression of the disease might be most effective.

ACKNOWLEDGMENTS

This chapter was supported in part by NIH grant AG12674 and by funds from the Medical Research Service of the Department of Veterans Affairs. The authors thank their many collaborators at the UCSD Alzheimer's Disease Research Center.

REFERENCES

Bayles, K.A. and Kaszniak, A.W. 1987. *Communication and cognition in normal aging and dementia*. Boston: College-Hill/Little, Brown and Company.

Blessed, G., Tomlinson, B.E. and Roth, M. 1968. The association between quantitative measures of dementia and of senile change in the cerebral grey matter of elderly subjects. *British Journal of Psychiatry*. 114: 797–811.

Bondi, M.W., Monsch, A.U., Butters, N., Salmon, D.P. and Paulsen, J.S. 1993. Utility of a modified version of the Wisconsin Card Sorting Test in the detection of dementia of the Alzheimer type. *Clinical Neuropsychologist*. 7: 161–170.

Bondi, M.W., Monsch, A.U., Galasko, D., Butters, N., Salmon, D.P. and Delis, D.C. 1994. Preclinical cognitive markers of dementia of the Alzheimer type. *Neuropsychology*. 8: 374–384.

Bondi, M.W., Salmon, D.P., Monsch, A.U., Galasko, D., Butters, N., Klauber, M.R., Thal, L.J. and Saitoh, T. 1995. Episodic memory changes are associated with the ApoE-ε4 allele in nondemented older adults. *Neurology*. 45: 2203–2206.

Braak, H. and Braak, E. 1991. Neuropathological staging of Alzheimer-related changes. *Acta Neuropathologica*. 82: 239–259.

Buschke, H. and Fuld, P.A. 1974. Evaluating storage, retention and retrieval in disordered memory and learning. *Neurology*. 24: 1019–1025.

Delis, D.C., Kramer, J.H., Kaplan, E. and Ober, B.A. 1987. *The California Verbal Learning Test*. New York: Psychological Corporation.

Delis, D.C., Massman, P.J., Butters, N., Salmon, D.P., Kramer, J.H. and Cermak, L. 1991. Profiles of demented and amnesic patients on the California Verbal Learning Test: Implications for the assessment of memory disorders. *Psychological Assessment*. 3: 19–26.

Diamond, R., White, R.F., Myers, R.H., Mastromauro, C., Koroshetz, W.J., Butters, N., Rothstein, D.M., Moss, M.B. and Vaterling, J. 1992. Evidence of presymptomatic cognitive decline in Huntington's disease. *Journal of Clinical and Experimental Neuropsychology*. 14: 961–975.

Eslinger, P.J., Damasio, A.R., Benton, A.L. and Van Allen, M. 1985. Neuropsychologic detection of abnormal mental decline in older persons. *Journal of the American Medical Association*. 253: 670–674.

Flicker, C., Ferris, S.H. and Reisberg, B. 1991. Mild cognitive impairment in the elderly: Predictors of dementia. *Neurology*. 41: 1006–1009.

Folstein, M.F., Folstein, S. and McHugh, P.R. 1975. Mini-Mental State: A practical method for grading the cognitive state of patients for the clinician. *Journal of Psychiatric Research*. 12: 189–198.

Foroud, T., Siemers, E., Kleindorker, D., Bill, D.J., Hodes, M.E., Norton, J.A., Conneally, P.M. and Christian, J.C. 1995. Cognitive scores in carriers of Huntington's disease gene compared to noncarriers. *Annals of Neurology*. 37: 657–664.

Fuld, P.A. 1977. *Fuld Object–Memory Evaluation*. Woodale, Il: Stoelting Company.

Fuld, P.A., Masur, D.M., Blau, A.D., Crystal, H. and Aronson, M.K. 1990. Object-memory evaluation for prospective detection of dementia in normal functioning elderly: Predictive and normative data. *Journal of Clinical and Experimental Neuropsychology*. 12: 520–528.

Giordani, B., Berent, S., Boivin, M.J., Penney, J.B., Lehtinen, S., Markel, D.S., Hollingsworth, Z., Butterbaugh, G., Hichwa, R.D., Gusella, J.F. and Young, A.B. 1995. Longitudinal neuropsychological and genetic linkage analysis of persons at risk for Huntington's disease. *Archives of Neurology*. 52: 59–64.

Gusella, J.F., Wexler, N., Conneally, P.M., Naylor, S.L. Anderson, M.A., Tanzi, R.E., Watkins, P.C., Ottina, K., Wallace, M.R., Sakaguchi, A.Y., Young, A.B., Shoulson, I., Bonilla, E. and Martin, J.B. 1983. A polymorphic DNA marker genetically linked to Huntington's disease. *Nature*. 306: 234–238.

Haxby, J.V., Grady, C.L., Duara, R., Schlageter, N.L., Berg, G. and Rapoport, S.I. 1986. Neocortical metabolic abnormalities precede non-memory cognitive deficits in early Alzheimer-type dementia. *Archives of Neurology*. 43: 882–885.

Haxby, J.V., Grady, C.L., Koss, E., Horwitz, B., Schapiro, M., Friedland, R.P. and Rapoport, S.I. 1988. Heterogeneous anterior-posterior metabolic patterns in Alzheimer's type dementia. *Neurology*. 38: 1853–1863.

Hom, J., Turner, M.B., Risser, R., Bonte, F.J. and Tintner, R. 1994. Cognitive deficits in asymptomatic first-degree relatives of Alzheimer's disease patients. *Journal of Clinical and Experimental Neuropsychology*. 16: 568–576.

Huntington's Disease Collaborative Research Group (MacDonald, M.E., Ambrose, C.M., Duyao, M.P., Myers, R.H., Lin, C., Srinidhi, L., Barnes, G., Taylor, S.A., James, M., Groot, N., MacFarlane, H., Jenkins, B. Anderson, M.A., Wexler, N.S. and Gusella, J.F.) 1993. A novel gene containing a trinucleotide repeat that is expanded and unstable on Huntington's disease chromosomes. *Cell*. 72: 971–983.

Hyman, B.T., Gomez-Isla, T., Briggs, M., Chung, H., Nichols, S., Kohout, F. and Wallace, R. 1996. Apolipoprotein E and cognitive change in an elderly population. *Annals of Neurology*. 40: 55–66.

Hyman, B.T., Van Hoesen, G.W., Damasio, A. and Barnes, C.L. 1984. Alzheimer's disease: Cell-specific pathology isolates the hippocampal formation. *Science*. 225: 1168–1170.

Jacobs, D.M., Sano, M., Dooneief, G., Marder, K., Bell, K.L. and Stern, Y. 1995. Neuropsychological detection and characterization of preclinical Alzheimer's disease. *Neurology*. 45: 957–962.

Jason, G.W., Pajurkova, E.M., Suchowersky, O., Hewitt, J., Hilbert, C., Reed, J. and Hayden, M.R. 1988. Presymptomatic neuropsychological impairment in Huntington's disease. *Archives of Neurology*. 45: 769–773.

Kaszniak, A.W., Wilson, R.S., Fox, J.H. and Stebbins, G.T. 1986. Cognitive assessment in Alzheimer's disease: Cross-sectional and longitudinal perspectives. *Canadian Journal of Neurological Sciences*. 13: 420–423.

Katzman, R. 1994. Apolipoprotein E and Alzheimer's disease. *Current Opinion in Neurobiology*. 4: 703–707.

Katzman, R., Aronson, M., Fuld, P., Kawas, C., Brown, T., Morgenstern, H., Frishman, W., Gidez, L., Eder, H. and Ooi, W.L. 1989. Development of dementing illness in an 80-year-old volunteer cohort. *Annals of Neurology*. 25: 317–324.

Katzman, R. and Kawas, C. 1994. The epidemiology of dementia and Alzheimer disease. In *Alzheimer disease*, ed. R. D. Terry, R. Katzman and K. L. Bick, pp. 105–122. New York: Raven Press.

Khachaturian, Z.S., Phelps, C.H. and Buckholtz, N.S. 1994. The prospect of developing treatments for Alzheimer disease. In *Alzheimer disease*, ed. R. D. Terry, R. Katzman and K. L. Bick, pp. 445–454. New York: Raven Press.

Knopman, D.S. and Ryberg, S. 1989. A verbal memory test with high predictive accuracy for dementia of the Alzheimer type. *Archives of Neurology*. 46: 141–145.

La Rue, A. 1992. *Aging and neuropsychological assessment*. New York: Plenum Press.

La Rue, A. and Jarvik, L. R. 1980. Reflections of biological changes in the psychological performance of the aged. *Age*. 3: 29–32.

La Rue, A. and Jarvik, L. R. 1987. Cognitive function and prediction of dementia in old age. *International Journal of Aging and Human Development*. 25: 79–89.

La Rue, A. and Markee, T. 1995. Clinical assessment research with older adults. *Psychological Assessment*. 7: 376–386.

La Rue, A., Matsuyama, S.S., McPherson, S., Sherman, J. and Jarvik, L.F. 1992. Cognitive performance in relatives of patients with probable Alzheimer disease: An age at onset effect? *Journal of Clinical and Experimental Neuropsychology*. 14: 533–538.

Linn, R.T., Wolf, P.A., Bachman, D.L., Knoefel, J.E., Cobb, J.L., Belanger, A.J., Kaplan, E.F. and D'Agostino, R.B. 1995. The 'preclinical phase' of probable Alzheimer's disease: A 13-year prospective study of the Framingham cohort. *Archives of Neurology*. 52: 485–490.

Manton, K.G. 1990. Mortality and morbidity. In *Handbook of aging and the social sciences*, 3rd ed., ed. R.H. Binstock and L.K. George, pp. 64–90. San Diego: Academic Press.

Masur, D.M., Fuld, P.A., Blau, A.D., Crystal, H. and Aronson, M.K. 1990. Predicting development of dementia in the elderly with the selective reminding test. *Journal of Clinical and Experimental Neuropsychology*. 12: 529–538.

Masur, D.M., Sliwinski, M., Lipton, R.B., Blau, A.D. and Crystal, H.A. 1994. Neuropsychological prediction of dementia and the absence of dementia in healthy elderly persons. *Neurology*. 44: 1427–1432.

Mattis, S. 1976. Mental status examination for organic mental syndrome in the elderly patient. In *Geriatric psychiatry: A handbook for psychiatrists and primary care physicians*, ed. L. Bellack and T.B. Karasu, pp. 77–121. New York: Grune and Stratton.

Mayeux, R., Saunders, A.M., Shea, S., Mirra, S., Evans, D., Roses, A.D., Hyman, B.T., Crain, B., Tang, M.-X. and Phelps, C.H. for the Alzheimer's Disease Centers Consortium on Apolipoprotein E and Alzheimer's Disease. 1998. Utility of the Apolipoprotein E genotype in the diagnosis of Alzheimer's disease. *New England Journal of Medicine*. 338: 506–511.

Monsch, A.U., Bondi, M.W., Butters, N., Salmon, D.P., Katzman, R. and Thal, L.J. 1992. Comparisons of verbal fluency tasks in the detection of dementia of the Alzheimer type. *Archives of Neurology*. 49: 1253–1258.

Morris, J.C., McKeel, D.W., Storandt, M., Rubin, E.H., Price, J.L., Grant, E.A., Ball, M.J. and Berg, L. 1991. Very mild Alzheimer's disease: Informant-based clinical, psychometric and pathologic distinction from normal aging. *Neurology*. 41: 469–478.

Myers, G.C. 1990. Demography of aging. In *Handbook of aging and the social sciences*, 3rd ed., ed. R.H. Binstock and L.K. George, pp. 19–44. San Diego: Academic Press.

Ohm, T., Müller, H., Braak, H. and Bohl, J. 1995. Close-meshed prevalence rates of different stages as a tool to uncover the rate of Alzheimer's disease-related neurofibrillary changes. *Neuroscience*. 64: 209–217.

Petersen, R.C., Smith, G., Ivnik, R.J., Kokmen, E. and Tangalos, E.G. 1994. Memory function in very early Alzheimer's disease. *Neurology*. 44: 867–872.

Petersen, R.C., Smith, G., Ivnik, R.J., Tangalos, E.G., Schaid, D.J., Thibodeau, S.N., Kokmen, E., Waring, S.C. and Kurland, L.T. 1995. Apolipoprotein E status as a predictor of the development of Alzheimer's disease in memory-impaired individuals. *Journal of the American Medical Association*. 273: 1274–1278.

Petersen, R.C., Waring, S.C., Smith, G., Tangalos, E.G. and Thibodeau, S.N. 1996. Predictive value of APOE genotyping in incipient Alzheimer's disease. *Annals of the New York Academy of Sciences*. 802: 58–69.

Poon, L.W., Kaszniak, A.W. and Dudley, W.N. 1992. Approaches in the experimental neuropsychology of dementia: A methodological and model review. In *Aging and mental disorders: International perspectives*, ed. M. Bergner, K. Hasegawa, S. Finkel and T. Nishimura, pp. 150–173. New York: Springer.

Rebeck, G.W., Perls, T.T., West, H.L., Sodhi, P., Lipsitz, L.A. and Hyman, B.T. 1994. Reduced apolipoprotein ε4 allele frequency in the oldest old Alzheimer's patients and cognitively normal individuals. *Neurology*. 44: 1513–1516.

Reed, T., Carmelli, D., Swan, G.E., Breitner, J.C.S., Welsh, K.A., Jarvik, G.P., Deeb, S. and Auwerx, J. 1994. Lower cognitive performance in normal older adult male twins carrying the apolipoprotein E ε4 allele. *Archives of Neurology*. 51: 1189–1192.

Reiman, E.M., Caselli, R.J., Yun, L.S., Chen, K., Bandy, D., Minoshima, S., Thibodeau, S.N. and Osborne, D. 1996. Preclinical evidence of Alzheimer's disease in persons homozygous for the ε4 allele for lipoprotein E. *New England Journal of Medicine*. 334: 752–758.

Rothlind, J.C., Brandt, J., Zee, D., Codori, A.M. and Folstein, S. 1993. Unimpaired verbal memory and oculomotor control in asymptomatic adults with the genetic marker for Huntington's disease. *Archives of Neurology*. 50: 799–802.

Salmon, D.P., Butters, N., Thal, L.J. and Jeste, D.V. In press. Alzheimer's disease: Analysis for the DSM-IV task force. In *DSM-IV Sourcebook*, vol. IV, ed. T.A. Widiger, A. Frances and H. Pincus. Washington, DC: American Psychiatric Association.

Small, G.W., Mazziotta, J.C., Collins, M.T., Baxter, L.R., Phelps, M.E., Mendelkern, M.A., Kaplan, A., LaRue, A., Adamson, C.F., Chang, L., Guze, B.H., Corder, E.H., Saunders, A.M., Haines, J.L., Pericak-Vance, M.A. and Roses, A.D. 1995. Apolipoprotein E type 4 allele and cerebral glucose metabolism in relatives at risk for Alzheimer disease. *Journal of the American Medical Association*. 273: 942–947.

Smalley, S.L., Wolkenstein, B.H., La Rue, A., Woodward, J.A., Jarvik, L.F. and Matsuyama, S.S. 1992. Commingling analysis of memory performance in offspring of Alzheimer patients. *Genetic Epidemiology*. 9: 333–345.

Smith, G.E., Petersen, R.C., Parisi, J.E., Ivnik, R.J., Kokmen, E., Tangalos, E.G. and Waring, S. 1996. Definition, course and outcome of mild cognitive impairment. *Aging, Neuropsychology and Cognition*. 2: 141–147.

Snowdon, D.A., Kemper, S.J., Mortimer, J.A., Greiner, L.H., Wekstein, D.R. and Markesbery, W.R. 1996. Linguistic ability in early life and cognitive function and Alzheimer's disease in late life: Findings from the Nun Study. *Journal of the American Medical Association*. 275: 528–532.

Snowdon, D.A., Ostwald, S.K. and Kane, R.L. 1989. Education, survival and independence in elderly Catholic sisters, 1936–1988. *American Journal of Epidemiology*. 180: 999–1012.

Soininen, H., Partanen, K., Pitkänen, A., Hallikainen, M., Hänninen, T., Helisalmi, S., Mennermaa, A., Ryynänen, M., Koivisto, K. and Riekkinen, P. 1995. Decreased hippocampal volume asymmetry on MRIs in nondemented elderly subjects carrying the apolipoprotein E ε4 allele. *Neurology*. 45: 391–392.

Soininen, H., Partanen, K., Pitkänen, A., Vainio, P., Hänninen, T., Hallikainen, M., Koivisto, K. and Riekkinen, P. 1994. Volumetric MRI analysis of the amygdala and the hippocampus in subjects with age-associated memory impairment: Correlation to visual and verbal memory. *Neurology*. 44: 1660–1668.

Squire, L.R., Knowlton, B. and Musen, G. 1993. The structure and organization of memory. *Annual Review of Psychology*. 44: 453–495.

Storandt, M., Botwinick, J., Danziger, W.L., Berg, L. and Hughes, C.P. 1984. Psychometric differentiation of mild senile dementia of the Alzheimer type. *Archives of Neurology*. 41: 497–499.

Strauss, M.E. and Brandt, J. 1990. Are there neuropsychological manifestations of the gene for Huntington's disease in asymptomatic, at risk individuals? *Archives of Neurology*. 47: 905–908.

Tierney, M.C., Szalai, J.P., Snow, W.G., Fisher, R.H., Nores, A., Nadon, G., Dunn, E. and St. George-Hyslop, P.H. 1996b. Prediction of probable Alzheimer's disease in memory-impaired patients: A prospective longitudinal study. *Neurology*. 46: 661–665.

Tierney, M.C., Szalai, J.P., Snow, W.G., Fisher, R.H., Tsuda, T., Chi, H., McLachlan, D.R. and St. George-Hyslop, P.H. 1996a. A prospective study of the clinical utility of ApoE genotype in the prediction of outcome in patients with memory impairment. *Neurology*. 46: 149–154.

Tröster, A.I., Moe, K.E., Vitiello, M.V. and Prinz, P.N. 1994. Predicting long-term outcome in individuals at risk for Alzheimer's disease with the Dementia Rating Scale. *Journal of Neuropsychiatry and Clinical Neurosciences*. 6: 54–57.

Welsh, K., Butters, N., Hughes, J., Mohs, R. and Heyman, A. 1991. Detection of abnormal memory decline in mild cases of Alzheimer's disease using CERAD neuropsychological measures. *Archives of Neurology*. 48: 278–281.

Zonderman, A.B., Giambra, L.M., Arenberg, D., Resnick, S.M., Costa, P.T. and Kawas, C.H. 1995. Changes in immediate visual memory predict cognitive impairment. *Archives of Clinical Neuropsychology*. 10: 111–123.

18 Clinical differentiation of memory disorders in neurodegenerative disease

KATHLEEN A. WELSH-BOHMER
AND PAULA K. OGROCKI

INTRODUCTION

Cognitive impairment in late life is a growing public health care problem. By the year 2050, conservative estimates indicate as many as 7 to 14 million individuals in the USA (US Census Figures) will be affected by some form of dementia requiring specialized care or institutionalization (Khachaturian 1994). Alzheimer's disease (AD) is by far the most prevalent of the disorders accounting for at least 60% of the progressive dementias. Vascular dementias are believed to account for 20% and a variety of other dementias account for the remaining 20%. Many of these 'other' dementias are treatable and some, if treated, are reversible (Breitner and Welsh 1995).

A challenge facing today's clinician is reliably detecting dementia in scenarios where the distinctions between early dementia and normal aging are quite difficult. Accurate diagnoses at this stage are important in allaying anxieties when dementia is not suspected. In the cases of dementia, diagnostic certainty as to the type of dementia can have consequences particularly if the disorder is treatable. In the future, should effective treatment strategies become available for AD and some of the other irreversible forms of dementia, early clinical intervention will be important in an effort to prevent the expression of fulminant symptoms.

At present there is no diagnostic test or biological marker for AD which will permit reliable prediction of who is likely to develop the disease (Roses 1995). Consequently, the diagnosis of this late onset dementia as well as some of the other common neurodegenerative conditions continues to rely on sound clinical methods. It is in this area that neuropsychology has made a significant contribution. The neuropsychological evaluation has helped to characterize the clinical expression of the various late onset illnesses producing dementia, including common diseases such as AD, vascular dementia, frontal lobe dementias, Parkinson's disease and some of the less common conditions of the elderly such as Huntington's disease (HD), progressive supranuclear palsy, diffuse Lewy body disease and infectious conditions such as AIDS and Creutzfeldt–Jakob disease. The neuropsychological evaluation is now a basic requisite for many of the diagnostic criteria for these disorders (e.g. McKhann et al. 1984).

This chapter briefly discusses the cognitive features of normal aging and considers the clinical distinctions between the major conditions that lead to primary progressive dementias in the elderly. The current place of neuropsychology in the clinical evaluation of the elderly patient with memory complaints is also considered. The discussion then focuses on the changing role of neuropsychology with the advances in other clinical technologies, such as neuroimaging and genetic testing.

COGNITIVE CHANGES OF AGING

Normal aging

A discussion of the clinical characteristics of the primary degenerative conditions cannot be entertained without first considering the changes in function that occur as a result of normal brain aging. Mentation change with aging is perhaps best considered to fall on a continuum with normal age related central nervous system change representing one end of the scale, brain diseases producing bona fide dementias falling on the other end and gradations of cognitive change due to a heterogenous mix of systemic or chronic diseases and prodromal dementias (e.g. early stage AD) falling between the two ends of the spectrum (Gutierrez et al. 1993). Indeed, by far the most common cause of memory complaints in the elderly is not brain disease but rather the normal aging of the nervous system. An understanding of the normal range of behavioral and cognitive change is of obvious importance to the examining clinician, but is also essential in research studies for accurate estimates of disease base rates or prevalence (Breitner and Welsh 1995).

Some fundamental findings should be noted when considering the distinctions between normal aging and brain disease. Studies of normal aging consistently report changes in very specific areas of cognitive function which contrast it to the patterns seen in pathological conditions such as AD. In normal aging, deficits are reported in retrieving information from secondary memory, i.e. memory for information recently learned minutes to days before. Immediate or primary memory is relatively unaffected (Siegler et al. 1995). In contrast to conditions such as AD, there is partial savings of information and less rapid forgetting from secondary memory (Hart et al. 1988). Other areas of cognition affected by normal aging include the ability to effectively divide attention between multiple demanding activities (McCrae et al. 1987), divergent thinking (Mc-Dowd and Craik 1988) and aspects of nonverbal problem solving and visuospatial functions (Koss et al. 1991). Although similar deficits are manifest in dementia, the impairments in normal aging are not considered disabling and seem to reflect a generalized inefficiency in cognitive processing.

A current hypothesis that effectively encompasses the various behavioral observations in aging is the idea that cognitive operations associated with the frontal lobes are particularly vulnerable to the effects of age (Van Gorp and Mahler 1990). Several lines of converging radiological, neuropsychological and neuropathological evidence support this notion. Reductions in frontal lobe blood flow are noted with advanced age (Welsh-Bohmer and Hoffman 1996), a pattern of decreased executive functions (diminished behavioral flexibility, decreased integrative capacity and difficulties with divergent thinking and working memory) are observed on neuropsychological examination (Salthouse et al. 1996) and neuropathological examination shows selective cell loss in the superior frontal, precentral and superior temporal gyri in the aged brain (Haug et al. 1983; Creasy and Rapoport 1985).

Age associated memory impairment

Some memory loss with age, particularly a decline in recent memory function, is now well recognized (for a review, see Verhaeghen et al. 1993). There remains considerable debate, however, as to whether these changes reflect a fundamental process of the aging nervous system or are reflective of co-occurring physical and medical changes (e.g. cardiovascular disease, diabetes, pulmonary conditions, etc.) that may be more frequent in aging (Paulsen et al. 1994). Regardless of the outcome of this line of inquiry into causation, considerable attention has been devoted to standardizing terminology, diagnostic criteria and the methods of memory assessment in aging to permit better cross laboratory comparisons and to assist clinicians in distinguishing between conditions of normal aging and specific disease states such as AD.

The notion of 'Age Associated Memory Impairment' (AAMI), a refinement of the terminology 'Benign Senescent Forgetfulness' (BSF) of Kral (1962), was proposed over a decade ago in an effort to standardize diagnostic criteria for at least a certain subset of memory problems occurring with age (Crook et al. 1986). The criteria for the AAMI diagnosis are presented in Table 18.1. Although similar in form to the types of criteria used in arriving at diagnoses of other neurodegenerative disorders, such as AD and vascular dementia (summarized later), the definition of AAMI differs in its specification of strict psychometric cut-points for the demonstration of memory loss and the absence of dementia. To this end, achieving criteria for AAMI requires the individual to perform at least one standard deviation below the mean for young adults on at least one standard memory test (e.g. Logical Memory from the Wechsler Memory Scale) and the absence of dementia defined by another psychometric measure, the Mini Mental State Examination (MMSE; a score of 24 or higher required).

This psychometric approach to defining the memory loss of aging has been challenged on numerous counts (Koivisto et al. 1995). With its reliance on classifying individuals as 'memory impaired' based on the results of a single memory test rather than on a consistent pattern of memory deficit, the criteria are vulnerable to unreliability and may include a high number of 'false positives'. The criteria do not take into account individual differences in performance or any of a variety of conditions that can alter performance and result in the mistaken impression of memory deficits, such as low education opportunities, age

Table 18.1. *Age Associated Memory Impairment diagnostic criteria*

1. *Inclusion criteria*

   a. Men and women at least 50 years of age

   b. Complaints of memory loss in the context of everyday activities such as difficulty remembering names, misplacing objects, or remembering to do multiple tasks. The onset of the memory difficulty is gradual in onset without sudden worsening in recent months

   c. The memory deficit is demonstrated on psychometric tests. Memory test performance is at least 1 SD below the mean established for young adults on a standardized test of recent (secondary) memory which has appropriate normative data for the population under investigation. Typically tests such as the Wechsler Memory Scale-Revised (Wechsler 1987) are recommended

   d. Adequate intellectual development determined by standardized testing, such as a scaled score of at least 9 on the Vocabulary subtest of the Wechsler Adult Intelligence Scale-Revised (Wechsler 1981)

   e. Absence of dementia as determined by a score of 24 or higher on the Mini-Mental State Examination (Folstein et al. 1975)

2. *Exclusion criteria*

   a. Evidence of disturbances in consciousness or delirium

   b. Any neurological disorder that could produce cognitive deterioration (e.g. AD, PD, stroke, tumor, etc.)

   c. History of infectious or inflammatory disease (viral, fungal or syphilitic)

   d. Evidence of significant cerebral vascular pathology as determined by a Hachinski Ischemia Scale score of 4 or higher (Hachinski et al. 1975)

   e. History of repeated minor head injury or a single injury resulting in a period of unconsciousness for one hour or more

   f. A current psychiatric diagnosis of depression, mania or other major psychiatric diagnosis using DSM criteria

   g. Current diagnosis of alcoholism or drug dependency

   h. Evidence of depression (e.g. exceeding a score of 13 on the Hamilton Depression Rating Scale (Hamilton 1967))

   i. Any medical disorder that can produce cognitive deterioration. The determination of such causes is based on complete medical history and clinical examination including appropriate laboratory studies

   j. Use of psychoactive drugs during the month prior to psychological testing

Note:
Summarized from Crook et al. (1986).

cohort effects, or test anxiety. Finally, because there is no lower limit to the psychometric cut-points in the criteria for AAMI, organic defects cannot be satisfactorily ruled out with MMSE scores of 24 or higher. The validity of the entire notion of AAMI has also been called into question (for a review see, Larrabee and McEntee 1995,) as the relationship between AAMI and AD is not clear. Whether AAMI is a benign entity (i.e. normal aging), a risk factor for AD or a prodromal stage of AD remains to be determined.

PROGRESSIVE NEURODEGENERATIVE DISEASES

Dementia defined

Dementia is defined as a syndrome of global cognitive decline from a previous level of function which leads to impairments in the ability to function in everyday life. The syndrome can be produced by any of numerous disorders and is a slowly evolving neurodestructive process (Breitner and Welsh 1995). The characteristics of the dementia syndrome vary with the underlying cause, but all of the dementing disorders share one defining feature, decline in *several* areas of cognitive function (e.g. memory, language, orientation, abstract reasoning, judgement, problem solving, calculation, spatial judgement and praxis). Several criteria have been forwarded for characterizing dementia; the most commonly used have been those of the *Diagnostic and Statistical Manual* (DSM; Table 18.2) and those proposed by Cummings and Benson (1983).

Diagnostic process for determining dementia

In evaluating a cognitive complaint in an elderly patient, the first task is to verify the presence and the extent of a cognitive disorder. In many instances the presence of symptoms may be obvious, requiring little in terms of formal mental status testing. In other situations, particularly in the early stages of brain disease, the mental status assessment alone will not be sufficient. Systematic testing for signs and symptoms is needed to clearly establish the extent of impairment and distinguish the problem from normal aging. The neuropsychological evaluation is particularly helpful in these instances (Chapter 17). The neuropsychological examination is an inferential process which provides a mechanism for establishing the presence of a brain disorder. It brings together a variety of well-developed tools of

Table 18.2 *DSM-IV Diagnostic criteria for dementia of the Alzheimer's type*

(1) Cognitive Criteria: The development of multiple cognitive impairments including memory impairment, defined as impaired ability to learn new information, and at least one of the following cognitive disorders:

a) impairment in language (*aphasia*)

b) impairment in the execution of planned motor acts despite normal motor and sensory function *(apraxia)*

c) failure to recognize or identify objects despite intact sensory function (*agnosia*)

d) disturbance in higher intellectual and so-called 'executive' functions. Typically this is manifest by impaired abstract thinking (e.g. similarities and differences), judgment, planning, organization, sequencing, and in ability to think flexibly and to 'multitask' (attend to multiple competing task demands). This problem often leads to interpersonal problems, family issues or job-related problems

(2) Functional Criteria: The impairments interfere with social or occupational function

(3) Course Criteria: Insidious onset with gradual and continual decline in cognitive function

(4) Exclusionary Criteria:

a) The cognitive disorder cannot be attributed to some other central nervous system disorder known to have cognitive effects, such as cerebrovascular disease, Parkinson's disease, normal pressure hydrocephalus, tumor, subdural hematoma, etc.

b) Systemic conditions, known to cause dementia, are excluded as causal (e.g. hypothyroidism, B12 deficiency, neurosyphilis, etc.)

c) Substance abuse conditions are ruled out

d) The impairment is not due to delirium

e) The impairment is not due to another Axis I disorder (e.g. Major Depressive Disorder, Schizophrenia)

Note:
Modified from the Diagnostic and Statistical Manual of Mental Disorders, Fourth Edition (DSM-IV). Washington DC, American Psychiatric Association, 1994, p 142–143. Note that the DSM-IV (1994) lists separately criteria for dementia by type or cause, unlike the previous version (DSM-III-R), which contained a more generic description of dementia.

cognitive function, normative information against which an individual's results can be compared and an empirical base of information regarding the brain bases of behavioral change and impairment which guides the interpretative process (Lezak 1995). A typical neuropsychological evaluation of an elderly individual with a memory complaint will include standardized assessments of at least six different cognitive domains: intelligence, language, learning and memory, visuospatial function, executive functions (including abstraction and attention) and sensorimotor function. Personality assessment, particularly an evaluation of mood, is critical as is some assessment of functional ability (Breitner and Welsh 1995).

The interpretation of the examination findings is made by considering the degree to which the performance in the neuropsychological examination conforms to known profiles of cognitive change associated with disease or with other conditions affecting test performance (e.g. anxiety). Critical to the interpretative process is the availability of relevant normative information against which an individual's performance can be compared. The age of the patient, educational background, cultural group and birth cohort can all have an impact on test performance and must be considered (Welsh et al. 1994, 1995; Chapter 16). Consequently, test selection in clinical practice must be guided by the availability of the appropriate normative information for the individual or group under investigation.

The 'cortical' and 'subcortical' classification of dementia

Once the presence of dementia is established, there are virtually hundreds of neurological conditions that must be entertained as potentially causal (Table 18.3). The most commonly occurring conditions include AD, ischemic vascular dementias, extrapyramidal disorders and several degenerative disorders such as frontal lobe dementia, diffuse Lewy body disease and progressive supranuclear palsy. For a fuller consideration of the atypical or rare dementias the reader is referred to other sources (Cummings and Benson 1992).

A contribution of neuropsychology to the clinical differentiation of memory disorders has been the recognition that dementia is not a unitary disorder of brain failure. In general, the cognitive profiles tend to sort into two patterns. One pattern, dominated by symptoms of amnesia and signs of language and perceptual or praxis disturbances, is

Table 18.3. *Conditions causing progressive dementia in the elderly*

Neurodegenerative	*Vascular*
Alzheimer's disease	Lacunar state
Frontal lobe dementias	Binswanger's disease
Picks disease	Multi-infarct dementia
Frontotemporal degeneration	Vasculitis
Amyotrophic lateral sclerosis (ALS) dementia	Arteriovenous malformations
Extrapyramidal syndromes	
Parkinson's disease	*Infectious*
Diffuse Lewy body disease	Human immunodeficiency virus (HIV) dementia
Progressive supranuclear palsy	Creutzfeldt–Jakob dementia
Huntington's disease	Brain abscess
Wilson's disease	Bacterial or fungal meningitis
Spinocerebellar degeneration	Postviral encephalitic conditions
Striatonigral degeneration	Neurosyphilis
Corticobasal ganglionic degeneration	Subacute sclerosing panencephalitis
Progressive subcortical gliosis	Whipples disease
Progressive myoclonic epilepsy (Kufs disease)	
Gerstmann–Sträussler syndrome	
Other	
Normal pressure hydrocephalus	
Multiple sclerosis	
Sarcoidosis	
Brain tumor	
Paraneoplastic effects	
Irradiation to frontal lobes	

Sources: Adapted from Whitehouse et al. (1993) and Merck Manual of Geriatrics (1995). Diseases that do not lead to progressive dementias, and inherited metabolic disorders, are excluded from this summary as their clinical course or age of disease onset are not easily confused with progressive dementing conditions of the elderly.

typically observed in conditions like AD which affect the medial temporal lobe cortices and the association cortices in the frontal, temporal and parietal lobes. Another pattern involves milder changes in memory, behavioral changes, impaired affect and mood, motor slowing and executive dysfunction and is commonly observed following damage to the diencephalon, basal ganglia, midbrain and brain stem structures. To capture these distinctions, the classification of dementias as *'cortical'* and *'subcortical'* was proposed by Albert and coworkers in 1974 and was further developed and refined by other investigators (Cummings and Benson 1984). The nomenclature has been debated on grounds of anatomical validity as neuronal loss, gliosis and other neuropathological changes may not respect strictly cortical or subcortical boundaries. Nonetheless, the terminology has some heuristic value and is useful as a short-hand

description of the two principal patterns of neuropsychological change seen in dementia.

CORTICAL DEMENTIAS

Alzheimer's disease

AD is characterized by an insidious onset and slow progression over time, lasting 10 years or more from the time of diagnosis to death. The average age of disease onset is in the mid to late seventies, although there is tremendous variability in both the age of onset and the rate of decline, likely owing to a host of factors including individual differences in genetic makeup and lifetime exposures to environmental risk factors.

    The clinical diagnosis of AD is based on the presenta-

Table 18.4. *NINCDS-ADRDA criteria for Alzheimer's disease*

Probable Alzheimer's disease
1. Dementia established by clinical examination and documented by mental status testing
2. Dementia confirmed by neuropsychological assessment
3. Deficits in two or more areas of cognition
4. Progression in symptoms over time
5. No disturbances in consciousness (no delirium)
6. Late onset and not developmentally acquired; Onset between ages 40–90 years
7. Absence of other conditions that are capable of producing dementia

Possible Alzheimer's disease
1. Atypical onset, presentation or progression of dementia symptoms, and/or
2. Presence of another systemic or other brain disease capable of producing dementia but not thought to be the cause in the case
    under consideration
3. Meets criteria for dementia as confirmed by clinical examination and neuropsychological testing
4. Progression in symptoms over time
5. No disturbances in consciousness
6. Absence of other identifiable causes

Definite Alzheimer's disease
1. Clinical criteria for probable Alzheimer's disease are fulfilled
2. Histopathological evidence of Alzheimer's disease by biopsy or postmortem examination

Source: Summarized from the criteria of McKhann et al. 1984. 'Clinical diagnosis of Alzheimer's disease: Report of the NINCDS-ADRDA Work Group, Department of Health and Human Services Task Force on Alzheimer's Disease,' *Neurology.* 34: 939–944. These criteria were developed by a consensus panel of two joint groups from the National Institute of Neurological and Communicative Disorders and Stroke (NINCDS) and the Alzheimer's Disease and Related Disorders Association (ADRDA).

tion of known clinical signs (as described below) and the exclusion of medical causes other than AD that might give rise to dementia (McKhann et al. 1984). Three categories, based on the level of diagnostic certainty, were proposed for the clinical diagnosis of AD: Probable AD, Possible AD and Definite AD. In this schema, the diagnosis of *Probable AD* requires that a series of conditions are met, as outlined in Table 18.4. The diagnostic classification of *Possible AD* is generally reserved for cases where the certainty of the AD diagnosis is less secure, such as in cases where there is an atypical presentation of dementia (e.g. prominent progressive aphasia) or another brain disease also capable of producing the dementia is present. The diagnosis of *Definite AD* requires pathological verification of the disease, such as brain biopsy in life or autopsy at the time of death. With adherence to these clinical criteria, the diagnostic reliability is generally reported to be between 80 and 90% in pathologically confirmed series of progressive dementia (Gearing et al. 1995). Diagnostic accuracy may be somewhat lower if early stage dementia cases or atypical

dementia presentations are included (Breitner et al. 1994).

The disease course of AD is often conceptualized as following three distinct phases in which higher cognitive functions are progressively lost in a fairly characteristic fashion (Hughes et al. 1982). *Stage 1*, lasting for 1–3 years is characterized by relatively mild cognitive impairments often with attendant personality changes of low mood or major depression. Neurodiagnostic tests, such as electro-encephalography (EEG), computed tomography (CT) and magnetic resonance imaging (MRI) may be essentially normal. In the middle stage of the illness (*Stage II*, lasting 2–10 years), dementia and concomitant changes on neuro-imaging (atrophy with ventricular dilatation) and on EEG (diffuse slowing) are now clearly apparent. By the late stage (*Stage III*, lasting 8–12 years), patients are essentially un-communicative and progress to a vegetative state.

Neuropsychology and cognitive psychology have been critically important in defining the cognitive profiles of AD. The disease is now considered the prototype for the so-called 'cortical' dementias and its cognitive presentation is now well characterized and easily recognized clinically (for a review, see Butters et al. 1995). Profound impairment in recent memory is usually the initial presenting sign and remains a constant feature throughout the duration of the disease. Early in the disease, this memory disorder involves specific impairments in the acquisition and retention of new information (Butters et al. 1988; Welsh et al. 1991; Robinson-Whelen and Storandt 1992; Larrabee et al. 1993). At this stage, working memory impairments (Baddeley et al. 1991; Becker et al. 1992) and a propensity to commit intrusions and false positive recognition errors on memory tests (Pillon et al. 1993) are also evident. Some other areas of memory function, such as procedural learning and immediate memory span, are relatively well preserved (Cherry et al. 1996). Mnemonic strategies, such as category cuing, associative strategies, repetition and recognition structuring, are ineffectual in facilitating recall of recent information in these patients (Butters et al. 1983). This unique profile of memory preservation and impairment in AD contrasts to the pattern seen in subcortical dementing conditions, such as Huntington's disease (HD; described later) where cuing and recognition techniques facilitate recall (Granholm and Butters 1988; Heindel et al. 1990; Massman et al. 1992), but procedural learning is deficient (Eslinger and Damasio 1986; Heindel et al. 1988).

Subtypes of Alzheimer's disease

The majority of cases of AD present in a typical fashion, with pronounced amnesic disorders accompanied by lesser impairments in expressive language and visuospatial function. A growing literature shows that the disease may be quite heterogenous in clinical presentation (Chui et al. 1985; Martin et al. 1986; Blennow and Wallin 1992). A small percentage of cases (under 10% of all AD cases) have been described with presentations of fairly circumscribed brain disease (Jagust et al. 1990) or signs suggestive of progressive posterior cortical atrophy (Victoroff et al. 1994). These patients tend to present with progressive transcortical sensory aphasia (Mesulam and Weintraub 1992) or progressive complex visual system disturbances evidenced by any of a combination of symptoms of Balint's syndrome, alexia, visual object agnosia, apraxia or Gerstmann's syndrome, which suggests a lateralization of their disease to the left or right posterior cerebrum (Ross et al. 1996; Ardila et al. 1997).

Some caution is necessary when diagnosing atypical variants of AD. Neuropathological investigations of these progressive posterior cortical conditions indicate that no single pathological entity accounts for all cases (Victoroff et al. 1994). The condition is etiologically heterogenous and may be any of a variety of conditions including AD, subcortical gliosis, Pick's disease, corticobasal degeneration, Creutzfeldt–Jakob disease or dementia lacking disinctive histopathology (Victoroff et al. 1994). Consequently, instances of unusual presentations of progressive dementia with fairly circumscribed language disturbance or visuospatial impairment should be viewed with suspicion as presumed Alzheimer's disease. In any of these instances, additional diagnostic testing, such as apolipoprotein genotyping (described later) may be particularly useful in clarifying the diagnostic assignment (Welsh-Bohmer et al. 1997).

GENETIC MARKERS AND THE DIFFERENTIAL DIAGNOSIS OF AD

Current findings particularly promising in enhancing diagnostic reliability come from the area of genetics (for a review, see Plassman and Breitner 1996). Several genetic mutations on chromosomes 1, 14 and 21 have been identified which account for some of the rare autosomal dominant forms of AD (Chapters 3 and 14). The amyloid precursor protein gene on chromosome 21 is likely responsible for only a few cases of early onset familial AD. The two other genes located on chromosomes 1 and 14 account for the majority of familial cases of AD (Sherrington et al. 1995). Genetic tests are available for the rare autosomal dominant forms of AD linked to chromosome 14 and 21. These tests are applicable in less than 1% of AD cases seen in clinical practice.

In the more common late onset, sporadic forms of AD, there is now a well-documented association between the apolipoprotein gene (APOE) on chromosome 19 and the occurrence of AD (Strittmatter et al. 1993). In contrast to the rare occurrence of the autosomal dominant disease, most clinical series of AD show that 60–75% of the cases carry at least one copy of the $\varepsilon 4$ form of the gene which is associated with a heightened risk of AD (Hyman et al. 1996). Thus, APOE genotyping is conceptualized as the first of a new paradigm of genetic testing in which the sensitivity to AD is high and more generally applicable to a larger group of patients (Relkin 1996). Supporting this supposition, recent investigations examining the sensitivity, specificity and positive predictive value of the APOE-ε4 allele in pathologically confirmed AD patients suggest that knowledge of APOE genotype may enhance diagnostic certainty (Saunders et al. 1996; Welsh-Bohmer et al. 1997). In each study, the positive predictive value of the ε4 allele for the diagnosis of AD was quite high (97%) and added to diagnostic confidence in over two-thirds of the AD patients assessed. In the future, the genetic information may prove particularly useful in diagnostically challenging situations, such as in cases of very early disease or in patients with atypical symptoms. Expanded study is ongoing in much larger patient samples with a broader range of non-AD diagnoses. Studies combining the use of APOE information and other phenotypic markers of disease, such as mental status and memory test results (Tierney et al. 1996; Chapter 17) or regional neuroimaging changes (Reiman et al. 1996; Chapter 6), hold promise for enhancing the early diagnosis of AD.

Pick's disease and frontal lobe dementias

A variety of conditions account for the nearly 20–30% of cases that are not AD in neuropathological series (Jackson and Lowe 1996). Of these non-AD dementias, a number of disorders grouped under 'frontal lobe' dementias account for approximately 8–10% of the progressive dementias within epidemiological series (Gustafson 1993) and may be responsible for perhaps as high as 12–20% of the cases of dementia coming to neuropathological examination in clinical series (Jackson and Lowe 1996). Until recently, frontal lobe dementia was considered synonymous with Pick's disease. Now, a variety of disorders are recognized under this heading. These disorders share behavioral symptomatology (e.g. personality change, impaired judgement, abstraction and executive functions) as well as neuropathology localized to the frontal lobe (Lund 1993). The most frequently occurring primary frontal disorder is 'frontal dementia of the non-Alzheimer type' or 'frontotemporal dementia'. This condition has a strong familial association and is characterized neuropathologically by mild gliosis and microvacuolation but neither Pick bodies, plaques, tangles nor amyloid deposition. Less common is presenile dementia associated with motor neuron disease, such as amyotrophic lateral sclerosis with dementia. There also exist a variety of degenerative conditions with 'secondary' frontal lobe effects. The manifest symptoms of degenerative vascular conditions, such as Binswanger's

disease, are often frontal lobe impairments believed to be secondary to the apparent disruption of subcortical white matter pathways (discussed later under Vascular dementia).

Several studies have independently confirmed that dementia of the frontal lobe type is distinct from AD based on clinical, neuropsychological and neuropathological grounds (Gustafson 1987; Neary et al. 1988). Diagnostic criteria have been suggested (Brun et al. 1994) as summarized in Table 18.5. In brief, the disorder is characterized early in its course by frank changes in personality and social conduct with these personality disorders running the gamut from behavioral disinhibition to apathy and inertia. Language is frequently disturbed but is characteristically unique from AD in that it tends to be adynamic in nature, progressing often to frank mutism. Paraphasic errors (semantic and phonemic types) classic of AD and vascular disorders are rare. In addition, visuospatial and motor functions are maintained until late in the course, a distinctive difference from the prototypical picture of AD (Locascio et al. 1995). Recent memory dysfunction, unlike in AD, is not a prominent feature of the frontal lobe dementias. On formal neuropsychological testing, deficits in acquisition and retention of new information are often demonstrable but these impairments are relatively mild compared to those evident in executive function and language (Moss et al. 1992).

There has been a recent attempt to systematically compare the neuropsychological profiles of frontal lobe type dementia and AD, controlling for disease severity (Pachana et al. 1996). The AD patients showed significantly more impaired memory performance when compared to the frontal lobe type dementia group, particularly on a nonverbal memory test (Rey Osterrieth Complex Figure Memory Test). The frontal lobe type dementia patients, in contrast, demonstrated more defective performance on executive tasks than did the AD patients (verbal fluency, Stroop). No group differences emerged on tests of confrontation naming, recognition memory or basic attentional processing in this study. More work is needed to further understand the distinctions between frontal lobe type dementia and other cortical conditions, such as AD. The results from this study show that careful attention to relative position of neuropsychological scores on memory and executive tasks may be instructive in the differential diagnosis. Ultimately, the diagnosis of frontal lobe type dementia or Pick's disease must take into account

Table 18.5. *Clinical diagnostic features of frontotemporal dementia*

Core diagnostic features

1. Behavioral disorder which is insidious in onset and slowly progressive. The disorder is characterized by any of the following early in the disease course:
   a) loss of personal awareness (neglect of personal hygiene or grooming)
   b) loss of social awareness (e.g. loss of social tact, misdemeanors, etc.)
   c) decreased awareness of pathologic changes in their own behavior or mental state
   d) disinhibition early in course (e.g. unrestrained sexuality)
   e) mental inflexibility
   f) hyperorality (oral/dietary changes such as overeating, food fads, excessive smoking or alcohol consumption, oral exploration of objects)
   g) stereotyped and perseverative behaviors (e.g. mannerisms such as clapping, singing, humming, or ritualistic fixations such as hoarding or preoccupations with toileting or dressing)
   h) utilization behavior (unrestrained exploration of objects in the environment)

2. Affective symptoms are common and include any of the following:
   a) depression, anxiety, sentimentality, suicidal and fixed ideation or delusions early in the disorder
   b) hypochondriasis or bizarre somatic preoccupations early in the illness
   c) emotional indifference or lack of empathy, sympathy, apathy
   d) amimia (inertia, aspontaneity)

3. Speech disturbances characteristic of the disorder uniquely identify it from other common dementias. Symptoms include:
   a) Progressive reduction of speech (aspontaneity, economy of utterance)
   b) Stereotyped speech (limited repertoire of words or themes)
   c) echolalia or perseveration
   d) late mutism

4. Frontal lobe signs and other physical signs
   a) Early primitive reflexes
   b) Early incontinence
   c) Late akinesia, rigidity, tremor
   d) low and labile blood pressure

5. Perceptual-spatial disorders are absent. Intact abilities to negotiate the environment.

6. Investigative findings include:
   a) Normal EEG despite clinically evident dementia
   b) Brain imaging (structural or functional or both) that show predominantly frontal or anterior temporal lobe abnormalities
   c) Neuropsychology findings of profound failure on frontal lobe tests in the absence of severe memory impairments, aphasic disorder, or perceptual spatial disturbance.

Supportive diagnostic features

1. Onset before age 65 years
2. Positive family history of a similar disorder in a first degree relative (parent, sibling)
3. Bulbar palsy, muscular weakness, wasting, fasciculations (motor neuron disease)

Exclusionary features

1. Abrupt onset with ictal events
2. Head trauma related to the onset
3. Early severe amnesia
4. Early spatial disorientation or other signs of agnosia
5. Early severe apraxia
6. Logoclonic speech with rapid loss of train of thought
7. Myoclonus

Table 18.5. (*cont.*)

8. Corticobulbar and spinal deficits
9. Cerebellar ataxia
10. Choreo-athetosis
11. Early, severe pathological EEG
12. Brain imaging with either predominant postcentral structural or functional defect or multifocal cerebral lesions on CT or MRI
13. Laboratory tests indicating brain involvement from inflammatory process

Relative diagnostic exclusions:
1. Typical history of chronic alcoholism
2. Sustained hypertension
3. History of vascular disease

Source: Summarized from Brun et al. 1994. Clinical and neuropathological criteria for frontotemporal dementia. *Journal of Neurology, Neurosurgery and Psychiatry*, 57 : 416–418.

not only the cognitive profile but also the history of behavioral and personality changes which may not be readily observable on neuropsychological testing (Benson 1993).

Vascular dementia

Vascular diseases leading to white matter ischemia or blatant infarction are estimated to account for 20–25% of the cases of progressive dementia (Tomlinson et al. 1970; Schoenberg 1988; Tatemichi et al. 1994a,b). The prevalence, the definition and even the existence of ischemic vascular dementia are debated (Meyer et al. 1995). Traditionally, the diagnosis of vascular dementia has been made using the Hachinski Ischaemia Scale (Hachinski et al. 1975) or DSM-III-R criteria; however, this has not proved satisfactory. Low scores, for example, on the Hachinski scale permit comfortable exclusion of vascular dementia; however, high scores do not rule out degenerative dementias. More recent attempts to hone diagnostic criteria for multi-infarct dementia and ischemic vascular dementia, such as the criteria proposed by the State of California Alzheimer's Disease Diagnostic and Treatment Centers (Chui et al. 1992), or those of an international workshop (Roman et al. 1993), appear promising. Both these proposals go beyond previous methods but neither can be considered definitive as each requires pathological validation and is constrained by our current understanding of the ischemic disorders. The emerging literature shows that drawing distinctions between AD and vascular dementias is not always a meaningful exercise, as it imposes a dichotomy which may not reflect the true nature and interaction of these disorders. Early neuropathological series

indicate that the occurrence of vascular changes alone in the context of dementia is fairly uncommon. Co-occurring AD with vascular changes is more commonly observed (Welsh et al. 1996). The association of the risk factor for AD, apolipoprotein E ε4 gene, with some forms of vascular dementia suggests that the two diseases may share common pathophysiology thereby accounting for their frequent co-occurrence (Saunders et al. 1993; Plassman and Breitner 1996).

Multi-infarct dementia is characterized by a dementia which follows a stepwise course, with acute changes in mentation occurring during periods of ischemia followed by periods of stability or improvement in cognition. The defining course of multi-infarct dementia does not easily confuse it with progressive dementias, such as AD, where the clinical course is one of relentless decline. Furthermore, the neuropsychological deficits of multi-infarct dementia are not easily confused with the patterns of cognitive impairment of AD. Deficits correspond to the regions of identified lesions or diaschisis in functionally related areas.

SUBCORTICAL DEMENTIAS

Fairly common forms of late onset subcortical dementias include Binswanger's disease, progressive supranuclear palsy, Parkinson's disease dementia and normal pressure hydrocephalus. Rarer disorders include human immunodeficiency virus (HIV)-associated dementia and Creutzfeldt–Jakob disease. Huntington's disease, more commonly observed in early to middle adulthood, is another classic form of subcortical dementia. The neuro-psychological profile in each of these subcortical disorders is typically one of memory inefficiency with disturbed spontaneous recall but relatively intact cued recall and recognition memory. Slowed information processing and retrieval, as well as concentration difficulties, are common. Motor functions are frequently impaired as well; however, unlike AD, language functions and praxis are generally well preserved (Cummings 1993). There are some neuro-psychological distinctions between the various forms of subcortical dementias (Robbins et al. 1994), as described in the text that follows.

The differential diagnosis of these disorders, of course, never rests on the neuropsychological examination alone but is based on the combined use of neurological and phys-ical examination findings, clinical history and the results of laboratory data including neuroimaging and neuropsycho-logical testing. The neuropsychological examination can be quite valuable in raising competing explanations for dementia causation when unexpected cognitive profiles emerge. For example, obtaining a subcortical profile in a case where AD was suspected instead of the more classic profile of memory and cognitive disturbance of this dis-order, may suggest another condition is operating (e.g. vas-cular disease, Parkinson's disease (PD), etc.).

Binswanger's disease

Binswanger's disease is a condition of chronic progressive subcortical dementia attributed to pronounced atrophy and diffuse lesions within the cerebral white matter. The disease has been recognized since 1894 when the neuro-pathology of eight cases of progressive dementia and severe atherosclerosis were described by Otto Binswanger. The diagnosis was rarely discussed until recently and its position as a unique clinicopathological entity has been the subject of debate (Tatemichi et al. 1994b). Reappearance of the diagnosis is largely due to the advent of advanced neuroimaging technologies, specifically magnetic reso-nance imaging (MRI), which has facilitated the visualiza-tion of white matter ischemic changes and demyelination. The appearance on CT or on T2 weighted MRI images of extensive patchy, diffuse white matter and low-density changes in the periventricular brain regions support the diagnosis. Recent studies have explored the clinical his-tological correlate of these changes and indicate a variety of distinct causes which depend on the location, size and shape and imaging characteristics of the lesions

(Tatemichi et al. 1994b). Causes include demyelination, axonal loss, dilation of perivascular spaces, incomplete infarction and lacunar infarcts. The condition is fre-quently accompanied by arteriosclerosis but the relation-ship of Binswanger's disease to the vascular dementias is still not completely understood.

The history of symptoms in Binswanger's disease gene-rally favors a gradually progressive decline and does not have the stepwise appearance of multi-infarct dementia. The dementia manifest in this disorder tends to display a patchy profile of cognitive impairment and is generally described as conforming to the 'subcortical' pattern. Some distinctive features of these vascular conditions include: (1) information retrieval deficits manifest as decreased verbal fluency and impaired spontaneous recall, (2) inefficiency in cognitive processing leading to attentional disturbances and (3) motor slowing. The profile of change has been ascribed to the structural brain injuries localized to the subcortical brain areas, an assertion finding support from a number of recent neuroimaging studies using MRI or CT (Rao et al. 1989; Tupler et al. 1992). In addition, functional imaging studies demonstrate decreased cere-bral perfusion localized to the frontal cortices (Sultzer et al. 1995) and the frontal white matter, thalamus and internal capsule (Meyer et al. 1995). The picture of hypo-metabolism in Binswanger's disease contrasts with the hypoperfusion of AD which tends to be more apparent in the temporal and parietal lobes.

Huntington's disease

Huntington's disease (HD) is an autosomal dominant, pro-gressive disorder recently localized to a gene defect on chromosome 4 (Huntington's Disease Collaborative Research Group 1993). The disease characteristically strikes within the fourth or fifth decades of life. Although there is high variability both in age at onset and in initial symptoms (Claes et al. 1995), the leading features of the condition are choreic movements, cognitive decline con-forming to a 'subcortical' dementia, personality change and psychiatric symptoms. Some patients will first present with movement symptoms, such as intermittent facial grimacing or tics, others may initially manifest solely psychiatric symptoms, depression or schizophrenia-like disorders (Folstein et al. 1979). Still other cases will demonstrate both neurological and psychiatric symptoms from the outset.

The cognitive profile of HD is considered a leading example of the so-called 'subcortical' dementias (Brandt and Butters 1986). The dementia is characterized by slowed mentation (bradyphrenia), impaired attention, poor retrieval on tests of verbal fluency and spontaneous recall but generally intact performance on recognition memory and naming tasks (Hodges et al. 1991; Jacobs and Huber 1992). The underlying brain defect mediating these symptoms is degeneration of the caudate nucleus. Eventually, structures beyond the caudate are involved including the frontal and parietal cortex, the globus pallidus, putamen, thalamus and substantia nigra (Myers et al. 1988).

The memory deficits distinguishing HD and AD are among the best studied areas in the neuropsychology of dementia (Brandt and Butters 1986; Butters 1992). Unlike AD where severe storage deficits occur in the processing of recent memory information, the memory impairment of HD is characterized by inefficient encoding and retrieval strategies from memory (Butters et al. 1985, 1986; Moss et al. 1986). Consequently, whereas the memory disorder of AD is primarily characterized by rapid forgetting, HD patients show relatively intact forgetting rates and savings scores (Tröster et al. 1993). Also unlike AD, patients with HD benefit from cuing strategies and other methods of retrieval support (Granholm and Butters 1988; Heindel et al. 1990). As a result, HD patients frequently show less impaired performance on recognition memory than on delayed recall and intrusions and false positive recognition errors are also less common in HD than in AD (Pillon et al. 1993).

Semantic memory, assessed through procedures such as fluency and naming tests, is relatively spared in HD when compared to AD (Chapter 11). On formal testing of verbal fluency, diminished output is seen in both HD and AD; however, a comparison of the deficits associated with each reveals consistent differences. In HD both lexical and category fluency are equally disturbed and naming is relatively intact except for perceptual errors (Butters et al. 1987; Hodges et al. 1991). In AD, category generation is much more severely affected than is lexical retrieval (Monsch et al. 1992) and naming problems are common (Bayles and Tomoeda 1983). These findings have provided further support of the hypothesis that HD patients suffer from a general retrieval deficit whereas AD patients demonstrate a breakdown in the structure and organization of semantic memory (Tröster et al. 1989).

Another area distinguishing AD and HD patients is skill learning (Chapter 12). In HD and in PD where the integrity of the corticostriatal circuits is compromised, impairments are reported on procedural motor tasks such as weight biasing (Heindel et al. 1991), motor skill learning (Heindel et al. 1988, 1989; Harrington et al. 1990) and on prism adaptation (Paulsen et al. 1993). Patients with AD generally demonstrate normal performances on motor skill learning (Eslinger and Damasio 1986; Heindel et al. 1989). This relatively selective impairment in motor learning in HD and PD can be valuable in the differential diagnosis of cortical and subcortical conditions. The presence of a subcortical neuropsychological profile on memory, language and perceptual testing, complemented by impairments in motor function, raise the strong suspicion of a disorder other than AD.

Progressive supranuclear palsy

Progressive supranuclear palsy is a relatively rare condition characterized by supranuclear oculomotor palsy (difficulty with voluntary upward gaze), bradykinesia and a parkinsonian syndrome with ataxia, postural instability and neck and truncal rigidity (Johnson et al. 1992). Neuronal loss is confined primarily to the subcortical structures such as the basal ganglia, upper brain stem and cerebellar nuclei; however, recent studies note pathological change in the hippocampus and neocortex as well (Hauw et al. 1990). The disorder is believed to result from disruption of the major output of the basal ganglia to the frontal lobes. This hypothesis is consistent with the neuropathological distribution of cellular change as well as neuroimaging data which shows reduced glucose metabolism and cerebral perfusion in the frontal lobes of these patients (Foster et al. 1988; Johnson et al. 1992).

Cognitive impairments are common in the disorder and the classic profile of neuropsychological deficits is the prototype on which the definition of subcortical dementia is based (Albert et al. 1974). The progressive supranuclear palsy disorder is characterized by a cluster of symptoms including memory impairment, bradyphrenia, difficulty with mental manipulations and emotional and personality changes. More recent neuropsychological investigations have provided further definition of the cognitive and memory disorders of progressive supranuclear palsy (Litvan 1994; Robbins et al. 1994; Grafman et al. 1995). Compared to AD patients, progressive supranuclear palsy patients show less severe impairments in learning of new information, retrieval and forgetting rates but greater impairments in procedural learning (Litvan 1994). Patients have more difficulty on word learning tests retrieving words across trials and then recalling these words without cues after delay intervals. Recognition memory, on the other hand, is qualitatively superior to free recall in these patients (Litvan 1994) and episodic memory performance in general is superior in progressive supranuclear palsy patients when compared to AD patients (Pillon et al. 1991).

Also distinguishing the neuropsychological impairments of progressive supranuclear palsy from other neurodegenerative disorders is the early and pronounced impairment in central executive function, principally in sustained attention, central processing speed and in the shifting of conceptual sets (Grafman et al. 1995). Patients perform poorly on tests involving concept formation (such as tests of proverbs) and behavioral flexibility (Pillion et al. 1986). Performance on verbal and nonverbal fluency tests involving systematic retrieval strategies is impaired as well (Grafman et al. 1995). While on the surface the performance of progressive supranuclear palsy patients on frontal executive tasks resembles that of other subcortical disorders, there are some qualitative and quantitative distinctions in information processing speed (Robbins et al. 1994). In progressive supranuclear palsy information processing speed is much slower even when care is taken to remove motor confounds. These patients also have more difficulty on tests of visual attention and vigilance (Grafman et al. 1995). The cognitive profile of subcortical compromise as described together with evidence from clinical examination of: (1) restricted vertical gaze, (2) extrapyramidal signs, (3) frequent falling, (4) pseudobulbar palsy and/or dystonic dysarthria, in the absence of focal lesions, almost always indicates a diagnosis of progressive supranuclear palsy (Pillon et al. 1991).

Parkinson's disease dementia

Parkinson's disease (PD), like progressive supranuclear palsy, is a subcortical neurodegenerative disorder. It is characterized by neuronal cell loss in the pigmented nuclei of the brain stem (Pujol et al. 1992) and results primarily in motor, cognitive and affective symptoms. Dementia is also observed in some cases. With the use of rigorous diagnostic criteria for PD, a rate of dementia between 20 and 30% is suggested (Gibb 1993; Quinn 1993; Aarsland et al. 1996).

The cognitive impairments accompanying PD are very similar to those of progressive supranuclear palsy. After controlling for motor impairment, depressed mood and

medication effects, clear patterns of impairments emerge that appear to be fundamental to PD and distinguish it from normal aging and other brain conditions (Boyd et al. 1991; Cooper et al. 1991). PD groups show specific deficits in immediate recall of verbal information, language production and verbal fluency, set formation, cognitive sequencing, working memory and visuomotor construction (Cooper et al. 1991). Some studies report procedural memory impairments in PD (e.g. on tasks such as rotary pursuit) which are not typically observed in patients with AD (Saint-Cyr et al. 1988). Other investigations suggest that such deficits are a function of disease severity and the presence or absence of dementia in PD (Heindel et al. 1989; Harrington et al. 1990). Unaffected by the disorder are memory span, long-term forgetting, naming, comprehension and visual perception (Cooper et al. 1991; Levin et al. 1992). This pattern of impaired and preserved functions in PD contrasts with AD where the forgetting rates are characteristically rapid (Welsh et al. 1991; Tröster et al. 1993) and where impairments in naming, praxis and visual perception are common (Welsh et al. 1992).

Diffuse Lewy body disease

Diffuse Lewy body disease can also produce progressive dementia with neuropsychological and behavioral features that mimic both cortical and subcortical dementias (Galasko et al. 1996; Salmon et al. 1996). There has not been general consensus as to whether this disorder is a unique condition or a variant of AD. Recent genetic evidence of an over-representation of the APOE ε4 allele in diffuse Lewy body disease (Galasko et al. 1994) and postmortem observations of combined pathological signs of both AD and Lewy bodies in cases of diffuse Lewy body disease, argue that the condition may be a phenotypic variant of AD (Katzman et al. 1995); however, occasionally cases are observed with subcortical and neocortical Lewy bodies but without significant AD pathology (Galasko et al. 1996). Consequently, until the relationship of AD and diffuse Lewy body disease is resolved, the illness is now often referred to as the 'Lewy body variant of AD' when pathological features of both conditions are present, but as 'pure diffuse Lewy body disease' when AD lesions are absent.

The characteristic clinical features of this illness include fluctuating cognitive impairment along with parkinsonian signs, psychotic features and episodes of falling with orthostatic hypotension (for a review, see Perry et al. 1996). Visual hallucinations are usually prominent early in this disorder. This unique feature contrasts diffuse Lewy body disease from other forms of progressive dementia where hallucinations, when they occur, do so late in the dementing illness.

The neuropsychological features of diffuse Lewy body disease have been poorly understood until fairly recently (for review, see Salmon and Galasko 1996). Detailed neurocognitive investigations in small samples (Hansen et al. 1990) and in single case designs (Wagner and Bachman 1996) note the presence of frontal lobe impairments, forgetfulness and motor slowing in diffuse Lewy body disease affected patients. Comparisons of individuals with clinically suspected Lewy body disease and patients with AD reveal that the diffuse Lewy body disease patients have greater deficits in attention, verbal fluency and visuospatial processing (Hansen et al. 1990). A recent retrospective study in neuropathologically confirmed cases of diffuse Lewy body disease and AD confirm and extend these previous results (Salmon et al. 1996). In this study, the neuropsychological profiles of five cases of diffuse Lewy body disease were contrasted to those obtained from five cases of AD matched for overall dementia severity at the clinical assessment. The results of this analysis indicate that pure diffuse Lewy body disease, like AD, can produce a global dementia with impairments in memory, language, attention, executive functions, visuospatial ability and psychomotor performance. The disorder differs from AD in that the diffuse Lewy body disease patients had more significant impairments on tests of visuoconstructive ability (Block Design, clock drawing tests) and psychomotor performance (Trail Making test) than the AD group. In contrast, their memory deficits on the California Verbal Learning Test (CVLT) were relatively mild when compared to those of the AD patients. Most of the diffuse Lewy body disease cases did not show the very poor retention and recognition discriminability deficits characteristic of AD, nor did they show the propensity to commit a large number of intrusion errors. On language testing, patients with disorder demonstrated deficits in confrontation naming and equally impaired performance on category and letter fluency procedures. The latter finding is in contrast to that observed in AD, where a greater deficit on category than letter fluency is frequently observed (Monsch et al. 1994). Considered within the 'cortical versus subcortical dementia' framework, the dementia associated with diffuse Lewy body disease is best conceptualized as

involving a 'superimposition' of both neuropsychological profiles, an interpretation consistent with the distribution of neuropathological changes seen in the hippocampus, association cortices, substantia nigra and other subcortical structures (Hansen et al. 1990; Salmon and Galasko 1996).

Normal pressure hydrocephalus

Normal pressure hydrocephalus or *communicating hydrocephalus* is also associated with a subcortical dementia, with its symptoms likely due to the distension of corticospinal axons and anterior cerebral arteries and capillaries running adjacent to the ventricular system and providing important blood flow to the frontal lobes (Stambrook et al. 1994). The disorder is potentially reversible with effective reduction of intraventricular volume of the cerebrospinal fluid (CSF) such as by lumbar puncture or shunt procedures to divert CSF (Mamo et al. 1987). Typically, gait disturbance is the symptom most likely to improve with surgical intervention, while dementia is the least likely symptom to resolve. When postsurgical improvement in mentation is reported, the changes can be global, but typically they are not observed across all affected functions (Stambrook et al. 1994).

Typically, the disorder presents with a triad of clinical symptoms (gait and balance disturbance, bladder incontinence, dementia) and radiographically there is evidence of ventricular dilatation (Adams et al. 1965). In many cases, however, the complete triad of symptoms is not observed and evidence of ventricular enlargement does not assure the diagnosis because similar ventriculomegaly is common in other neurological diagnoses including progressive dementias such as AD.

The neuropsychological profile of hydrocephalus is less well recognized and documented than that of the more prevalent dementing conditions. As a result of the low prevalence of the condition, the reported clinical series often include samples of patients with differing disease severities making the appreciation of the natural history of the disorder difficult. Despite these limitations, systematic investigations have advanced the understanding of the neuropsychological profile of this disorder. The typical presentation of normal pressure hydrocephalus is now understood to be one of frontal deficits characterized by prominent impairments in attention and concentration, mental tracking and flexibility, bradyphrenia and loss of behavioral initiative (Stambrook et al. 1994). In contrast to AD, anterograde memory deficits are not prominent in the early stages of normal pressure hydrocephalus. As the condition progresses, memory problems are often profound and noted in at least half of the patients (Fisher 1977). In the few studies which compared normal pressure hydrocephalus to other dementias, patients with hydrocephalus were reported to have less impaired memory functions compared to AD and multi-infarct dementia patients with similar dementia severity (Cooke 1981, in Stambrook et al. 1994), but to show tendencies toward response confabulation (Berglund et al. 1979).

Dementias of infectious etiology

There are a variety of infectious agents that may give rise to dementia or delirium. Although infections are not among the common causes of dementia in the elderly, familiarity with the various presenting signs of these disorders is critical as these dementias virtually all have high rates of mortality and morbidity and because at least some of these disorders are treatable. The two most well-known infectious dementias are human immunodeficiency virus (HIV) associated dementia and Creutzfeldt–Jakob disease. General paresis, the late sequel of syphilis, is another infectious dementia but is no longer considered a prevalent cause of dementia in Western societies because of the general availability of penicillin and the improvements in early identification of sexually transmitted diseases (Simon 1985). Less common infectious causes for dementia include tuberculous meningitis, fungal meningitis and viral encephalitis (Whitehouse et al. 1993). Unlike slowly progressive dementias, such as AD, these disorders tend to be rapidly progressive over a period of months and have other associated symptoms such as fever, signs of inflammation elsewhere in the body, neurological signs including focal impairments, headache, nausea or seizures. Occasionally, patients develop dementia as a result of infection with Lyme disease; however, this disorder is also accompanied by other neurological signs and either a clear history of arthropod bite or the classic skin rash accompanying this disorder (Logigian et al. 1990).

HIV associated dementia

Although not considered a major cause of dementia in the elderly, HIV associated dementia is occurring more frequently in the elderly segment of the population (Janssen et al. 1992; Kernutt et al. 1993). The under-recognition of HIV as an etiological factor in older patients presenting with memory complaints leads to the potential confusion

of HIV associated dementia for more prevalent causes of memory loss in the older patient, such as AD (Perry and Marotta 1987; Scharnhorst 1992). Clinical criteria for HIV associated dementia, as well as for milder forms of neurocognitive disorders associated with HIV positivity, have been proposed and these criteria can be applied to patients regardless of their age (Grant et al. 1995).

HIV associated dementia is often said to be characterized by a *subcortical* dementia profile. The cognitive features of early HIV associated dementia include partial forgetting and impairments in sustained attention and concentration. Verbal memory deficits are noted in some, but not all, HIV cases (Peavy et al. 1994). Specific impairments in acquisition, retention of new information over brief delays and the use of semantic clustering strategies to facilitate retrieval are noted. When compared to the pattern of performance seen in HD and in AD, the memory profile of HIV patients most closely approximates that of the HD group, thus supporting the typology of a subcortical dementia. In a comprehensive examination of possible subcortical cognitive dysfunction patterns in HIV infection (for a review, see Martin 1994), specific discriminating patterns were noted involving tests typically associated with either frontal lobe or striatal function but less reliant on parietal-cortical integrity. Impairments were noted in tests of simple and choice reaction time, visual attention, egocentric spatial judgement (which emphasizes spatial localization relative to the observer) and on some tests of motor performance, such as the pursuit rotor test.

Activities of daily living are affected in HIV associated dementia, particularly performance on sequential tasks or in activities involving the splitting of attentional resources amongst multiple competing task demands. Mild word finding difficulties and dysarthria are also noted. Typical signs of cortical dysfunction (apraxia, agnosia and aphasia) are usually entirely absent or less pronounced. As the disease progresses, more global dysfunction emerges affecting many aspects of memory function, abstract thinking and components of expressive language. During the end stages, mutism and hypersomnolence result. In these later stages of illness, the cognitive dysfunction has a mixed cortical/subcortical appearance.

Creutzfeldt–Jakob disease

Creutzfeldt–Jakob disease is a clinically well recognized, but very rare, transmissible neurodegenerative disorder with an estimated worldwide incidence of one case per million per year (Tabrizi et al. 1996). The disease is generally characterized by a rapidly progressive dementia with an average age of disease onset typically in the early sixties, with the range of disease onsets varying from age 45 to 75 years (Bendheim 1984; Brown et al. 1986, 1987). Although generally rapid in its course, a more indolent form of the illness has been described. This form has an earlier age of disease onset and is many times familial (Collinge et al. 1992).

The clinical characteristics of Creutzfeldt–Jakob disease are diverse, involving various combinations of neurological signs. This has led to a confusing literature with an array of many different subtypes proposed; however, typically, the illness involves personality change (such as depression) as the earliest sign of the illness. Later, a pervasive and profound dementia is identifiable. The presence of a triad of symptoms (subacute dementia in a middle age adult, myoclonus and characteristic electroencephalogram findings of diffuse slowing with periodic sharp waves or spikes) and a rapid course allow the reliable diagnosis of the illness in the majority of cases. The common clinical subtypes that clinicians need to be aware of are: (1) the ataxic or cerebellar form of the disease which presents with gait disturbances or intention tremor sometimes in the absence of mental status changes, (2) the rapidly progressive dyskinetic subtype, which is characterized by the presence of basal ganglia signs (such as rigidity, bradykinesia, tremor, dystonic posturing or choreoathetosis) and includes a dementia with subcortical features, (3) the amyotrophic form, which is less common and is characterized by loss of anterior horn cells causing muscle atrophy and weakness, (4) the rare 'Heidenhain's variant', which by its visual symptoms (e.g. visual agnosia or cortical blindness) suggests occipitoparietal lobe involvement in the dementia.

The most challenging clinical differentiation of Creutzfeldt–Jakob disease from other dementias occurs with the indolent form of the disease. This slowly progressive form of Creutzfeldt–Jakob disease can be virtually indistinguishable from AD and often requires neuropathological verification through biopsy or autopsy at the time of death (Brown et al. 1984). Even in this ambiguous situation the disorder can usually be distinguished from AD by the early appearance of motor or reflex changes on the neurological examination and periodic EEG abnormalities (Mendez et al. 1994; Tabrizi et al. 1996). At neuropathological examination, the illness is easily differentiated from AD by prominent spongiform

changes and gliosis throughout the cerebral cortex along with dendritic swelling, axonal and dendritic loss and the accumulation of abnormal cytoskeletal protein (Harrison and Roberts 1991).

CONCLUSIONS

Systematic neuropsychological studies of aging and the various neurodegenerative dementias of the elderly have highlighted some of the unique features of these various conditions permitting more accurate differential diagnoses. These studies have also indicated variability in symptom presentations within each of these conditions. This observation underscores the limits of the neuropsychological examination. The examination is helpful in detecting the presence of subtle disorders and in providing neuropsychological profiles which may guide the conceptualization of the case and permit exclusion of some competing neurobehavioral syndromes. The examination by itself is insufficient to delineate the cause of a dementing disorder. The differential diagnosis of progressive degenerative conditions requires a clear history of the presenting problem, neurological examination, neuropsychological and psychiatric history and a diagnostic workup which includes neuroimaging, and other laboratory studies and tests to exclude other medical conditions. The continuing progress in neuroimaging technologies and in the identification of promising biomarkers of disease, such as apolipoprotein E, may enhance early differential diagnosis in the future. In addition, the advances in neuropsychology, particularly in the area of memory processing, may also prove valuable in enhancing reliable disease identification. In disorders such as AD, attention to memory changes along with biological markers of disease (e.g. APOE) appears to be a promising method for detecting and verifying early stages of the illness.

Until there are reliable diagnostic tests for AD and the other forms of dementia, however, the members of the multidisciplinary teams evaluating elderly patients will need to rely on the clinical examination of these patients. It is the responsibility of the neuropsychologist, as a member of this team, to be knowledgeable about the clinical features, cognitive profiles and base rates of neurodegenerative disorders that can compromise physical, cognitive and emotional function in the elderly. Even with refinements in other diagnostic methods, the neuropsychological evaluation will continue to serve an important function in the clinical diagnosis and management of neurodegenerative disease. The neuropsychological evaluation provides unique neurobehavioral data which are essential in diagnosis, tracking of disease course and the development of effective behavioral, cognitive, emotional and environmental interventions.

ACKNOWLEDGMENT

This work was supported in part by federal research grants from the National Institutes of Aging (AG-09997 and AG-05128).

REFERENCES

Aarsland, D., Tandberg, E., Larsen, J.P. and Cummings, J.L. 1996. Frequency of dementia in Parkinson disease. *Neurology*. 53: 538–542.

Adams, R.D., Fisher, C.M, Hakim, S., Ojemann, R.G. and Sweet, W.H. 1965. Symptomatic occult hydrocephalus with 'normal' cerebrospinal fluid pressure. *New England Journal of Medicine*. 273: 117–126.

Albert, M.L., Feldman, R.G. and Willis, A.L. 1974. The 'subcortical dementia' of progressive supranuclear palsy. *Journal of Neurology, Neurosurgery and Psychiatry*. 37: 121–134.

American Psychiatric Association. 1994. *Diagnostic and Statistical Manual of Mental Disorders - Fourth Edition (DSM-IV)*. Washington, DC: American Psychiatric Association.

Ardila, A., Rosselli, M., Arvizu, L. and Kuljis, R.O. 1997. Alexia and agraphia in posterior cortical atrophy. *Neuropsychiatry, Neuropsychology and Behavioral Neurology*. 10: 52–59.

Baddeley, A.D., Bressi, S., Dalla Salla, S., Logie, R. and Spinnler, H. 1991. The decline of working memory in Alzheimer's disease. A longitudinal study. *Brain*. 114: 2521–2542.

Bayles, K.A. and Tomoeda, C.K. 1983. Confrontation naming impairment in dementia. *Brain and Language*. 19: 98–114.

Becker, J.T., Bajulaiye, O. and Smith, C. 1992. Longitudinal analysis of a two component model of the memory deficit in Alzheimer's disease. *Psychological Medicine*. 22: 437–445.

Bendheim, P.E. 1984. Human spongiform encephalopathies. Symposium on neurovirology. *Neurologic Clinics*. 2: 281–298.

Benson, D.F. 1993. Progressive frontal dysfunction. *Dementia*. 4: 149–153.

Berglund, M., Gustafson, L. and Hagberg, B. 1979. Amnestic-confabulatory syndrome in hydrocephalic patients and Korsakoff's psychosis in alcoholism. *Acta Psychiatrica Scandinavica*. 60: 323–333.

Binswanger, O. 1894. Abgrenzung der allgemeinen progressiven Paralyse. *Berliner Klinische Wochenschrift*. 31: 1102–1105, 1137–1139, 1180–1186.

Blennow, K. and Wallin, A. 1992. Clinical heterogeneity of probable Alzheimer's disease. *Journal of Geriatric Psychiatry and Neurology*. 5: 106–113.

Boyd, J.L, Cruickshank, C.A., Kenn, C.W., Madeley, P., Mindham, R.H.S., Oswald, A.G., Smith, R.J. and Spokes, E.G.S. 1991. Cognitive impairment and dementia in Parkinson's disease: A controlled study. *Psychological Medicine*. 21: 911–921.

Brandt, J. and Butters, N. 1986. The neuropsychology of Huntington's disease. *Trends in Neurosciences*. 118–120.

Breitner, J.C.S. and Welsh, K.A. 1995. An approach to diagnosis and management of memory loss and other cognitive syndromes of aging. *Psychiatric Services: A Journal of the American Psychiatric Association*. 46: 29–35.

Breitner, J.C.S., Welsh, K.A., Robinette, C.D., Gau, B.A., Folstein, M.F. and Brandt, J. 1994. Alzheimer's disease in the National Academy of Sciences Registry of Aging Twin Veterans. II. Longitudinal findings in a pilot series. *Dementia*. 5: 99–105.

Brown, P., Cathala, F., Castaigne, P. and Gajdusek, D.C. 1986. Creutzfeldt–Jakob disease: Clinical analysis of a consecutive series of 230 neuropathologically verified cases. *Annals of Neurology*. 20: 597–602.

Brown, P., Cathala, F., Raubertas, R.F., Gajdusek, D.C. and Castaigne, P. 1987. The epidemiology of Creutzfeldt–Jakob disease: Conclusion of a 15 year investigation in France and review of the world literature. *Neurology*. 37: 895–904.

Brown, P., Rodgers-Johnson, P., Cathala, F., Gibbs, C.J. and Gajdusek, D.C. 1984. Creutzfeldt-Jakob disease of long duration: Clinicopathological characteristics, transmissibility and differential diagnosis. *Annals of Neurology*. 16: 295–304.

Brun, A., Englund, B., Gustafson, L., Passant, U., Mann, D.M.A., Neary, D. and Snowden, J.S. 1994. Clinical and neuropathological criteria for frontotemporal dementia. *Journal of Neurology, Neurosurgery and Psychiatry*. 57: 416–418.

Butters, N. 1992. Memory remembered: 1970–1991. *Archives of Clinical Neuropsychology*. 7: 285–295.

Butters, N., Albert, M.S., Sax, D.S., Miliotis, P., Nagode, J. and Sterste, A. 1983. The effect of verbal mediators on the pictorial memory of brain-damaged patients. *Neuropsychologia*. 21: 307–323.

Butters, N., Delis, D.C. and Lucas, J.A. 1995. Clinical assessment of memory disorders in amnesia and dementia. *Annual Review of Psychology*. 46: 493–523.

Butters, N., Granholm, E., Salmon, D.P., Grant, I. and Wolfe, J. 1987. Episodic and semantic memory: A comparison of amnesic and demented patients. *Journal of Clinical and Experimental Neuropsychology*. 9: 479–497.

Butters, N., Salmon, D.P., Cullum, C., Cairns, P., Tröster, A.I., Jacobs, D., Moss, M. and Cermak, L.S. 1988. Differentiation of amnesic and demented patients with the Wechsler Memory Scale - Revised. *Clinical Neuropsychologist*. 2: 133–148.

Butters, N., Wolfe, J., Granholm, E. and Martone, M. 1986. An assessment of verbal recall, recognition and fluency abilities in patients with Huntington's disease. *Cortex*. 22: 11–32.

Butters, N., Wolfe, J., Martone, M., Granholm, E. and Cermak, L.S. 1985. Memory disorders association with Huntington's disease: Verbal recall, verbal recognition and procedural memory. *Neuropsychologia*. 23: 729–744.

Cherry, B., Buckwalter, J. and Henderson, V. 1996. Memory span procedures in Alzheimer's disease. *Neuropsychology*. 10: 286–293.

Chui, H.C., Teng, E.L., Henderson, V.W. and Moy, A.C. 1985. Clinical subtypes of dementia of the Alzheimer type. *Neurology*. 35: 1544–1550.

Chui, H.C., Victoroff, J.I., Margolin, D., Jagust, W., Shankle, R. and Katzman, R. 1992. Criteria for the diagnosis of ischemic vascular dementia proposed by the State of California Alzheimer's Disease Diagnostic and Treatment Centers. *Neurology*. 42: 473–480.

Claes, S., Van And, K., Legius, E., Dom, R., Malfroid, M., Baro, F., Godderis, J. and Cassiman, J.J. 1995. Correlations between triplet repeat expansion and clinical features in Huntington's disease. *Archives of Neurology*. 113: 749–753.

Collinge, J., Brown, J., Hardy, J., Mullan, M., Rossor, M.N., Baker, H., Crow, T.J., Lofthouse, R., Poulter, M., Ridley, R., Owen, F., Bennett, C., Dunn, G., Harding, A.E., Quinn, F., Doshi, B., Roberts, G.W., Honavar, M., Janota, I. and Lantos, P.L. 1992. Inherited prion disease with 144 base pair gene insertion. 2. Clinical and pathological features. *Brain*. 115: 687–710.

Cooper, J.A., Sagar, H.J., Jordan, N., Harvey, N.S. and Sullivan, E.V. 1991. Cognitive impairment in early untreated Parkinson's disease and its relationship to motor disability. *Brain*. 114: 2095–2122.

Creasy, H. and Rapoport, S.I. 1985. The aging human brain. *Annals of Neurology*. 17: 2–10.

Crook, T., Bartus, R.T., Ferris, S.H., Whitehouse, P., Cohen, G.D. and Gershon, S. 1986. Age-Associated Memory Impairment: Proposed diagnosis criteria and measures of clinical change- Report of a National Institute of Mental Health Work Group. *Developmental Neuropsychology*. 2: 261–276.

Cummings, J.L. 1993. Frontal-subcortical circuits and human behavior. *Archives of Neurology*. 50: 873–880.

Cummings, J.L. and Benson, D.F. 1983. *Dementia: A clinical approach*. Boston: Butterworth.

Cummings, J.L. and Benson, D.F. 1984. Subcortical dementia: Review of an emerging concept. *Archives of Neurology*. 41: 874–879.

Cummings, J.L. and Benson, D.F. 1992. *Dementia: A clinical approach*, 2nd ed. Boston: Butterworth-Heinemann.

Eslinger, P.J. and Damasio, A.R. 1986. Preserved motor learning in Alzheimer's disease: Implications for anatomy and behavior. *Journal of Neuroscience*. 6: 3006–3009.

Fisher, C.M. 1977. The clinical picture in occult hydrocephalus. *Clinical Neurosurgery*. 24: 270–284.

Folstein M.F., Folstein S.E. and McHugh P.R. 1975. 'Mini-Mental State': A practical method for grading the cognitive state of patients for the clinician. *Journal of Psychiatric Research*. 12: 189–198.

Folstein, S.E., Folstein, M.F. and McHugh P.R. 1979. Psychiatric syndromes in Huntington's disease. *Advances in Neurology*. 23: 281–289.

Foster, N.L., Gilman, S., Berent, S., Morin, E.M., Brown, M.B. and Koeppe, R.A. 1988. Cerebral hypometabolism in progressive supranuclear palsy studied with positron emission tomography. *Annals of Neurology*. 24: 399–406.

Galasko, D., Katzman, R., Salmon, D.P. and Hansen, L. 1996. Clinical and neuropathological findings in Lewy body dementias. *Brain and Cognition*. 31: 166–175.

Galasko, D., Saitoh, T., Xia, Y., Thal, L.J., Katzman, R., Hill, L.R. and Hansen, L. 1994. The apolipoprotein E allele ε4 is overrepresented in patients with the Lewy body variant of Alzheimer's disease. *Neurology*. 44: 1950–1951.

Gearing, M., Mirra, S.S., Hedreen, J.C., Sumi, S.M., Hansen, L.A. and Heyman, A. 1995. Consortium to Establish a Registry for Alzheimer's Disease (CERAD). Part X. Neuropathology confirmation of the clinical diagnosis of Alzheimer's disease. *Neurology*. 45: 461–466.

Gibb, W.R.G. 1993. Cortical dementia in Parkinson's disease. In *Mental dysfunction in Parkinson's disease*, ed. E.C. Wolters and P. Scheltens, pp. 211–220. Amsterdam, Netherlands: Vrije Universiteit.

Grafman, J., Litvan, I. and Stark, M. 1995. Neuropsychological features of progressive supranuclear palsy. *Brain and Cognition*. 28: 311–320.

Granholm, E. and Butters, N. 1988. Associative encoding and retrieval in Alzheimer's disease and Huntington's disease. *Brain and Cognition*. 7: 335–347.

Grant, I., Heaton, R.K. and Atkinson, J.H. 1995. Neurocognitive disorders in HIV–1 infection. HNRC Group. HIV Neurobehavioral Research Center. *Current Topics in Microbiology and Immunology*. 202: 11–32.

Gustafson, L. 1987. Frontal lobe degeneration of the non-Alzheimer type. II. Clinical picture and differential diagnosis. *Archives of Gerontology and Geriatrics*. 6: 209–223.

Gustafson, L. 1993. Clinical picture of frontal dementia of non-Alzheimer type. *Dementia*. 4: 143–148.

Gutierrez, R., Atkinson, J.H. and Grant, I. 1993. Mild neurocognitive disorder: Needed addition to the nosology of cognitive impairment (organic mental) disorders. *Journal of Neuropsychiatry and Clinical Neurosciences*. 5: 161–177.

Hachinski, V.C., Iliff, L.D., Zilhka, E., DuBoulay, G.H., McAllister, V.L., Marshall, J., Russell, R.W.R. and Symon, L. 1975. Cerebral blood flow in dementia. *Archives of Neurology*. 32: 632–637.

Hamilton, M. 1967. Development of a rating scale for primary depressive illness. *British Journal of Social and Clinical Psychology*. 6: 278–296.

Hansen, L., Salmon, D., Galasko, D., Masliah, E., Katzman, R., DeTeresa, R., Thal, L., Pay, M., Hofstetter, R., Klauber, M, Rice, V., Butters, N. and Alfore, M. 1990. The Lewy body variant of Alzheimer's disease: A clinical and pathological entity. *Neurology*. 40: 1–8.

Harrington, D.L., Haaland, K.Y., Yeo, R.A. and Marder, E. 1990. Procedural memory in Parkinson's disease: Impaired motor but not visuo-perceptual learning. *Journal of Clinical and Experimental Neuropsychology*. 12: 323–339.

Harrison, P.J. and Roberts G.W. 1991. 'Life, Jim, but not as we know it'? Transmissible dementias and the prion protein. *British Journal of Psychiatry*. 158: 457–470.

Hart, R.P., Kwentus, J.A., Harkins, S.W. and Taylor, J.R. 1988. Rate of forgetting in mild Alzheimer's type dementia. *Brain and Cognition*. 7: 31–38.

Haug, H., Barmwater, U., Eggers, R., Fischer, D., Kuhl, S. and Sass, N.L. 1983. Anatomical changes in aging brain: Morphometric analysis of the human prosencephalon. In *Neuropharmacology*, vol 21, ed. J. Cervos-Navarro and H.I. Sarkander, pp. 1–12. New York: Raven Press.

Hauw, J.J., Verny, M., Delaere, P., Cervera, P., He, Y. and Duyckaerts, C. 1990. Constant neurofibrillary changes in the neocortex in progressive supranuclear palsy: Basic differences with Alzheimer's disease and aging. *Neuroscience Letters*. 119: 182–186.

Heindel, W.C., Butters, N. and Salmon, D.P. 1988. Impaired learning of a motor skill in patients with Huntington's disease. *Behavioral Neuroscience*. 102: 141–147.

Heindel, W.C., Salmon, D.P. and Butters, N. 1990. Pictorial priming and cued recall in Alzheimer's and Huntington's disease. *Brain and Cognition*. 13: 282–295.

Heindel, W.C., Salmon, D.P. and Butters, N. 1991. The biasing of weight judgments in Alzheimer's and Huntington's disease: A priming or programming phenomenon? *Journal of Clinical and Experimental Neuro-psychology*. 13: 189–203.

Heindel, W.C., Salmon, D.P., Shults, C.W., Walicke, P.A. and Butters, N. 1989. Neuropsychological evidence for multiple implicit memory systems: A comparison of Alzheimer's disease, Huntington's disease, and Parkinson's disease patients. *Journal of Neuroscience.* 9: 582–587.

Hodges, J.R., Salmon, D.P. and Butters, N. 1991. The nature of the naming deficit in Alzheimer's and Huntington's disease. *Brain.* 114: 1547–1558.

Hughes C.P., Berg, L., Danziger W.L., Coben, L.A. and Martin, R.L. 1982. A new clinical scale for the staging of dementia. *British Journal of Psychiatry.* 140: 566–572.

Huntington's Disease Collaborative Research Group. 1993. A novel gene containing a trinucleotide repeat that is expanded and unstable on Huntington's disease chromosomes. *Cell.* 72: 971–983.

Hyman, B.T., Gomez-Isla, T., Briggs, M., Chung, H., Nichols, S., Kohout, F. and Wallace, R. 1996. Apolipoprotein E and cognitive change in an elderly population. *Annals of Neurology.* 40: 55–66.

Jackson M. and Lowe, J. 1996. The new neuropathology of degenerative frontotemporal dementias. *Acta Neuropathologica.* 91: 127–134.

Jacobs, D.H. and Huber, S.J. 1992. The role of the caudate in nonmotor behaviors in Huntington's disease. *Behavioural Neurology.* 5: 205–214.

Jagust, W.J., Davies, P., Tiller-Borcich, J.K. and Reed, B.R. 1990. Focal Alzheimer's disease. *Neurology.* 40: 14–19.

Janssen, R.S., Nwanyanwu, O.C., Selik, R.M. and Stehr-Green, J.K. 1992. Epidemiology of human immuno-deficiency virus encephalopathy in the United States. *Neurology.* 42: 1472–1476.

Johnson, K.A., Sperling, R.A., Holman, B.L., Nagel, J.S. and Growdon, J.H. 1992. Cerebral perfusion in progressive supranuclear palsy. *Journal of Nuclear Medicine.* 3: 704–709.

Katzman, R., Galasko, D., Saitoh, T., Thal, L.J. and Hansen, L. 1995. Genetic evidence that the Lewy body variant is indeed a phenotypic variant of Alzheimer's disease. *Brain and Cognition.* 28: 259–265.

Kernutt, G.J., Price, A.J., Judd, F.K. and Burrows, G.D. 1993. Human immunodeficiency virus infection, dementia and the older patient. *Australian and New Zealand Journal of Psychiatry.* 27: 9–19.

Khachaturian, Z.S. 1994. Scientific opportunities for developing treatments for Alzheimer's disease: Proceedings of Research Planning Workshop 1. *Neurobiology of Aging.* 15: S11-S15.

Koivisto, K., Reinikainen, K.J., Hanninen, T., Vanhanen, M., Helkala, E-L., Mykkanen, L., Laakso, M., Pyorala, K. and Riekkinen, P.J. 1995. Prevalence of age-associated memory impairment in a randomly selected population from eastern Finland. *Neurology.* 45: 741–747.

Koss, E., Haxby, J.V., DeCarli, C., Schapiro, M.B., Friedland, R.P. and Rapoport, S.I. 1991. Patterns of performance preservation and loss in healthy aging. *Developmental Neuropsychology.* 7: 99–113.

Kral, V.A. 1962. Senescent forgetfulness: Benign and malignant. *Journal of the Canadian Medical Association.* 86: 257–260.

Larrabee, G.J. and McEntee, W.J. 1995. Age-associated memory impairment: Sorting out the controversies. *Neurology.* 45: 611–614.

Larrabee, G.J., Youngjohn, J.R., Sudilovsky, A. and Crook, T.H. 1993. Accelerated forgetting in Alzheimer type dementia. *Journal of Clinical and Experimental Neuropsychology.* 15: 701–712.

Levin, B.E., Tomer, R. and Rey, G.J. 1992. Cognitive impairments in Parkinson's disease. *Neurologic Clinics.* 2: 471–485.

Lezak, M.D. 1995. *Neuropsychological assessment,* 3rd ed. New York: Oxford University Press.

Litvan, I. 1994. Cognitive disturbances in progressive supranuclear palsy. *Journal of Neural Transmission.* 42 (Suppl.): 69–78.

Locascio, J.J., Growdon, J.H. and Corkin, S. 1995. Cognitive test performance in detecting, staging and tracking Alzheimer's disease. *Archives of Neurology.* 52: 1087–1099.

Logigian, E.L., Kaplan, R.F. and Steere, A.C. 1990. Chronic neurologic manifestations of Lyme disease. *New England Journal of Medicine.* 323: 1438–1444.

Lund, A. 1993. Dementia of the frontal type. *Dementia.* 4: 125.

Mamo, H.L., Meric, P.C., Ponsin, J.C., Rey, A.C., Luft, A.G. and Seylaz, J.A. 1987. Cerebral blood flow in normal pressure hydrocephalus. *Stroke.* 18: 1074–1080.

Martin A. 1994. HIV, cognition and the basal ganglia. In *Neuropsychology of HIV infection,* ed. I. Grant and A. Martin, pp. 234–259. New York: Oxford University Press.

Martin, A., Brouwers, P., Lalonde, F., Cox, C., Teleska, P. and Fedio, P. 1986. Towards a behavioral typology of Alzheimer's patients. *Journal of Clinical and Experimental Neuropsychology*. 8: 594–610.

Massman, P.J., Delis, D.C., Butters, N., Dupont, R.M. and Gillin, J.C. 1992. The subcortical dysfunction hypothesis of memory deficits in depression: Neuropsychological validation in a subgroup of patients. *Journal of Clinical and Experimental Neuropsychology*. 14: 687–706.

McCrae, R.R., Arenberg, D. and Costa, P.T., Jr. 1987. Declines in divergent thinking with age: Cross-sectional, longitudinal and cross sequential analyses. *Psychology and Aging*. 2: 130–137.

McDowd, J.M. and Craik, F.I.M. 1988. Effects of aging and task difficulty on divided attention performance. *Journal of Experimental Psychology (Human Perception)*. 14: 267–280.

McKhann, G., Drachman, D., Folstein, M., Katzman, R., Price, D. and Stadlan, E.M. 1984. Clinical diagnosis of Alzheimer's disease: Report of the NINCDS-ADRDA Work Group under the auspices of the Department of Health and Human Services Task Force on Alzheimer's Disease. *Neurology*. 34: 939–944.

Mendez, M.F., Selwood, A. and Frey, W.H. 1994. Clinical characteristics of chronic Creutzfeldt–Jakob disease. *Journal of Geriatric Psychiatry and Neurology*. 7: 206–208.

Merck and Co. 1995. *Merck manual of geriatrics*, 2nd ed. Whitehouse Station, NJ: Merck and Co., Inc.

Mesulam, M.M. and Weintraub, S. 1992. Spectrum of primary progressive aphasia. *Clinical Neurology*. 1: 583–609.

Meyer, J.S., Muramatsu, K., Mortel, K.F., Obara, K. and Shirai, T. 1995. Prospective CT confirms differences between vascular and Alzheimer's dementia. *Stroke*. 26: 735–742.

Monsch, A.U., Bondi, M.W., Butters, N., Salmon, D.P., Katzman, R. and Thal, L.J. 1992. Comparisons of verbal fluency tasks in the detection of dementia of the Alzheimer type. *Archives of Neurology*. 49: 1253–1258.

Monsch, A.U., Bondi, M.W., Paulsen, J.S., Brugger, P., Butters, N., Salmon, D.P. and Swenson, M. 1994. A comparison of category and letter fluency in Alzheimer's disease and Huntington's disease. *Neuropsychology*. 8: 25–30.

Moss, M.B., Albert, M.S., Butters, N. and Payne, M. 1986. Differential patterns of memory loss among patients with Alzheimer's disease, Huntington's disease and alcoholic Korsakoff syndrome. *Archives of Neurology*. 43: 239–246.

Moss, M.B., Albert, M.S. and Kemper, T.L. 1992. Neuropsychology of frontal lobe dementia. In *Clinical syndromes in adult neuropsychology: The practitioner's handbook*, ed. R.F. White, pp. 287–303. New York: Elsevier.

Myers, R.H., Vonsattel, J.P., Stevens, T.J., Cupples, L.A., Richardson, E.P., Martin, J.B. and Bird, E.D. 1988. Clinical and neuropathologic assessment of severity in Huntington's disease. *Neurology*. 38: 341–347.

Neary, D., Snowden, J.S., Northen, B. and Goulding, P. 1988. Dementia of frontal lobe type. *Journal of Neurology, Neurosurgery and Psychiatry*. 51: 353–361.

Pachana, N.A., Boone, K.B., Miller, B.L., Cummings, J.L. and Berman, N. 1996. Comparison of neuro-psychological functioning in Alzheimer's disease and fronto-temporal dementia. *Journal of the International Neuropsychological Society*. 2: 1–6.

Paulsen, J.S., Butters, N., Salmon, D.P., Heindel, W.C. and Swenson, M.R. 1993. Prism adaptation in Alzheimer's and Huntington's disease. *Neuropsychology*. 7: 73–81.

Paulsen, J.S., Weisstein, C.C. and Heaton, R.K. 1994. The neuro-psychology of aging. *Current Opinion in Psychiatry*. 7: 347–353.

Peavy, G., Jacobs, D., Salmon, D.P., Butters, N., Delis, D.C., Taylor, M., Massman, P., Stout, J.C., Heindel, W.C., Kirson, K., Atkinson, J.H., Chandler, J.L., Grant, I. and the HNRC Group. 1994. Verbal memory performance of patients with human immunodeficiency virus infection: Evidence of subcortical dysfunction. *Journal of Clinical and Experimental Neuropsychology*. 16: 508–523.

Perry, R., McKeith, I. and Perry, E. (eds.) 1996. *Dementia with Lewy bodies: Clinical, pathological and treatment issues*. Cambridge: Cambridge University Press.

Perry, S.W. and Marotta, R.F. 1987. AIDS dementia: A review of the literature. *Alzheimer Disease and Associated Disorders*. 1: 221–235.

Pillon, B., Deweer, B., Agid, Y. and Dubois, B. 1993. Explicit memory in Alzheimer's, Huntington's and Parkinson's diseases. *Archives of Neurology*. 50: 374–379.

Pillon, B., Dubois, B., Lhermitte, F. and Agid, Y. 1986. Heterogeneity of cognitive impairment in progressive supranuclear palsy, Parkinson's disease and Alzheimer's disease. *Neurology*. 36: 1179–1185.

Pillon, B., Dubois, B., Ploska, A. and Agid, Y. 1991. Severity and specificity of cognitive impairment in Alzheimer's, Huntington's, Parkinson's disease and progressive supranuclear palsy. *Neurology*. 41: 634–643.

Plassman, B.L. and Breitner, J.C.S. 1996. Recent advances in the genetics of Alzheimer's disease and vascular dementia with an emphasis on gene environment interactions. *Journal of the American Geriatrics Society*. 44: 1242–1250.

Pujol, J., Junque, C., Vendrell, P., Grau, J.M. and Capdevila, A. 1992. Reduction of the substantia nigra width and motor decline in aging and Parkinson's disease. *Archives of Neurology*. 49: 1119–1122.

Quinn, N.P. 1993. Dementia and Parkinson's disease. In *Mental dysfunction in Parkinson's disease*, ed. E.C. Wolters and P. Scheltens, pp. 113–122. Amsterdam, Netherlands: Vrije Universiteit.

Rao, S.M., Mittenberg, W., Bernardin, L., Haughton, V. and Leo, G.J. 1989. Neuropsychologic test findings in subjects with leukoaraiosis. *Archives of Neurology*. 46: 40–44.

Reiman, E.M., Caselli, R.J., Yun, L.S., Chen, K., Bandy, D., Minoshima, S., Thibodeau, S.N. and Osborne, D. 1996. Preclinical evidence of Alzheimer's disease in persons homozygous for the ε4 allele for Apolipoprotein E. *New England Journal of Medicine*. 334: 752–758.

Relkin, N.R. 1996. Apolipoprotein E genotyping in Alzheimer's disease. *Lancet*. 347: 1091–1095.

Robbins, T.W., James, M., Owen, A.M., Lange, K.W., Lees, A.J., Leigh, P.N., Marsden, C.D., Quinn, N.P. and Summers, B.A. 1994. Cognitive deficits in progressive supranuclear palsy, Parkinson's disease and multiple system atrophy in tests sensitive to frontal lobe dysfunction. *Journal of Neurology, Neurosurgery and Psychiatry*. 57: 79–88.

Robinson-Whelen, S. and Storandt, M. 1992. Immediate and delayed prose recall among normal and demented adults. *Archives of Neurology*. 49: 32–34.

Roman, G.C., Tatemichi, T.K., Erkinjuntti, T. and Cummings, J.L. 1993. Vascular dementia: diagnostic criteria for vascular studies. *Neurology*. 43: 250–260.

Roses, A.D. 1995. Apolipoprotein E genotyping in the differential diagnsosis, not prediction, of Alzheimer's disease. *Annals of Neurology*. 38: 6–14.

Ross, S.K., Graham, N., Stuartgreen, L., Prins, M., Xuereb, J., Patterson, K. and Hodges, J.R. 1996. Progressive bilateral atrophy: An atypical presentation of Alzheimer's disease. *Journal of Neurology, Neurosurgery and Psychiatry*. 61: 388–395.

Saint-Cyr, J.A., Taylor, A.E. and Lang, A.E. 1988. Procedural learning and neostriatal dysfunction in man. *Brain*. 111: 941–959.

Salmon, D.P. and Galasko, D. 1996. Neuropsychological aspects of Lewy body dementia. In *Dementia with Lewy bodies: Clinical, pathological and treatment issues*, ed. R. Perry, I. McKeith and E. Perry, pp. 99–113. Cambridge: Cambridge University Press.

Salmon, D.P., Galasko, D., Hansen, L.A., Masliah, E., Butters, N., Thal, L.J. and Katzman, R. 1996. Neuropsychological deficits associated with diffuse Lewy body disease. *Brain and Cognition*. 31: 148–165.

Salthouse, R.A., Fristoe, N. and Rhee S.H. 1996. How localized are age-related effects on neuropsychological measures? *Neuropsychology*. 10: 272–285.

Saunders, A.M., Hulette, C., Welsh-Bohmer, K.A., Schmechel, D.E., Crain, B., Burke, J.R., Alberts, M.A., Strittmatter, W.J., Breitner, J.C.S., Earl, N., Clark, C., Heyman, A., Gaskell, P.C., Pericek-Vance, M.A. and Roses, A.D. 1996. Specificity and sensitivity of apolipoprotein E genotyping in a prospectively ascertained series of probable Alzheimer disease patients with autopsy-confirmed diagnoses. *Lancet*. 348: 90–93.

Saunders, A.M., Schmader, K., Breitner, J.C., Benson, M.D., Brown, W.T., Goldfarb, L., Goldgaber, D., Manwaring, M.G., Szymanski, M.H., McCown, N., Dole, K.C., Schmechel, D.E., Strittmatter, W.J., Pericak-Vance, M.A. and Roses, A.D. 1993. Apolipoprotein E- ε4 allele distributions in late onset Alzheimer's disease and in other amyloid forming diseases. *Lancet*. 342: 710–711.

Scharnhorst, S. 1992. AIDS dementia complex in the elderly. Diagnosis and management. *Nurse Practitioner*. 17: 37–43.

Schoenberg, B.S. 1988. Epidemiology of vascular dementia and multi-infarct dementia. In *Vascular and multi-infarct dementia*, ed. J.S. Meyer, H. Lechner, J. Marshall and J.F. Toole, pp. 47–59. Mt Kisco, NY: Futura Publishing Company, Inc.

Sherrington, R., Rogaev, E.I., Liang, Y., Rogaeva, E.A., Levesque, G., Ikeda, M., Chi, H., Lin, C., Li, G. and Holman, K. 1995. Cloning of a gene bearing mis-sense mutations in early onset Alzheimer's disease. *Nature*. 375: 754–760.

Siegler, I.C., Poon, L.W., Madden, D.J. and Welsh, K.A. 1995. Psychological aspects of normal aging. In *Textbook of geriatric psychiatry*, 2nd ed., ed. E.W. Busse and D.G. Blazer, pp. 105–127. Washington DC: American Psychiatric Press, Inc.

Simon, R.P. 1985. Neurosyphilis. *Archives of Neurology*. 42: 606–613.

Stambrook, M., Gill, D.D., Cardoso, E.R. and Moore, A.D. 1994. Communicating (normal pressure) hydrocephalus. In *Neuropsychology of Alzheimer's disease and other dementias*, ed. R.W. Parks, R.F. Zec and R.S. Wilson, pp. 283–307. New York: Oxford University Press.

Strittmatter, W.J., Saunders, A.M., Schmechel, D., Pericak-Vance, M., Enghild, J., Salvesen, G.S. and Roses, A.D. 1993. Apolipoprotein E: High avidity binding to beta amyloid and increased frequency of type 4 allele in late-onset familial Alzheimer's disease. *Proceedings of the National Academy of Sciences*. 90: 1977–1981.

Sultzer, D.L., Mahler, M.E., Cummings, J.L., Van Gorp, W.G., Hinkin, C.H. and Brown, C. 1995. Cortical abnormalities associated with subcortical lesions in vascular dementia. Clinical and positron emission tomographic findings. *Archives of Neurology*. 52: 773–780.

Tabrizi S.J., Howard R.S., Collinge J., Rossor M.N. and Scaravilli F. 1996. Creutzfeldt–Jakob disease in a young woman. *Lancet*. 347: 945–948.

Tatemichi, T.K., Desmond, D.A., Stern, Y., Paik, M., Sano, M. and Bagiella, E. 1994a. Cognitive impairment after stroke: Frequency, patterns and relationships to functional abilities. *Journal of Neurology, Neurosurgery and Psychiatry*. 57: 202–207.

Tatemichi, T.K. Sacktor, N. and Mayeux, R. 1994b. Dementia associated with cerebrovascular disease, other degenerative disease and metabolic disorders. In *Alzheimer disease*, ed. R.D. Terry, R. Katzman and K.L. Bick, pp. 123–166. New York: Raven Press.

Tierney M.C., Szalai J.P., Snow W.G., Fisher R.H., Tsuda T., Chi H., McLachlan, D.R. and St.George-Hyslop, P.H. 1996. A prospective study of the clinical utility of ApoE genotype in the prediction of outcome in patients with memory impairment. *Neurology*. 46: 149–154.

Tomlinson, B.E., Blessed, G. and Roth, M. 1970. Observations of the brains of demented old people. *Journal of Neurological Science*. 11: 205–242.

Tröster, A.I., Butters, N., Salmon, D.P., Cullum, C.M., Jacobs, D., Brandt, J. and White, R.F. 1993. The diagnostic utility of savings scores: Differentiating Alzheimer's and Huntington's diseases with the Logical Memory and Visual Reproduction tests. *Journal of Clinical and Experimental Neuropsychology*. 15: 773–788.

Tröster, A.I., Salmon, D.P., McCullough, D. and Butters, N. 1989. A comparison of the category fluency deficits associated with Alzheimer's and Huntington's disease. *Brain and Language*. 37: 500–513.

Tupler, L.A., Coffey, E., Logue, P.E., Djang, W.T. and Fagan, S.M. 1992. Neuropsychologic importance of subcortical white mater hyperintensity. *Archives of Neurology*. 49: 1248–1252.

Van Gorp, W.G. and Mahler, M. 1990. Subcortical features of normal aging. In *Subcortical dementia*, ed. J.L. Cummings, pp. 231–250. New York: Oxford University Press.

Verhaeghen, P., Marcoen, A. and Goossens, L. 1993. Facts and fiction about memory aging: A quantitative integration of research findings. *Journal of Gerontology: Psychological Sciences*. 48: P157-P171.

Victoroff, J., Ross, W., Benson, D.F., Verity, M.A. and Vinters, H.V. 1994. Posterior cortical atrophy: Neuropathological correlations. *Archives of Neurology*. 51: 269–274.

Wagner, M.T. and Bachman, D.L. 1996. Neuropsychological features of diffuse Lewy body disease. *Archives of Clinical Neuropsychology*. 11: 175–184.

Wechsler, D. 1981. *Wechsler Adult Intelligence Scale – Revised*. San Antonio, TX: The Psychological Corporation.

Wechsler, D. 1987. *Manual for the Wechsler Memory Scale-Revised*. San Antonio: The Psychological Corporation.

Welsh, K.A., Butters, N., Hughes, J.P., Mohs, R.C. and Heyman, A. 1991. Detection of abnormal memory decline in mild Alzheimer's disease using CERAD neuropsychological measures. *Archives of Neurology*. 48: 278–281.

Welsh, K.A., Butters, N., Hughes, J., Mohs, R. and Heyman, A. 1992. Detection and staging of dementia in Alzheimer's disease: Use of neuropsychological measures developed for the Consortium to Establish a Registry for Alzheimer's Disease (CERAD). *Archives of Neurology*. 49: 448–452.

Welsh, K.A., Butters, N., Mohs, R.C., Beekly, D., Edland, S., Fillenbaum, G. and Heyman, A. 1994. The Consortium to Establish a Registry of Alzheimer's disease (CERAD) Part V: A normative study of the neuro-psychological battery. *Neurology*. 44: 609–614.

Welsh, K.A., Fillenbaum, G., Wilkinson, W., Heyman, A., Mohs, R.C., Stern, Y. and Harrell, L. 1995. Neuro-psychological performance of black and white patients with Alzheimer's disease. *Neurology*. 45: 2207–2211.

Welsh, K.A., Mirra, S., Fillenbaum, G., Gearing, M., Beekly, D. and Edland, S. 1996. Neuropsychological and neuropathological differentiation of Alzheimer's disease from other dementias: The CERAD experience. *Journal of the International Neuropsychological Society*. 2: 12.

Welsh-Bohmer, K.A. and Hoffman, J.M. 1996. Positron emission tomography neuroimaging in dementia. In *Neuroimaging II: Clinical applications*, ed. E. Bigler, pp. 185–222. New York: Plenum Press.

Welsh-Bohmer, K.A., Gearing, M., Saunders, A.M., Roses, A.D. and Mirra, S.M. 1997. Apolipoprotein E genotypes in a neuropathological series from the Consortium to Establish a Registry for Alzheimer's Disease (CERAD). *Annals of Neurology*. 42: 319–325.

Whitehouse, P.J., Lerner, A. and Hedera, P. 1993. Dementia. In *Clinical neuropsychology*, 3rd ed., ed. K.M. Heilman and E. Valenstein, pp. 603–645. New York: Oxford University Press.

19

The impact of depression on memory in neurodegenerative disease

JULIE A. FIELDS, SUZANNE NORMAN,
KRISTY A. STRAITS-TRÖSTER
AND ALEXANDER I. TRÖSTER

INTRODUCTION

The widely held notion that depression exerts a negative impact on cognition is not novel: ancient Egyptian writings already noted the coexistence of mood disorders and impaired cognition (Loza and Milad 1990). Despite extensive study, however, the extent, nature and underlying mechanisms of depression's influence on cognition remain relatively poorly understood. If one views the effects of depression on cognition as falling on a continuum, it is generally evident that individuals with dysthymia or only mild-to-moderate depressive symptomatology, despite their subjective complaints of memory impairment, demonstrate little, if any, objectively verifiable cognitive impairment. At the other extreme of the continuum, major depression can lead to such pervasive cognitive dysfunction, accompanied by impairments in occupational and social functioning, that an individual is diagnosed as having a dementia syndrome.

This dementia syndrome associated with depression is known by a plethora of appellations (e.g. dementia syndrome of depression, pseudo-dementia, depressive dementia, reversible dementia caused by depression). Not typically considered under the rubric of neurodegenerative diseases and not per se the focus of this chapter, the dementia syndrome of depression nonetheless raises some important issues concerning the etiology, diagnosis and treatment of memory impairment in neurodegenerative diseases. In particular, given the apparent coexistence of depression and neurodegenerative diseases, as well as an overlap in the cognitive impairments associated with major depression and neurodegenerative diseases, several questions of practical importance arise: Is depression a risk factor for, or harbinger of dementia? Is depression a consequence of neurodegeneration, or is it a reaction to the diagnosis and/or limitations in activities of daily living brought about by the disease? If depression is primarily biological in etiology, do depression and cognitive impairment in neurodegenerative diseases have a common biological substrate? Does depression alter the extent or quality of cognitive impairment in neurodegenerative disease? If so, might dementia be overdiagnosed in individuals with a neurodegenerative disease and depression? How best might one differentiate whether a memory impairment is related to the neurodegenerative disease and/or depression? Does memory improve if depression is adequately treated?

In an attempt to address these questions, research has sought to document the incidence and prevalence of coexisting depression and neurodegenerative diseases, to characterize the cognitive manifestations of depression in neurodegenrative disorders, to identify the biological correlates of depression and cognitive impairment and to refine and evaluate diagnostic and treatment methods for depression in neurodegenerative disease. It is this research which is the focus of this chapter. After providing a brief overview of the effects of depression on memory in individuals without neurodegenerative disease, research findings are discussed separately for Alzheimer's disease (AD; a so called 'cortical' dementia) and 'subcortical' (basal ganglia) dementias. Although the distinction between 'cortical and subcortical dementia' has been criticized on neuroanatomical grounds, it remains a useful clinical short-hand for describing the patterns of cognitive and behavioral disturbances associated with different dementias which early in their course are associated predominantly with either cortical or subcortical pathology. Furthermore, the distinction is of particular relevance to a discussion of depression and memory because it has been suggested that severe depression is associated with memory impairments that qualitatively resemble those observed in 'subcortical' dementias and because depression is more prevalent in subcortical than cortical dementias.

DEPRESSION AND MEMORY IN ELDERLY INDIVIDUALS WITHOUT NEURODEGENERATIVE DISEASE

Incidence and prevalence

The incidence and prevalence estimates of depression in the elderly vary, depending upon case ascertainment methods (diagnostic criteria and assessment measures employed). Major depression is relatively rare among community-living elderly (about 1–6%) and, in fact, the 1-year and lifetime prevalence of depression is probably lower among elderly than younger populations (McGuire and Rabins 1994). Although the prevalence of cognitive impairment in major depression is unknown, about 20% of elderly with severe depression suffer cognitive impairment sufficiently severe to qualify them for a diagnosis of dementia (LaRue et al. 1986b); however, because some of these dementia patients will eventually be diagnosed with a neurodegenerative disorder, the true prevalence of dementia syndrome of depression remains elusive.

Nature of the memory impairment in depression

Numerous methodological differences among studies might account for the vastly discordant findings concerning the effects of depression on memory. These include, but are not limited to, sample characteristics (age, severity and duration of depression, type of affective disorder, treatment type and setting, co-existence of other psychiatric or neurological disorders), diagnostic criteria employed and the instruments used to assess depression and memory. Given this array of methodological differences, it is not surprising that some studies have found depression to be associated with memory impairment whereas other studies have not. The central question, then, is whether the preponderance of evidence favors an association between depression and cognitive impairment and, if so, which factors might account for the discordant findings reported in the literature.

Burt et al. (1995) recently meta-analysed data from studies examining the effects of depression on memory, with the aim of identifying whether there is a reliable effect of depression on memory and which factors might mediate this relationship. A search of three literature databases (Medline, Psychological Abstract and ERIC) using the key terms 'depression' and 'memory' yielded 590 studies between 1966 and 1991. From these studies, 99 studies of recall and 48 studies of recognition met criteria for inclusion in the meta-analysis. The studies included had to (1) have samples of controls and adults with naturally occurring depression (i.e. mood induction studies were excluded), (2) use at least one dependent variable involving recall or recognition, and (3) report pretreatment comparisons between groups if the study involved treatment of depression.

Almost all meta-analyses yielded significant associations between memory and depression (with small to moderate effect sizes); however, Burt et al. (1995) found that the impact of depression on memory varies as a function of the type of retention test (i.e. recall versus recognition), the interval imposed between stimulus presentation and retention testing, the valence of the memoranda and the type of patients studied. Specifically, depression was found to impact recognition particularly after the imposition of a delay interval between stimulus presentation and retention testing. In contrast, depression exerted a more negative influence on immediate than delayed recall. Depression more detrimentally affected retention of memoranda of positive than negative or neutral valence. Memory impairment was consistently more pronounced in depressed inpatients than outpatients.

Of greatest relevance to the present discussion is Burt et al.'s finding concerning the mediating effect which age might exert on the depression–memory relationship. Contrary to predictions (but consistent with the observation of Watts 1995) the association between recall and depression and between recognition (hit-rate) and depression, was consistently greater for younger (less than 60 years) than older (more than 60 years) samples. Kindermann and Brown (1997) in their meta-analysis also found younger (less than 45 years of age) groups to be more impaired in memory than older groups. Although Burt et al. found a stronger association between depression and memory impairment in young than elderly groups, this is not to say that depression does not negatively affect memory in the elderly. As Burt et al. themselves point out, potential floor effects on memory measures in the elderly might limit the strength of the association between depression and memory. There might also be differences in

Table 19.1. *Characteristics of memory dysfunction in Major Depression and Alzheimer's disease*

Characteristic	Depression	Alzheimer's disease	Sample references
Recall	Impaired	Impaired	Des Rosiers et al. 1995 Massman et al. 1992
Spontaneous Strategy Use (Clustering) / Provision of Organizational Structure	Impaired/ Helpful	Impaired/ Not Helpful	Weingartner et al. 1981 Massman et al. 1992
Recall Intrusion Errors	Uncommon	Common	Gainotti and Marra 1994 LaRue et al. 1986a
Forgetting Rate	Normal	Accelerated	Des Rosiers et al. 1995 Gainotti and Marra 1994 Hart et al. 1987a King et al. 1998 Kopelman, 1986
Recognition	Normal or Slightly Impaired	Impaired	Hart et al. 1987b Massman et al. 1992
Bias on Recognition Testing	Negative	Positive	Gainotti and Marra 1994 Miller and Lewis 1977
Remote Memory	Normal	Impaired	Kopelman 1986
'Metamemory'	Overestimate Impairment	Overestimate Ability	Kotler-Cope and Camp 1995 McGlynn and Kaszniak 1991 Williams et al. 1987

depression patterns, etiology and severity among young and elderly groups, for which the meta-analysis did not control. As noted earlier, major depression might be less prevalent among elderly than younger populations and only the severely depressed might evidence cognitive impairment of practical significance (LaRue 1992). Consequently, if the meta-analysis included predominantly less severely depressed elderly samples, a bias exists against finding a strong association between depression and cognitive impairment.

A further factor that might hinder detection of a strong relationship between depression and memory in the elderly involves the apparent heterogeneity of memory impairment in depressed elderly (King and Caine 1996). For example, only a subgroup of depressed elderly might have impairments in recall and a different subgroup might demonstrate recognition impairments. The work of Massman et al. (1992, 1994) is particularly informative in this regard. Three variables from the California Verbal Learning Test (CVLT) were particularly helpful in separating patients with Alzheimer's (AD) and Huntington's disease (HD) from normal controls (total recall across five learning trials) and AD from HD patients (cued recall intrusions and the difference between recall on the fifth

learning trial and recognition discriminability). Massman and colleagues used these three variables to derive a discriminant function maximally separating AD, HD and normal control subjects. When the same discriminant function was applied to samples with unipolar and bipolar depression, the discriminant function classified approximately 65% of the depressed subjects as 'normal control' and 35% as 'HD'. None of the depressed patients was classified on the basis of their memory impairment as having AD. In other words, only a minority of patients with depression demonstrated a verbal memory impairment, but when they did, the pattern of impairment resembled that seen in 'subcortical' rather than 'cortical' dementias.

The heterogeneity of memory impairment in depression is an important consideration in determining whether memory impairment is a manifestation of depression or neurodegenerative disease. Some of the qualitative characteristics of memory impairment differentiating between depression and AD (Table 19.1) should thus be used as a guide rather than a prescriptive menu of absolute differences that are invariant (see Christensen et al. 1997).

In general, patients with depression perform relatively well on short-term memory tasks such as digit span

(LaRue 1992; Watts 1995). Deficits become apparent on long-term memory tasks and, in particular, on unstructured tasks, i.e. depressed patients' recall, unlike that of AD patients, is likely to benefit from the provision of an organizing framework (e.g. semantic organization of word lists) (Weingartner et al. 1981). Patients with depression tend to demonstrate relatively preserved (albeit not always intact) recognition memory relative to free recall (Massman et al. 1992). False positive recognition errors are more likely to be seen in AD than depression and, conversely, depression is often associated with a negative response bias (e.g. Gainotti and Marra 1994). Forgetting rate is relatively normal in depression (e.g. Hart et al. 1987a), but markedly accelerated in AD (Tröster et al. 1993). Unlike patients with AD, those with depression tend to make few intrusion errors (LaRue et al. 1986a). Remote memory is impaired in AD (Chapter 10), but typically preserved in depression (Kopelman 1986). Whereas depressed patients frequently overestimate their objectively verified memory impairment (Williams et al. 1987), AD patients typically underestimate their memory difficulties (McGlynn and Kaszniak 1991). Thus, although both patient groups demonstrate difficulties with knowledge of their memory (i.e. metamemory), AD and depressed groups make errors in opposite directions.

Biological correlates of cognitive impairment in depression

Neuroimaging and functional neuroimaging studies in particular, have provided insights into the pathophysiology of depression and cognitive impairment. Structural computed tomography (CT) and magnetic resonance imaging (MRI) neuroimaging studies have generally revealed only nonspecific changes in elderly with major depression (Nasrallah et al. 1989). Such nonspecific findings include cortical atrophy, sulcal prominence and ventricular enlargement. Pearlson et al. (1989) reported that even patients with 'reversible pseudodementia', who did not develop a nonreversible dementia within 2-year follow-up, demonstrated ventricular enlargement and diminished attenuation on CT comparable to that of patients with AD.

Subcortical (white matter) hyperintensities also are not specific to the depressed elderly (Nussbaum 1994) and have been reported to occur in normal elderly and in patients with vascular dementia and AD (Stoudemire et al. 1989; O'Brien et al. 1996). Nonetheless, recent MRI studies show that white matter hyperintensities are more

likely to occur in the elderly with late- than early-onset depression and that such hyperintensities are associated with greater cognitive impairment (Lesser et al. 1996; Salloway et al. 1996), worse functioning in activities of daily living (Cahn et al. 1996) and increased risk for the development of cognitive impairment over a 2-year follow-up (Nussbaum et al. 1995).

Functional (e.g. single positron emission computed tomography (SPECT) and positron emission tomography (PET)) imaging studies have been more fruitful than structural imaging studies in revealing the potential cerebral abnormalities underlying depression and cognitive impairment. The systematic studies of Bench and colleagues have been particularly revealing in this regard. Bench et al. (1992) reported that relative to a normal control group, patients with depression demonstrated decreased regional cerebral blood flow (rCBF) in the left anterior cingulate and dorsolateral prefrontal cortex. Patients with depression-related cognitive impairment, relative to patients without cognitive impairment but with similarly severe depression, demonstrated additional rCBF reductions in the left medial frontal gyrus and increased rCBF in the cerebellar vermis (Dolan et al. 1992). The left medial prefrontal rCBF reduction, in particular, related more strongly to cognitive impairment ratings than to depressed mood, anxiety and psychomotor retardation (Bench et al. 1993; Dolan et al. 1994). Further evidence for a relationship between depression and frontal rCBF abnormalities comes from the observation that dorsolateral and medial prefrontal rCBF increases with remission of depression (Bench et al. 1995), although it is unclear how such a reversal of rCBF abnormalities relates to resolution of cognitive and, more particularly, memory impairment.

Treatment of depression and changes in cognition

It is generally held that successful treatment of depression also results in recovery from cognitive impairments. Unfortunately, as LaRue (1992) points out, data supporting this assertion generally pertain to younger patient populations and rarely to the elderly (and even more rarely to the dementia syndrome of depression). Issues which remain poorly addressed include the extent to which cognitive recovery occurs, the persistence of this recovery and whether antidepressant treatment might in fact have adverse effects on memory.

There is some suggestion that depression and cognitive dysfunction respond favorably to treatment. LaRue et al. (1986b) found that depression in groups of elderly inpatients with and without cognitive impairment responded similarly to treatment (various antidepressants and electroconvulsive therapy (ECT)), although the group with cognitive impairment required lengthier hospitalization. Memory was not evaluated, but depressed patients with and without cognitive impairment showed comparable gains (of unknown clinical significance) on an idiosyncratic 'dementia' factor score after treatment. Whether cognition or memory recover to normal levels after treatment of depression is questionable. For example, Abas et al. (1990) observed visual memory impairment in 70% of their depressed, elderly inpatients. Although cognitive improvement occurred with antidepressant treatment, memory did not recover to the level of performance evidenced by the normal control group.

Potential adverse effects of antidepressant treatment on memory in the elderly remain debated, but the limited empirical literature suggests that such adverse effects are minimal and probably not of practical significance. In general, controlled studies have shown tricyclics to negatively impact memory, but naturalistic studies have found little if any relationship between antidepressant treatment and memory impairment (LaRue 1992). For example, LaRue et al. (1992) found no correlation between antidepressant dosage and memory test performance, despite the fact that the majority of this elderly sample had cognitive impairment. Even when an association between antidepressant treatment and memory impairment is demonstrated, the variance in memory scores attributable to antidepressant treatment is typically small. For example, relative to unmedicated patients with depression of similar severity, patients treated with one of a variety of antidepressants for 2–3 weeks showed only mild memory deficits and the grouping variable (medicated versus unmedicated) accounted for less than 7% of the variance in a composite memory score (Marcopulos and Graves 1990). It is imperative to point out, however, that none of the patients in this study had dementia and less than half the sample met criteria for *major* affective disorder.

ECT is widely perceived to adversely impact memory. Although transient memory disturbance has been documented following ECT and some patients have subjective complaints of memory disturbance more than 6 months after ECT treatment, there is little objective evidence of memory impairment persisting beyond 6 months after treatment (Squire 1986). Potential cognitive changes accompanying ECT treatment of depression in individuals with dementia have rarely been the subject of systematic investigation. Only one study has prospectively investigated cognitive function in patients with the dementia syndrome of depression specifically, before and after ECT treatment (Stoudemire et al. 1995). In this sample of eight patients, the Mattis Dementia Rating Scale's Memory and Initiation/Perseveration scores showed consistent improvement and this improvement was maintained over 4-year follow-up. This finding parallels reports by the same authors that cognition improved in ECT-treated patients who had major depression and cognitive impairment before treatment (Stoudemire et al. 1991, 1993).

Other reports of ECT treatment in patients with dementia and depression have generally been retrospective, not well controlled and samples have generally included patients with cognitive impairment due to a variety of disorders. Nonetheless, with few exceptions (Liang et al. 1988) these reports also provide tentative evidence of improved cognitive function in patients with dementia and depression following ECT (Price and McAllister 1989; Mulsant et al. 1991). As not all patients with depression and dementia respond well to ECT (Greenwald et al. 1989; Mulsant et al. 1991) it will be important for future research to identify the best prognostic indicators for ECT in patients with dementia and depression.

THE EFFECTS OF DEPRESSION ON MEMORY IN ALZHEIMER'S DISEASE

Incidence and prevalence

In autopsy-confirmed AD, 12–22% of cases are reported to have experienced depression during the course of the disease (Alexopoulos and Nambudiri 1994). Clinical studies of AD have most commonly reported depression prevalence rates between about 15% (Kral 1983; Rovner et al. 1989; Pearlson et al. 1990) and 30% (Reifler et al. 1986), but estimates vary from 0% to 86% (Loreck and Folstein 1993). These large variations likely reflect differences in sampling and case ascertainment methods across studies. Studies reporting zero prevalence (Knesevich et al. 1983; Burke et al. 1988b) likely suffer from selection bias by excluding patients with a history of major affective disorder at study entry. It is also possible that timepoint of assessment influences prevalence estimates: Starkstein and Robinson (1996) proposed that *depression* often has an onset before AD, whereas *dysthymia* most often has its onset soon after AD.

Debate continues about whether dementia with Lewy bodies (or diffuse Lewy body disease) is a variant of AD or a unique entity. Small sample sizes and controversy concerning diagnostic criteria notwithstanding, it is acknowledged that depression is common in diffuse Lewy body disease (Filley 1995). Indeed, there is preliminary evidence that depression might be more common in diffuse Lewy body disease than AD, with prevalence estimated at about 40% (McKeith et al. 1992; Ballard et al. 1993; Klatka et al. 1996; Weiner et al. 1996).

Nature of the memory impairment in Alzheimer's disease with depression

Comparisons among the cognitive, and especially memory deficits, of AD patients with and without depression have received very little attention. While comparisons among patients with either depression or AD address the important issue of differential diagnosis, comparisons between AD with and without depression are needed before statements can be made about the effects of depression upon cognition in AD. The few studies of memory in AD with and without depression suggest that depression has minimal, if any impact, on memory.

Very few differences on memory tests were found in a study of depressed and nondepressed AD groups equated for overall severity of cognitive impairment (Des Rosiers et al. 1995). Whereas the AD group without depression demonstrated more rapid forgetting of the Wechsler Memory Scale (WMS) Logical Memory passages than did the depressed AD group, the depressed AD group performed significantly more poorly on the Kendrick Digit Copying test.

Breen et al. (1984), despite finding a depressed AD group to have a lower Full Scale IQ than a nondepressed AD group, found the two groups to have similar WMS memory quotients (MQ). Furthermore, no differences were found between the two groups' scores on any of the WMS subtests. Rubin et al. (1991) also found mildly demented AD groups with and without depression to perform similarly on a psychometric test battery, including several WMS subtests and the Benton Visual Retention Test. Only on WMS digit span backward did the mildly demented and depressed group perform more poorly than the group with only mild dementia. Similarly, Lopez et al. (1990) found no differences, either at baseline or 1 year later, between depressed and nondepressed AD groups on memory measures including the prose passages from the WMS, Rey-Osterrieth Complex Figure and two paired associate tasks. Fitz and Teri (1994) found no differences among depressed and non-depressed AD groups on the Mattis Dementia Rating Scale, including the Memory subtest. Although Fitz and Teri (1994) found that depression exacerbated cognitive impairment in a mildly, but not in a moderately demented group, it was not reported whether depression exerted a differential impact on *memory* in mildly and moderately demented groups.

The apparent lack of a robust effect of depression on memory in AD parallels the findings with respect to the effects of depression on the severity and progression of AD-associated cognitive impairment in general. The preponderance of studies has either failed to find a significant effect of depression on cognition in AD, or found depressed AD groups to be less cognitively impaired than nondepressed AD groups (for a review, see Ballard et al. 1996).

Several explanations can be advanced for the apparent lack of a relationship between cognitive impairment and depression in AD. First, it is possible that depression affects cognition in only a subset of AD patients. Perhaps, as Fitz and Teri (1994) have found, depression exacerbates cognitive impairment only in early AD. Second, floor effects in cognitive test scores (especially when only cognitive screening instruments are used), might obscure depression effects in more advanced AD. Third, because insight into cognitive and behavioral deficits is likely to decline with advancing disease, one might speculate that impaired insight leads to less frequent depression later in the disease, so that group studies are less apt to find associations between depression and cognitive impairment later in the course of AD. That depression and its influence on cognition might be mediated by awareness of deficits has not, however, been convincingly supported (for opposing views, see Sevush and Leve 1993; Cummings et al. 1995; Seltzer et al. 1995). Finally, it is possible that global measures of depression and cognition fail to reveal the effects of depression on cognition in AD because only some symptoms of depression relate to severity of cognitive impairment (Haupt et al. 1995).

Biological correlates of depression in Alzheimer's disease

The neural basis of depression in AD remains debated, largely because empirical findings are ambiguous. Fairly consistent reports have been made of more pronounced loss of neurons in the locus coeruleus of depressed than nondepressed AD patients, which suggests that noradrenergic dysfunction might relate to depression in AD (Zweig et al. 1988; Zubenko et al. 1990; Förstl et al. 1992). Dopaminergic and serotonergic dysfunction have also been implicated, either via observed cell loss in the substantia nigra and the dorsal raphe nuclei, respectively, or reductions in these neurotransmitters and their metabolites in a variety of brain regions (Zweig et al. 1988; Zubenko et al. 1990; Mulsant and Zubenko 1994). The noradrenergic findings are more robust than those pertaining to dopaminergic and serotonergic dysfunction.

A relative preservation of cholinergic neurons in the nucleus basalis of Meynert (Förstl et al. 1992) and of choline acetyltransferase (ChAT) activity in thalamus, caudate and amygdala (Zubenko et al. 1990) have been observed in depressed relative to nondepressed AD patients. This has been variously interpreted to suggest that at least some cholinergic integrity is necessary for the expression of depressed mood (Loreck and Folstein 1993), that cholinergic deficiency protects against depression (Cummings 1992) or that a cholinergic/noradrenergic imbalance underlies depression in AD (Burns and Förstl 1996). Parenthetically, the observation that depression is more likely to occur early than late in the course of AD (Fischer et al. 1990) has been interpreted as possibly supporting the view that depression in AD is a reaction to the diagnosis of AD or AD-associated disability (Teri and Wagner 1992). Given that cholinergic deficits are least pronounced early in AD, one might reinterpret the observed higher prevalence of depression early in AD as indirect support for the cholinergic hypotheses of depression in AD.

Although much attention has been devoted to functional neuroimaging in AD and major affective disorders, less has been reported about functional neuroimaging changes in AD with depression. Typically, AD alone is associated early on with particular CBF reductions in temporo–parietal regions and these changes are not seen in patients with only major depression (for a review, see Mayberg 1994a). Although disinhibition, agitation and personality change in AD have been associated with frontal hypometabolism (Sultzer et al. 1995), and although one study reported a relationship between frontal lobe hypometabolism and depression in AD (Hirono et al. 1998), Grady et al. (1990) found depression to be *less* common in AD patients with than without frontal hypometabolism. This finding might be interpreted as consistent with the findings of two studies which suggest that depression in AD is associated with posterior (superior temporal and/or parietal) hypometabolism. Sultzer et al. (1995) found dep-

ression/anxiety to be related to parietal hypometabolism. A study of particular significance by virtue of including AD groups with major depression, dysthymia and without mood disturbance, was reported by Starkstein et al. (1995). In this SPECT study, depressed relative to nondepressed AD patients demonstrated left superior temporal and parietal hypometabolism. Dysthymic and nondepressed AD groups' cerebral metabolism was similar. It thus appears that major depression, but not dysthymia, is associated with altered posterior cerebral metabolism in AD.

Treatment of depression in Alzheimer's disease

Clinical lore holds that depression in AD be treated much like depression in the elderly with major depression; however, surprisingly few studies have examined in a methodologically rigorous manner the effects of antidepressant or ECT treatment in AD and fewer studies yet have evaluated the impact of such therapies on memory. Most studies are difficult to interpret due to a variety of methodological limitations: inclusion of heterogeneous 'dementia' groups (i.e. multi-infarct, AD, etc.), small sample sizes, heterogeneity of treatment (combination of ECT with multiple other treatments, types of antidepressants used, duration of treatment, variations in antidepressant dosages, number and frequency of ECT treatments) and use of cognitive screening examinations which might not be sensitive to subtle cognitive changes.

With respect to ECT, Price and McAllister (1989) in their review of treatment outcome in 135 cases with depression and either 'organic dementia', depressive dementia, or leukoencephalopathy, reported that 21% of patients experienced transient memory dysfunction after ECT, but that 45% of patients with dementia demonstrated improvement in cognitive function and/or memory after ECT. Although Reynolds et al. (1987), Liang et al. (1988), Greenwald et al. (1989) and Mulsant et al. (1991) provide data tentatively supporting the efficacy of ECT in treating depression in patients with dementia, conclusions about the potential effects of this treatment on cognitive function in AD cannot be drawn with confidence given that these studies suffer from many methodological limitations.

The impact of antidepressant treatment on cognition and memory in AD is very sparsely documented: only two methodologically sound studies have examined the impact of antidepressants on cognition and only one of these two studies evaluated memory. Teri et al. (1991) evaluated the effects of imipramine on memory and cognition in 28 patients with AD and depression and 33 patients with AD only. In this double-blind study, subjects were randomly assigned to 8-week trials of either imipramine or placebo treatment. Imipramine-treated, but not placebo treated subjects showed a small decline on a cognitive screening examination (Dementia Rating Scale; DRS), with a tendency for the decline to be most obvious on the Conceptualization scale of this instrument. No treatment effects were observed on a variety of memory tests (Fuld Object Memory Evaluation, WMS Logical Memory and Paired Associates).

Petracca et al. (1996) randomly assigned 21 patients with AD and depression to 6-week trials of clomipramine or placebo in a double-blind, cross-over study. The effect of treatment on cognition was evaluated with the Mini Mental State Exam (MMSE) only and is somewhat difficult to interpret. In the overall analysis, clomipramine adversely impacted MMSE performance. However, the clomipramine-to-placebo group showed an increase in MMSE scores after the full 12 weeks of treatment, whereas the placebo-to-clomipramine group showed no significant change in MMSE score. Together, the two studies suggest that antidepressant treatment in AD may not be benign in terms of cognitive side-effects; however, these adverse effects are likely subtle and may not extend to memory.

THE IMPACT OF DEPRESSION ON MEMORY IN SUBCORTICAL (BASAL GANGLIA) DEMENTIAS

Incidence and prevalence

Depression is a frequent finding in patients with neurodegenerative diseases of the basal ganglia (i.e. diseases affecting with predilection one or more of the caudate, putamen, globus pallidus, subthalamic nucleus and substantia nigra). Indeed, mood disturbance is considered a cardinal feature of the 'subcortical' dementias of Parkinson's disease (PD), HD and progressive supranuclear palsy. The frequency of depression in progressive supranuclear palsy remains unknown, as mood changes in this disease have typically been the subject of case studies (Litvan et al. 1996). On the basis of clinical studies, the prevalence of depression is estimated most often to be approximately 40% in both PD and HD (Folstein et al. 1983; Gotham et al. 1986; Shoulson 1990; Cummings

1992). The range of depression prevalence estimates is narrower in HD (4%–44%; Peyser and Folstein 1993) than in PD (7%–90%; Tröster in press).

Variability in the reported prevalence of depression stems in part from methodological inconsistencies across studies and from difficulties in diagnosing depression in basal ganglia diseases. Two recent studies show that major depression might be far less common in PD than previously thought and that the majority of 'depressed' PD patients have minor depression (Hantz et al. 1994; Tandberg et al. 1996). The difficulty in diagnosing depression in basal ganglia disease is further compounded by the overlap of cognitive and neurovegetative symptoms in depression and basal ganglia disease. Specifically, Gotham et al. (1986) and Taylor et al. (1988) noted that coexisting depression may be difficult to detect in some patients with basal ganglia diseases because psychomotor retardation, impaired cognition, apathy and disturbed frontal lobe function, which are characteristics of PD, HD and progressive supranuclear palsy (Albert et al. 1974; Cantello et al. 1989; Pillon and Dubois 1992; Peyser and Folstein 1993; Mayberg 1994b), can also be present in idiopathic depression. Litvan et al. (1996) recently provided compelling data that apathy (which correlated significantly with executive dysfunction) is very common in progressive supranuclear palsy (observed in 91% of the sample), but that dysphoria is relatively uncommon (occurring in 18% of the sample). This finding further highlights the potential for misattributing behavioral changes (apathy) to depression and thus overdiagnosing depression, when in fact the behavioral changes might relate to cognitive impairment.

Nature of the memory impairment in subcortical (basal ganglia) dementias with depression

Lundervold and Reinvang (1991) suggested that symptoms of depression and cognitive dysfunction (concentration impairment) in HD might have a similar pathophysiological basis; however, no studies have specifically examined the effects of depression on memory in HD or progressive supranuclear palsy. Consequently, this section of the chapter focuses on the limited research which has examined the effects of depression on cognitive function and memory in PD.

Early studies yielded contradictory findings about the effects of depression on cognition in PD. One potential explanation for these discordant findings is that subtypes of

PD exist: one with, the other without depression. Such subtypes might reflect two distinct disease processes, a hypothesis which would be supported by the observation that membership in depressed and nondepressed PD groups remains relatively stable over the course of the disease (Cummings 1992). Alternatively, there might be a threshold effect, such that certain cognitive and affective symptoms do not appear until a critical amount of frontocortical deafferentation has occurred (Starkstein et al. 1989a), or disease burden exceeds the brain's functional reserve capacity (Boone et al. 1992). Another explanation of the discordant findings concerning the association between depression and cognition in PD concerns methodological variance across studies. In general, cross-sectional studies with small sample sizes often fail to uncover an association between depression and cognitive impairment, whereas more recent longitudinal and better-controlled, cross-sectional studies do find such a relationship (Bondi and Tröster 1997).

Recent studies yield rather compelling evidence that depression might be a risk factor not only for PD (Hubble et al. 1993), but for the evolution of dementia in PD (Stern et al. 1993; Marder et al. 1995), although risk for dementia might be modified by education (Glatt et al. 1996; Chapter 14). Furthermore, it has been proposed that depression may accelerate the rate of progression of both PD itself and its attendant cognitive decline (Sano et al. 1989; Starkstein et al. 1990a) and adversely impact functional ability (Cole et al. 1996).

Several studies using cognitive screening examinations (Starkstein et al. 1990a,b; 1992) have been particularly fruitful in demonstrating that initial depression score strongly predicts subsequent declines in cognitive function and the ability to carry out activities of daily living and that the severity of depression is related to the severity of cognitive impairment. Expanding upon this research, Tröster et al. (1995a) found that a depressed PD group was significantly more cognitively impaired than a nondepressed PD group, even once the two groups were matched for age, education, gender, age at disease onset, disease duration and severity of motor symptoms. More specifically, Starkstein et al. (1989d) and Tröster et al. (1995a) found that depression exerts an especially detrimental effect upon memory. Tröster et al.'s (1995a) finding that a depressed PD group also performed more poorly on conceptualization and initiation tasks than a nondepressed PD group raises the possibility that depression's effect on

memory might be mediated by increased fronto-subcortical dysfunction manifesting itself in poorer executive control over memory processes.

The notion that PD memory impairments are secondary to executive deficits mediated by fronto-striatal dysfunction is not novel (Taylor et al. 1986a; Taylor and Saint-Cyr 1995; Tröster and Fields 1995) and two lines of research support the possibility that depression impacts memory in PD by exacerbating this frontal-subcortical dysfunction. First, functional neuroimaging studies (reviewed later) provide evidence that depression in PD is associated with frontal CBF and metabolic changes above and beyond those observed in PD alone. Second, a few neuropsychological studies which have compared in detail the memory performance of depressed and nondepressed PD patients, suggest that the quality or pattern of memory impairments in PD with depression resembles that observed in individuals with frontal lobe dysfunction.

Wertman et al. (1993) found not only that the memory impairment in PD with depression is more pronounced than that in either depression or PD alone, but that the pattern of memory impairment in PD with depression resembles that of patients with frontal dysfunction (i.e. poor acquisition of information, poor recall consistency and an inability to develop a systematic recall strategy from selective reminding, accompanied by normal rates of forgetting and delayed recognition). Furthermore, although potential associations between measures of memory and set shifting were not evaluated, the depressed PD group had more pronounced set shifting impairments than the nondepressed PD group, which suggests again that depression in PD might exacerbate executive (frontal) deficits. Taylor et al. (1986b) found neither depressed nor nondepressed PD groups to be impaired on a series of memory tasks (WAIS-R Digit Span, Arithmetic and WMS Logical Memory, Visual Reproduction and Paired Associate Learning) when memory performance was evaluated relative to subjects' own WAIS-R Vocabulary scores. However, the finding that the depressed PD group performed relatively more poorly than the non-depressed group on what the study's authors defined as 'ordered recall tasks' (i.e. Digit Span and Arithmetic), suggests that depression might exacerbate fronto-striatal dysfunction in mild PD.

It is important to emphasize, however, that although depression affects cognition (and especially executive functions and memory) (Starkstein et al. 1989c; Kuzis et al. 1997), this effect might be a function of disease severity.

For example, Starkstein et al. (1989a) found that depression impacts performance on frontal-tasks (e.g. Wisconsin Card Sorting Test – WCST) in severe, but not mild PD, and Tröster et al. (1995b) also failed to find differences between depressed and nondepressed groups with mild PD on the WCST. If the effect of depression on cognition is a function of disease severity, then an important question is whether the effects of depression on cognition are a matter of quantity or quality, i.e. does depression merely exacerbate cognitive deficits or does it alter or produce novel patterns of cognitive deficits?

Tröster et al. (1995b), utilizing a broad neuropsychological test battery, found that a depressed PD group had more severe immediate verbal recall impairments than a nondepressed PD group, but when the groups were matched for overall severity of cognitive impairment, all differences among test scores disappeared. This supports Starkstein et al.'s (1990a) finding that depression exerts a quantitative rather than a qualitative effect on cognition.

Biological correlates of depression in subcortical (basal ganglia) dementias

Neuroimaging studies provide evidence that depression influences fronto-subcortical blood flow and metabolism not only in indiopathic depression, but also in basal ganglia diseases (Mayberg 1994b). Bilateral hypometabolism of orbital-inferior prefrontal cortex and anterior temporal cortex has been reported in both PD and HD with depression (Mayberg et al. 1990; 1992), as well as in patients with unipolar depression (Mayberg 1993, 1994b). Ring et al. (1994) recently found that PD with depression, relative to PD without depression, is associated with medial frontal and cingulate cortex hypometabolism, an abnormality also observed in idiopathic depression. This pattern of cerebral pathophysiology revealed by PET imaging studies implicates in depression the paralimbic pathways linking frontal cortex, temporal cortex and striatum (Mayberg 1994b), which are known to be important in the expression and modulation of mood and affect (Salloway and Cummings 1994).

Although there are commonalities among the patterns of cerebral hypometabolism observed in idiopathic depression and PD and HD with depression, it is likely that different neurochemical systems and brain structures are associated with depression in HD and PD, i.e. frontal lobe metabolic changes reported in functional neuroimaging studies might represent a 'final common pathway' down-stream from changes in other neuroanatomical and chemical systems (i.e. result from frontal deafferentation from different subcortical structures in HD and PD). In HD, the medial anterior caudate has been implicated in depression (Peyser and Folstein 1993), because this is the site of the earliest neuronal loss in HD (VonSattel et al. 1985) and depression is an early feature which can precede other manifestations of HD by many years. Furthermore, medial anterior caudate damage, or caudate atrophy (Starkstein et al. 1989b), would disrupt the limbic-caudate-frontal system. It remains unclear to what extent GABAergic, enkephalinergic and gultamatergic abnormalities might contribute to depression. Noradrenergic and serotonergic abnormalities are thought at this time to play a minimal role in depression in HD (Peyser and Folstein 1993). Specifically, Zweig et al. (1992) failed to find differences in the locus coeruleus and dorsal raphe nuclei (the major sources of norepinephrine and serotonin, respectively) of depressed and never-depressed HD patients.

Affective changes in PD, in contrast, have been most strongly linked to serotonergic abnormalities. For example, reductions in cerebrospinal fluid of the serotonin metabolite 5-hydroxy-indoleacetic acid (5-HIAA) have been found in depressed but not nondepressed PD patients (Mayeux et al. 1984, 1988) and improvement of depression has been associated with increases in 5-HIAA levels in response to treatment with 5-hydroxy-tryptophan and 1-tryptophan (Mayeux et al. 1986). Noradrenergic system involvement in depression has been largely inferred from the observation that depression in PD responds to tricyclic antidepressants (for a review, see Klaassen et al. 1995).

The potential role of dopaminergic abnormalities in PD depression is best supported by the finding that depressed PD patients demonstrate particularly pronounced degeneration of dopaminergic neurons in the ventral tegmentum (Torack and Morris 1988), although entorhinal cortical and hippocampal pathology was also pronounced. The predominant finding that treatment with dopamine agonists does not alleviate depression (but, see Miyoshi et al. 1996) should not be taken to discount entirely the role of dopaminergic abnormalities because it is possible that such therapies might improve dopaminergic function in the nigrostriatal system to a greater extent than in the mesolimbic system (Kelly et al. 1975) which is more likely to be involved in depression.

These biological correlates of depression in HD and PD do not imply causation. For example, an already diseased fronto–striatal system could represent a diathesis for the genesis of depression in basal ganglia dementias. Indeed, Brown and Jahanshahi (1995) have provided a complex biopsychosocial model of how depression is caused and modified in PD, the discussion of which is not feasible within the confines of this chapter. Similarly, although the potential role of psychosocial factors in the etiology of depression in HD is hard to deny, readers are referred to Brandt and Butters (1996) for a discussion of why psychosocial explanations alone cannot satisfactorily account for depression in HD.

Treatment of depression in subcortical (basal ganglia) dementias

Depression in PD has been demonstrated to respond to a variety of antidepressants, including tricyclics and selective serotonin-reuptake inhibitors, although there are very few adequately controlled studies (Klaassen et al. 1995). Unfortunately, none of the studies has examined the impact of antidepressant therapy on cognition and more specifically, memory. Starkstein et al. (1992) provided preliminary data that antidepressant therapy might improve cognitive function, or at least retard further cognitive deterioration. Similarly, ECT has been reported to improve depression in PD (Burke et al. 1988a), but the cognitive effects of this treatment modality in PD have not been adequately addressed. ECT can lead to delirium in PD patients (Oh et al. 1992), but whether this side-effect is more common in PD than in other elderly depressed patients remains to be established. Similarly, although a variety of antidepressant agents and ECT have been shown to be efficacious in treating depression in HD (Peyser and Folstein 1993), few of these studies are well controlled and none reports the effects of these therapies on memory. One case study reported beneficial effects of amitriptyline in progressive supranuclear palsy (Asanuma et al. 1993), but the effects of this treatment on cognition were not reported.

THE EFFECTS OF DEPRESSION ON MEMORY IN HIV DISEASE AND HIV-ASSOCIATED DEMENTIA

Incidence and prevalence

Time-point prevalence estimates of major depression among outpatients infected with the human immuno-deficiency virus (HIV+) are somewhat (about two times)

higher than in the general community, but comparable to those reported for other groups with chronic medical illnesses, ranging from 5% to 8% (Perry et al. 1990; Williams et al. 1991; Atkinson and Grant 1994). However, lifetime prevalence of depression and the prevalence of depression among HIV-infected cohorts participating in longitudinal studies, might be considerably higher than in community samples. Some longitudinal studies have found that up to 25% of outpatient HIV+ homosexual men developed depressive syndromes within 2 years of study enrollment (Atkinson and Grant 1994), with no differences in incidence noted according to disease status (asymptomatic, mildly symptomatic or frank AIDS) and lifetime prevalence estimates of depression have similarly been reported to be approximately 25–35% (Robins et al. 1984; Atkinson and Grant 1994). The high rates of lifetime psychiatric disorders (Perry et al. 1990), alcohol and other substance abuse disorders in those *at risk* for HIV suggests that many cases of depression in HIV might represent recurrences rather than new onset of depression and that the relatively high lifetime prevalence of depression in HIV might be associated with psychosocial factors preceding HIV infection.

Mood disturbance continues to be the most frequent neuropsychiatric complication also among *hospitalized* AIDS patients (Perry and Tross 1984; Atkinson and Grant 1997); and depression is diagnosed in up to 40% of hospitalized HIV+ patients (Perry and Tross 1984). Particularly in the case of the severely ill or demented HIV-infected patient, the diagnosis (and thus, also prevalence estimation) of depression is complicated by somatic symptoms associated with physical illness, side-effects from antiretroviral medications and protease inhibitors, and neurobehavioral symptoms of HIV-associated dementia (Navia et al. 1986; Boccellari et al. 1988).

Nature of the memory impairment in HIV disease and depression

About 75% of the patients who die with AIDS have some evidence of central nervous system (CNS) pathology, but it is not clear at what point during the disease the CNS becomes involved and how HIV affects memory and cognition across the disease spectrum (Wiley 1994). The annual incidence of dementia among AIDS patients is estimated to be about 7% and median survival from time of diagnosis of dementia is approximately 6 months (McArthur et al. 1993).

No studies have directly assessed the relationship between HIV-associated dementia and depression, and several good reasons probably underlie this omission. First, criteria for the diagnosis of HIV-associated dementia have only recently been proposed by the American Academy of Neurology (AAN) (Working Group of the American Academy of Neurology AIDS Task Force 1991) and by Grant and Martin (1994), and the first published attempt to evaluate the utility of the diagnostic algorithm proposed by the AAN excluded all patients with clinical depression (Dana Consortium 1996). Second, the differentiation between dementia and depression can be difficult in HIV-spectrum disease. The AAN recommended criteria for diagnosis of HIV-associated dementia include an acquired impairment of at least 1 month's duration in at least two cognitive domains, a decline in motor function and/or social or emotional behavior and the *absence* of another cause of the cognitive, motor or behavioral symptoms and signs. Unfortunately, establishing the absence of another cause for signs and symptoms can be complicated because such symptoms are frequently evidenced in active CNS opportunistic infections (e.g. toxoplasmosis, histoplasmosis), or other CNS disorders sometimes confirmable only by brain biopsy or at autopsy (e.g. progressive multifocal leukoencephalopathy). Third, McArthur and Selnes (1997) reported that the most common presenting symptoms in their large sample of HIV dementia patients were memory impairment, gait difficulty, mental slowing and depressive symptoms (especially social withdrawal and apathy). These symptoms, especially in their early stages, may be overlooked entirely or confused with depression. Fourth, the apparently short survival of individuals with HIV-associated dementia makes recruitment of these individuals into studies difficult. Finally, the majority of subjects with HIV-associated dementia fatigue easily, may forget appointments and may lose interest in participating in studies requiring them to perform tasks which often frustrate them.

The relationship between depression and memory impairment in HIV-associated dementia has not been fully investigated, but numerous studies have examined neuropsychological test performance as a function of depression in HIV+ groups. The vast majority of studies has failed to find a significant relationship between depression and objectively verified cognitive impairment in HIV (van Gorp et al. 1991; Wilkins et al. 1991; Hinkin et al. 1992; Levin et al. 1992; Grant et al. 1993; Mapou et al. 1993; Pace

et al. 1993; Beason-Hazen et al. 1994; Marsh and McCall 1994; Bix et al. 1995; Harker et al. 1995; Silvestre et al. 1995; Poutiainen and Elovaara 1996) even though there might be a relationship between subjective complaints of cognitive difficulties and affective disturbance (van Gorp et al. 1991; Wilkins et al. 1991; Mapou et al. 1993) and between such subjective complaints and neuropsychological test performance (Bornstein et al. 1993; Mapou et al. 1993; Beason-Hazen et al. 1994; Poutiainen and Elovaara 1996). Only a minority of studies has found a relationship between depression and memory impairment in HIV. Comparing cognitive performance in HIV+ groups with major depression and no depression, Goggin et al. (1997) found that the depressed group performed more poorly on two measures of verbal and nonverbal memory. Hinkin et al. (1992) reported poorer performance by depressed HIV+ subjects on the final trial of a word list learning task.

The largely negative findings pertaining to the relationship between depression and memory in HIV disease might reflect that many studies of neuropsychological function in HIV treat depression as a potential confound and exclude patients with depression. Alternatively, depression might influence memory in only a subgroup of HIV+ individuals. Although Peavy et al. (1994) did not examine the influence of depression on memory per se, these authors found a symptomatic HIV+ group, but not an asymptomatic one, to perform more poorly than a normal control group on a word list learning and memory task. Finally, depression might account for only a small proportion of the variance in memory test scores of individuals with HIV. For example, Heaton et al. (1995) found that HIV+ subjects with global neuropsychological impairment were significantly more likely to have syndromic major depression, as diagnosed by the Structured Clinical Interview for Depression (SCID), than were those without such neuropsychological impairment; however, because greater levels of cognitive impairment were evident in the HIV+ cohort even once subjects with syndromal depression and significantly depressed mood were excluded, the investigators concluded that cognitive deficits in HIV disease could not be explained by depressed mood alone.

Biological correlates of depression in HIV-associated dementia

Whether depression in HIV has a biological basis, or represents a natural reaction to diagnosis, limitations in the activities of daily living and other stressors, has been debated. The observation that depression is more common among HIV+ individuals with histories of personality disorders and depression (often predating HIV infection) than in those individuals without such histories (e.g. Perkins et al. 1994), suggests that HIV-related neuropathology alone cannot adequately account for emergence of depression in HIV disease. On the other hand, Perry (1994) convincingly argues that depression in HIV disease should not be seen simply as an understandable and 'normal' reaction to the illness.

It remains plausible that neuropathology exacerbates a susceptibility to depression because the basal ganglia and related structures have been shown to be the brain regions most affected by pathology in AIDS patients (Aylward et al. 1993; Martin 1994). Possible mechanisms for neuronal death include secretion of neurotoxins from HIV–1 infected macrophages (Epstein and Gendelman 1993). It is also possible that other factors may predispose HIV+ patients to dementia, depression or both. For example, neurosyphilis is extremely difficult to eradicate in HIV+ patients and symptoms may include memory problems and fatigue. Nutritional and vitamin deficiencies are prevalent in HIV disease and some studies have reported that 25–50% of HIV+ patients demonstrate impaired absorption of vitamin B_{12} (Beach et al. 1992), which can impact cognition.

Future studies closely examining the nature of depressive symptoms across the HIV disease course are needed if a better understanding of the pathogenesis of depression in this disease is to be gained. Such studies would also have to take into account the difficulty in documenting depression in HIV disease because it appears that disease-related somatic and cognitive symptoms significantly influence scores on self-report measures of depression (Drebing et al. 1994).

Treatment of depression in HIV disease and HIV-associated dementia

Treatment of depression in HIV disease is relatively straightforward, but the effects of such treatment on memory have rarely been examined. Generally, clinicians have had success treating depression with psychotherapy, tricyclics with low anticholinergic profiles (e.g. desipramine) and selective serotonin reuptake inhibitors (SSRIs) such as fluoxetine, sertraline or paroxetine (Markowitz et al. 1994; Atkinson and Grant 1997). The potential adverse

effects of tricyclic treatment in AIDS patients include delirium (Storch 1991). Indeed, as is the case in the treatment of older adults, antidepressant dosing might need to be modified in AIDS patients and agents with strong anticholinergic properties are probably better avoided (Atkinson and Grant 1997). Severely impaired patients with both depression and dementia who have not responded to traditional pharmacological therapies, may respond positively to ECT (Schaerf et al. 1989).

Fernandez and Levy (1994) recommend considering psychostimulants (methylphenidate, dextroamphetamine and pemoline) for depressed HIV+ patients, and particularly for those patients whose affect is more apathetic than depressed, who have failed to maintain good nutrition and who have cognitive impairments. In their review, Masand and Tesar (1996) concluded that a substantial proportion of patients demonstrated improvements in depressive symptomatology, and some also in cognition, after treatment with psychostimulants. These authors, however, also caution that most of the studies reviewed did not differentiate between depressed mood and clinical depression and that many studies had small sample sizes and lacked blinding, placebo controls, controls for practice effects on cognitive tests and female patients.

A BRIEF NOTE CONCERNING THE EFFECTS OF DEPRESSION ON MEMORY IN MULTIPLE SCLEROSIS

There may be no single pattern of cognitive impairment which characterizes multiple sclerosis (see Beatty 1995), but, when dementia does occur in multiple sclerosis, it often manifests in a 'subcortical' pattern of cognitive dysfunction. This is not surprising, because multiple sclerosis affects with proclivity the subcortical white matter, particularly in the periventricular area (Salloway and Cummings 1994). The multiple sclerosis lesions' proximity to projection fibers connecting cortical and subcortical structures would lead one to expect that individuals afflicted with multiple sclerosis would be especially vulnerable to cognitive dysfunction and depression, and this expectation is confirmed by empirical research.

Depression prevalence estimates in multiple sclerosis range from 27% to 54% (Minden and Schiffer 1990), and this variability in estimates probably reflects methodological differences among studies and the general failure of studies to distinguish depressive symptoms from major depressive illness (Schiffer and Wineman 1990). Studies indicate that depression has a negligible effect on memory and cognition in multiple sclerosis (Huber and Rao 1993), but most of these studies have considered the influence on memory of depressive symptoms (often of mild-to-moderate severity), rather than of major depression. Although some researchers have found that depression symptoms relate to memory difficulties in multiple sclerosis (Rao et al. 1984; Beatty et al. 1988), most studies have failed to find direct correlations between depression and memory dysfunction (Surridge 1969; Grafman et al. 1990; Rao et al. 1991; Schiffer and Caine 1991; Grossman et al. 1994). As Beatty (1995) points out, even when depression is found to influence memory, the amount of variance attributable to depression is small.

The etiology of depression in multiple sclerosis remains unknown, but several lines of evidence suggests that depression might in part be attributable to neuropathology. MRI studies have found that total lesion load, while an important factor in cognitive impairment (Huber et al. 1987; Rao et al. 1989), is not related to depression (Honer et al. 1987; Ron and Logsdail 1989). Instead, the distribution (location) of lesions is an important determinant of affective disturbance. The observation that especially temporal lobe involvement is related to affective disturbance suggests that the disconnection of frontal lobes from limbic structures might be a critical biological determinant of depression (Rao et al. 1984). That depression might be of pathophysiological origin in multiple sclerosis is also supported by the finding that depression appears to be more prevalent in multiple sclerosis than other disorders involving chronic physical disability (Rao et al. 1992). A genetic basis for depression in multiple sclerosis has recently been explored, but not supported (Sadovnick et al. 1996).

Few studies have examined the treatment of depression in multiple sclerosis and how it might affect memory and other cognitive functions. Rao et al. (1984) found that 68% of patients presenting with mild memory impairments were likely to be taking psychoactive medication. In a study of the effectiveness of desipramine in patients with multiple sclerosis, Schiffer and Wineman (1990) found that this tricyclic was more effective in alleviating depressive symptoms than no treatment, but the observed side-effects led the authors to conclude that only a modest benefit was derived from this treatment. Scott et al. (1996) reported

that multiple sclerosis patients tolerate antidepressants relatively well, but that the relapse rate is high once medication is discontinued. Interestingly, Rodgers et al. (1996) reported preliminary data indicating that, in comparison to a wait-list multiple sclerosis control group, multiple sclerosis patients receiving cognitive therapy over 24 weeks demonstrated significantly greater improvements not only in depressive symptoms, but also in verbal abstraction and memory.

CONCLUSIONS

Common themes of methodological concerns emerge in reviewing studies of depression and memory in neurodegenerative diseases. Studies differ in their use of diagnostic criteria for depression, assessment instruments and sampling methods. Furthermore, it is often unclear whether studies are referring to a depression syndrome or to depressed mood, and to what extent potential symptoms of depression might reflect somatic symptoms of medical illness or the side-effects of treatment. These methodological concerns might account for inconsistent findings concerning depression and memory in a given disease, but are less likely to account for differences in findings across different neurodegenerative conditions as these differences emerge consistently.

The research reviewed in this chapter allows one to draw not only the conclusion that depression is more common in PD and HD than in AD, but also that depression reliably exacerbates memory impairment only in PD. Given the neuropathology of PD and HD, and the observation that lesions of the pallidum and caudate are more likely to be associated with secondary depression than are lesions of other subcortical structures (Starkstein et al., 1988; Brumback, 1993; Lauterbach et al., 1997), it is not surprising that PD and HD are associated with a high prevalence of depression. More remarkable is the convergence of neuropsychological and functional imaging data, which is beginning to shed light on how depression influences memory in PD. Specifically, it appears that depression exacerbates the subcortical-frontal circuit pathophysiology of PD, thus leading to difficulties with encoding, retrieval and executive control over memory processes. Depression in AD, on the other hand, appears to be related to metabolic and blood flow changes in the posterior cortical regions.

The critical role of frontal-subcortical circuits in depression is also supported by studies of the effects of severe depression on otherwise healthy elderly individuals' memory and CBF. Unfortunately, the opportunity to corroborate the role of frontal-subcortical pathophysiology in depression and memory dysfunction by studying the effects of depression on memory in HD and HIV-associated dementia has not been realized. Indeed, not one such study was found in searches of major psychological and medical literature databases. The finding that depression in HIV infected individuals appears not to impact memory significantly should not be taken as refuting the probable role of the basal ganglia in memory dysfunction and depression. It is likely that basal ganglia pathology sufficiently extensive to cause clinically remarkable depression and memory dysfunction probably does not arise until the individual with HIV has developed at least an incipient dementia.

Few studies have rigorously evaluated the effects of antidepressant treatment on memory in neurodegenerative diseases. The limited data available allows one to tentatively conclude that well-chosen antidepressants have minimal adverse effect on cognition and, indeed, that treatment of depression alleviates (but, rarely reverses) cognitive impairments in at least some patients with neurodegenerative disease.

REFERENCES

Abas, M.A., Sahakian, B.J. and Levy, R. 1990. Neuropsychological deficits and CT scan changes in elderly depressives. *Psychological Medicine*. 20: 507–520.

Albert, M., Feldman, R. and Willis, A. 1974. The subcortical dementia of progressive supranuclear palsy. *Journal of Neurology, Neurosurgery and Psychiatry*. 37: 121–130.

Alexopoulos, G.S. and Nambudiri, D.E. 1994. Depressive dementia: Cognitive and biologic correlates and the course of illness. In *Dementia: Presentations, differential diagnosis and nosology*, ed. V.O.B. Emery and T.E. Oxman, pp. 321–335. Baltimore: Johns Hopkins University Press.

Asanuma, M., Hirata, H., Kondo, Y. and Ogawa, N. 1993. A case of progressive supranuclear palsy showing marked improvements of frontal hypoperfusion, as well as parkinsonism with amitriptyline. *Rinsho-Shinkeigaku*. 33: 317–321.

Atkinson, J.H. and Grant, I. 1994. Natural history of neuropsychiatric manifestations of HIV disease. *Psychiatric Clinics of North America*. 17: 17–33.

Atkinson, J.H. and Grant, I. 1997. Neuropsychiatry of human immunodeficiency virus infection. In *AIDS and the nervous system, 2nd ed.*, ed. J.R. Berger and R.M. Levy, pp. 419–449. Philadelphia: Lippincott-Raven Publishers.

Aylward, E.H., Henderer, J.D., McArthur, J.C., Brettschneider, P.D., Harris, G.J., Barta, P.E. and Pearlson, G.D. 1993. Reduced basal ganglia volume in HIV–1-associated dementia: Results from quantitative neuroimaging. *Neurology*. 42: 2099–2104.

Ballard, C.G., Bannister, C. and Oyebode, F. 1996. Depression in dementia sufferers. *International Journal of Geriatric Psychiatry*. 11: 507–515.

Ballard, C.G., Mohan, R.N.C., Patel, A. and Bannister, C. 1993. Idiopathic clouding of consciousness: Do the patients have cortical Lewy body disease? *International Journal of Geriatric Psychiatry*. 8: 571–576.

Beach, R.S., Morgan, R., Wilkie, F., Mantero-Atienza, E., Blaney, N., Shor-Posner, G., Lu, Y., Eisdorfer, C. and Baum, M.K. 1992. Plasma B^{12} level as a potential cofactor in studies of human immunodeficiency virus type 1-related cognitive changes. *Archives of Neurology*. 49: 501–506.

Beason-Hazen, S., Nasrallah, H.A. and Bornstein, R.A. 1994. Self-report of symptoms and neuropsychological performance in asymptomatic HIV-positive individuals. *Journal of Neuropsychiatry and Clinical Neurosciences*. 6: 43–49.

Beatty, W.W. 1995. Multiple sclerosis. In *Neuropsychology for clinical practice: Etiology, assessment and treatment of common neurological disorders*, ed. R.L. Adams, O.A. Parsons, J.L. Culbertson and S.J. Nixon, pp. 225–242. Washington, DC: American Psychological Association.

Beatty, W.W., Goodkin, D.E., Monson, E., Beatty, P.A. and Hertsgaard, D. 1988. Anterograde and retrograde amnesia in patients with chronic progressive multiple sclerosis. *Archives of Neurology*. 45: 611–619.

Bench, C.J., Frackowiak, R.S. and Dolan, R.J. 1995. Changes in regional cerebral blood flow on recovery from depression. *Psychological Medicine*. 25: 247–261.

Bench, C.J., Friston, K.J., Brown, R.G., Frackowiak, R.S. and Dolan, R.J. 1993. Regional cerebral blood flow in depression measured by positron emission tomography: The relationship with clinical dimensions. *Psychological Medicine*. 23: 579–590.

Bench, C.J., Friston, K.J., Brown, R.G., Scott, L.C., Frackowiak, R.S. and Dolan, R.J. 1992. The anatomy of melancholia: Focal abnormalities of cerebral blood flow in major depression. *Psychological Medicine*. 22: 607–615.

Bix, B.C., Glosser, G., Holmes, W., Ballas, C., Meritz, M., Hutelmyer, C. and Turner, J. 1995. Relationship between psychiatric disease and neuropsychological impairment in HIV seropositive individuals. *Journal of the International Neuropsychological Society*. 1: 581–588.

Boccellari, A., Dilley, J.W. and Shore, M.D. 1988. Neuropsychiatric aspects of AIDS dementia complex: A report on a clinical series. *NeuroToxicology*. 9: 381–390.

Bondi, M.W. and Tröster, A.I. 1997. Parkinson's disease: Neurobehavioral consequences of basal ganglia dysfunction. In *Handbook of neuropsychology and aging*, ed. P.D. Nussbaum, pp. 216–245. New York: Plenum.

Boone, K., Miller, B., Lesser, I., Mehringer, C.M., Hill-Gutierrez, E., Goldberg, M.A. and Berman, N.G. 1992. Neuropsychological correlates of white matter lesions in healthy elderly subjects: A threshold effect. *Archives of Neurology*. 49: 549–554.

Bornstein, R.A., Pace, P., Rosenberger, P., Nasrallah, H.A., Para, M.F., Whitacre, C.C. and Fass, R.J. 1993. Depression and neuropsychological performance in asymptomatic HIV infection. *American Journal of Psychiatry*. 150: 922–927.

Brandt, J. and Butters, N. 1996. Neuropsychological characteristics of Huntington's disease. In *Neuropsychological assessment of neuropsychiatric disorders*, 2nd ed., ed. I. Grant and K.M. Adams, pp. 312–341. New York: Oxford University Press.

Breen, A.R., Larson, E.B., Reifler, B.V., Vitaliano, P.P. and Lawrence, G.L. 1984. Cognitive performance and functional competence in coexisting dementia and depression. *Journal of the American Geriatrics Society*. 32: 132–137.

Brown, R. and Jahanshahi, M. 1995. Depression in Parkinson's disease: A psychosocial viewpoint. In *Behavioral neurology of movement disorders. Advances in neurology*, vol 45, ed. W.J. Weiner and A.E. Lang, pp. 61–84. New York: Raven Press.

Brumback, R.A. 1993. Is depression a neurologic disease? *Neurologic Clinics*. 11: 79–104.

Burke, W.J., Peterson, J. and Rubin, E.H. 1988a. Electroconvulsive therapy in the treatment of combined depression and Parkinson's disease. *Psychosomatics*. 29: 341–346.

Burke, W.J., Rubin, E.H., Morris, J.C. and Berg, L. 1988b. Symptoms of depression in senile dementia of the Alzheimer's type. *Alzheimer Disease and Associated Disorders*. 2: 356–362.

Burns, A. and Förstl, H. 1996. The Institute of Psychiatry Alzheimer's disease cohort: Part 2: Clinicopathological observations. *International Journal of Geriatric Psychiatry*. 11: 321–327.

Burt, D.B., Zembar, M.J. and Niederehe, G. 1995. Depression and memory impairment: A meta-analysis of the association, its pattern and specificity. *Psychological Bulletin*. 117: 285–305.

Cahn, D.A., Malloy, P.F., Salloway, S., Rogg, J., Gillard, E., Kohn, R., Tung, G., Richardson, E.D. and Westlake R. 1996. Subcortical hyperintensities on MRI and activities of daily living in geriatric depression. *Journal of Neuropsychiatry and Clinical Neurosciences*. 8: 404–411.

Cantello, R., Aguaggia, M., Gilli, M., Delsedime, M., Chiardo-Cutin, I., Riccio, A. and Mutano, R. 1989. Major depression in Parkinson's disease and the mood response to intravenous methylphenidate: Possible role of the 'hedonic' dopamine synapse. *Journal of Neurology, Neurosurgery and Psychiatry*. 52: 724–731.

Christensen, H., Griffiths, K., Mackinnon, A. and Jacomb, P. 1997. A quantitative review of cognitive deficits in depression and Alzheimer-type dementia. *Journal of the International Neuropsychological Society*. 3: 631–651.

Cole, S.A., Woodard, J.L., Juncos, J.L., Kogos, J.L., Youngstrom, E.A. and Watts, R.L. 1996. Depression and disability in Parkinson's disease. *Journal of Neuropsychiatry and Clinical Neurosciences*. 8: 20–25.

Cummings, J.L. 1992. Depression and Parkinson's disease: A review. *American Journal of Psychiatry*. 149: 443–454.

Cummings, J.L., Ross, W., Absher, J., Gornbein, J. and Hadjiaghai, L. 1995. Depressive symptoms in Alzheimer disease: Assessment and determinants. *Alzheimer Disease and Associated Disorders*. 9: 87–93.

Dana Consortium on Therapy for HIV Dementia and Related Cognitive Disorders. 1996. Clinical confirmation of the American Academy of Neurology algorithm for HIV–1–associated cognitive/motor disorder. *Neurology*. 47: 1247–1253.

Des Rosiers, G., Hodges, J.R. and Berrios G. 1995. The neuropsychological differentiation of patients with very mild Alzheimer's disease and/or major depression. *Journal of the American Geriatrics Society*. 43: 1256–1263.

Dolan, R.J., Bench, C.J., Brown, R.G., Scott, L.C. and Frackowiak, R.S. 1994. Neuropsychological dysfunction in depression: The relationship to regional cerebral blood flow. *Psychological Medicine*. 24: 849–857.

Dolan, R.J., Bench, C.J., Brown, R.G., Scott, L.C., Friston, K.J. and Frackowiak, R.S. 1992. Regional cerebral blood flow abnormalities in depressed patients with cognitive impairment. *Journal of Neurology, Neurosurgery and Psychiatry*. 55: 768–773.

Drebing, C.E., VanGorp, W.G., Hinkin, C., Miller, E.N., Satz, P., Kim, D.S., Holston, S. and D'Elia, L.F. 1994. Confounding factors in the measurement of depression in HIV. *Journal of Personality Assessment*. 62: 68–83.

Epstein, L.G. and Gendelman, H.E. 1993. Human immunodeficiency virus type–1 infection of the nervous system: Pathogenetic mechanisms. *Annals of Neurology*. 33: 429–436.

Fernandez, F. and Levy, J.K. 1994. Psychopharmacology in HIV spectrum disorders. *Psychiatric Clinics of North America*. 17: 135–148.

Filley, C.M. 1995. Neuropsychiatric features of Lewy body disease. *Brain and Cognition*. 28: 229–239.

Fischer, P., Simamyi, M. and Danielczyk, W. 1990. Depression in dementia of the Alzheimer type and in multi-infarct dementia. *American Journal of Psychiatry*. 147: 1484–1487.

Fitz, A.G. and Teri, L. 1994. Depression, cognition and functional ability in patients with Alzheimer's disease. *Journal of the American Geriatrics Society*. 42: 186–191.

Folstein, S.E., Abbott, M.H., Chase, G.A., Jensen, B.A. and Folstein, M.F. 1983. The association of affective disorder with Huntington's disease in a case series and in families. *Psychological Medicine*. 13: 537–542.

Förstl, H., Burns, A., Luthert, P., Cairns, N., Lantos, P. and Levy, R., 1992. Clinical and neuropathological correlates of depression in Alzheimer's disease. *Psychological Medicine*. 22: 877–884.

Gainotti, G. and Marra, C. 1994. Some aspects of memory disorders clearly distinguish dementia of the Alzheimer's type from depressive pseudo-dementia. *Journal of Clinical and Experimental Neuropsychology*. 16: 65–78.

Glatt, S.L., Hubble, J.P., Lyons, K., Paolo, A., Tröster, A.I., Hassanein, R.E.S. and Koller, W.C. 1996. Risk factors for dementia in Parkinson's disease: Effect of education. *Neuroepidemiology*. 15: 20–25.

Goggin, K.J., Zisook, S., Heaton, R.K., Grant, I., Atkinson, J.H., Marshall, S., McCutchan, J.A., Chandler, J.L. Grant, I. and the HNRC Group. 1997. Neuropsychological correlates of HIV-associated depression. *Journal of the International Neuropsychological Society*. 3: 457–464.

Gotham, A.M., Brown, R.G. and Marsden, C.D. 1986. Depression in Parkinson's disease: A quantitative and qualitative analysis. *Journal of Neurology, Neurosurgery, and Psychiatry*. 49: 381–389.

Grady, C.L., Haxby, J.V., Schapiro, M.B., Gonzalez-Aviles, A., Kumar, A., Ball, M.J., Heston, L. and Rapoport, S.I. 1990. Subgroups in dementia of the Alzheimer type identified using positron emission tomography. *Journal of Neuropsychiatry and Clinical Neurosciences*. 2: 373–384.

Grafman, J., Rao, S.M. and Litvan, I. 1990. Disorders of memory. In *Neurobehavioral aspects of multiple sclerosis*, ed. S.M. Rao, pp. 102–117. New York: Oxford University Press.

Grant, I. and Martin, A. (ed.) 1994. *Neuropsychology of HIV infection*. New York: Oxford University Press.

Grant, I., Olshen, R.A., Atkinson, J.H., Heaton, R.K., Nelson, J., McCutchan, J.A. and Weinrich, J.D. 1993. Depressed mood does not explain neuropsychological deficits in HIV-infected persons. *Neuropsychology*. 7: 53–61.

Greenwald, B.S., Kramer-Ginsberg, E., Marin, D.B., Laitman, L.B., Hermann, C.K., Mohs, R.C. and Davis, K.L. 1989. Dementia with coexistent major depression. *American Journal of Psychiatry*. 146: 1472–1478.

Grossman, M., Armstrong, C., Onishi, K., Thompson, H., Schaefer, B., Robinson, K., D'Esposito, M., Cohen, J., Brennan, D., Rostami, A., Gonzalez-Scarano, F., Kolson, D., Constantinescu, C. and Silberberg, D. 1994. Patterns of cognitive impairment in relapsing-remitting and chronic progressive multiple sclerosis. *Neuropsychiatry, Neuropsychology and Behavioral Neurology*. 7: 194–210.

Hantz, P., Caradoc-Davies, G., Caradoc-Davies, T., Weatherall, M. and Dixon, G. 1994. Depression in Parkinson's disease. *American Journal of Psychiatry*. 151: 1010–1014.

Harker, J.O., Satz, P., Jones, F.DeL., Verma, R.C., Gan, M.P., Poer, H.L., Gould, B.D. and Chervinsky, A.B. 1995. Measurement of depression and neuropsychological impairment in HIV–1 infection. *Neuropsychology*. 9: 110–117.

Hart, R.P., Kwentus, J.A., Hamer, R.M. and Taylor, J.R. 1987b. Selective reminding procedure in depression and dementia. *Psychology and Aging*. 2: 111–115.

Hart, R.P., Kwentus, J.A., Taylor, J.R. and Harkins, S.W. 1987a. Rate of forgetting in dementia and depression. *Journal of Consulting and Clinical Psychology*. 55: 101–105.

Haupt, M., Kurz, A. and Greifenhagen, A. 1995. Depression in Alzheimer's disease: Phenomenological features and association with severity and progression of cognitive and functional impairment. *International Journal of Geriatric Psychiatry*. 10: 469–476.

Heaton, R.K., Grant, I., Butters, N., White, D.A., Kirson, D., Atkinson, J.H., McCutchan, J.A., Taylor, M.J., Kelly, M.D., Ellis, R.J., Wolfson, T., Velin, R., Marcotte, T.D., Hesselink, J.R., Jernigan, T.L., Chandler, J., Wallace, M., Abramson, I. and the HNRC Group. 1995. The HNRC 500-Neuropsychology of HIV infection at different disease stages. *Journal of the International Neuropsychological Society*. 1: 231–251.

Hinkin, C.H., Van Gorp, W.G., Satz, P., Weisman, J.D., Thommes, J. and Buckingham, S. 1992. Depressed mood and its relationship to neuropsychological test performance in HIV–1 seropositive individuals. *Journal of Clinical and Experimental Neuropsychology*. 14: 289–297.

Hirono, N., Mori, E., Ishii, K., Ikejiri, Y., Imamura, T., Shimomura, T., Hashimoto, M., Yamashita, Y. and Sasaki, M. 1998. Frontal lobe hypometabolism and depression in Alzheimer's disease. *Neurology*. 50: 380–383.

Honer, W.G., Hurwitz, T., Li, D.K.B., Palmer, M. and Paty, D.W. 1987. Temporal lobe involvement in multiple sclerosis patients with psychiatric disorders. *Archives of Neurology*. 44: 187–190.

Hubble, J.P., Cao, T., Hassanein, R.E.S., Neuberger, J.S. and Koller, W.C. 1993. Risk factors for Parkinson's disease. *Neurology*. 43: 1693–1697.

Huber, S.J. and Rao, S.M. 1993. Depression in multiple sclerosis. In *Depression in neurologic disease*, ed. E.S. Starkstein and R.E. Robinson, pp. 85–96. Baltimore: Johns Hopkins University Press.

Huber, S.J., Paulson, G.W., Shuttleworth, E.C., Chakeres, D., Clapp, L.E., Pakalnis, A., Weiss, K., and Rammohan, K. 1987. Magnetic resonance imaging correlates of dementia in multiple sclerosis. *Archives of Neurology*. 44: 732–736.

Kelly, P.H., Seviour, P.W. and Iversen, S.D. 1975. Amphetamine and apomorphine responses in the rat following 6-OHCA lesions of the nucleus accumbens septi and corpus striatum. *Brain Research*. 94: 507–522.

Kindermann, S.S. and Brown, G.G. 1997. Depression and memory in the elderly: A meta-analysis. *Journal of Clinical and Experimental Neuropsychology*. 19: 625–642.

King, D.A. and Caine E.D. 1996. Cognitive impairment and major depression: Beyond the pseudo-dementia syndrome. In *Neuropsychological assessment of neuropsychiatric disorders*, 2nd edn., I. Grant and K.M. Adams, pp. 200–217. New York: Oxford University Press.

King, D.A., Cox, C., Lyness, J.M., Conwell, Y. and Caine, E.D. 1998. Quantitative and qualitative differences in the verbal learning performance of elderly depressives and healthy controls. *Journal of the International Neuropsychological Society*. 4: 115–126.

Klaassen, T., Verhey, F.R.J., Sneijders, G.H.J.M., Rozendaal, N., deVet, H.C.W. and vanPraag, H.M. 1995. Treatment of depression in Parkinson's disease: A meta-analysis. *Journal of Neuropsychiatry and Clinical Neurosciences*. 7: 281–286.

Klatka, L.A., Louis, E.D. and Schiffer, R.B. 1996. Psychiatric features in diffuse Lewy body disease: A clinico-pathologic study using Alzheimer's disease and Parkinson's disease comparison groups. *Neurology*. 47: 1148–1152.

Knesevich, J.W., Martin, R.L., Berg, L. and Danziger, W. 1983. Preliminary report on affective symptoms in the early stages of senile dementia of the Alzheimer type. *American Journal of Psychiatry*. 140: 233–235.

Kopelman, M.D. 1986. Clinical tests of memory. *British Journal of Psychiatry*. 148: 517–525.

Kotler-Cope, S. and Camp, C.J. 1995. Anosognosia in Alzheimer disease. *Alzheimer Disease and Associated Disorders*. 9: 52–56.

Kral, V. 1983. The relationship between senile dementia (Alzheimer type) and depression. *Canadian Journal of Psychiatry*. 28: 304–306.

Kuzis, G., Sabe, L., Tiberti, C., Leiguarda, R. and Starkstein, S.E. 1997. Cognitive functions in major depression and Parkinson disease. *Archives of Neurology*. 54: 982–986.

LaRue, A. 1992. *Aging and neuropsychological assessment*. New York: Plenum.

LaRue, A., D'Elia, L.F., Clark, E.O., Spar, J.E. and Jarvik, L.F. 1986a. Clinical tests of memory in dementia, depression and healthy aging. *Journal of Psychology and Aging*. 1: 69–77.

LaRue, A., Goodman, S. and Spar, J.E. 1992. Risk factors for memory impairment in geriatric depression. *Neuropsychiatry, Neuropsychology and Behavioral Neurology*. 5: 178–184.

LaRue, A., Spar, J. and Hill, C.D. 1986b. Cognitive impairment in late-life depression: Clinical correlates and treatment implications. *Journal of Affective Disorders*. 11: 179–184.

Lauterbach, E.C., Jackson, J.G., Wilson, A.N., Dever, G.E.A. and Kirsh, A.D. 1997. Major depression after left posterior globus pallidus lesions. *Neuropsychiatry, Neuropsychology and Behavioral Neurology*. 10: 9–16.

Lesser, I.M., Boone, K.B., Mehringer, C.M., Wohl, M.A., Miller, B.L. and Berman, N.G. 1996. Cognition and white matter hyperintensities in older depressed patients. *American Journal of Psychiatry*. 153: 1280–1287.

Levin, B.E., Berger, J.R., Didona, T. and Duncan, R. 1992. Cognitive function in asymptomatic HIV–1 infection: The effects of age, education, ethnicity and depression. *Neuropsychology*. 6: 303–313.

Liang, R.A., Lam, R.W. and Ancill, R.J. 1988. ECT in the treatment of mixed depression and dementia. *British Journal of Psychiatry*. 152: 281–284.

Litvan, I., Mega, M.S., Cummings, J.L. and Fairbanks, L. 1996. Neuro-psychiatric aspects of progressive supranuclear palsy. *Neurology*. 47: 1184–1189.

Lopez, O.L., Boller, F., Becker, J.T., Miller, M. and Reynolds, C.F. 1990. Alzheimer's disease and depression: Neuropsychological impairment and progression of the illness. *American Journal of Psychiatry*. 147: 855–860.

Loreck, D.J. and Folstein M.F. 1993. Depression in Alzheimer disease. In *Depression in neurologic disease*, ed. E.S. Starkstein and R.E. Robinson, pp. 50–62. Baltimore: Johns Hopkins University Press.

Loza, N. and Milad, G. 1990. Notes from ancient Egypt. *International Journal of Geriatric Psychiatry*. 5: 403–405.

Lundervold, A.J. and Reinvang, I. 1991. Neuropsychological findings and depressive symptoms in patients with Huntington's disease. *Scandinavian Journal of Psychology*. 32: 275–283.

Mapou, R.L., Law, W.A., Martin, A., Kampen, D., Salazar, A.M. and Rundell, J.R. 1993. Neuro-psychological performance, mood and complaints of cognitive and motor difficulties in individuals infected with the human immunodeficiency virus. *Journal of Neuropsychiatry and Clinical Neurosciences*. 5: 86–93.

Marcopulos, B.A. and Graves, R.E. 1990. Antidepressant effect on memory in depressed older persons. *Journal of Clinical and Experimental Neuro-psychology*. 12: 655–663.

Marder, K., Tang, M.X., Côté, L., Stern, Y. and Mayeux, R. 1995. The frequency and associated risk factors for dementia in patients with Parkinson's disease. *Archives of Neurology*. 52: 695–701.

Markowitz, J.C., Rabkin, J.G. and Perry, S.W. 1994. Treating depression in HIV-positive patients. *AIDS*. 8: 403–412.

Marsh, N.V. and McCall, D.W. 1994. Early neuropsychological change in HIV infection. *Neuropsychology*. 8: 44–48.

Martin, A. 1994. HIV, cognition and the basal ganglia. In *Neuropsychology of HIV infection*, ed. I. Grant and A. Martin, pp. 234–259. New York: Oxford University Press.

Masand, P.S. and Tesar, G.E. 1996. Use of stimulants in the medically ill. *Psychiatric Clinics of North America*. 19: 515–547.

Massman, P.J., Butters, N.M. and Delis, D.C. 1994. Some comparisons of the verbal learning deficits in Alzheimer dementia, Huntington disease and depression. In *Dementia: Presentations, differential diagnosis and nosology*, ed. V.O.B. Emery and T.E. Oxman, pp. 232–248. Baltimore: Johns Hopkins University Press.

Massman, P.J., Delis, D.C., Butters, N., Dupont, R.M. and Gillin, C. 1992. The subcortical dysfunction hypothesis of memory deficits in depression: Neuropsychological validation in a subgroup of patients. *Journal of Clinical and Experimental Neuropsychology*. 14: 687–706.

Mayberg, H.S. 1993. Neuroimaging studies of depression in neurologic disease. In *Depression in neurologic disease*, ed. E.S. Starkstein and R.E. Robinson, pp. 186–216. Baltimore: Johns Hopkins University Press.

Mayberg, H.S. 1994a. Clinical correlates of PET- and SPECT-identified defects in dementia. *Journal of Clinical Psychiatry*. 55 (Suppl.): 12–21.

Mayberg, H.S. 1994b. Frontal lobe dysfunction in secondary depression. *Journal of Neuropsychiatry and Clinical Neurosciences*. 6: 428–442.

Mayberg, H.S., Starkstein, S.E., Peyser, C.E., Brandt, J., Dannals, R.F. and Folstein, S.E. 1992. Paralimbic frontal lobe hypometabolism in depression associated with Huntington's disease. *Neurology*. 42: 1791–1797.

Mayberg, H.S., Starkstein, S.E., Sadzot, B., Preziosi, T., Andrezejewski, P.L., Dannals, R.F., Wagner, Jr, H.N. and Robinson, R.G. 1990. Selective hypometabolism in the inferior frontal lobe in depressed patients with Parkinson's disease. *Annals of Neurology*. 28: 57–64.

Mayeux, R., Stern, Y., Côté, L. and Williams, J.B. 1984. Altered serotonin metabolism in depressed patients with Parkinson's disease. *Neurology*. 34: 642–646.

Mayeux, R., Stern, Y., Sano, M., Williams, J.B. and Côté, L.J. 1988. The relationship of serotonin to depression in Parkinson's disease. *Movement Disorders*. 3: 237–244.

Mayeux, R., Stern, Y., Williams, J.B.W., Côté, L., Frantz, A. and Dyrenfurth, I. 1986. Clinical and biochemical features of depression in Parkinson's disease. *American Journal of Psychiatry*. 143: 756–759.

McArthur, J.C., Hoover, D.R., Bacellar, M.A., Miller, E.N., Cohen, B.A., Becker, J.T., Graham, N.M.H., McArthur, J.H., Selnes, O.A., Jacobson, L.P., Visscher, B.R., Concha, M. and Saah, A. for the Multicenter AIDS Cohort Study. 1993. Dementia in AIDS patients: Incidence and risk factors. *Neurology*. 43: 2245–2252.

McArthur, J.C. and Selnes, O.A. 1997. Human immunodeficiency virus-associated dementia. In *AIDS and the nervous system*, ed. J.R. Berger and R.M. Levy, pp. 527–567. Philadelphia: Lippincott-Raven.

McGlynn, S.M. and Kaszniak, A.W. 1991. When metacognition fails: Impaired awareness of deficit in Alzheimer's disease. *Journal of Cognitive Neuroscience*. 3: 183–189.

McGuire, M.H. and Rabins, P.V. 1994. Mood disorders. In *Textbook of geriatric neuropsychiatry*, ed. C.E. Coffey and J.L. Cummings, pp. 243–260. Washington, DC: American Psychiatric Press.

McKeith, I.G., Perry, R.H., Fairbairn, A.F., Jabeen, S. and Perry, E.K. 1992. Operational criteria for senile dementia of the Lewy body type. *Psychological Medicine*. 22: 911–922.

Miller, E. and Lewis, P. 1977. Recognition memory in elderly patients with depression and dementia: A signal detection analysis. *Journal of Abnormal Psychology*. 86: 84–86.

Minden, S.L. and Schiffer, R.B. 1990. Affective disorders in multiple sclerosis: Review and recommendations for clinical research. *Archives of Neurology*. 47: 98–104.

Miyoshi, K., Ueki, A. and Nagano, O. 1996. Management of psychiatric symptoms of Parkinson's disease. *European Neurology*. 36 (Suppl. 1): 49–54.

Mulsant, B.H., Rosen, J., Thornton, J.E. and Zubenko, G.S. 1991. A prospective naturalistic study of electroconvulsive therapy in late-life depression. *Journal of Geriatric Psychiatry and Neurology*. 4: 3–13.

Mulsant, B.H. and Zubenko, G.S. 1994. Clinical, neuropathologic and neurochemical correlates of depression and psychosis in primary dementia. In *Dementia: Presentations, differential diagnosis and nosology*, ed. V.O.B. Emery and T.E. Oxman, pp. 336–352. Baltimore: Johns Hopkins University Press.

Nasrallah, H.A., Coffman, J.A. and Olson, S.C. 1989. Structural brain imaging findings in affective disorders: An overview. *Journal of Neuropsychiatry and Clinical Neurosciences*. 1: 21–26.

Navia, B.A., Jordan, B.D. and Price, R.W. 1986. The AIDS dementia complex: 1. Clinical features. *Annals of Neurology*. 19: 517–524.

Nussbaum, P.D. 1994. Pseudodementia: A slow death. *Neuropsychology Review*. 4: 71–90.

Nussbaum, P.D., Kaszniak, A.W., Allender, J. and Rapcsak, S. 1995. Depression and cognitive decline in the elderly: A follow-up study. *The Clinical Neuropsychologist*. 9: 101–111.

O'Brien, J.T., Ames, D. and Schwietzer, I. 1996. White matter changes in depression and Alzheimer's disease: A review of magnetic resonance imaging studies. *International Journal of Geriatric Psychiatry*. 11: 681–694.

Oh, J.J., Rummans, T.A., O'Conner, M.K. and Ahlskog, J.E. 1992. Cognitive impairment after ECT in patients with Parkinson's disease and psychiatric illness (letter). *American Journal of Psychiatry*. 149: 271.

Pace, P.L., Rosenberger, P., Nasrallah, H.A. and Bornstein, R.A. 1993. Depression and neuropsychological performance in symptomatic HIV infection (abstract). *Journal of Clinical and Experimental Neuropsychology*. 15: 95.

Pearlson, G.D., Rabins, P.V., Kim, W.S., Speedie, L.J., Moberg, P.J., Burns, A. and Bascom, M.J. 1989. Structural brain CT changes and cognitive deficits in elderly depressives with and without reversible dementia ('pseudodementia'). *Psychological Medicine*. 19: 573–584.

Pearlson, G.D., Ross, C.A., Lohr, W.D., Rovner, B.W., Chase, G.A. and Folstein, M.F. 1990. Association between family history of affective disorder and the depressive syndrome of Alzheimer's disease. *American Journal of Psychiatry*. 147: 452–456.

Peavy, G., Jacobs, D., Salmon, D.P., Butters, N., Delis, D.C., Taylor, M., Massman, P., Stout, J.C., Heindel, W.C., Kirson, D., Atkinson, J.H., Chandler, J.L., Grant, I. and the HNRC Group. 1994. Verbal memory performance of patients with human immunodeficiency virus infection: Evidence of subcortical dysfunction. *Journal of Clinical and Experimental Neuropsychology*. 16: 508–523.

Perkins, D.O., Stern, R.A., Golden, R.N., Murphy, C., Naftolowitz, D. and Evans, D.L. 1994. Mood disorders in HIV infection: Prevalence and risk factors in a nonepicenter of the AIDS epidemic. *American Journal of Psychiatry*. 151: 233–236.

Perry, S., Jacobsberg, L.B., Fishman, B., Frances, A., Bobo, J. and Jacobsberg, B.K. 1990. Psychiatric diagnoses before serological testing for the human immunodeficiency virus. *American Journal of Psychiatry*. 147: 89–93.

Perry, S.W. 1994. HIV-related depression. *Research Publications – Association for Research in Nervous and Mental Disease*. 72: 223–238.

Perry, S.W. and Tross, S. 1984. Psychiatric problems of AIDS inpatients at the New York Hospital: Preliminary report. *Public Health Reports*. 99: 200–205.

Petracca, G., Tesón, A., Chemerinski, E., Leiguarda, R. and Starkstein, S.E. 1996. A double-blind placebo-controlled study of clomipramine in depressed patients with Alzheimer's disease. *Journal of Neuropsychiatry and Clinical Neurosciences*. 8: 270–275.

Peyser, C.E. and Folstein, S.E. 1993. Depression in Huntington disease. In *Depression in neurologic disease*, ed. E.S. Starkstein and R.G. Robinson, pp. 117–138. Baltimore: Johns Hopkins University Press.

Pillon, B. and Dubois, B. 1992. Cognitive and behavioral impairments. In *Progressive supranuclear palsy: Clinical and research approaches*, ed. I. Litvan and Y. Agid, pp. 223–239. Oxford: Oxford University Press.

Poutiainen, E. and Elovaara, I. 1996. Subjective complaints of cognitive symptoms are related to psychometric findings of memory deficits in patients with HIV–1 infection. *Journal of the International Neuropsychological Society*. 2: 219–225.

Price, T.R. and McAllister, T.W. 1989. Safety and efficacy of ECT in depressed patients with dementia: A review of clinical experience. *Convulsive Therapy*. 5: 61–74.

Rao, S.M., Hammeke, T.A., McQuillen, M.P., Khatri, B.O. and Lloyd, D. 1984. Memory disturbance in chronic progressive multiple sclerosis. *Archives of Neurology*. 41: 625–631.

Rao, S.M., Huber, S.J. and Bornstein, R.A. 1992. Emotional changes with multiple sclerosis and Parkinson's disease. *Journal of Consulting and Clinical Psychology*. 60: 369–378.

Rao, S.M., Leo, G.L., Bernardin, L. and Unverzagt, F. 1991. Cognitive dysfunction in multiple sclerosis. I. Frequency, patterns and prediction. *Neurology*. 41: 685–691.

Rao, S.M., Leo, G.H., Haughton, V.M., St. Aubin-Faubert, P. and Bernardin, L. 1989. Correlation of magnetic resonance imaging with neuropsychological testing in multiple sclerosis. *Neurology*. 39: 161–166.

Reifler, B.V., Larson, E., Teri, L. and Poulsen, M. 1986. Dementia of the Alzheimer's type and depression. *Journal of the American Geriatrics Society*. 34: 855–859.

Reynolds, C.F., Perel, M.M., Kupfer, D.J., Zimmer, B., Stack, J.A. and Hoch, C.C. 1987. Open-trial response to antidepressant treatment in elderly patients with mixed depression and cognitive impairment. *Psychiatry Research*. 21: 111–122.

Ring, H.A., Bench, C.J., Trimble, M.R., Brooks, D.J., Frackowiak, R.S.J. and Dolan, R.J. 1994. Depression in Parkinson's disease: A positron emission study. *British Journal of Psychiatry*. 165: 333–339.

Robins, L.N., Helzer, J.E., Weissman, M.M., Orvaschel, H., Gruenberg, E., Burke, J.D. and Regier, D.A. 1984. Lifetime prevalence of specific psychiatric disorders in three sites. *Archives of General Psychiatry*. 41: 949–958.

Rodgers, D., Khoo, K., MacEachen, M., Oven, M. and Beatty, W.W. 1996. Cognitive therapy for multiple sclerosis: A preliminary study. *Alternative Therapies in Health and Medicine*. 2: 70–74.

Ron, M.A. and Logsdail, S.J. 1989. Psychiatric morbidity in multiple sclerosis: A clinical and MRI study. *Psychological Medicine*. 19: 887–895.

Rovner, B.W., Broadhead, J., Spencer, M., Carson, K. and Folstein, M.F. 1989. Depression and Alzheimer's disease. *American Journal of Psychiatry*. 146: 350–353.

Rubin, E.H., Kinscherf, D.A., Grant, E.A. and Storandt, M. 1991. The influence of major depression on clinical and psychometric assessment of senile dementia of the Alzheimer type. *American Journal of Psychiatry*. 148: 1164–1171.

Sadovnick, A.D., Remick, R.A., Allen, J., Swartz, E., Yee, M.L., Eisen, K., Farquhar, R., Hashimoto, S.A., Hooge, J., Kastrukoff, L.F., Morrison, W., Nelson, J., Oger, J. and Paty, D.W. 1996. Depression and multiple sclerosis. *Neurology*. 46: 628–632.

Salloway, S. and Cummings, J. 1994. Subcortical disease and neuro-psychiatric illness. *Journal of Neuropsychiatry and Clinical Neurosciences*. 6: 93–99.

Salloway, S., Malloy, P., Kohn, R., Gillard, E., Duffy, J., Rogg, J., Tung, G., Richardson, E., Thomas, C. and Westlake, R. 1996. MRI and neuro-psychological differences in early- and late-life-onset geriatric depression. *Neurology*. 46: 1567–1574.

Sano, M., Stern, Y., Williams, J. Côté, L., Rosenstein, R. and Mayeux, R. 1989. Coexisting dementia and depression in Parkinson's disease. *Archives of Neurology*. 46:1284–1286.

Schaerf, F.W., Miller, R.R., Lipsey, J.R. and McPherson, R.W. 1989. ECT for major depression in four patients infected with human immuno-deficiency virus. *American Journal of Psychiatry*. 146: 782–784.

Schiffer, R.B. and Caine, E.D. 1991. The interaction between depressive affective disorder and neuro-psychological test performance in multiple sclerosis patients. *Journal of Neuropsychiatry and Clinical Neurosciences*. 3: 28–32.

Schiffer, R.B. and Wineman, N.M. 1990. Antidepressant pharmacotherapy of depression associated with multiple sclerosis. *American Journal of Psychiatry*. 147: 1493–1497.

Scott, T.F., Allen, D., Price, T.R.P., McConnell, H. and Lang, D. 1996. Characterization of major depression symptoms in multiple sclerosis patients. *Journal of Neuropsychiatry and Clinical Neurosciences*. 8: 318–323.

Seltzer, B., Vasterling, J.J., Hale, M.A. and Khurana, R. 1995. Unawareness of memory deficit in Alzheimer's disease: Relation to mood and other disease variables. *Neuropsychiatry, Neuro-psychology and Behavioral Neurology*. 8: 176–181.

Sevush, S. and Leve, N. 1993. Denial of memory deficit in Alzheimer's disease. *American Journal of Psychiatry*. 150: 748–751.

Shoulson, I. 1990. Huntington's disease: cognitive and psychiatric features. *Neuropsychiatry, Neuropsychology and Behavioral Neurology*. 3: 15–22.

Silvestre D., Linard, F., Desi, M., Seibel, N., Korezlioglu, J., Pequart, C. and Saimot, A.G. 1995. Statut anxio-depressif et deficit cognitif au cours de l'infection par le VIH. *Encephale*. 21: 285–288.

Squire, L.R. 1986. Memory functions as affected by electroconvulsive therapy. *Annals of the New York Academy of Sciences*. 462: 307–314.

Starkstein, S.E., Bolduc, P.L., Mayberg, H.S., Preziosi, T.J. and Robinson, R.G. 1990a. Cognitive impairments and depression in Parkinson's disease: A follow-up study. *Journal of Neurology, Neurosurgery and Psychiatry*. 53: 597–602.

Starkstein, S.E., Bolduc, P.L., Preziosi, T.J. and Robinson, R.G. 1989a. Cognitive impairments in different stages of Parkinson's disease. *Journal of Neuropsychiatry and Clinical Neurosciences*. 1: 243–248.

Starkstein, S.E., Folstein, S.E., Brandt, J., Pearlson, G.D., McDonnell, A. and Folstein, M. 1989b. Brain atrophy in Huntington's disease. *Neuroradiology*. 31: 156–159.

Starkstein, S.E., Mayberg, H.S., Leiguarda, R., Preziosi, T.J. and Robinson, R.G. 1992. A prospective longitudinal study of depression, cognitive decline and physical impairments in patients with Parkinson's disease. *Journal of Neurology, Neurosurgery and Psychiatry*. 55: 377–382.

Starkstein, S.E., Preziosi, T.J., Berthier, M.L., Bolduc, P.L., Mayberg, H.S. and Robinson, R.G. 1989d. Depression and cognitive impairments in Parkin-son's disease. *Brain*. 112: 1141–1153.

Starkstein, S.E., Preziosi, T.J., Bolduc, P.L. and Robinson, R.G. 1990b. Depression in Parkinson's disease. *Journal of Nervous and Mental Disease*. 178: 27–31.

Starkstein, S.E., Rabins, P.V., Berthier, M.L., Cohen, B.J., Folstein, M.F. and Robinson, R.G. 1989c. Dementia of depression among patients with neurological disorders and functional depression. *Journal of Neuropsychiatry and Clinical Neurosciences*. 1: 263–268.

Starkstein, S.E. and Robinson, R.G. 1996. Mood disorders in neurodegenerative diseases. *Seminars in Clinical Neuropsychiatry*. 1: 272–281.

Starkstein, S.E., Robinson, R.G., Berthier, M.L., Parikh, R.M. and Price, T.R. 1988. Differential mood changes following basal ganglia vs thalamic lesions. *Archives of Neurology*. 45: 725–730.

Starkstein, S.E., Vázquez, S., Migliorelli, R., Tesón, A., Petracca, G. and Leiguarda, R. 1995. A SPECT study of depression in Alzheimer's disease. *Neuropsychiatry, Neuropsychology and Behavioral Neurology*. 8: 38–43.

Stern, Y., Marder, K., Tang, M.S. and Mayeux, R. 1993. Antecedent clinical features associated with dementia in Parkinson's disease. *Neurology*. 43: 1690–1692.

Storch, D.D. 1991. Caution with use of tricyclics in patients with AIDS. *American Journal of Psychiatry*. 148: 1750.

Stoudemire, A., Hill, C., Gulley, L.R. and Morris, R. 1989. Neuropsychological and biomedical assessment of depression-dementia syndromes. *Journal of Neuropsychiatry and Clinical Neurosciences*. 1: 347–361.

Stoudemire, A., Hill, C.D., Morris, R. and Dalton, S.T. 1995. Improvement in depression-related cognitive dysfunction following ECT. *Journal of Neuropsychiatry and Clinical Neurosciences*. 7: 31–34.

Stoudemire, A., Hill, C.D., Morris, R., Martino-Saltzman, D. and Lewison, B. 1993. Long-term affective and cognitive outcome in depressed older adults. *American Journal of Psychiatry*. 150: 896–900.

Stoudemire, A., Hill, C.D., Morris, R., Martino-Saltzman, D., Markwalter, H. and Lewison, B. 1991. Cognitive outcome following tricyclic and electroconvulsive treatment of major depression in the elderly. *American Journal of Psychiatry*. 148: 1336–1340.

Sultzer, D.L., Mahler, M.E., Mandelkern, M.A., Cummings, J.L., VanGorp, W.G., Hinkin, C.H. and Berisford, M.A. 1995. The relationship between psychiatric symptoms and regional cortical metabolism in Alzheimer's disease. *Journal of Neuropsychiatry and Clinical Neurosciences*. 7: 476–484.

Surridge, D. 1969. An investigation into some psychiatric aspects of multiple sclerosis. *British Journal of Psychiatry*. 115: 749–764.

Tandberg, E., Larsen, J.P., Aarsland, D. and Cummings, J.L. 1996. The occurrence of depression in Parkinson's disease: A community-based study. *Archives of Neurology*. 53: 175–179.

Taylor, A.E. and Saint-Cyr, J.A. 1995. The neuropsychology of Parkinson's disease. *Brain and Cognition*. 28: 281–296.

Taylor, A.E., Saint-Cyr, J.A. and Lang, A.E. 1986a. Frontal lobe dysfunction in Parkinson's disease: The cortical focus of the neostriatal outflow. *Brain*. 109: 845–883.

Taylor, A.E., Saint-Cyr, J.A. and Lang A.E. 1988. Idiopathic Parkinson's disease: Revised concepts of cognitive and affective status. *Canadian Journal of Neurological Sciences*. 15: 106–113.

Taylor, A.E., Saint-Cyr, J.A., Lang, A.E. and Kenny, F.T. 1986b. Parkinson's disease and depression: A critical re-evaluation. *Brain*. 109: 279–292.

Teri, L. and Wagner, A. 1992. Alzheimer's disease and depression. *Journal of Consulting and Clinical Psychology*. 60: 379–391.

Teri, L., Reifler, B.V., Veith, R.C., Barnes, R., White, E., McLean, P. and Raskind, M. 1991. Imipramine in the treatment of depressed Alzheimer's patients: Impact on cognition. *Journal of Gerontology*. 46: P372-P377.

Torack, R.M. and Morris, J.C. 1988. The association of ventral tegmental area histopathology with adult dementia. *Archives of Neurology*. 45: 211–218.

Tröster, A.I. In press. Assessment of movement and demyelinating disorders. In *Clinical neuropsychology: A pocket handbook for assessment*, ed. P.J. Snyder and P.D. Nussbaum. Washington, DC: American Psychological Association.

Tröster, A.I. and Fields, J.A. 1995. Frontal cognitive function and memory in Parkinson's disease: Toward a distinction between prospective and declarative memory impairments? *Behavioural Neurology*. 8: 59–74.

Tröster, A.I., Butters, N., Salmon, D.P., Cullum, C.M., Jacobs, D., Brandt, J. and White, R.F. 1993. The diagnostic utility of savings scores: Differentiating Alzheimer's and Huntington's diseases with the Logical Memory and Visual Reproduction tests. *Journal of Clinical and Experimental Neuropsychology*. 15: 773–788.

Tröster, A.I., Paolo, A.M., Lyons, K.E., Glatt, S.L., Hubble, J.P. and Koller, W.C. 1995a. The influence of depression on cognition in Parkinson's disease: A pattern of impairment distinguishable from Alzheimer's disease. *Neurology*. 45: 672–676.

Tröster, A.I., Stalp L.D., Paolo, A.M., Fields, J.A. and Koller, W.C. 1995b. Neuropsychological impairment in Parkinson's disease with and without depression. *Archives of Neurology*. 52: 1164–1169.

VanGorp, W.G., Satz, P., Hinkin, C., Selnes, O., Miller, E.N., McArthur, J., Cohen, B., Paz, D. and the Multicenter AIDS Cohort Study. 1991. Meta-cognition in HIV–1 seropositive asymptomatic individuals: Self-ratings versus objective neuropsychological performance. *Journal of Clinical and Experimental Neuropsychology*. 13: 812–819.

VonSattel, J.P., Ferrante, R.J., Stevens, T.J. and Richardson, E.P. 1985. Neuropathologic classification of Huntington's disease. *Journal of Neuropathology and Experimental Neurology*. 44: 559–577.

Watts, F.N. 1995. Depression and anxiety. In *Handbook of memory disorders*, ed. A.D. Baddeley, B.A. Wilson and F.N. Watts, pp. 293–317. Chichester: John Wiley.

Weiner, M.F., Risser, R.C., Cullum, C.M., Honig, L., White, C., Speciale, S. and Rosenberg, R.N. 1996. Alzheimer's disease and its Lewy body variant: A clinical analysis of postmortem verified cases. *American Journal of Psychiatry*. 153: 1269–1273.

Weingartner, H., Cohen, R.M., Murphy, D.L., Martello, J. and Gerdt, C. 1981. Cognitive processes in depression. *Archives of General Psychiatry*. 38: 42–47.

Wertman, E., Speedie, L., Shemesh, Z., Gilon, D., Raphael, M. and Stessman, J. 1993. Cognitive disturbances in Parkinsonian patients with depression. *Neuropsychiatry, Neuropsychology and Behavioral Neurology*. 6: 31–37.

Wiley, C.A. 1994. Pathology of neuro-logic disease in AIDS. *Psychiatric Clinics of North America*. 17: 1–15.

Wilkins, J.W., Robertson, K.R., Snyder, C.R., Robertson, W.K., van der Horst, C. and Hall, C.D. 1991. Implications of self-reported cognitive and motor dysfunction in HIV-positive patients. *American Journal of Psychiatry*. 148: 641–643.

Williams, J.B.W., Rabkin, J.G., Remien, R.H., Gorman, J.M. and Ehrhardt, A.A. 1991. Multidisciplinary baseline assessment of homosexual men with and without human immunodeficiency virus infection. *Archives of General Psychiatry*. 48: 124–130.

Williams, J.M., Little, M.M., Scates, S. and Blockman, N. 1987. Memory complaints and abilities among depressed older adults. *Journal of Consulting and Clinical Psychology*. 55: 595–598.

Working Group of the American Academy of Neurology AIDS Task Force 1991. Nomenclature and research case definitions for neuro-logical manifestations of human immunodeficiency virus type–1 (HIV–1) infection. *Neurology*. 41: 778–785.

Zubenko, G.S., Moossy, J. and Kopp, Y. 1990. Neurochemical correlates of major depression in primary dementia. *Archives of Neurology*. 47: 209–214.

Zweig, R.M., Ross, C.A., Hedreen, J.C., Peyser, C., Cardillo, J.E., Folstein, S.E. and Price D.L. 1992. Locus coeruleus involvement in Huntington's disease. *Archives of Neurology*. 49: 152–156.

Zweig, R.M., Ross, C.A., Hedreen, J.C., Steele, C., Cardillo, J.E., Whitehouse, P.J., Folstein, M.F. and Price, D.L. 1988. The neuropathology of the aminergic nuclei in Alzheimer's disease. *Annals of Neurology*. 24: 233–242.

20 Preserved cognitive skills in neurodegenerative disease

JONI R. GRABER, ROBERT H. PAUL,
JULIE A. TESTA, DAVID C. BOWLBY,
MICHAEL J. HARNISH
AND WILLIAM W. BEATTY

INTRODUCTION

Progressive dementing diseases, regardless of their etiology, are associated with a relentless loss of cognitive capability in many domains, which in turn is associated with demonstrable and varied neuropathological changes, most of which are irreversible. From this perspective, it is not surprising that extensive research effort has been devoted to the careful description of the various cognitive and neuropathological changes that occur in both Alzheimer's disease and in vascular dementia. Because the changes that occur in the brain with these diseases are cumulative and eventually result in marked tissue loss, current conceptions about the nature of cognitive deficits have implicitly or explicitly assumed that these deficits arise because the necessary information to perform the cognitive functions is simply 'gone', on account of the neural substrate being either absent or hopelessly 'scrambled'.

Against this background, demonstrations that some demented patients retain the ability to perform some complicated activities quite well even though they apparently can no longer perform simpler functions competently pose fascinating theoretical questions, which in turn may have important practical implications. In this chapter we review the literature on preserved cognitive skills in dementia. As a prelude, it is desirable to consider what is known about the status of everyday cognitive skills in normal aging and in amnesia. Finally, the literature on savants is also reviewed briefly because savants, like some demented elderly patients, also exhibit exceptional cognitive abilities against a background of globally impaired intellectual functioning.

NORMAL AGING

Age-related declines in performance have been carefully documented on tests of sensory acuity, psychomotor speed, recent memory, attention, visuospatial and visuoperceptual abilities and forming novel concepts (Flicker et al. 1986; Salthouse 1989, 1990).

Most work on problem solving has used problems that are unfamiliar to the solver in order to eliminate possibly confounding effects of prior experience. On such tasks, older people consistently perform poorly (Arenberg 1968; Heaton et al. 1986). Differences in memory capacity, education and the use of inefficient search strategies may all contribute to the poor performance by the elderly (Charness 1985).

In contrast to the usual pattern of age-related deficits, little or no influence of age has been found in the solution of anagrams (Hayslip and Sterns 1979). This is probably so because vocabulary, knowledge of letter sequence frequencies and fluency for generating words to letter cues, the components of language necessary for anagram solution, are relatively stable with age (Eysenck 1975; Gardner and Monge 1977; Albert 1988). Familiarity with the task may also contribute to relatively normal performance by older persons on anagram problems. Anagrams and other word puzzles are found in most daily newspapers; other work indicates that age-related differences in problem-solving are minimized when subjects have experience with and some prior skill at the task (Charness 1981a; Salthouse 1989).

Games such as chess and bridge offer an interesting arena for studying problem-solving that approximates the demands of everyday life (Anders Ericsson and Charness

1994). Both games require the player to have acquired an extensive set of rules and strategies and to apply these rules and strategies appropriately to the current novel game situation.

Cross-sectional studies of competitive chess players indicate that playing skill increases rapidly up to age 35 years and slowly declines; by age 75 years average performance is slightly less than one standard deviation lower than at age 35 years. To study the effects of age and skill on measures of the cognitive components of chess skill, Charness (1981a, 1981b) selected players so that age and skill were uncorrelated. Skill, but not age, affected the selection of best moves and accuracy in evaluating endgame positions. By contrast, older players were less accurate than younger players in recalling meaningful game configurations of chess pieces, although they did recall more of these meaningful configurations than did young chess-naive subjects (Charness 1981c).

Similar approaches have been used to study the influence of age and skill on components of skill at bridge. Skill, but not age, influenced the accuracy with which players produced an opening bid and summed the number of honor points in a predealt hand. Older players did, however, bid more slowly (Charness 1983). Age also influenced recall of previously presented bridge hands. Older players recalled less than comparably skilled younger players. Skill also affected memory; highly skilled players recalled more information than less skilled players and skill attenuated the age-related memory loss (Charness 1979). In a task designed to measure skill at playing the hand, the more highly skilled players produced more elaborate and diverse plans for play and were more likely to perceive the critical problem in making the bid (Charness 1989).

In general, the findings for skilled chess and bridge players are quite similar. Greater knowledge of the games seems to permit skilled players to recognize critical patterns in board positions (chess) and card distribution (bridge). Recognizing these patterns seems to evoke more sophisticated plans for play of the game which depend on vastly greater stored knowledge of probable outcomes of one line of play against major alternatives. In this way, Charness (1989) suggests that older bridge and chess players are able to compensate for their more limited working memory capacities and maintain high skill at actual play.

The nature of the hypothesized compensation and its limits are poorly understood at present. Most of the 'old' subjects in the studies of bridge and chess were in their fifties and sixties. Little is known about how well skill at complex games is maintained in older individuals whose working memory and other cognitive capabilities can be expected to be more limited. A second consideration is that all of the participants in the reviewed studies were rather highly skilled (sufficiently skilled to have established ratings). Most older chess and bridge players never achieved such a high level of skill, so the applicability of the findings, particularly the extent to which more limited skill can compensate for age-related losses in cognitive efficiency, is not presently known.

AMNESIA

Unfortunately, there is almost no systematic research on preserved cognitive skills in amnesia. There are probably several reasons for this. First, it is widely believed that amnesics can acquire new procedural and implicit memory tasks and retain premorbidly acquired procedural knowledge normally (Cermak 1976; Kolb and Whishaw 1990). If preserved cognitive skills are entirely the result of intact remote procedural memory as some researchers believe, then demonstrating their existence in amnesics is not theoretically interesting. Second, some theorists have argued that semantic memory (knowledge memory) is also intact in amnesia (Cermak 1984). If one accepts this point of view, then the display of any premorbidly acquired cognitive skill by an amnesic is again uninteresting.

The most convincing demonstration of preserved skill learning in amnesia would be if a patient acquired competence at a complex game such as bridge or chess after the onset of amnesia. The closest approximation is the report of Hirst et al. (1988) of an amnesic patient who acquired an unfamiliar foreign language normally despite severe deficits when tested for learning and memory for other verbal materials.

Sacks (1995) described a patient who was diagnosed with amnesia in 1975 following removal of a large midline tumor that destroyed the pituitary gland, the optic chiasm and tracts, much of the diencephalon, parts of the ventral and orbito-frontal regions and portions of the medial temporal lobes. Despite his blindness and other neural and endocrine disturbances, the patient continued to play favorite tunes from the 1960s on his guitar and he retained much factual knowledge about the rock bands of that era. He apparently failed to acquire new information about public events after 1970 and he could not remember that his father had died in 1990. Nevertheless, he acquired new guitar playing skills from a music therapist who worked at the hospital where he lived. He also learned and remembered the lyrics to 'hundreds' of jingles that he heard on television. His improved guitar playing could be attributed to the operation of procedural memory systems that were not damaged by the tumor, but his ability to learn jingles requires the ability to encode, store and retrieve factual information that is not usually considered to be procedural memory. This spared ability is especially surprising because the basal forebrain, medial diencephalon and medial temporal lobes, which are the major components of the explicit memory system, were severely damaged.

Two other amnesic patients appear to have retained certain complex cognitive skills despite losses in procedural and/or semantic memory abilities. M.R.L., who developed amnesia after an hypoxic episode and was subsequently shown to have bilateral hippocampal atrophy, continued to solve crossword puzzles after the onset of his amnesia. No formal assessment of his skill was undertaken and it is not known what, if any, losses of premorbid ability he may have experienced. This case is interesting, however, because M.R.L. showed deficits in learning certain procedural memory tasks (Beatty et al. 1987b) and he also showed temporally graded retrograde amnesia and impaired knowledge of his own profession, an aspect of semantic memory (Beatty et al. 1987a).

Wilson et al. (1994) described a patient who developed amnesia after a bout of herpes encephalitis. Despite severe anterograde and retrograde amnesia, he was able to conduct a choir competently through several selections from memory. Several other amnesic patients with retained skills are known: an amnesic typist who lost her job, not because of her typing skill, but because she kept typing the same letter over again; an amnesic t-shirt maker who can still run the appropriate machinery; bridge players who cannot remember the bid, but play competently otherwise; and chess players who can still play but may have trouble recalling and planning ahead more than one or two moves (L.S. Cermak, personal communication). Some, but possibly not all, of these examples can be explained as instances of preserved procedural memory.

It is unfortunate that more detailed information about the extent of the skills exhibited by amnesic patients is not available. An explanation of such abilities as preserved procedural memory seems to ignore the amnesics' capacity to modify their abilities in new situations, which involves considerably greater complexity than pursuit rotor tasks or mirror image drawing.

DEMENTIA

Perhaps the first report of a demented patient with a preserved cognitive skill came from Alajouanine (1948), a neurologist who studied the French composer Maurice Ravel. Ravel developed a progressive neurodegenerative disorder of uncertain diagnosis which resulted in a loss of his ability to read, write or play music. His ability to recognize and evaluate musical pieces remained intact and memories of his own compositions were perfect. A second case study from the early literature was reported by Sacks (1985), who described a patient who presented with severe memory loss and visual agnosia, but could nonetheless still recite from memory long passages of literature and continued to teach vocal lessons at a school of music. In both of these cases, neither neuropsychological evaluations nor autopsy results are available, thus making it difficult to determine either the extent of cognitive impairment or the cause of the dementia.

Since 1984, when the NINCDS-ADRDA criteria (McKhann et al. 1984) for the diagnosis of probable Alzheimer's disease (AD) were proposed, there have been several other case reports of preserved cognitive skills in demented patients for which comprehensive neuropsychological and medical examinations were conducted.

In 1987, Cummings and Zarit studied an artist with probable AD who, early in the course of his disease, continued to paint with great skill despite exhibiting significant cognitive deficits. Nevertheless, as his disease progressed the quality of his paintings declined, corresponding closely with his worsening visuospatial capacity. Two other case studies (Beatty et al. 1988; Crystal et al. 1989) involved AD patients who were skilled musicians prior to disease onset. One patient (Crystal et al. 1989) had 12 years of formal musical training and had worked as a musical editor for 40 years, while the other (Beatty et al. 1988) had a Master's degree in music with emphasis in piano. In both cases, the patients could play, from memory, various songs but were unable to either recall or recognize the titles or composers of these songs. The patient studied by Beatty et al. (1988)

could not learn the pursuit rotor task, a measure of skill learning, but Crystal et al.'s (1989) patient learned to read mirror reversed text normally. The patient studied by Beatty et al. (1988) was able to transfer her piano skills to an unfamiliar instrument, the xylophone, without practice.

More recently, Polk and Kertesz (1993) studied musical skill in two musicians, a male guitarist and a female pianist, both of whom presented with a progressive neurodegenerative disease described as possible AD. The guitarist was aphasic and amusic and magnetic resonance (MR) images showed enlarged ventricles and cortical atrophy with greater left hemisphere involvement. While he could still play the guitar well, he could no longer read music notation, replicate rhythm patterns or write or copy music. An MRI scan of the female pianist showed parieto–occipital atrophy with greater right hemisphere involvement. While she had lost the ability to play piano, she was not aphasic and could replicate rhythmic patterns presented to her.

The case studies recounted above all concern patients with progressive dementia (most often AD) who exhibited preserved skills pertaining to artistic or musical endeavors. The first research done with patients exhibiting a broad range of preserved skills was conducted by Beatty et al. (1994), with five patients who met NINCDS-ADRDA criteria for probable AD. The preserved skills for these five patients included contract bridge, canasta, dominoes, jigsaw puzzles and playing trombone. The patients were given standard neuropsychological tests as well as individualized tests on their preserved skill. Despite deficits in recent memory and other cognitive domains that were severe enough to interfere with daily functioning, all five patients were competitive with normal adult controls at their chosen skill. Three of these case studies are described in more detail below.

Patient B was an 80-year-old man with a Mini-Mental State Examination (MMSE; Folstein et al. 1975) score of 10, who continued to play contract bridge. His ability to play competitively was confirmed by one of the authors, who engaged in several games with him and two other normal control players. After compiling the scores from the series of matches, patient B ranked third of the four players. Of interest is the fact that upon later questioning, the patient was unable to answer elementary questions about how to bid a hand, how to play a hand and the basic rules of bridge; for example, he could not name the four suits or rank them when given the names.

A second patient, patient T, was a man with probable AD who continued to play trombone in a Dixieland jazz band without sheet music or other memory aids despite impaired intelligence, naming, visuospatial function and memory demonstrated by extensive neuropsychological testing. His ability to play trombone was only slightly affected by his dementia; this conclusion was confirmed by both a professional jazz musician and nonprofessional musician raters who were asked to compare a premorbid recording (made approximately 25 years before the onset of dementia) and a recording made after the diagnosis of dementia. Although the professional musician detected subtle differences in the patient's trombone play, these were not evident to the nonmusician raters. This patient was able to learn the pursuit rotor task normally, but suffered a form a dressing apraxia in that he could not tie his necktie or his shoes and had difficulty putting on his jacket.

A third patient, J.S., was a retired engineer who at the time of study was in a nursing home where he regularly solved adult jigsaw puzzles. He refused to complete neuropsychological testing, but he did complete the Object Assembly puzzles from the Wechsler Adult Intelligence Scale-Revised (Wechsler 1981). Comparison of his scores on this measure from original testing when he was evaluated for dementia and from retest 4 years later showed that his performance remained stable even though other cognitive functions deteriorated significantly during this time. Only on the most difficult puzzles was there evidence of deterioration. Most remarkably, J.S. did not engage in jigsaw puzzle solving until after he developed dementia.

The above discussion indicates that a wide range of complex cognitive skills may be preserved in demented patients, long after performances of seemingly simpler abilities have significantly deteriorated. A central question that remains to be answered is what underlying mechanisms might be responsible for the preservation of these skills. Two possible contributing factors might be the general level of the premorbid functioning possessed by such patients and the severity of dementia. The majority of published cases of dementia patients with preserved skills had college degrees. Dementia appears to be more prevalent in persons with lower levels of education (Berkman 1986) and it has been suggested that the retention of certain cognitive skills might be due in part to a greater 'reserve capacity' in the brains of more highly educated people (Beatty et al. 1994; Chapter 14).

Recent cases from our studies demonstrate clearly that dementia patients with very little formal education may retain their ability at complex games. One patient, an 80-year-old woman with a third grade education and an MMSE of 19 remained a skillful domino player. A second patient, an 88-year-old man with a fourth grade education and an MMSE of 11, won 14 of 16 checkers games against three opponents (two PhDs and a neuropsychology graduate student), who collectively had more than 58 years of formal education. In addition to emphasizing the point that education is no substitute for skill, these observations indicate that the preservation of certain cognitive skills may be a general phenomenon in dementia which is certainly not limited to patients presumed to have had high premorbid ability.

Regarding severity of dementia, the majority of patients demonstrating a preserved skill have been mildly to moderately demented, but we have observed preserved skill at playing dominoes in a patient with an MMSE score of eight. The only two severely demented patients studied longitudinally (Cummings and Zarit 1987; Crystal et al. 1989), showed a loss of skill that closely corresponded to their loss of other cognitive functions. Level of premorbid functioning and severity of dementia may play some role in preserved skill, but they are not absolute determinants.

The most popular theoretical explanation for preserved skills in demented patients is that these behaviors are simply remote procedural memory. Several researchers (Crystal et al. 1989; Polk and Kertesz 1993) have embraced this theory and attributed their patients' skilled behaviors to a form of procedural memory, part of which is presumably stored in regions of the brain spared until the later stages of the dementing process. Of the preserved cognitive skills that have been described thus far, almost all of them are activities that the patients had engaged in throughout their adult lives (Cummings and Zarit 1987; Beatty et al. 1988; Crystal et al. 1989) and as a result are highly-practiced and well-learned. Research with normal elderly subjects has demonstrated that well-learned abilities such as vocabulary and solving familiar problems are resistant to age-related decline (Albert 1988; Gardner and Monge 1977). As described earlier, performance on complex games such as chess and bridge is relatively resistant to age-associated deficits. Furthermore, a majority of even moderately demented AD patients demonstrate normal acquisition of tasks that require certain perceptuomotor skills, such as mirror reading and pursuit rotor tracking

(Eslinger and Damasio 1986; Dick 1992). In effect, the argument is that because demented patients can acquire some new motor skills normally, their remote procedural or implicit memories must also be intact. There are no standard tests of remote procedural memory, but measures of praxis assess some aspects of these memories.

From this perspective it should be noted that the skills that are preserved in dementia patients are at least as complex if not more complex than skills that the same patients have lost. For example, the female pianist studied by Beatty et al. (1988) was apraxic, required verbal prompts to dress herself and was sometimes incontinent. The demented trombonist (Beatty et al. 1994) was also apraxic, being unable to tie his necktie or shoes and oftentimes unable to put on his jacket. Nevertheless, both of these patients demonstrated considerable ability when playing their respective instruments. Furthermore, if their abilities were due only to remote procedural memory, it is doubtful that the trombonist could coordinate his improvised solos with the band as well as play background for other solos, or that the female pianist could transfer her playing to the xylophone, which she did immediately. This degree of flexibility is not typical of implicit memory systems, which are characterized by performance losses if the testing conditions are changed between original learning and retention testing (Graf and Gallie 1992). Remote procedural memory also cannot easily account for the ability to play bridge, dominoes and other games that differ each time they are played, requiring the application of knowledge to novel situations.

A second theory proposed to account for preserved cognitive skills in dementia posits that these patients exhibit a relative sparing of right hemisphere function (Polk and Kertesz 1993); it applies primarily to patients who demonstrate preserved musical abilities. The theory behind this hypothesis is based on numerous research studies (Botez and Wertheim 1959; Gordon and Bogen 1974) demonstrating that right hemisphere lesions disrupt artistic skills such as painting and musical ability to a significant degree while leaving language relatively unaffected. Conversely, patients with comparable lesions of the left hemisphere show significant deficits in language, but frequently show either a partial or a complete sparing of artistic abilities (Alajouanine 1948; Smith 1966; Basso and Capitani 1985). Furthermore, studies on cerebral metabolism of glucose in subgroups of AD patients have demonstrated asymmetrical patterns of metabolism correlating significantly with

Table 20.1. *Mean performances of controls and dementia patients of differing musical skill*

| | Controls | Dementia patients | | |
		Musically Skilled	Never Skilled	Formerly Skilled
N	32	12	12	7
Age	75.1	74.7	78.0	78.6
Education	12.8	14.9	14.3	13.6
MMSE	28.7	18.8	17.3	19.3
BNT/30	26.1	17.0	13.6	11.4
BNT, Z-score	−0.51	−5.27	−7.26	−7.58
BNT, % Det.	−0	−39.3	−50.2	−58.6
BD/69	41.21	−18.25	12.42	7.86
BD, Z-score	−0.04	−2.77	−2.91	−2.94
BD, % Det.	−0	−52.8	−58.0	−81.6

Note:

BD: Block Design; BNT: Boston Naming Test; Det: Deterioration; MMSE: Mini Mental State Examination.

asymmetry of neuropsychological performance (Haxby et al. 1985). Furthermore, it has been shown that the patterns of performance by AD patients on the Boston Naming Test (BNT; Kaplan et al. 1983), a test that mainly taps left hemisphere functions and the WISC-R Block Design (Wechsler 1974), a test that mainly taps right hemisphere functions, can be used to predict performance on tests of attention that favor the left or right hemisphere (Delis et al. 1992).

From this it can be predicted that dementia patients who retained musical skill would show relatively better performance on Block Design than patients of comparable overall dementia severity who were never musically skilled or were once musically skilled, but could no longer display musical skill (i.e. formerly skilled patients). Table 20.1 summarizes performances by musically skilled, formerly skilled and never (musically) skilled dementia patients and elderly controls on the MMSE, BNT and WISC-R Block Design tests. Each dementia group contained some individuals presumed to have AD and others thought to have vascular dementia, but there were no differences related to type of dementia so the data were combined. Musical skill was verified by recording performances by patients and controls which were evaluated independently for quality of performance by two raters who were blind to the status of the performers. Preliminary analyses indicate no differences

between controls who were or were not musically skilled so their data were pooled.

There were no significant differences among the four groups in terms of age or education; the three dementia groups were comparable in terms of dementia severity as indexed by the MMSE. With dementia severity equated, there were also no differences among the three dementia groups in terms of degree of impairment on the BNT or the Block Design test. This conclusion applies regardless of whether performance is expressed as raw scores, Z-scores relative to an independent group of age- and education- matched controls or in terms of percentage possible deterioration (which corrects for the fact that variability in performance by elderly controls is four to five times greater on Block Design than on BNT).

Further evidence against the right hemisphere hypothesis comes from MR images taken of patient T, the demented trombonist described by Beatty et al. (1994). These scans revealed bilateral atrophy in the hippocampus and the parietal and temporal cortices, which was greater in the right hemisphere (Figure 20.1). Although based on a single case, the imaging data from patient T solidly refute anatomical sparing of the right hemisphere as a basis for preserved trombone playing in this AD patient.

A third explanation proposed to account for preserved cognitive skills in patients with AD is that these behaviors represent enhanced access to semantic memory. The essence of this theory is that semantic memory is relatively intact but inaccessible in AD, as opposed to the notion that semantic knowledge is irreversibly lost in this disease. Evidence for an actual loss of knowledge in AD includes studies demonstrating that AD patients perform poorly on tests of confrontational naming and word finding and show greater impairment on category fluency than on letter fluency (Butters et al. 1987; Tröster et al. 1989; Martin 1992). According to Martin (1992), these findings suggest a loss of specific information due to an actual degradation of the semantic memory store.

An alternative to the claim of a loss of semantic memory is that the semantic memory store remains relatively intact but inaccessible. Nebes (1989) suggests that semantic memory deficits in AD are the result of impaired access; he believes that demented patients perform poorly on certain cognitive tests due to global deficits in cognitive functions such as decision making and attention, rather than due to a degradation of semantic knowledge.

The strongest evidence for this hypothesis comes from

Figure 20.1. Coronal T1 weighted MR image of the brain of Patient T, who remained a skilled trombonist despite his dementia, which was probably of the Alzheimer type (Beatty et al. 1994). Note that the hippocampi are atrophied and the parietal and temporal sulci and ventricles are enlarged. The temporal lobe atrophy appears greater on the right side of the brain (left side of photograph). Reprinted from Beatty et al. (1995) with permission.

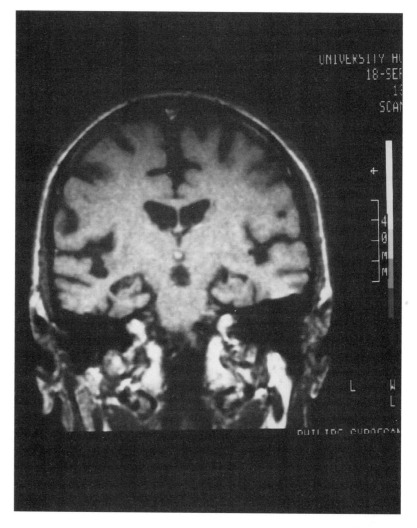

studies of dementia patients who retain skill at playing dominoes. When tested on measures of knowledge of the game that required choosing the best move among several legal moves and verbally explaining the reasons for their choices, 70% of 23 patients we have studied performed within the range of comparably skilled elderly control players. Yet when knowledge of dominoes was probed with questions in the usual format of explicit memory tests, these patients performed no better than students who were unfamiliar with the game. Compared to patients of comparable dementia severity who did not retain any cognitive skill, the skilled domino players had no advantage on conventional semantic memory tests like naming and verbal fluency (Greiner et al. 1997).

SAVANTS

Savants, once called autistic or idiot savants, are described as persons having some degree of mental handicap but possessing one or more outstanding talents (O'Conner and Hermelin 1984). These talents often take the form of unique cognitive abilities that exceed the savants' normal functional level and appear similar to the cognitive skills that are preserved in some demented individuals. Two similarities between savants and demented individuals with preserved cognitive skills can be noted. First, both groups are able to perform a repetitive, highly overlearned skill in a manner that seems outside the range of their usual cognitive level (Lewis 1985). Second, savants are often socially withdrawn and have difficulty relating to others emotionally; demented patients may also have difficulty interacting with people.

A brief review of the savant syndrome may be helpful because of these apparent similarities. Among mentally retarded individuals, the savant syndrome is more prevalent in autistic than among nonautistic individuals. Rimland and Hill (1984) reported that 9.8% of 5400 autistic individuals were found to have savant abilities; conversely, only 0.06% of a nonautistic handicapped population was found to have savant abilities (Hill 1977). Sacks (1995) reported similar conclusions. A report by Rimland and Hill (1984) on the abilities seen in autistic savants found that among 119 savants, 53% had musical abilities, 40% had memory skills, 9% were artistic, 6% were described as 'pseudoverbal' (e.g. reading aloud), 14% had mathematical abilities, 12% had special abilities in either mechanical realms, coordination, directions or calendar calculations and 3% were claimed to have some form of extrasensory perception.

As with savants, musical abilities are retained by some dementia patients, but no patient has yet been shown to be capable of learning to perform a musical composition that was known to be unfamiliar premorbidly. The first account of an AD patient with a preserved skill was a graphic artist (Cummings and Zarit 1987), but he did not exhibit unusual visuospatial abilities. Finally, we know of no dementia patients with exceptional mathematical abilities including calendar calculations. Although reading without comprehension does persist in dementia (Bayles and Kaszniak 1987), exceptional anterograde memory abilities similar to those described for some savants are obviously not seen in dementia.

In summary, the similarities between preserved cognitive skills in dementia and the exceptional abilities shown by some autistic savants, at present, seem more superficial than fundamental. In addition to the differences noted above, preserved cognitive skills in demented patients survive in persons with once normal brains, while savants acquire their exceptional abilities with brains that were abnormal, perhaps from the beginning of neural differentiation. Although this point is certainly valid, the implications are not absolutely clear. We have now encountered three dementia patients, who as best can be told from interviewing family members, acquired or at least substantially enhanced their 'preserved' skill after they developed dementia. These limited observations suggest that the plasticity of the demented brain may be greater than has been assumed.

IMPLICATIONS OF PRESERVED SKILL IN DEMENTIA

The study of preserved skills in demented patients has important theoretical significance for understanding cognition in dementia and it may suggest interventions that have immediate practical applications. For example, if evidence is found to support the possibility that semantic memory systems that govern 'lost' behaviors are relatively intact but inaccessible, then treatments that foster access to this lost knowledge might be devised. Second, anecdotal evidence indicates that engaging patients in skilled activities may help manage the disruptive behaviors they often exhibit and improve the quality of life for these persons and their carers. These behavioral approaches may serve as substitutes for or adjuncts to the pharmacological therapies typically employed to manage disruptive behaviors.

The study of preserved abilities in dementia patients is obviously in its infancy, but this much is clear. Under appropriate circumstances, patients are able to solve complex problems related to their retained skill (e.g. playing dominoes) and provide precise and correct verbal explanations for their behavior. When the same or simpler knowledge is tested by conventional explicit memory methods, it is unavailable. Such findings do not easily fit within the compartments of implicit, explicit or semantic memory as defined by contemporary cognitive psychology. Perhaps the taxonomy will have to be revised.

Except for some aspects of musical skill, nothing is known about the brain mechanisms subserving the other skilled activities that may be retained in dementia. The complexity of games like bridge and dominoes, which appear to require many different cognitive abilities, suggests that multiple brain systems are probably involved. Perhaps this is a clue to understanding the phenomenon of preserved cognitive skills.

ACKNOWLEDGMENTS

This work was supported by Grant HR 4-087 from the Oklahoma Center for the Advancement of Science and Technology. We thank P. Winn, K. Dean and K. Olson for their assistance.

REFERENCES

Alajouanine, T. 1948. Aphasia and artistic realization. *Brain.* 71: 229–241.

Albert, M.S. 1988. Cognitive function. In *Geriatric neuropsychology*, ed. M.S. Albert and M.B. Moss, pp. 33–56. New York: Guilford Press.

Anders Ericsson, K. and Charness, N. 1994. Expert performance: Its structure and acquisition. *American Psychologist.* 49: 725–747.

Arenberg, D. 1968. Concept problem solving in young and old adults. *Journal of Gerontology.* 23: 279–282.

Basso, A. and Capitani, E. 1985. Spared musical abilities in a conductor with global aphasia and ideomotor apraxia. *Journal of Neurology, Neurosurgery and Psychiatry.* 48: 407–412.

Bayles, K.A. and Kaszniak, A.W. 1987. *Communication and cognition in normal aging and dementia.* Boston: Little, Brown.

Beatty, W.W., Salmon, D.P., Bernstein, N. and Butters, N. 1987b. Remote memory in a patient with amnesia due to hypoxia. *Psychological Medicine.* 17: 657–665.

Beatty, W.W., Salmon, D.P., Bernstein, N., Martone, M., Lyon, L. and Butters, N. 1987a. Procedural learning in a patient with amnesia due to hypoxia. *Brain and Cognition.* 6: 386–402.

Beatty, W.W., Scott, J.G., Wilson, D.A., Prince, J.R. and Williamson, D.J. 1995. Memory deficits in a demented patient with probable corticobasal degneration. *Journal of Geriatric Psychiatry and Neurology.* 8: 132–136.

Beatty, W.W., Winn, P., Adams, R.L., Allen, E.W., Wilson, D.A., Prince, J.R., Olson, K.A., Dean, K. and Littleford, D. 1994. Preserved cognitive skills in dementia of the Alzheimer type. *Archives of Neurology.* 51: 1040–1046.

Beatty, W.W., Zavadil, K.D., Bailly, R.C., Rixen, G.J., Zavadil, L.E., Farnham, N. and Fisher, L. 1988. Preserved musical skill in a severely demented patient. *International Journal of Clinical Neuropsychology.* 10: 158–164.

Berkman, L.F. 1986. The association between educational attainment and mental status examinations: Of etiologic significance for senile dementia or not? *Journal of Chronic Diseases.* 39: 171–174.

Botez, M.I. and Wertheim, N. 1959. Expressive aphasia and amnesia following right frontal lesion in a right-handed man. *Brain.* 82: 186–202.

Butters, N., Granholm, E.L., Salmon, D.P., Grant, I. and Wolfe, J. 1987. Episodic and semantic memory: A comparison of amnesic and demented patients. *Journal of Clinical and Experimental Neuropsychology.* 9: 479–497.

Cermak, L.S. 1976. The encoding capacity of a patient with amnesia due to encephalitis. *Neuropsychologia.* 14: 311–326.

Cermak, L.S. 1984. The episodic-semantic distinction in amnesia. In *Neuropsychology of memory*, ed. L.R. Squire and N. Butters, pp. 55–62. New York: Guilford Press.

Charness, N. 1979. Components of skill in bridge. *Canadian Journal of Psychology.* 33: 1–16.

Charness, N. 1981a. Aging and skilled problem solving. *Journal of Experimental Psychology (General).* 110: 21–38.

Charness, N. 1981b. Search in chess: age and skill differences. *Journal of Experimental Psychology (Human Perception and Performance).* 7: 467–476.

Charness, N. 1981c. Visual short-term memory and aging in chess players. *Journal of Gerontology.* 36: 615–619.

Charness, N. 1983. Age, skill and bridge bidding: a chronometric analysis. *Journal of Verbal Learning and Verbal Behavior.* 22: 406–416.

Charness, N. 1985. Aging and problem-solving performance. In, *Aging and human performance*, ed. N. Charness, pp. 225–259. New York: Wiley.

Charness, N. 1989. Expertise in chess and bridge. In *Complex information processing: The impact of Herbert A. Simon*, ed. D. Klahr and K. Kotovsky, pp. 183–208. Hillsdale, NJ: Erlbaum.

Crystal, H.A., Grober, E. and Masur, D. 1989. Preservation of musical memory in Alzheimer's disease. *Journal of Neurology, Neurosurgery and Psychiatry.* 52: 1415–1416.

Cummings, J.L. and Zarit, J.M. 1987. Probable Alzheimer's disease in an artist. *Journal of the American Medical Association.* 258: 2731–2734.

Delis, D.C., Massman, P.J., Butters, N. Salmon, D.P., Shear, P.K. Demadura, T. and Filoteo, J.V. 1992. Spatial cognition in Alzheimer's disease: Subtypes of global–local impairment. *Journal of Clinical and Experimental Neuropsychology.* 14: 463–477.

Dick, M.B. 1992. Motor and procedural learning in Alzheimer's disease. In *Memory functioning in dementia*, ed. L. Bäckman, pp. 135–150. Amsterdam, Netherlands: Elsevier.

Eslinger, P.J. and Damasio, A.R. 1986. Preserved motor learning in Alzheimer's disease: Implications for anatomy and behavior. *Journal of Neuroscience*. 6: 3006–3009.

Eysenck, M.W. 1975. Retrieval from semantic memory as a function of age. *Journal of Gerontology*. 30: 174–180.

Flicker, C. Ferris, S.H., Crook, T., Bartus, R.T. and Reisberg, B. 1986. Cognitive decline in advanced age: Future directions for the psychometric differentiation of normal and pathological age changes in cognitive function. *Developmental Neuropsychology*. 2: 309–322.

Folstein, M.F., Folstein, S.E. and McHugh, P.R. 1975. 'Mini-Mental State': A practical method of grading the cognitive state of patients for the clinician. *Journal of Psychiatric Research*. 12: 189–198.

Gardner, E.F. and Monge, R.H. 1977. Adult age differences in cognitive abilities and educational background. *Experimental Aging Research*. 3: 337–383.

Gordon, H.W. and Bogen, J.E. 1974. Hemispheric lateralization of singing after intracarotid sodium amylobarbitone. *Journal of Neurology, Neurosurgery and Psychiatry*. 37: 727–738.

Graf, P. and Gallie, K.A. 1992. A transfer-appropriate processing account for memory and amnesia. In *Neuropsychology of memory*, ed. L. R. Squire and N. Butters, 2nd ed., pp. 241–248. New York: Guilford Press.

Greiner, F., English, S., Dean, K., Olson, K.A., Winn, P. and Beatty, W.W. 1997. Expression of game-related and generic knowledge by dementia patients who retain skill at playing dominoes. *Neurology*. 49: 518–523.

Haxby, J.V., Duara, R., Grady, C.L., Cutler, N.R. and Rapoport, S.I. 1985. Relations between neuropsychological and cerebral metabolic asymmetries in early Alzheimer's disease. *Journal of Cerebral Blood Flow and Metabolism*. 5: 193–200.

Hayslip, B. and Sterns, H.L. 1979. Age differences in relationships between crystallized and fluid intelligences and problem solving. *Journal of Gerontology*. 34: 404–414.

Heaton, R.K., Grant, I. and Mathews, C.C. 1986. Differences in neuropsychological test performance associated with age, education and sex. In *Neuropsychological assessment of neuropsychiatric disorders*, ed. I. Grant and K.M. Adams, pp. 100–120. New York: Oxford University Press.

Hill, A.L. 1977. Idiot savants: Rate of incidence. *Perceptual and Motor Skills*. 44: 161–162.

Hirst, W., Phelps, E.A., Johnson, M.K. and Volpe, B.T. 1988. Amnesia and second language learning. *Brain and Cognition*. 8: 105–116.

Kaplan, E., Goodglass, H. and Weintraub, S. 1983. *Boston Naming Test*. Philadelphia: Lea & Febiger.

Kolb, B. and Whishaw, I.Q. 1990. *Fundamentals of human neuropsychology*, 3rd ed. New York: W.H. Freeman.

Lewis, M. 1985. Gifted or dysfunctional: The child savant. *Pediatric Annals*. 14: 733–742.

Martin, A. 1992. Semantic knowledge in patients with Alzheimer's disease: Evidence for degraded representations. In *Memory functioning in dementia*, ed. L. Bäckman, pp. 119–134. Amsterdam, Netherlands: Elsevier.

McKhann, G., Drachman, D., Folstein, M., Katzman, R., Price, D. and Stadlan, E.M. 1984. Clinical diagnosis of Alzheimer's disease: Report of the NINCDS-ADRDA work group under the auspices of Department of Health and Human Services Task Force on Alzheimer's disease. *Neurology*. 34: 939–944.

Nebes, R.D. 1989. Semantic memory in Alzheimer's disease. *Psychological Bulletin*. 106: 377–394.

O'Conner, N. and Hermelin, B. 1984. Idiot savant calendrical calculators: Math or memory? *Psychological Medicine*. 14: 801–806.

Polk, M. and Kertesz, A. 1993. Music and language in degenerative disease of the brain. *Brain and Cognition*. 22: 98–117.

Rimland, B. and Hill, A.L. 1984. Idiot savants. In *Mental retardation and developmental disabilities*, vol. 13, ed. J. Wortis, pp. 155–169. New York: Plenum Press.

Sacks, O. 1985. *The man who mistook his wife for a hat and other clinical tales*. New York: Summit Books.

Sacks, O. 1995. *An anthropologist on Mars: Seven paradoxical tales*. New York: Alfred A. Knopf.

Salthouse, T.A. 1989. Ageing and skilled performance. In *The acquisition and performance of cognitive skills*, ed. A. Colley and J. Beech, pp. 247–264. New York: Wiley.

Salthouse, T.A. 1990. Cognitive competence and expertise in aging. In *Handbook of the psychology of aging*, ed. J. E. Birren and K. W. Schaie, 3rd ed., pp. 310–319. San Diego: Academic Press.

Smith, A. 1966. Speech and other functions after left (dominant) hemispherectomy. *Journal of Neurology, Neurosurgery and Psychiatry*. 29: 467–471.

Tröster, A.I., Salmon, D.P., McCullough, D. and Butters, N. 1989. A comparison of category fluency deficits associated with Alzheimer's and Huntington's diseases. *Brain and Language*. 37: 500–513.

Wechsler, D. 1974. *Wechsler Intelligence Scale for Children - Revised manual*. San Antonio: Psychological Corporation.

Wechsler, D. 1981. *Wechsler Adult Intelligence Scale - Revised manual*. San Antonio: Psychological Corporation.

Wilson, B., Baddeley, A. and Kapur, N. 1994. Dense amnesia and preserved musical ability in a professional musician following herpes simplex virus encephalitis. Presented at Memory Disorders Research Society, Sixth Annual Meeting, 27–28 October 1994. Cambridge, MA.

21

Drug treatment of cognitive impairment in neurodegenerative disease: rationale, current experience and expectations for the future

LOUIS T. GIRON, JR AND WILLIAM C. KOLLER

INTRODUCTION

Treatment of cognitive impairment of neurodegenerative diseases has developed late in comparison to treatment of motor impairment. Many reasons apply. Cognitive impairment in Parkinson's disease (PD) has not been regarded as an intrinsic feature of the disease, probably because of Parkinson's original dictum, until relatively recently in the English language literature. Furthermore, also until relatively recently, cognitive impairment has not been studied widely or rigorously enough to permit ready or valid comparisons among investigators. Therapy of cognitive impairment has been neglected perhaps also because it had been indulgently regarded as the universal heritage of age and not as a result of pathological processes which can be compensated, halted or reversed by treatment. While therapeutic nihilism now appears in abeyance, clinical experience has tempered recent enthusiasm.

In this chapter, we offer clinical perspectives of current pharmacological treatment and its effects, intended and otherwise, on cognition and especially memory, in Age-Associated Memory Impairment, Alzheimer's disease (AD) and PD. We speculate about future therapies.

GENERAL PHARMACOLOGICAL PRINCIPLES OF THERAPY

Current pharmacological theory posits that the most specific agents offer the greatest likelihood of efficacy and the least likelihood of adverse effects. To design a highly specific drug requires not only technical knowledge about structure–activity relations, (i.e. *molecular* structure, *biological* activity) but also the specific identification of the biochemical defect which is to be corrected by the drug. Development of potent specific agents for dementia (a potentially undifferentiated clinical state) is limited at a crucial juncture by our lack of identification of specific defects which cause dementia. Many (e.g. Growdon 1993) believe that current agents treat dementia epiphenomena poorly and fundamental causes not at all. The most critical admit that the clearest rationale for drug treatment occurs in disorders involving specific biochemical deficits.

Another pharmacological principle is that drugs exert their most specific effects (and the fewest side-effects) when they are administered at the lowest effective dose. For example, botulinum toxoid when injected in small doses for dystonia may selectively destroy local nerve terminals without systemic effects, but when ingested in large quantity may cause whole body paralysis. Higher doses of cholinesterase inhibitors used to treat memory impairment can cause nausea, vomiting and liver toxicity.

GENERAL CLINICAL CONCERNS

Clinicians do not have the advantage of treating cognitive impairments in patients who have been carefully diagnosed and selected according to inclusion and exclusion criteria. Rather, they treat all patients, including those with a variety of systemic medical disorders which, especially in the elderly, may impair cognitive function. Other conditions, for example multi-infarct state, alcoholism and depression may obscure diagnoses and complicate treatment. Medications such as sedatives, hypnotics, neuroleptics, histamine antagonists, anticonvulsants and homeopathic or over-the-counter medications can contribute to cognitive impairment; then, as ailments mount, the likelihood of drug interactions leading to cognitive impairment multiplies. In the following section, we briefly describe the major clinical entities contributing to memory impairment, their most likely correctable biochemical defects and the rationale and current clinical experience with treatments.

AGE-ASSOCIATED MEMORY IMPAIRMENT

The hypothesis that progressive memory loss is a normal consequence of aging is consistent with popular wisdom but, because of methodological issues, has been difficult to test (Chapter 18). Until recently, normative data for cognitive function in the elderly had been extrapolated from data acquired from younger populations. Even with new, more appropriate normative data (Chapter 16), the definition of what constitutes normal memory in aging eludes consensus. Kral (1958) coined the term *benign senescent forgetfulness* to refer to a group of forgetful elderly with otherwise preserved and stable global functioning whose survival clearly differed from that of the demented. The National Institute of Mental Health (NIMH) working group (Crook et al. 1986) defined Age-Associated Memory Impairment (AAMI) to include: (1) subjective memory complaint, (2) absence of memory-impairing medical conditions, and (3) scores on one memory test more than one standard deviation below the mean of younger adults. Blackford and LaRue (1989) revised the AAMI criteria and added two subgroups: one, with age-consistent memory scores (Age-Consistent Memory Impairment); and the second, with memory scores impaired in comparison to young adults and in the borderline range relative to age-matched peers (Late-Life Forgetfulness). Ignoring the requirement for a subjective complaint of memory impairment, Smith et al. (1991) applied the various criteria to a group of age- and gender-matched control subjects for an AD population study and to a group of predominantly community-dwelling elderly who were more nearly representative of the elderly population at large. By the original NIMH criteria, 98% of the control group and 77% of the community-dwelling group had AAMI. Applying the criteria of Blackford and LaRue (1989), Smith et al. found that AAMI

was present in 31% of the control subjects and in 8% of the community-dwelling group. The incidence of Age-Consistent Memory Impairment was 52% in the control group and 30% in the community-dwelling elderly; Late-Life Forgetfulness was diagnosed in none of the control subjects, but in 31% of the community-dwelling group. By this study, both the original and revised criteria lack specificity. Preparation of more sensitive test instruments (Youngjohn et al. 1992; Gomez de Caso et al. 1994) and their wider application, may enhance the selectivity of AAMI diagnosis.

Considerable risk attends misdiagnosing a 'normal' condition as pathological. Nonetheless, because it may contain individuals with indolent AD, the population characterized to have either AAMI or its more severe subtype, Late-Life Forgetfulness, deserves investigation. This population should be followed prospectively by psychometric, neurological, biochemical, genetic and physiological testing (Grady et al. 1988) to determine the natural history of 'normality' and the risk factors for the development of AD. Furthermore, if some of this population eventually develops AD (Hanninen et al. 1996), then the predictive validity of psychometric tests may be evaluated in this group (Tierney et al. 1996).

The relation of normal aging to AAMI and of AAMI to AD, may be intimate. This notion gains credence by the demonstration of neuronal loss, neurofibrillary tangles and granulovacuolar degeneration in the cortex of normal elderly (Ball 1977) and the similarity of distribution of these markers in nondemented elderly compared to those with AD (Arriagada et al. 1991). Other studies, such as that of Parnetti et al. (1996), employing magnetic resonance imaging (MRI) hippocampal volumetry, magnetic resonance spectroscopy and single positron emission computed tomography (SPECT) scanning, have also suggested a continuum between AAMI and AD. A spectrum of increasing burdens of pathological alterations would then show itself first by preserved memory, then by faulty but serviceable memory and then lastly by unequivocal dementia.

The implications for treatment are these: it is axiomatic that prevention is preferred to treatment. Logically then, the AAMI population has the greatest potential to benefit from preventive and restorative therapy. As specific neurochemical deficits have not, however, been identified in this population, it is reasonable now to discuss the use of nootropics, which do not rectify specific biochemical defects.

NOOTROPICS

Nootropics, by definition, improve cognition and have essentially no side-effects. As 'general tonics' they do not correct known biochemical defects, i.e. as a class they violate the first pharmacological principle set forth earlier. They are typically regarded as 'metabolic enhancers', although many have cholinergic activity (Sarter 1991). Agents in the nootropic category include hydergine, piracetam, acetyl-l-carnitine (Thal et al. 1996), thiamine and the vasodilators papaverine and cyclandelate. In general, nootropics are of theoretical interest, but appear to have limited clinical benefit (Table 21.1). For example, a recent meta-analysis (Schneider and Olin 1994) of the cognitive effects of hydergine, considered now a largely outdated drug combination (Thompson et al. 1990), suggests that while hydergine may be statistically superior to placebos in enhancing memory, its clinical effects are not significant.

Piracetam has been found to facilitate learning of a variety of tasks in experimental animals (e.g. Sara et al. 1979) and, in combination with a memory training program, to be effective in those AAMI subjects with the poorest recall (Israel et al. 1994). Phosphatidylserine has similarly shown promise in treating AAMI subjects who perform at a relatively low level before treatment (Crook et al. 1991). Unfortunately, piracetam has generally been found to be ineffective in clinical trials (Growdon et al. 1988). Sarter (1991) has attributed the typical lack of success in the transition of nootropic from experimental animal to human, to inappropriate reliance on behavioral tasks of unproved validity and generalizability in animal studies.

CHOLINERGIC THERAPY IN ALZHEIMER'S DISEASE

The cholinergic therapy of the memory impairment of AD has a sound experimental basis in both animal and human studies (Bartus et al. 1982; Thal 1994). Cholinergic structures, such as the nucleus basalis of Meynert, the major cholinergic input to the cortex, have been shown to bear the brunt of the degenerative process (Chapters 3 and 4). Cholinergic therapy has been attempted by: (1) increasing the amount of a precursor, as by choline, phosphatidylcholine, or lecithin, (2) direct cholinergic receptor stimulation, as by arecoline, and (3) blocking cholinesterase activity, thereby increasing the amount of acetylcholine

available for synaptic transmission. The first method has been nearly uniformly unsuccessful in clinical trials (Corkin 1981; Crook 1985; Thal 1994). Choline availability is either not the rate-limiting step in the production of acetylcholine, or else, a decline in the numbers or function of the presynaptic cholinergic terminals may explain this failure. The second method has been limited by the short half-life of arecoline and by peripheral side-effects of this and other direct cholinergic agonists.

The third method showed promise early on. Intravenous physostigmine improved performance on verbal and nonverbal memory tasks in double-blind trials. If patients with the most severe dementia were excluded, physostigmine was also of benefit when administered orally in escalating doses (Thal 1994). One major drawback to treatment with physostigmine is its short half-life; a longer-acting preparation has been developed. Tacrine, another anticholinesterase, in doses up to 80 mg/day yielded modest effects on AD patients' memory, but not on their global level of functioning (Davis et al. 1992; Farlow et al. 1992). When given at a higher dose (up to 160 mg/day) in a randomized, double-blind, placebo-controlled trial, tacrine improved objectively measured memory in a dose-related fashion while both clinicians and caregivers saw global improvement (Knapp et al. 1994). At these doses, asymptomatic increases in liver transaminases and gastrointestinal complaints were the chief causes for stopping treatment in about one-fourth and one-sixth of cases, respectively. Consequently, the clinician must exclude pre-existing liver disease, as well as those conditions in which enhanced cholinergic tone may be harmful, such as active peptic ulcer disease, bradycardia and sick-sinus syndrome. Treatment is not advised in the severely demented (a Mini Mental Status Exam score of less than 10) as benefit would be predicted not to occur. Practical limitations include the necessity and cost of weekly liver function tests. The family must understand the requirement for regular four times-a-day dosing, the chances for improvement and the limited efficacy and duration of treatment. A written contract may clarify treatment objectives and expectations. The clinician and family must also be alert to drug interactions, especially with drugs metabolized by the cytochrome–450 system, such as theophylline, cimetidine and succinylcholine.

The most recently released anticholinesterase, donepezil (Aricept) has been shown to be well-tolerated in doses of 5–10 mg/day and statistically significant improvements in cognition and quality of life have been demonstrated

Table 21.1. *Selected drugs with clinical effects on memory in neurodegenerative disorders*

Drug	Class	Rationale	Mode of action	Side-effects and draw-backs	Population	Effect on memory
Piracetam	Nootropics	'Metabolic enhancer'	? Stimulates cholinergic function	Few or none	AAMI / Alzheimer's disease	Disappointing; some benefit in AAMI when combined with memory training
Hydergine	Nootropics	As above	As above	Few or none	Alzheimer's disease	Some statistically but probably not clinically significant benefit
Choline and lecithin	Acetylcholine precursors	Restore acetylcholine	Converts to acetylcholine	Few	Alzheimer's disease	No benefit
Arecholine	Cholino-mimetic	Enhance cholinergic tone	Stimulates cholinergic receptor	Short-half life; nausea and vomiting	Alzheimer's disease	Very limited
Tacrine and Donepezil (E2020)	Acetylcholin-esterases	Enhance cholinergic tone	Improves efficiency of cholinergic transmission	Nausea, vomiting, liver toxicity	Alzheimer's disease	Modest but definite
					Parkinson's disease	Worsens motor impairment
Levodopa	Dopamine precursor	Restore dopamine depletion	Converts to dopamine	Dyskinesias, hallucinations, hypotension	Parkinson's disease	Mixed effects; no consensus
Deprenyl	Selective MAO-B inhibitor	Prolong dopaminergic activity	Prevents breakdown of dopamine	As above	Parkinson's disease	Probably no effect; in early stages, none
		Possibly acts as a 'neuro protective' agent	Prevents formation of endogenous toxins		Alzheimer's disease	Possible benefit depending on selection of patients

Note:
AAMI: Age-Associated Memory Impairment.

in a relatively small number of patients (Rogers et al. 1996). Even with the latter drug, effective delivery of anticholinesterases to the nervous system may not yet have been optimized and further refinements in anticholinesterase therapies can be expected.

The efficacy of cholinergic therapy in AD cannot approach that of levodopa in PD. While the neurons characteristically affected in AD are predominantly cholinergic, other neurotransmitters including glutamate, serotonin and somatostatin are also reduced from normal (Hedera and Whitehouse 1994). The acetylcholine deficiency in AD is more complicated than the near singularity of dopamine deficiency in PD. Furthermore, because anticholinergics (e.g. scopolamine) administered to healthy volunteers do not produce the full range of memory impairments (especially remote memory loss) evident in AD (Kopelman and Corn 1988; Tröster et al. 1989), cholinergic treatment may be expected to improve only certain aspects of memory. More importantly, while synaptic transmission may be made more efficient by cholinergic therapies, the numbers of synapses are progressively declining (Terry et al. 1991). As no current therapy halts or reverses synaptic and neuronal loss, the clinician may enter a tortoise versus hare race – but, unlike in the fable, the winner is foreordained.

DOPAMINERGIC AND OTHER PHARMACOLOGICAL TREATMENT OF COGNITIVE IMPAIRMENT IN PARKINSON'S DISEASE

Cognitive impairment is common in PD. Overall, among recent and methodologically sounder studies, the average prevalence of dementia in PD falls into the 25–30% range (Mohr et al. 1995). It is not the purpose of this chapter to debate the relation of PD to Lewy body disease, but it is appropriate to emphasize that in North America, Lewy body disease (the pathological substratum that may extend to cortex as well as to, or instead of, brain stem) may be a more frequent cause of dementia than even vascular disease (for a review, see Kalra et al. 1996).

In PD, a profound deficit of dopamine has been documented in the striatum at postmortem examination (Ehringer and Hornykiewicz 1960). The pathological basis of this dopaminergic deficit is the loss of pigmented neurons in the pars compacta of the substantia nigra (Chapters 3 and 4). While other monoamine neurotransmitters, namely

serotonin (Jellinger 1990) and norepinephrine (Chui et al. 1986; Chan-Palay 1991) are also reduced, the decline in dopamine is considerably greater and the degree of akinesia correlates with the extent of dopamine depletion (Hornykiewicz 1988). The levels of acetylcholine in the striatum may actually be increased in PD and aggravate motor symptoms (Hornykiewicz and Kish 1986).

These biochemical data form the rationale for treating motor symptoms in PD by restoring dopaminergic tone. The usual means is to furnish levodopa, the immediate precursor to dopamine. Levodopa is nearly universally administered with a peripheral dopa-decarboxylase inhibitor, such as carbidopa, which prevents the peripheral conversion of levodopa to dopamine. Amantadine, which is thought primarily to speed synthesis and release of dopamine, is often used as an adjunct. Other alternative and adjunctive agents are the direct dopaminergic agonists, such as bromocriptine and pergolide; and the anticholinergics, such as trihexyphenidyl and benztropine mesylate. In addition, deprenyl or, as it is often termed, selegiline, a monoamine oxidase B inhibitor, is often used to prolong the activity of dopamine; it is used as a presumptive neuroprotective agent (Parkinson Study Group 1993).

Levodopa treatment

Dopamine deficiency may contribute to the cognitive impairment in PD. The strongest evidence for this proposal is the finding that patients with 1-methyl–4-phenyl–1,2,3,6-tetrahydropyridine (MPTP)-induced parkinsonism have cognitive deficits resembling those seen in idiopathic PD (Stern and Langston 1985). As MPTP causes highly specific lesions depleting striatal dopamine, and because cognitive impairment may be detectable before the motor symptoms after MPTP poisoning (Stern et al. 1990), the hypothesis that dopaminergic deficits contribute to cognitive dysfunction in PD would seem supported. If dopamine deficiency does cause cognitive impairment, then repletion of dopamine ought to ameliorate the impairment. Although early studies reported that cognitive function improved after dopaminergic therapy, their methodology has been criticized (Riklan et al. 1976).

Later studies have yielded conflicting data. Some investigators found no effect of exogenous levodopa on cognitive function (Pillon et al. 1989). Gotham et al. (1988) suggested that alterations of both dopaminergic and nondopaminergic functions contribute to cognitive defects in PD; they also concluded that memory dysfunction can occur because of both dopamine depletion and dopamine overstimulation. Other investigators reported minimal benefit of exogenous levodopa on cognitive function (Stern et al. 1990), or else only on simultaneously performed tasks (Malapani et al. 1994). Some improvement in cognitive function may be 'state-dependent', varying with 'on' versus 'off' condition (Huber et al. 1989). The 'on' state refers to a period of clinical dopaminergic activity, usually with clear antiparkinsonian effects or possibly with peak dose dyskinesias; the 'off', to a period of hypodopaminergic activity with marked immobility; they are related, respectively, to high and low levels of plasma levodopa. Delis and Massman (1992) reviewed the literature on the relation between alteration in dopamine levels and cognitive function. They concluded that the differences in performance between 'on' and 'off' states were less than the similarities; recall seemed best when the dopaminergic status was the same during learning and retrieval of memoranda.

Still other workers have shown an adverse effect of levodopa on PD patients' performance on demanding, high-speed memory scanning (Poewe et al. 1991) and executive tasks (Kulisevsky et al. 1996). Withdrawal of levodopa, however, may result in confusion (Lang 1987) and in selective impairments on psychological tests sensitive to frontal lobe dysfunction (Lange et al. 1992).

Amantadine

Amantadine enhances the activity of levodopa by speeding the conversion of levodopa to dopamine and the release of dopamine from the presynaptic terminal. It likely also has anticholinergic properties as well as antagonist activity at the glutamate N-methyl-D-aspartate (NMDA) receptor (Lange and Riederer 1994). Anticholinergic side-effects are common. In doses greater than 300 mg/day and in conjunction with other dopaminergic agents, amantadine may cause hallucinations. In comparison with conventional anticholinergics administered to healthy volunteers, amantadine causes less adverse effect on memory (Gelenberg et al. 1989). A 'neuroprotective' effect, presumably related to its NMDA antagonism, is suspected clinically, based on a recent report comparing patient survival with and without amantadine (Uitti et al. 1996); however, a relation between amantadine treatment and the subsequent course of cognitive function has not been documented.

Dopaminergic agonists

The dopaminergic agonists bromocriptine, pergolide, lisuride and mesulergine, can be predicted to have similar therapeutic and adverse effects to levodopa. As a result of

their potency, additional activity at nondopamine receptors and their frequent concurrent use with levodopa, they are even more likely to cause adverse reactions. In fact, psychiatric symptoms have been the chief reason for discontinuation of dopaminergic agents in several studies (LeWitt 1992), although these complications may be dose-related (Simonetta et al. 1987). Some workers insist that severe dementia is an indication not to begin bromocriptine treatment because of the high incidence of confusion and hallucinations (Grimes and Hassan 1983). No change in intellect or cognitive function was found in a series of patients treated with pergolide (Stern et al. 1984).

Anticholinergics

Until the advent of levodopa, the anticholinergics have been the mainstays of the treatment of PD. It has been proposed that a disturbed balance between cholinergic and dopaminergic activity (i.e. cholinergic hyperactivity and dopaminergic underactivity) causes the motor symptoms in PD. This interpretation is consistent with the neurochemical data cited earlier and provides a broad theoretical basis for the use of anticholinergics in PD. Several complexities attend the use of anticholinergics in PD. As cell loss in the nucleus basalis of Meynert in patients with PD and dementia has been correlated with the severity of dementia (Perry et al. 1985), one might expect anticholinergics to aggravate memory and cognitive impairments. Indeed, patients with PD with dementia do appear to be more sensitive to the anticholinergic drugs and become more readily confused than do patients without dementia (deSmet et al. 1982). Even PD patients unselected in relation to dementia (Sadeh et al. 1982), or else without dementia (Koller 1984), develop memory deficits in response to anticholinergic drugs. Relative youth does not protect against this effect, as patients younger than 50 years of age will also experience memory impairment. Some authorities assert that anticholinergic agents should never be given to patients with mental impairment (Obeso and Martinez-Lage 1992). The mechanism by which anticholinergics produce memory and cognitive impairments is probably more complex than previously thought because both benztropine and trihexyphenidyl, the most widely used of these agents in this country, also have dopamine reuptake-blocking properties (Coyle and Snyder 1969).

Deprenyl and selective MAO-B inhibition

Deprenyl (selegiline), at the usual daily dose of 10 mg/day, is a selective inhibitor of monoamine oxidase-B (MAO-B).

The latter is a predominantly glial-based enzyme that catalyzes the breakdown of dopamine. Thus, inhibition of MAO-B can prolong the action of dopamine. This inhibition is the basis for the use of deprenyl in the symptomatic, usually adjunctive treatment of PD. In addition, selective MAO-B inhibition has been shown to block the toxic effect of MPTP in monkeys (Cohen et al. 1984), raising the possibility that the agent may protect the nervous system against a similar, yet unidentified toxic agent (such as a metabolite of dopamine) which causes PD by means of excessive oxidative stress (Olanow 1992). The DATATOP study (Parkinson Study Group 1989, 1993) showed that in patients with early PD the time between diagnosis and the need for levodopa treatment was extended for deprenyl- as opposed to placebo-treated subjects. The DATATOP study has been criticized, but the notion of neuroprotection in PD by deprenyl has some clinical respectability. As, at the usual doses, deprenyl does not release other amines from the nerve terminals, the dangerous 'cheese effect' of other MAO inhibitors can be avoided. The agent can therefore be safely used in combination with other antiparkinsonian drugs.

Deprenyl has been reported to have either beneficial or no effects on memory. Tarczy and Szirmai (1995) reported that deprenyl (5 mg twice a day) improved memory (as measured with the MMSE) in patients with PD who had dementia and frontal lobe hypoperfusion on single positron emission computed tomography (SPECT) scanning, but not in groups with other SPECT-hypometabolism patterns. Finali et al. (1994) reported that deprenyl, at a dose of 10 mg a day, had a statistically significant effect on verbal and visuospatial learning in nondemented patients with PD; however, Dalrymple-Alford et al. (1995) found that deprenyl at 5 mg twice a day, improved 20 young, levodopa-naive PD patients' mentation/mood scores on the Unified Parkinson's Disease Rating Scale, but not their scores on specific neuropsychological measures. In a group of 18 patients, Haitenen (1991) found that deprenyl (30 mg a day) improved recall of easy word associations. The authors attributed this finding to a nonspecific arousal effect because effects on other specific cognitive functions were not observed. At doses of 10–40 mg per day, deprenyl may improve reaction time, depression and subjective feelings of vitality (Lees 1991); at these doses, deprenyl probably acts as an antidepressant, like members of the class of nonspecific MAO inhibitors.

Unfortunately, reports of cognitive improvements associated with deprenyl treatment are difficult to interpret due to: (1) small numbers of patients studied, (2) variability in the disease stage of included patients, (3) heterogeneity in neuropsychological assessment methods and the breadth of cognitive functions assessed, (4) the possible inclusion of patients with coexistent AD, and (5) variability in deprenyl dosages. In the most comprehensive study to date of the effects of deprenyl, no significant effect on memory or cognition was observed. The DATATOP study included the results of extensive standardized testing performed on 800 patients with early untreated PD; it utilized doses of deprenyl which can be expected to be more nearly specific and more typical of the usual doses. None of these patients was judged to be demented or depressed on entry to the study. The investigators concluded that in early untreated PD: (1) cognitive performance is stable and appears unrelated to motor deterioration, and (2) deprenyl caused no significant effect on cognitive test performance (Kieburtz et al. 1994).

DRUGS DEVELOPED FOR TREATMENT OF ONE DISORDER AND APPLIED TO ANOTHER

Tacrine and other cholinomimetics

It seems logical to use cholinomimetics to treat the memory deficit in PD because of the known alterations in the nucleus basalis in this disorder. Nonetheless, clinical trials with large numbers of patients cannot be anticipated: the case study of Ott and Lannon (1992) shows that exacerbation of parkinsonism may preclude such trials.

Amantadine

Amantadine has been used in traumatically brain-injured patients because it fosters alertness and sustained attention; however, a consistent effect of the drug on memory has not been observed (Nickels et al. 1994).

Dopamine agonists

In a case of mediobasal forebrain injury studied with a blinded, controlled protocol, Dobkin and Hanlon (1993) found that bromocriptine significantly improved verbal learning, functional memory and day-to-day recall. In a crossover trial with patients with vascular dementia, bromocriptine either failed to improve or worsened performance on multiple measures of cognition (Nadeau et al. 1988).

MAO-B inhibitors

An apparent augmenting benefit occurred when deprenyl was added to fluoxetine in the treatment of a patient with Huntington's disease (HD) (Patel et al. 1996); in this case, the dose of deprenyl was low and the improvement was predominantly affective and behavioral.

Deprenyl may eventually prove to have a role in the treatment of AD. In Italian trials, deprenyl was more effective than oxiracetam, a nootropic with good penetration into the central nervous system, in improving higher cortical function and everyday living skills (Falsaperla et al. 1990); and more effective than a placebo (Piccinin et al. 1990). Improvement in 'cognitive efficiency' was also reported in another pilot study of deprenyl in AD (Agnoli et al. 1992). In Tariot et al.'s (1987) study of 17 patients with AD, deprenyl, at a dose of 10 mg per day, appeared to enhance performance on tasks requiring attention and sustained conscious effort, but it did not alter intrusion errors or other cognitive deficits (Tariot et al. 1987). When AD patients are especially selected for an early onset and for memory impairment, deprenyl appears to facilitate verbal memory (Finali et al. 1991, 1992). In a double-blind cross-over study that compared acute physostigmine infusions with either placebo or deprenyl, neither physostigmine nor deprenyl resulted in significant improvement of test performance (Marin et al. 1995). In a 15-month trial of patients with mild AD, deprenyl at a low dose appeared to have a significant effect on only one measure, the Brief Psychiatric Rating Scale, specifically on disorientation (Burke et al. 1993). Part of the behavioral improvement that deprenyl confers in AD might result from a mild disinhibiting effect (Schneider et al. 1991).

Even though deprenyl has not consistently been shown to improve cognitive and especially, memory performance, a recent study suggests that deprenyl may slow the progression of moderately severe AD. Sano et al. (1997) randomly assigned 341 patients with moderately severe AD to receive either deprenyl, alpha-tocopherol (vitamin E), a combination of deprenyl and alpha-tocopherol, or placebo for 2 years. Deprenyl and alpha-tocopherol delayed time to the primary outcome (any one of death, institutionalization, progression to severe dementia, or inability to carry out activities of daily living), which suggests that deprenyl may slow the progression of AD.

THE FUTURE

Considering the relatively modest benefits of current drug treatments on memory and cognition, the prospects for agents or techniques conferring more meaningful benefit must be viewed with cautious optimism. Presymptomatic detection of PD and AD might permit earlier treatment and render current neuroprotective agents more effective. Undoubtedly, in the future, more research will also address the prevention of neurodegenerative diseases. For example, estrogen might facilitate verbal memory and new learning in elderly women and estrogen replacement therapy in postmenopausal women might provide some protection against AD (Henderson 1997). The value of estrogen replacement therapy in the prevention and treatment of AD remains debated, however, as there is a lack of adequately controlled, randomized clinical trials (Birge 1997). A recent, large scale, prospective study (but without randomization) nonetheless provides encouraging data about the value of estrogen replacement therapy (Kawas et al. 1997).

Regardless of whether agents are designed to treat or protect against neurodegenerative diseases, the development of more effective agents will require advances in the understanding of neuronal cell biology, molecular biology and molecular genetics of these disorders. Recent experimentation (Phelps et al. 1989; Hefti et al. 1992) shows that the most promising prospects for the correction of disruption of fundamental neuronal function and for enhanced neuronal survival in the neurodegenerative disorders, lie in specific neurotrophic treatments. It is encouraging that glia-derived neurotrophic factor (GDNF) when injected into the carotid artery of MPTP-treated rhesus monkeys reduces the symptomatology of parkinsonism and improves the decline in immunocytochemical markers of dopaminergic neurons (Gash et al. 1996). The current treatment of amyotrophic lateral sclerosis by a neurotrophic factor suggests that this modality has definite promise. As in the simpler case of the anticholinesterases, the uncomplicated delivery of these agents to the pharmacologically protected central nervous system will undoubtedly be problematic. Clinical safety trials of recombinant human nerve growth factor (Petty et al. 1994; Yuen and Mobley 1996) also show that myalgia and hyperalgesia may limit their effectiveness. One hopes that these impediments are resolvable by 'technical' advances.

REFERENCES

Agnoli, A., Fabrinni, G., Fioravanti, M. and Martucci, N. 1992. CBF and cognitive evaluation of Alzheimer type patients before and after IMAO-B treatment: A pilot study. *European Neuropsychopharmacology*. 2: 31–35.

Arriagada, P.V., Marzloff, K. and Heyman, B.T. 1991. Distribution of Alzheimer-type pathologic changes in nondemented elderly individuals matches the pattern in Alzheimer's disease. *Neurobiology of Aging*. 12: 295–312.

Ball, M.J. 1977. Neuronal loss, neurofibrillary tangles and granulovacuolar degeneration in the hippocampus with ageing and dementia. *Acta Neuropathologica*. 37: 111–118.

Bartus, R.T., Dean, R.L., Beer, B. and Lippa, A.S. 1982. The cholinergic hypothesis of geriatric memory dysfunction. *Science*. 217: 406–417.

Birge, S.J. 1997. The role of ovarian hormones in cognition and dementia. *Neurology*. 48 (Suppl. 7): S1.

Blackford, R.C. and LaRue, A. 1989. Criteria for diagnosing age-associated memory impairment: Proposed improvements from the field. *Developmental Neuropsychology*. 5: 295–306.

Burke, W.J., Roccaforte, W.H., Wengel, S.P., Bayer, B.L., Fanno, A.E. and Willcockson, N. K. 1993. L-deprenyl in the treatment of mild dementia of the Alzheimer type: Results of a 15-month trial. *Journal of the American Geriatrics Society*. 41: 1219–1225.

Chan-Palay, V. 1991. Alterations in the locus coeruleus in dementias of Alzheimer's and Parkinson's disease. *Progress in Brain Research*. 88: 626–630.

Chui, H.C., Mortimer, J.A., Slager, V., Zarow C., Bondareff, W. and Webster, D.D. 1986. Pathologic correlates of dementia in Parkinson's disease. *Archives of Neurology*. 43: 991–995.

Cohen, G., Pasik, P., Cohen, B., Leist, A., Mytilineou, C. and Yahr, M.D. 1984. Pargyline and (-)deprenyl prevent the neurotoxicity of 1-methyl–4-phenyl–1,2,3,6-tetrahydropyridine (MPTP) in monkeys. *European Journal of Pharmacology*. 106: 209–210.

Corkin, S. 1981. Acetylcholine, aging and Alzheimer's disease: Implications for treatment. *Trends in Neurosciences*. 4: 287–290.

Coyle, J.T. and Snyder, S.H. 1969. Antiparkinsonian drugs: Inhibition of dopamine uptake in the corpus striatum as a possible mechanism of action. *Science*. 166: 899–901.

Crook, T. 1985. Clinical trials in Alzheimer's disease. *Annals of the New York Academy of Sciences*. 444: 428–436.

Crook, T.H., Bartus, R.T., Ferris, S.H., Whitehouse, P., Cohen, G.D. and Gershon, S. 1986. Age-associated memory impairment. Proposed diagnostic criteria and measurement of clinical change – Report of a National Institute of Mental Health work group. *Developmental Neuropsychology*. 24: 261–276.

Crook, T.H., Tinklenberg, J., Yesavage, J., Petrie, W., Nunzi, M.G. and Massari, D.C. 1991. Effects of phosphatidylserine in age-associated memory impairment. *Neurology*. 41: 644–649.

Dalrymple-Alford, J.C., Jamieson, C.F. and Donaldson, I.M. 1995. Effects of selegiline (deprenyl) on cognition in early Parkinson's disease. *Clinical Neuropharmacology*. 18: 348–359.

Davis, K.L., Thal, L.J., Gamzu, E.F., Davis, C.S., Woolson, R.F., Gracon, S.I., Drachman, D.A., Schneider, L.S., Whitehouse, P.J., Hoover, T.M. and The Tacrine Collaborative Study Group. 1992. A double-blind, placebo-controlled multicenter study of tacrine for Alzheimer's disease. *New England Journal of Medicine*. 327: 1253–1259.

Delis, D.C. and Massman, P.J. 1992. The effects of dopamine fluctuation on cognition and affect. In *Parkinson's disease: Neurobehavioral aspects*, ed. S.J. Huber and J.L. Cummings, pp. 288–302. New York: Oxford University Press.

DeSmet, Y., Ruberg, M., Serdaru, M, Dubois, B., Lhermitte, F. and Agid, Y. 1982. Confusion, dementia and anticholinergics in Parkinson's disease. *Journal of Neurology, Neurosurgery and Psychiatry*. 45: 1161–1164.

Dobkin, B.H. and Hanlon, R. 1993. Dopamine agonist treatment of anterograde amnesia from a mediobasal forebrain injury. *Annals of Neurology*. 33: 313–316.

Ehringer, H. and Hornykiewicz, O. 1960. Verteilung von Noradrenalin und Dopamin (3-hydroxytyramin) im Gehirn des Menschen und ihr Verhalten bei Erkrankungen des extrapyramidalen Systems. *Wiener Klinische Wochenschrift*. 38: 1236–1260.

Falsaperla, A., Monici-Preti, P.A. and Oliani, C. 1990. Selegiline versus oxiracetam in patients with Alzheimer-type dementia. *Clinical Therapeutics*. 12: 376–384.

Farlow, M., Gracon, S.I., Hershey, L.A., Lewis, K.W., Sadowsky, C.H. and Dolan-Ureno, J. 1992. A controlled trial of tacrine in Alzheimer's disease. *Journal of the American Medical Association*. 268: 2523–2529.

Finali, G., Piccirilli, M., Oliani, C. and Piccinin, G.L. 1991. L-deprenyl therapy improves verbal memory in amnesic Alzheimer patients. *Clinical Neuropharmacology*. 14: 523–536.

Finali, G., Piccirilli, M., Oliani, C. and Piccinin, G.L. 1992. Alzheimer-type dementia and verbal memory performances: influence of selegiline therapy. *Italian Journal of Neurological Sciences*. 13: 141–148.

Finali, G., Piccirilli, M. and Piccinin, G.L. 1994. Neuropsychological correlates of L-deprenyl therapy in idiopathic parkinsonism. *Progress in Neuropsychopharmacology and Biological Psychiatry*. 18: 115–128.

Gash, D.M., Zhang, Z., Ovadia, A., Cass, W.A., Yi, A., Simmerman, L., Russell, D., Martin, D., Lapchak, P.A., Collins, F., Hoffer, B.J. and Gerhardt, G.A. 1996. Functional recovery in parkinsonian monkeys treated with GDNF. *Nature*. 388: 252–255.

Gelenberg, A.J., Van Putten, T., Lavori, P.W., Wojcik, J.D., Falk, W.E., Marder, S., Galvin-Nadeau, M., Spring, B., Mohs, R.C. and Brotman, A.W. 1989. Anticholinergic effects on memory: Benztropine versus amantadine. *Journal of Clinical Psycho-pharmacology*. 9: 180–185.

Gomez de Caso, J.A., Rodriguez-Artalejo, F., Claveria, L.E. and Coria, F. 1994. Value of Hodkinson's test for detecting dementia and mild cognitive impairment in epidemiological surveys. *Neuroepidemiology*. 13: 64–68.

Gotham, A.M., Brown, R.G. and Marsden, C.D. 1988. 'Frontal' cognitive function in patients with Parkinson's disease 'on' and 'off' levodopa. *Brain*. 111: 299–321.

Grady, C.L., Haxby, J.V., Horwitz, B., Sundaram, M., Berg, G., Shapiro, M., Friedland, R.P. and Rapoport, S.I. 1988. Longitudinal study of the early neuropsychological and cerebral metabolic changes in dementia of the Alzheimer type. *Journal of Clinical and Experimental Neuropsychology*. 10: 576–596.

Grimes, J.D. and Hassan, M.N. 1983. Bromocriptine in the long-term management of advanced Parkinson's disease. *Canadian Journal of Neurological Sciences*. 10: 86–90.

Growdon, J.H. 1993. Biologic therapies for Alzheimer's disease. In *Dementia*, ed. P. J. Whitehouse, pp. 375–399. Philadelphia: FA Davis Company.

Growdon, J.H., Corkin, S., Huff, F.J. and Rosen, T.J. 1988. Piracetam combined with lecithin in the treatment of Alzheimer's disease. *Neurobiology of Aging*. 7: 269–276.

Haitenen, M.H. 1991. Selegiline and cognitive function in Parkinson's disease. *Acta Neurologica Scandinavica*. 84: 407–410.

Hanninen, T., Hallikainen, M., Koivisto, K., Helkala, E.L., Reinikainen, K.J., Soininen, H., Mykkanen, L., Laakso, M., Pyorala, K. and Riekkinen, J. 1996. A follow-up of age-associated memory impairment: Neuro-psychological predictors of dementia. *Journal of the American Geriatrics Society*. 43: 1007–1015.

Hedera, P. and Whitehouse, P.J. 1994. Neurotransmitters in neuro-degeneration. In *Neurodegenerative diseases*, ed. D.B. Calne, pp. 97–126. Philadelphia: W.B. Saunders Company.

Hefti, F., Lapchak, P.A. and Denton, T.L. 1992. Growth factors and neurotrophic factors in neuro-degenerative diseases. In *Alzheimer's disease: New treatment strategies*, ed. Z. K. Khachaturian and J.P. Blass, pp. 87–101. New York: Marcel Dekker.

Henderson, V.W. 1997. The epidemiology of estrogen replacement therapy and Alzheimer's disease. *Neurology*. 48 (Suppl. 7): S27–S35.

Hornykiewicz, O. 1988. Neurochemical pathology and the etiology of Parkinson's disease: Basic facts and hypothetical possibilities. *Mount Sinai Journal of Medicine*. 55: 11–20.

Hornykiewicz, O. and Kish, S.J. 1986. Biochemical pathophysiology of Parkinson's disease. *Advances in Neurology*. 45: 19–34.

Huber, S.J., Shulman, H.G., Paulson, G.W. and Shuttleworth, E.C. 1989. Dose-dependent memory impairment in Parkinson's disease. *Neurology*. 39: 438–440.

Israel, L., Melac, M., Milinkevitch, D. and Dubos, G. 1994. Drug therapy and memory training programs: a double-blind randomized trial of general practice patients with age-associated memory impairment. *International Psychogeriatrics*. 6: 155–170.

Jellinger, K. 1990. New developments in the pathology of Parkinson's disease. *Advances in Neurology*. 22: 1–16.

Kalra, S., Bergeron, D. and Lang, A.E. 1996. Lewy body disease and dementia: A review. *Archives of Internal Medicine*. 156: 487–493.

Kawas, C., Resnick, S., Morrison, A., Brookmeyer, R., Corrada, M., Zonderman, A., Bacal, C., Lingle, D.D. and Metter, E. 1997. A prospective study of estrogen replacement therapy and the risk of developing Alzheimer's disease: The Baltimore Longitudinal Study of Aging. *Neurology*. 48: 1517–1521.

Kieburtz, K., McDermott, M., Como, P., Growdon, J., Brady, J., Carter, J., Huber, S., Kanigan, B., Landow, E., Rudolph, A., Saint-Cyr, J., Stern, Y., Tennis, M., Thelen, J., Shoulson, I. and Parkinson Study Group. 1994. The effect of deprenyl and tocopherol on cognitive performance in early untreated Parkinson's disease. *Neurology*. 44: 1756–1759.

Knapp, M.J., Knopman, D.S., Solomon, P.R., Pendlebury, W.W., Davis, C.S. and Gracon, S.I. 1994. A 30-week randomized controlled trial of high-dose tacrine in patients with Alzheimer's disease. *Journal of the American Medical Association*. 271: 985–991.

Koller, W.C. 1984. Disturbance of recent memory function in parkinsonian patients on anticholinergic therapy. *Cortex*. 20: 307–311.

Kopelman, M.D. and Corn, T.H. 1988. Cholinergic 'blockade' as a model for cholinergic depletion: a comparison of the memory deficits with those of Alzheimer-type dementia and the alcoholic Korsakoff syndrome. *Brain*. 111: 1079–1100.

Kral, V.C. 1958. Neuro-psychiatric observations in an old people's home. *Journal of Gerontology*. 13: 239–243.

Kulisevsky, J., Avila, A., Barbanoj, M., Antonijoan, R., Berthier, M.L. and Gironell, A. 1996. Acute effects of levodopa on neuropsychological performance in stable and fluctuating Parkinson's disease patients at different levodopa plasma levels. *Brain*. 119: 2121–2132.

Lang, A.E. 1987. Sudden confusion with levodopa withdrawal (letter). *Movement Disorders*. 2: 223.

Lange, K.W. and Riederer, P. 1994. Glutaminergic drugs in Parkinson's disease. *Life Sciences*. 55: 2067–2075.

Lange, K.W., Robbins, T.W., Marsden, C.D., James, M., Owen, A.M. and Paul, G.M. 1992. L-dopa withdrawal in Parkinson's disease selectively impairs cognitive performance in tests sensitive to frontal lobe dysfunction. *Psychopharmacology*. 107: 394–404.

Lees, A.J. 1991. Selegiline hydrochloride and cognition. *Acta Neurologica Scandinavica*. 136 (Suppl.): 91–94.

LeWitt, P. 1992. Dopaminergic drugs in Parkinson's disease. In *Handbook of Parkinson's disease*, 2nd ed., ed. W.C. Koller, pp. 469–507. New York: Marcel Dekker.

Malapani, C., Pillon, B., Dubois, B. and Agid, Y. 1994. Impaired simultaneous cognitive task performance in Parkinson's disease: A dopamine-related dysfunction. *Neurology*. 44: 319–326.

Marin, D.B., Biere, L.M., Lawlor, B.A., Ryan, T.M., Jacobson, R., Schmeidler, J., Mohs, R.C. and Davis, K.L. 1995. L-deprenyl and physostigmine for the treatment of Alzheimer's disease. *Psychiatry Research*. 58: 181–189.

Mohr, E., Mendis, T. and Grimes, J.D. 1995. Late cognitive changes in Parkinson's disease with an emphasis on dementia. In *Behavioral neurology of movement disorders*, ed. W.J. Weiner and A.E. Lang, pp. 97–113. New York: Raven Press.

Nadeau, S.E., Malloy, P.F. and Andrew, M.E. 1988. A crossover trial of bromocriptine in the treatment of vascular dementia. *Annals of Neurology*. 24: 270–272.

Nickels, J.L., Schneider, W.N., Dombovy, M.L. and Wong, T.M. 1994. Clinical use of amantadine in brain injury rehabilitation. *Brain Injury*. 8: 709–718.

Obeso, J.A. and Martinez-Lage, J.M. 1992. Anticholinergics and amantadine. In *Handbook of Parkinson's disease*, 2nd ed., ed. W.C. Koller, pp. 383–390. New York: Marcel Dekker.

Olanow, C.W. 1992. Protective treatment of Parkinson's disease. In *The scientific basis for the treatment of Parkinson's disease*, ed. C.W. Olanow and A.N. Lieberman, pp. 225–256. Park Ridge, New Jersey: Parthenon Publishing Group.

Ott, B.R. and Lannon, M.C. 1992. Exacerbation of parkinsonism by tacrine. *Clinical Neuropharmacology*. 15: 322–325.

Parkinson Study Group. 1989. Effect of (-)deprenyl in the progression of disability in early Parkinson's disease. *New England Journal of Medicine*. 321: 1364–1371.

Parkinson Study Group. 1993. Effects of tocopherol and deprenyl on the progression of disability in early Parkinson's disease. *New England Journal of Medicine*. 328: 176–183.

Parnetti, L., Lowenthal, D.T., Presciutti, O., Pellicccioli, G.P., Palumbo, R., Gobbi, G., Chiarinin, P., Palumbo, B., Tarducci, R. and Senin, U. 1996. 1H-MRS, MRI-based hippocampal volumetry and 99mTc-MPAO-SPECT in normal aging, age-associated memory impairment and probable Alzheimer's disease. *Journal of the American Geriatrics Society*. 44: 133–138.

Patel, S.V., Tariot, P.N. and Asnis, J. 1996. L-deprenyl augmentation of fluoxetine in a patient with Huntington's disease. *Annals of Clinical Psychiatry*. 8: 23–26.

Perry, E.K., Curtis, M., Dick, D.J., Candy, J.M., Atack, J.R., Bloxham, C.A., Blessed, G., Fairbairn, A., Tomlinson, B.E. and Perry, R.H. 1985. Cholinergic correlates of cognitive impairment in Parkinson's disease: Comparisons with Alzheimer's disease. *Journal of Neurology, Neurosurgery and Psychiatry*. 48: 413–421.

Petty, B.G., Cornblath, D.R., Adornato, B.T., Chaudhry, V., Flexner, C., Wachsman, M., Sinicropi, D., Burton, L.E. and Peroutka, S.J. 1994. The effect of systemically administered recombinant human nerve growth factor in healthy human subjects. *Annals of Neurology*. 36: 244–246.

Phelps, C.H., Gage, F.H., Growdon, J.H., Hefti, F., Harbaugh, R., Johnston, M.V., Khachaturian, Z.S., Mobley, W.C., Price, D.L., Raskind, M., Simpkins, J., Thal, L.J. and Woodcock, J. 1989. Potential use of nerve growth factor to treat Alzheimer's disease. *Neurobiology of Aging*. 10: 205–207.

Piccinin, G.L., Finali, G. and Piccirilli, M. 1990. Neuropsychological effects of L-deprenyl in Alzheimer's type dementia. *Clinical Neuropharmacology*. 13: 147–163.

Pillon, B., Dubois, B., Bonnet, A.-M., Esteguy, M., Guimaraes, J., Vigouret, J.M., Lhermitte, F. and Agid, Y. 1989. Cognitive slowing in Parkinson's disease fails to respond to levodopa treatment: the 15-objects test. *Neurology*. 39: 762–768.

Poewe, W., Berger, W., Benke, T. and Schelosky, L. 1991. High-speed memory scanning in Parkinson's disease: Adverse effects of levodopa. *Annals of Neurology*. 29: 670–673.

Riklan, M., Whelihan, W. and Cullinan, T. 1976. Levodopa and psychometric test performance in parkinsonism: 5 years later. *Neurology*. 26: 173–179.

Rogers, S.L., Doody, R., Mohs, R. and Friedhoff, L.T. 1996. E2020 produces both clinical global and cognitive test improvement in patients with mild to moderately severe Alzheimer's disease: results of a 30-week phase III trial. *Neurology*. 46: A217 (abstract).

Sadeh, M., Braham, J. and Modan, M. 1982. Effects of anticholinergic drugs on memory in Parkinson's disease. *Archives of Neurology*. 39: 666–667.

Sano, M., Ernesto, C., Thomas, R.G., Klauber, M.R., Schafer, K., Grundman, M., Woodbury, P., Growdon, J., Cotman, C.W., Pfeiffer, E., Schneider, L.S. and Thal, L.J. for the Members of the Alzheimer's Disease Cooperative Study. 1997. A controlled trial of selegiline, alpha-tocopherol or both as treatment for Alzheimer's disease. *New England Journal of Medicine*. 336: 1216–1222.

Sara, S.J., David-Remacle, M., Weyers, M. and Giurgea, C.E. 1979. Piracetam facilitates retrieval but does not impair extinction of bar-pressing in rats. *Psychopharmacology*. 61: 71–75.

Sarter, M. 1991. Taking stock of cognition enhancers. *Trends in Pharmacological Sciences*. 12: 456–461.

Schneider, L.S. and Olin, J.T. 1994. Overviews of clinical trials of hydergine in dementia. *Archives of Neurology*. 51: 787–798.

Schneider, L.S., Pollock, V.E., Zemansky, M.F., Gleason, R.P., Palmer, R. and Sloane, R.B. 1991. A pilot study of low-dose l-deprenyl in Alzheimer's disease. *Journal of Geriatric Psychiatry and Neurology*. 4: 143–148.

Simonetta, M., Schmitt, L., Montastruc, J.L. and Rascol, A. 1987. Neuropsychic side-effects of bromocriptine in Parkinson's disease. *Revue Neurologique*. 143: 608–611.

Smith, G., Ivnik, R.J., Petersen, R.C., Malec, J.F., Kokmen, E. and Tangalos, E.G. 1991. Age-associated memory impairment diagnoses: Problems of reliability and concerns for terminology. *Psychology and Aging*. 6: 551–558.

Stern, Y. and Langston, W. 1985. Intellectual changes in patients with MPTP-induced parkinsonism. *Neurology*. 35: 1506–1509.

Stern, Y., Mayeux, R., Ilson, J., Fahn, S. and Côté, L. 1984. Pergolide therapy for Parkinson's disease: Neurobehavioral changes. *Neurology*. 34: 201–204.

Stern, Y., Tetrud, J.W., Martin, W.R.W., Kutner, S.J. and Langston, J.W. 1990. Cognitive change following MPTP exposure. *Neurology*. 40: 261–264.

Tarczy, M. and Szirmai, I. 1995. Failure of dopamine metabolism: borderline of parkinsonism and dementia. *Acta Biomedica De L Ateneo Parmense*. 66: 93–97.

Tariot, P.N., Sunderland, T., Weingartner, H., Murphy, D.L. and Wolkowitz, J.A. 1987. Cognitive effects of L-deprenyl in Alzheimer's disease. *Psychopharmacology*. 91: 489–495.

Terry, R.D., Masliah, E., Salmon, D.P., Butters, N., DeTeresa, R., Hill, F., Hansen, L.A. and Katzman, R. 1991. Physical basis of cognitive alterations in Alzheimer's disease: Synapse loss is the major correlate of cognitive impairment. *Annals of Neurology*. 30: 572–580.

Thal, L.J. 1994. Clinical trials in Alzheimer's disease. In *Alzheimer disease*, ed. R.D. Terry, R. Katzman and K.L. Bick, pp. 431–444. New York: Raven Press.

Thal, L.J., Carta, A., Clarek, W.R., Ferris, S.H., Friedland, R.P., Petersen, R.C., Pettegrew, J.W., Pfeiffer, E., Raskind, M.A., Sano, M., Tuszynki, M.H. and Woolson, R.F. 1996. A 1-year multicenter placebo-controlled study of acetyl–1–carnitine in patients with Alzheimer's disease. *Neurology*. 47: 705–711.

Thompson, T.L., Filley, C.M., Mitchell, W.D., Culig, K.M., LoVerde, M. and Byyny, R.L. 1990. Lack of efficacy of hydergine in patients with Alzheimer's disease. *New England Journal of Medicine*. 323: 445–458.

Tierney, M.C., Szalai, J.P., Snow, W.G., Fisher, R.H., Nores, A., Nadon, G., Dunn, E. and St. George-Hyslop, P.H. 1996. Prediction of probable Alzheimer's disease in memory-impaired patients: A prospective longitudinal study. *Neurology*. 46: 661–665.

Tröster, A.I., Beatty, W.W., Staton, R.D. and Rorabaugh, A.G. 1989. Effects of scopolamine on anterograde and remote memory in humans. *Psychobiology*. 17: 12–18.

Uitti, R.J., Rajput, A.H., Ahlskog, J.E., Offord, K.P., Schroeder, D.R., Ho, M.M., Prasad, M., Rajput, A. and Basran, P. 1996. Amantadine treatment is an independent predictor of improved survival in Parkinson's disease. *Neurology*. 46: 1551–1556.

Youngjohn, J.R., Larrabee, G.J. and Crook, T.H. 1992. Discriminating age-associated memory impairment from Alzheimer's disease. *Psychological Assessment*. 1: 54–59.

Yuen, E.C. and Mobley, W.C. 1996. Therapeutic potential of neurotrophic factors for neurologic disorders. *Annals of Neurology*. 40: 346–354.

22

Surgical interventions in neurodegenerative disease: impact on memory and cognition

STEVEN B. WILKINSON
AND ALEXANDER I. TRÖSTER

INTRODUCTION

Surgical interventions for neurodegenerative diseases can be conceived as falling into three broad categories: ablative procedures, transplantation procedures and procedures involving cerebral implantation of chronic electrical stimulation devices. Procedures involving the implantation of drug delivery systems are better considered 'augmentative procedures', because signs and symptoms of the disease are not alleviated by the surgical intervention per se. All surgical interventions for neurodegenerative diseases are typically considered potential therapeutic options only after medical therapies either have failed to adequately control a patient's signs and symptoms, or have brought about intolerable side-effects.

Functional neurosurgical treatments have been attempted in numerous neurodegenerative conditions, including Alzheimer's disease (AD), Huntington's disease (HD), Parkinson's disease (PD), multiple sclerosis and amyotrophic lateral sclerosis. Attempts to improve or restore functioning in AD by experimental means such as intracranial implantation of cholinergic drug delivery systems (Harbaugh et al. 1984), or chronic electrical stimulation of the nucleus basalis of Meynert (Turnbull et al. 1985), have failed and been abandoned. AD, amyotrophic lateral sclerosis, multiple sclerosis, HD and PD are among neurodegenerative conditions envisioned as potentially treatable by transplantation of a variety of tissues and cells, including perhaps cells from the patient genetically engineered ex vivo, or genetically engineered cells from other species (xenografts) (e.g. Ffrench-Constant et al. 1994; Aebischer et al. 1996). Research using genetically engineered cells remains directed almost exclusively at experimental animal models of these disorders.

Autologous adrenal tissue transplantation in PD patients has been largely abandoned due to unsatisfactory results, but the efficacy of fetal tissue grafts is currently being evaluated in PD and HD. These fetal tissue transplantation studies indicate that many hurdles still need to be overcome before such treatments become commonplace. Preclinical and clinical issues requiring resolution are too numerous to review here and readers are referred to a recent review by Olanow et al. (1997).

Neurosurgical interventions for neurodegenerative conditions involving ablation and electrical stimulation are most often used to treat movement disorders. As PD is the most widely surgically treated neurodegenerative disorder, this chapter will primarily address this topic. After briefly reviewing the history of the surgical treatment of movement disorders, we describe different surgical procedures and their underlying rationale and indications. The chapter concludes with a review of the effects which surgical interventions have on memory.

A BRIEF OVERVIEW OF THE HISTORY OF MOVEMENT DISORDERS SURGERY

Neurosurgical interventions for movement disorders were already undertaken in the late nineteenth and early twentieth centuries. Early ablative procedures typically targeted the pyramidal motor system. For example, Horsley extirpated motor cortex to treat athetosis as early as 1890 (Laitinen 1995), although his first report was not published until 1909. Open, ablative procedures targeting the extrapyramidal system were first carried out in the early 1940s, but were associated with considerable morbidity. The results of apparently safer stereotactic procedures tar-

geting the ansa lenticularis, globus pallidus and thalamus were not reported until the 1950s. Meyers, Talairach, Leksell and Spiegel and Wycis, among others, pioneered the stereotactic surgical treatment of PD and other movement disorders. Not only did their initiative bring to the forefront procedures yielding functional improvement to patients who had failed to benefit from all other therapy, but the study of these patients yielded important insights into the role of the thalamus and basal ganglia in movement and cognition. The popularity of movement disorder surgeries peaked in the 1950s and 1960s, but decreased dramatically with the introduction in the late 1960s of levodopa for the treatment of parkinsonism (e.g. van Manen et al. 1984).

Several factors account for the recent renaissance of surgical treatment of movement disorders and particularly PD. These include an acknowledgment of the limitations and complications of medical treatments, the development of new neuroimaging, stereotactic and electrophysiological recording and stimulation techniques, and a burgeoning understanding of basal ganglia physiology.

PATHOPHYSIOLOGY OF PARKINSON'S DISEASE AND THE RATIONALE FOR SURGICAL INTERVENTIONS

A detailed discussion of the pathophysiology of movement disorders is beyond the scope of this chapter and readers are referred to reviews by Albin (1995) and Vitek (1997). In extremely simplified terms, the basal ganglia and cerebellum send outputs via the thalamus to cortical motor and premotor areas. Basal ganglia pathophysiology underlying PD is related to a reduction in striatal dopamine. This reduction in dopamine is thought to have opposite effects on transmission in the direct and indirect (via globus pallidus externa and subthalamic nucleus) pathways between striatum and globus pallidus interna. Specifically, there is reduced transmission in the direct pathway between the striatum and globus pallidus interna, manifesting in decreased inhibition of globus pallidus interna and increased transmission in the indirect pathway, resulting in increased stimulation of globus pallidus interna. The net effect of alterations in transmission in the direct and indirect pathways is the same, namely, an overactivity of globus pallidus interna. This overactivity results in excessive tonic and phasic inhibition by globus pallidus interna of the thalamocortical neurons.

Given even this oversimplified account of basal ganglia pathophysiology in PD, the theoretical rationale for increasing striatal dopamine by implanting in the striatum either catecholamine-secreting adrenal chromaffin cells or dopamine-producing embryonic mesencephalic tissue, seems obvious. Similarly obvious, at least on a superficial level, is the surgical targeting of globus pallidus interna, thalamus and subthalamus, given the role of these structures in the pathophysiology of PD. It is worth emphasizing at this point, however, that even detailed models of basal ganglia physiology and movement disorders have considerable difficulty in accounting for the observed clinical effects of surgical interventions. For example, the paradox that globus pallidus interna and thalamic lesions enhance voluntary and reduce unwanted movements in PD, when in fact such lesions would be predicted to have the opposite effect, remains to be explained (Marsden and Obeso 1994). Similarly, current models of movement disorders cannot adequately account for the clinical observations that parkinsonian signs respond differentially to thalamic, subthalamic and pallidal lesions; that subthalamic lesions, for example, do not typically result in hyperkinetic conditions such as ballism; and that stimulation of globus pallidus interna by different electrical poles (only millimeters apart on a quadripolar electrode) can have variable and even opposite effects on movements (Kuntzer et al. 1996). It would appear, then, that basal ganglia physiology is considerably more complex than envisioned by current theoretical models and that theoretical models and clinical studies of movement disorder surgery might come to enjoy a symbiotic relationship. Whereas the evolution of basal ganglia physiology and movement disorder models has in part provided the impetus for modern neurosurgical treatments of movement disorders, clinical outcome studies of such treatments might dictate and drive the re-evaluation and refinement of theoretical models.

SURGICAL INTERVENTIONS AND THEIR INDICATIONS

Transplant procedures and their potential indications are not described here. Although autologous adrenal medulla and sympathetic ganglion were used for neural transplantation in PD, these procedures have essentially been discontinued as the improvements in motor function are not maintained and graft survival is poor (Goetz et al.

Table 22.1. *Summary of indications for current surgical therapies for movement disorders*

	Thalamotomy	Thalamic stimulation	Pallidotomy	Pallidal stimulation
Parkinson's disease – tremor	I	A (especially second side)	C (especially if other procedures fail)	NI
Parkinson's disease – motor fluctuations and dyskinesias	C (especially if other procedures fail)	NI	I	A (especially for second side)
Parkinson's disease – gait imbalance, swallowing dysfunction	NI	NI	NI	NI
Essential tremor	I	I (especially for second side)	NI	NI
Other tremor unresponsive to medication	I	C (especially for second side)	NI	NI

Note:
A: alternative therapy; C: consider this therapy in certain situations; I: indicated; NI: not indicated.

1990; Itakura et al. 1994). Fetal mesencephalic tissue grafts are being carried out on an experimental basis for PD (Lindvall 1995) and HD (Madrazo et al. 1995), but despite the technique's promise, considerable practical and ethical problems remain to be resolved.

General considerations

Potential candidates for any of the surgical procedures described below should always be first evaluated by a neurologist experienced in movement disorders. This evaluation serves to rule out parkinson-plus syndromes (which do not respond to surgery) and to ensure that the patient has been properly treated from a medical standpoint (i.e. further medical treatment appears unwarranted). Evaluation should also indicate whether a patient can medically tolerate the surgery. As the major risk in all stereotactic surgery is hemorrhage, either on the surface of the brain (subdural hematoma) or in the brain parenchyma (intraparenchymal hematoma), patients should be screened for bleeding disorders. Finally, the patient and family should be made aware of the objectives and limitations of surgery and of the possible complications. As a rule, the outcome of lesioning procedures is thought to be more satisfactory in younger and cognitively intact patients.

Considerations in anatomical target selection

Multiple targets (thalamus, subthalamus, globus pallidus) have been lesioned or stimulated in an effort to improve movement disorders (for a review, see Obeso et al. 1997). As these surgical procedures typically ameliorate different aspects of the movement disorder (e.g. tremor, rigidity, akinesia and/or dyskinesia), different surgical interventions are indicated by the patient's predominant motor signs. As a rule, lesioning and stimulation of a given anatomical structure affect the same motor signs. Table 22.1 summarizes current indications for different surgical procedures in essential tremor and PD.

Procedures targeting the thalamus are principally used to treat extremity tremor (Alesch 1995; Alesch et al. 1995), although some investigators have also reported improvement of levodopa-induced dyskinesias, rigidity and bradykinesia with thalamotomy in PD. The tremor in PD and essential tremor responds to thalamotomy in 95% of patients (and, typically, the more distal the tremor, the better the response), while tremor secondary to multiple sclerosis, cerebrovascular disease and trauma responds less reliably (Burchiel 1995). The functional improvement conveyed by tremor control in essential tremor and PD might, however, differ. Functional improvement in essen-

tial tremor might be greater than in PD (except in a subset of 'tremor-predominant' PD patients) because the tremor in severe essential tremor is the sole determinant of marked functional limitations. Most PD patients, in contrast, are more functionally limited by rigidity, akinesia, motor fluctuations and dyskinesias than by tremor.

Levodopa-induced dyskinesias are the primary symptom alleviated by procedures targeting the globus pallidus interna, although rigidity, bradykinesia, tremor and gait dysfunction have occasionally also been reported to improve after pallidotomy (Dogali et al. 1995; Iacono et al. 1995; Johansson et al. 1997; Laitinen et al. 1992). The best candidate for pallidotomy is probably the younger PD patient with severe dyskinesia. Siegfried and Lippitz (1994) reported that pallidal deep brain stimulation conveys a functional benefit similar to pallidotomy but without significant morbidity. A.M. Lozano (personal communication) has extensive, favorable experience with pallidal deep brain stimulation, but mostly in the context of pallidal deep brain stimulation contralateral to successful prior pallidotomy. At our center we recently reported the favorable outcome in five PD patients treated with pallidal deep brain stimulation (three bilateral, two unilateral) (Pahwa et al. 1997).

Subthalamic stimulation has recently received increasing attention as a treatment for refractory PD. As the reported patient series are small (e.g. Limousin et al. 1995), the apparent efficacy of this procedure in alleviating parkinsonian akinesia and rigidity remains to be confirmed.

Considerations in selecting ablation versus stimulation procedures

Unfortunately there is a finality to ablation procedures: motor and behavioral effects of the surgical lesion cannot be reversed. If inadequate improvement is conferred by the procedure, further surgery might only occasionally augment the minimal initial improvement in motor signs. Furthermore, although surgical treatment can improve motor function bilaterally, the most profound effect is observed contralateral to the side of the surgery. In the case of patients with significant residual motor dysfunction on the side ipsilateral to the initial surgery, there is often a desire to perform surgery on the second side. Unfortunately, there is an increased risk of cognitive deficits after bilateral relative to unilateral lesioning procedures and this fact has to be weighed in deciding whether to recommend a second operation.

The development of deep brain stimulation procedures promises to address the problems of potential inadequate benefit or adverse side-effects associated with lesioning operations. Stimulation parameters can be modified to produce different responses or eliminate side-effects. The potential reversibility of side-effects is a feature deemed especially desirable in patients undergoing bilateral surgery. For example, there is tentative evidence that thalamic deep brain stimulation might be preferable to thalamotomy (Tasker, 1998) and that pallidal deep brain stimulation entails little if any morbidity relative to pallidotomy (Kumar et al. 1997). Stimulation procedures have the added appeal that, should restorative therapies become available, such therapies' potential utility would not be compromised by a surgical lesion in the basal ganglia. The potential disadvantages of stimulation involve device failure, the need for electrode repositioning, the cost of the device and the need to replace stimulator batteries. If further work confirms the initially reported efficacy and safety of deep brain stimulation, it may become a very attractive alternative to lesioning operations.

General description of surgical procedures targeting thalamus and pallidum

A localizing device (stereotactic frame) is attached to the head of the patient before undergoing brain imaging. Computed tomography (CT), magnetic resonance imaging (MRI) and ventriculography are used by different centers. CT and MRI are as reliable as ventriculography in locating the initial target and they avoid patient confusion and discomfort associated with intraventricular air and contrast studies (Alterman et al. 1995). From the obtained image, the anterior commissure-posterior commissure (AC-PC) line is found and the initial target location is calculated based in part on AC-PC line length to take into account anatomical variation from one patient to another. It is debated whether imaging studies alone are sufficient to reliably determine the precise target location and additional physiological target confirmation is sought by most surgeons.

Two means of intraoperative physiological target confirmation are commonly used: macro- and/or microelectrode recording and/or stimulation. A lack of comparative studies precludes resolution of the debate about which of these techniques is preferable. Macroelectrode techniques are fast and easy to use, but less reliable in locating specific nuclei. Microelectrode techniques, in contrast, allow very accurate localization of different nuclei and their borders, but are more time consuming and

difficult to perform because of electrical interference in the operating room.

In locating the thalamic target, transient paresthesias and decreased tremor in the affected extremity in response to high frequency macroelectrode stimulation are sought to physiologically confirm the exact location within the thalamus. Low frequency macroelectrode stimulation of the same site may drive the tremor. Microelectrode recordings allow recognition of individual thalamic nuclei. The ventral intermediate nucleus of the thalamus is the commonest target for tremor control and can be located by finding cells that respond to deep muscle stimulation and cells that fire in synchrony with the tremor. The ventral intermediate nucleus is bounded posteriorly by the ventral posterior medial and lateral nuclei (ventral caudal nucleus) and the recognition of cells that respond to tactile stimulation signify this nuclear complex and thus, the ventral intermediate nucleus posterior border.

Micro-electrode recording is also useful in locating the posterior ventral globus pallidus interna, the typical target in pallidotomy and pallidal stimulation. The globus pallidus interna is bounded by the optic tract inferiorly, the internal capsule posteriorly and medially and by the globus pallidus externa laterally. Microelectrode recording techniques accurately differentiate cells in the internal and external globus pallidus by their inherent firing patterns. Areas of white matter, such as the optic tract and the lamina between the external and internal pallidum, can also be readily delineated by microelectrode recording. Microstimulation can be used to identify the optic tract and internal capsule. Differentiation of gray from white matter is also achieved by recording changes in impedance with a macroelectrode. Responses to macrostimulation are commonly used to avoid visual field cuts and hemiparesis/hemisensory losses associated with optic tract and internal capsule lesions, respectively.

The thalamotomy and pallidotomy lesion is usually made with a radio-frequency probe. After a thalamic lesion is produced (usually in the ventral intermediate nucleus) there should be immediate tremor reduction. Persistence of tremor reduction 3 months after operation suggests that the tremor will probably not recur. If the tremor returns within 3 months, reoperation to increase the size of the lesion may be warranted. In the case of pallidotomy, the lesion is most often placed in globus pallidus interna as lesions exclusively of globus pallidus externa may worsen PD symptoms. Some, however, have proposed making the primary lesion

in this area (L.V. Laitinen, personal communication) and debate continues regarding the optimal site and size of pallidal lesions (Favre et al. 1996).

Complications from thalamotomy can be divided into those that are inherent to stereotactic procedures and those that are related to the lesion itself. Hemorrhage, infection and seizures are risks inherent to all stereotactic procedures. Lesioning complications result from lesions made too far laterally (resulting in damage to the internal capsule and thus hemiparesis), too far posteriorly (resulting in sensory deficit), too medially (resulting in hypophonia) or too far inferiorly (resulting in hemiballismus). Fortunately, the rate of such complications is low (Burchiel 1995), although bilateral lesions increase the risk of complications and especially of cognitive dysfunction. To minimize this risk, bilateral operations are often staged, with most surgeons waiting a year between operating on the two sides.

Stereotactic pallidotomy entails risks similar to those of thalamotomy, but the risk of hemorrhage may be greater because the pallidal region is more vascularized than the thalamus (R.G. Grossman, personal communication). Complications related to pallidal lesions include visual field loss (the lesion is too inferior to the target), hemiparesis or hemisensory loss (the lesion is too medial or posterior) and worsening of parkinsonian symptoms (the lesion, theoretically, is too lateral). The risks involved in bilateral relative to unilateral pallidotomies remains debated. Whereas some groups perform bilateral procedures in stages, others perform them simultaneously (Iacono et al. 1997).

Thalamic and pallidal stimulation

The procedure for deep brain stimulation device implantation is similar to the lesioning procedures, except that instead of creating a lesion in the desired area, an electrode is implanted. This electrode can be controlled by an external stimulation system, or by an internalized system (as used with cardiac pacemakers or dorsal column stimulation systems for pain control). The stimulation lead most often used has four individual electrode contacts spaced over a distance of 10 mm. Different electrode pairs, or groups of electrodes, can be chosen as the anode or cathode. The stimulator case can also act as the cathode. Stimulation amplitude, rate and pulse width can all be adjusted by interrogating the device with a programming wand held over the implanted stimulator.

EFFECTS OF MOVEMENT DISORDER SURGERY ON MEMORY AND COGNITION

We focus here on the effects of movement disorder surgeries on memory. Readers interested in, for example, an overview of the effects of surgical treatments on language, are referred to other sources (e.g. Crosson 1984).

Thalamotomy

Burchiel (1995) estimates that speech/language and memory difficulties occur in up to 39% of movement disordered patients after thalamotomy and that these changes are more common after bilateral than unilateral thalamotomy (60% and 31%, respectively). Cognitive outcome in early and modern thalamotomy series might be different, but direct comparisons are complicated, if not precluded, by several factors. Early and modern thalamotomy studies differ in at least three important respects: patient characteristics, surgical target and procedure and the extent to which cognitive outcome was formally evaluated.

Patients undergoing thalamotomy three or four decades ago are different from the patients undergoing thalamotomy today. Patients today probably represent a much more select group, namely that group with the most advanced and medically refractory disease. Early studies included not only patients with idiopathic PD (not treated with levodopa), but in some instances also patients with 'arteriopathic' and postencephalitic parkinsonism (Selby 1967), two conditions which are clinically and neuropathologically distinct from idiopathic PD.

The target for lesioning or stimulation in today's operations is different and much smaller. Furthermore, lesion parameters were sometimes varied in early thalamotomies not to 'tailor' the lesion to the patient's primary symptoms, but in an attempt to empirically establish the effects of different lesion parameters on tremor and other aspects of PD. Early studies also used both thermal and chemical lesioning techniques and there is an indication that chemical lesioning might be accompanied by greater cognitive impairment (Levita et al. 1964).

Estimates of the incidence of cognitive morbidity associated with early thalamotomy are typically based on subjective ratings by the physician and/or patient and the early studies were not usually designed to discern subtle changes in cognition and memory. Interpretive difficulties inherent in the subjective assessment of cognition are compounded by the use of inconsistent and vague terminology. Spiegel et al. (1955) already noted disturbances in memory, orientation and time sense (chronotaraxis) after bilateral thalamotomy, but the precise meaning of other authors' subsequent terminology (e.g. 'psycho organic syndrome', 'cognitive defects' or 'disorientation') is unclear. Detailed neuropsychological evaluations, when carried out, were often limited to small samples. Many studies suffer from significant subject attrition at follow-up, thus subjecting them to selection biases.

Early studies of memory in thalamotomized PD patients most often reported declines in memory (especially verbal memory) after left and bilateral thalamotomy, although these declines in memory typically were transient and more likely to be observed soon after surgery. In contrast, right thalamotomy was typically associated with no change or an improvement in memory, although it is frequently unclear whether statistically significant improvements in average test scores were clinically significant and in excess of any expected practice effects. Shapiro et al. (1973) administered, among other tests, the Wechsler Memory Scale (WMS) to 44 PD patients before and 2 weeks after unilateral thalamotomy and again to 25 of the 44 patients an average of 17 months after surgery. Two weeks after surgery, relative to preoperative baseline, left thalamotomy patients evidenced significant declines in memory quotient and, in particular, in the Mental Control (attention), Logical Memory (prose recall), Verbal Paired Associates and 'delayed memory' scores. In contrast, the right thalamotomy group showed significant gains in memory quotient and Logical Memory score. By long-term follow-up, however, the only remaining significant finding was the left thalamotomy group's decline on the Logical Memory subtest of the WMS.

Similar findings were reported by Krayenbühl et al. (1965). Using the German version of the WMS, they found that a group of 10 PD patients who underwent thalamotomy in the 'dominant' hemisphere evidenced declines in memory quotient, Logical Memory and Verbal Paired Associates scores which were evident 6 months after surgery. In contrast, a group of 10 PD patients who underwent thalamotomy in the 'nondominant' hemisphere, demonstrated postsurgical improvements in immediate visual memory (presumably Visual Reproduction scores). Perret and Siegfried (1969) evaluated 28 PD patients before, 6 and 18 months after unilateral thalamotomy. Unlike others, they found both right and left thalamotomy to be associated with declines on several subtests of a

German version of the WMS: immediate and delayed recall of prose passages, immediate recall of verbal paired associates (which improved, but not significantly, 18 months after surgery), delayed recall of easy verbal paired associates (significant in the left thalamotomy group) and delayed recall of hard verbal paired associates (with slight recovery in both groups 18 months after surgery). Furthermore, immediate recognition of nonsense figures declined in both groups (slightly more so in the right thalamotomy group), although delayed recognition of the figures declined only in the right thalamotomy group. (*See also* Asso et al. 1969.)

Left and/or bilateral thalamotomy has also been associated with declines on verbal memory tasks other than the WMS: the Peterson and Peterson short-term memory task (Ojemann et al. 1971); sentence learning (McFie 1960); digit span (McFie 1960; Riklan et al. 1960); and paired associates (Almgren et al. 1969; *see also* Kocher et al. 1982). The effects of thalamotomy on nonverbal memory measures have been less studied and the findings are inconsistent. Several studies reported no declines in nonverbal memory after thalamotomy. Vilkki and Laitinen (1974, 1976), despite finding right thalamotomy to be associated with visuoperceptual (facial matching) deficits, did not find impairments in facial recognition memory. Similarly, in Shapiro et al.'s (1973) study, although right thalamotomy patients showed declines in 'nonverbal performance' measures from an intelligence scale, they did not evidence declines on nonverbal memory measures of the WMS. In Riklan et al.'s (1966) report, no post-operative deficits were reported in memory for pictures and pure tones. Other studies, in contrast, reported either improvements in visual memory after nondominant (usually right) hemisphere thalamotomy (Krayenbühl et al. 1965), declines in visual memory after left thalamotomy (Jurko and Andy 1964), or declines in visual memory after both left and right thalamotomy (Perret and Siegfried 1969). Several other studies' findings are difficult to interpret because specific enough results were not reported (Riklan and Levita 1970) or only pre-operative results were reported (McFie 1960).

Exactly when memory deficits might resolve in thalamotomized PD patients remains unclear, although the preponderance of studies seems to show that deficits, when present, certainly resolve earlier than 1.5 years after surgery. Most of the memory deficits observed by Shapiro et al. (1973) had resolved by an average of 17 months after surgery. The deficits in paired associate learning observed by Almgren et al. (1969) were found to have resolved by 10

months after surgery (Almgren et al. 1972) and Hays et al. (1966) failed to find declines in paired associate learning (albeit a different version than that used by others) even 4 months after surgery. Jurko and Andy (1973), in a series of thalamotomy patients (with a variety of diagnoses including PD), found that verbal paired associate learning deficits persisted up to a year after surgery, but that only lesions outside the centromedian nucleus were associated with such declines. At the other extreme are reports by Perret and Siegfried (1969) who found memory deficits in their patients still 18 months after surgery. Van Buren et al. (1973) reported that among 78 unilateral thalamotomy PD patients, four left thalamotomy patients, despite some recovery, had sufficiently severe memory problems to preclude independent functioning up to 7 years after surgery.

In the more recent thalamotomy series memory complications seem to be rarer. One factor that might account for this is that more extensive intraoperative cognitive and motor function testing is performed and this may alter where and how large a lesion is made. Furthermore, careful preoperative neuropsychological evaluations are probably more commonly undertaken to exclude from surgical treatment those patients at greatest risks for poor cognitive outcome (i.e. older patients and patients with pre-existing or incipient dementia). Rossitch et al. (1988) attempted to identify factors which might predispose to cognitive impairment after thalamotomy. They concluded that more profound or bilateral neurological involvement, prior thalamotomy and CT-evident tissue loss were associated with poorer memory and language outcomes. The conclusions drawn do, however, need to be viewed with circumspection due to rather serious methodological limitations of the study. As the sample is small (18 patients), several potential confounding variables cannot be held constant or controlled for while examining the influence of a given variable on memory and language. Specifically, patients were heterogeneous in diagnosis (including PD, post-traumatic movement disorders, multiple sclerosis, congenital dystonia and 'postapoplectic' movement disorder), follow-up interval was variable (ranging from 2 days to 40 weeks), and the test battery was idiosyncratic. Although a decline in three tests of the 'memory and language protocol' was defined as constituting a significant decline, it was not specified what constituted a significant change in a given test score. It is apparent that of the seven of 18 patients experiencing significant memory and/or language declines, only one had PD. As most of the seven patients with cognitive decline had multiple sclerosis or post-traumatic tremor, one might conclude that possibly significant preoperative cognitive impairment predisposes to further cognitive declines after thalamotomy. Poor cognitive outcome in multiple sclerosis was also observed in two other studies (Blumetti and Modesti 1980; Wester and Hauglie-Hanssen 1990).

In a series of 36 PD patients followed-up for an average of 33 months after thalamotomy (one bilateral, 35 unilateral), Fox et al. (1991) found that five patients had persistent postoperative morbidity (dyspraxia, dysarthria, dysphasia, cognitive dysfunction); however, the morbidity was severe enough to curtail functional independence in only two patients. One of the patients had cognitive impairment and cerebral atrophy before surgery. It is noteworthy that the lesions produced in this series are somewhat smaller than in the older series and lesion location was adjusted if speech problems were detected during intraoperative testing. In a recent study detailing formal neuropsychological evaluation results, Lund-Johansen et al. (1996) reported no decrements in memory in 53 PD patients 3 months after unilateral thalamotomy (28 right, 25 left). Indeed, relative to their preoperative performance, both right and left thalamotomy groups demonstrated an improvement on a dichotic verbal memory test, but only for words presented to the left ear. No changes were observed on a facial recognition memory test.

Thalamotomy effects on memory in nonparkinsonian patients (e.g. multiple sclerosis, post-traumatic tremor, essential tremor, intention tremor) have not been well studied or documented. Blumetti and Modesti (1980) found that among five familial tremor and five multiple sclerosis patients, declines were observed 3–4 weeks after surgery in verbal and nonverbal memory, with left thalamotomy associated with verbal declines and right thalamotomy with nonverbal memory declines. By 12–24 months follow-up the familial tremor patients' cognitive difficulties had resolved and, in fact, some improvement in cognition relative to baseline was observed. The five multiple sclerosis patients, however, were found to have suffered marked and persistent cognitive (including memory) declines. The cognitive declines observed in multiple sclerosis patients after thalamotomy would be consistent with the observations of Rossitch et al. (1988) and Wester and Hauglie-Hanssen (1990). In Goldman et al.'s (1992) series of eight essential tremor patients, two patients had a postoperative 'verbal cognitive deficit' (one transient, one persistent), described as clinically nonsymptomatic and

detectable only on formal psychometric evaluation. Goldman and Kelly (1992), reporting thalamotomy outcome in patients with refractory intention tremor due to either multiple sclerosis, trauma or stroke, observed transient postoperative 'cognitive dysfunction' in one of 14 patients and this deficit was again described as mild and detectable only on psychometric testing. Overall, it appears that modern thalamotomy, especially unilateral operation, carries relatively little risk for memory dysfunction; however, in patients who have pre-existing or progressive cognitive impairment, the risk for postoperative memory dysfunction might be greater.

Thalamic and subthalamic stimulation

Findings pertaining to cognitive outcome of thalamic stimulation are considered highly preliminary, as only two reports with small numbers of PD patients have been published (Caparros-Lefebvre et al. 1992; Tröster et al. 1997b). Average neuropsychological test scores of nine patients did not change significantly from baseline to 10–14 days after surgery in the Caparros-Lefebvre et al. study. On almost all tests, however, some patients showed slight declines, others no change and yet others showed mild improvements. Tröster et al. (1997b) also found outcome to be variable in their series of nine patients evaluated before and 3 months after deep brain stimulation electrode implantation. When average scores were examined, no significant declines were observed. Significant improvements were found in delayed recognition (discriminability) of a word list and delayed recall of prose passages. There was also a trend toward improved visual confrontation naming. Examining individual patient test score changes, Tröster et al. (1997b) found changes of one standard deviation to be rare and changes of two standard deviations to be even rarer, which suggests that changes in cognition are typically not of clinical significance; however, improvements in scores were more common than decrements. It is unclear, if effects of deep brain stimulation electrode implantation on cognition are observed, whether they represent effects of a 'micro thalamotomy', or the effects of stimulation per se. On the basis of a single case tested rather extensively with the stimulator turned on and off, Tröster et al. (1997a) raised the hypothesis that stimulation itself might be associated with subtle improvements in semantic memory, but subtle decrements in episodic memory.

The effects of subthalamic stimulation on memory and cognition remain to be adequately evaluated and documented. In a preliminary report, Limousin et al. (1995)

observed that, among three PD patients, one developed transient confusion and hallucinations and one a frontal syndrome (ascribed to thalamic infarction) after bilateral subthalamic stimulator implantation. Von Falkenhayn et al. (1997) reported that subthalamic and pallidal stimulation might disrupt aspects of procedural learning and memory.

Pallidotomy

The neuropsychological outcome of pallidotomy remains understudied (Kuntzer et al. 1996). There are no reports of formally evaluated cognitive outcome in large series of pallidotomy patients. Among early studies, Spiegel and Wycis (1954) reported a 21% incidence of transitory disturbances in consciousness. Ten per cent of patients had postoperative 'psychic' disturbances, consisting of confusion, memory disturbance, emotional instability/depression and apraxia. Based on patient report, Svennilson et al. (1960) found that among 78 unilateral pallidotomy cases four had persistent mild dementia and 11 had severe memory impairment. All three bilateral pallidotomy cases are reported to have had 'disorders of this type'. The proportion of cases in which memory disturbances reflected the effects of the operation as opposed to progressing disease is unclear.

Memory evaluation data were not reported by Laitinen et al. (1992) in the study credited with the renaissance of pallidotomy. A large number of preliminary studies are beginning to now appear about the cognitive effects of pallidotomy. In the first published pilot study, Baron et al. (1996) reported neuropsychological evaluation data for 12 of 15 unilateral pallidotomy patients. They found that the Dementia Rating Scale memory score, as well as the California Verbal Learning Test delayed recognition (discriminability) score declined from baseline to 1-year follow-up. These changes are probably not clinically remarkable however, and furthermore, once the data from two patients experiencing postoperative complications (small frontal subdural hematomas) were excluded, memory changes were no longer evident in the remaining sample. Although Fazzini et al. (1995) did not present memory data, their study is noteworthy for inclusion of a control group and it highlights an important issue. While the operated PD group did not show significant changes on a cognitive screening examination (Mini Mental Status Exam) 3 months after pallidotomy, the group did not demonstrate the improvements (presumably practice effects) on the MMSE shown by an unoperated PD control group. Thus, an important interpretive issue for any surgi-

cal outcome study becomes whether an absence of changes in measures of cognitive function reflects a true lack of change, or actually a mild deterioration. (*See also* Alterman and Kelly 1998; Louw and Burchiel 1998.)

Several recent papers and conference presentations based on small samples indicate that unilateral pallidotomy may carry with it relatively little risk for memory dysfunction, particularly if patients are carefully screened for pre-existing cognitive impairment. It appears that centers generally are not finding significant changes in memory in patients after unilateral pallidotomy, regardless of whether or not physiological recording is used to define the surgical target (Cahn et al. 1997, in press; Cullum et al. 1997; Green et al. 1997; Soukup et al. 1997; Uitti et al. 1997). Significant changes in cognition (including memory and verbal fluency) have been reported by a center which does not exclude patients from surgery on the basis of age or significant pre-existing cognitive impairment (Riordan et al. 1997). Whereas motor outcome in that patient series was independent of age or baseline cognitive impairment, it was not reported whether cognitive outcome was a function of age or baseline cognitive impairment. This raises the possibility that the clinician faces a vexing issue in treating the elderly, cognitively impaired patient, namely, do benefits of motor improvement outweigh the cost of cognitive deterioration?

Separation of patient groups into those having undergone left and right pallidotomy may yield findings which are not evident in combined groups (Kumar et al. 1997; Riordan et al. 1997). In a sizeable cohort (40 patients), pallidotomy was associated with significant laterality-specific memory impairments (often resolving within 6 months), meaning that left pallidotomy lead to verbal memory decrements whereas right pallidotomy lead to nonverbal memory impairments (Kumar et al. 1997). Another unresolved issue concerns the cognitive risk posed by bilateral pallidotomy. Iacono et al. (1997) reported statistically significant improvements in mean Wechsler Memory Scale-Revised (WMS-R) index scores in 10 bilateral pallidotomy patients after surgery. Unfortunately, because mean scores were not presented and WMS-R index score changes have to be of considerable magnitude before being considered clinically significant, it remains unclear whether score changes were meaningful, or if they even approached the magnitude of the typical practice (test-retest) gain. Others (e.g. Gálvez-Jiménez et al. 1996) have reported considerable cognitive morbidity after bilateral pallidotomy.

Pallidal stimulation

The effects of pallidal stimulation on memory and cognition are only beginning to be documented. Fields et al. (1997) and Tröster et al. (1997d) evaluated nine patients undergoing unilateral (six left, three right) pallidal deep brain stimulation electrode implantation before and 3 months after surgery. Patients were tested while in their self-reported 'best on' state and with the stimulator on after surgery. As a group, the patients showed significant decrements only in semantic (categorical) verbal fluency and on a visuo-constructional task. In examining changes in test scores of individual patients, one patient demonstrated a decline in semantic verbal fluency score of two standard deviations and four patients a decrement between 1.00 and 1.99 standard deviations. Although no significant changes were observed in average scores on episodic memory tests, individual patients were more likely to demonstrate improvements than declines. While one patient evidenced a two standard deviation decline on a nonverbal recognition test (WMS-R Figural Memory), another patient demonstrated a gain of two standard deviations. In addition, two-standard deviation improvements were shown by one patient on delayed prose recall (Logical Memory), by one patient on delayed wordlist (CVLT) recall and by two patients on delayed word list recognition.

Among three patients having undergone staged bilateral pallidal deep brain stimulation electrode implantation, Tröster et al. (1997c) found that one patient demonstrated poorer word list recognition whereas another patient showed an improvement in word list recognition after surgery. Two patients showed possible improvements (1.00–1.99 standard deviations) in recall of prose passages. Kumar et al. (1997) reported that no neuropsychological morbidity was observed among four unilateral and four bilateral pallidal stimulation patients. Tronnier et al. (1997) reported that dysarthria occurred in two of six patients after bilateral pallidal stimulation; however, the dysarthria was evident only at high intensity stimulation and was fully reversible. Although these preliminary reports support the cognitive safety of pallidal stimulation, these reports remain to be empirically supported by controlled studies in larger patient series.

Transplantation

Few neuropsychological outcome data have been reported for adrenal medullary or fetal tissue transplant procedures. Although adrenal medullary tissue transplants are no longer being performed for PD, given disappointing re-sults, two studies did report cognitive outcome. Ostrosky-Solis et al. (1988) reported that seven PD patients, at least as a group, demonstrated improvements 3 months after surgery on memory tasks requiring 'an active organization of the response'. No changes were observed in immediate and delayed recall of words and sentences. Goetz et al. (1990), although not examining memory specifically, found no post-operative changes in overall level of cognitive functioning (measured with the MMSE).

Very few studies have examined cognitive outcome of fetal tissue grafting in PD, although it is now clear that such grafts are viable and survive (for up to 5 years in the study by López-Lozano et al. 1997). Sass et al. (1995) evaluated three patients who had tissue implanted in the right caudate and one who had tissue grafted into both caudate nuclei. Although some improvement was observed in these patients' verbal memory (WMS Logical Memory) 12 and 24 months after surgery, these improvements did not persist to 36 months. Leroy et al. (1996) evaluated five PD patients before and 12 months after unilateral striatal grafting. Four patients had tissue implanted into the right striatum, the other into the left striatum. All five patients had tissue implanted into the putamen and four patients had tissue implanted also into the head of the caudate nucleus. Although no significant changes in average scores were observed across the test battery, outcome was heterogeneous across individual tests and patients. Only one patient demonstrated rather global cognitive decline, but that patient likely had significant pre-existing cognitive impairments. With respect to memory, one patient demonstrated an improvement on a nonverbal memory test. Whereas one patient's prose recall improved, that of another declined. Two patients demonstrated poorer word list recall after surgery. Thompson et al. (1996) evaluated 14 PD patients from three to 18 months before surgery and from seven to 13 months after surgery. There was individual variability in outcome. Although there tended to be decreases in verbal fluency after surgery, verbal memory measures yielded contradictory results, with improvements noted on one measure (Logical Memory), but decrements on another measure (CVLT Total recall). The authors observed that patients with no more than mild cognitive impairment before surgery tended to show little cognitive change after surgery. In contrast, patients with more than mild cognitive impairment showed further cognitive declines after surgery. Together, the studies of Thompson et al. (1996) and Leroy et al. (1996) show that patients with notable cognitive impairment are probably not good candidates for tissue grafting, at least from a neurobehavioral perspective. This conclusion must be offered tentatively, as studies are based on small sample sizes and in the Thompson et al. (1996) study the surgical procedure was changed during the course of the study. Furthermore, only 14 of 22 patients returned for follow-up in the study by Thompson et al. (1996), raising the possibility of bias due to selective attrition.

Little is known about the cognitive effects of fetal tissue grafting in HD, likely because this procedure has only recently been attempted in this patient group. Madrazo et al. (1995) reported no significant cognitive changes in their two patients. Kurth et al. (1997) reported that neuropsychological functioning in three HD patients improved in the first 6 months after implantation of fetal lateral ganglionic eminence tissue into the basal ganglia, but specific results are still to be published. One study reported no consistent cognitive changes in three patients with HD who underwent fetal tissue grafts (Philpott et al. 1997). Similarly, porcine fetal tissue xenografts for HD and PD are being experimentally evaluated, but effects on cognition and behavior are undocumented.

CONCLUSIONS

Outcomes of early (pre-levodopa era) and modern thalamotomy and pallidotomy for movement disorders are difficult to compare given differences in patient populations, surgical targets and techniques and the rigor with which cognitive outcome was evaluated. It appears, nonetheless, that modern surgeries carry relatively little risk for cognitive morbidity. This risk appears to increase in cases of bilateral operations, for older patients and for patients with significant preoperative cognitive impairment. Cognitive morbidity associated with thalamotomy in multiple sclerosis appears, except in few series, considerable. It is unclear what factors might account for this morbidity, but because advanced stage patients were often included in surgical series, it might be speculated that results are biased by the inclusion of patients who probably already have significant and progressive, preoperative cognitive impairment.

The effects on cognition of deep brain stimulation are only beginning to be studied, although some preliminary findings show that these procedures might be relatively safe from a cognitive standpoint and perhaps even lead to mild improvements in some aspects of memory. Stimulation studies, aside from their potential benefits on functional capacity, also provide an avenue for cognitive neuroscientists to interrogate with precision subcortical nuclei as to their roles in cognition. This is a particularly exciting development as findings about the role of subcortical structures in human cognition are based almost exclusively on studies of patients with vascular and neurodegenerative pathology affecting multiple thalamic or basal ganglia nuclei. Efforts are also underway to refine and develop transplantation/grafting technologies for the treatment of a variety of neurodegenerative conditions. Insufficient is known about the potential cognitive effects of transplants/grafts, but fetal tissue grafts in PD might lead to transient improvements in memory or perhaps a slowing of the progression of cognitive impairment.

As operative therapy for different disorders is likely to increase in the coming years, it will become increasingly important for multidisciplinary teams to evaluate surgical candidates (Fernandez and Dujovny 1996). Such evaluation serves not only to minimize surgical morbidity, but also to carefully document whether 'functional' neurosurgery indeed does lead to significant functional improvements in neurodegenerative conditions.

REFERENCES

Aebischer, P., Schluep, M., Deglon, N., Joseph, J.M., Hirt, L., Heyd, B., Goddard, M., Hammang, J.P., Zurn, A.D., Kato, A.C., Regli, F. and Baetge, E.E. 1996. Intrathecal delivery of CNTF using encapsulated genetically modified xenogenic cells in amyotrophic lateral sclerosis patients. *Nature Medicine.* 2: 696–699.

Albin, R.L. 1995. The pathophysiology of chorea/ballism and parkinsonism. *Parkinsonism and Related Disorders.* 1: 3–11.

Alesch, F. 1995. Neurochirurgische Verfahren bei Morbus Parkinson. *Wiener Medizinische Wochenschrift.* 145: 305–309.

Alesch, F., Pinter, M.M., Helscher, R.J., Fertl, L., Benabid, A.L. and Koos, W.T. 1995. Stimulation of the ventral intermediate thalamic nucleus in tremor dominated Parkinson's disease and essential tremor. *Acta Neurochirurgica.* 136: 75–81.

Almgren, P.E. Andersson, A.L. and Kullberg, G. 1969. Differences in verbally expressed cognition following left and right ventrolateral thalamotomy. *Scandinavian Journal of Psychology*. 10: 243–249.

Almgren, P.E. Andersson, A.L. and Kullberg, G. 1972. Long-term effects on verbally expressed cognition following left and right ventrolateral thalamotomy. *Confinia Neurologica*. 34: 162–168.

Alterman, R.L., Kall, B.A., Cohen, H. and Kelly, P.J. 1995. Stereotactic ventrolateral thalamotomy: Is ventriculography necessary? *Neurosurgery*. 37: 717–722.

Alterman, R.L. and Kelly, P.J. 1998. Pallidotomy technique and results: the New York University experience. *Neurosurgery Clinics of North America*. 9: 337–343.

Asso, D., Crown, S., Russell, J.A. and Logue, V. 1969. Psychological aspects of the stereotactic treatment of parkinsonism. *British Journal of Psychiatry*. 115: 541–553.

Baron, M.S., Vitek, J.L., Bakay, R.A.E., Green, J., Kaneoke, Y., Hashimoto, T., Turner, R.S., Woodard, J.L., Cole, S.A., McDonald, W.M. and DeLong, M.R. 1996. Treatment of advanced Parkinson's disease by posterior GPi pallidotomy: 1-year results of a pilot study. *Annals of Neurology*. 40: 355–366.

Blumetti, A.E. and Modesti, L.M. 1980. Long term cognitive effects of stereotactic thalamotomy on non-parkinsonian dyskinetic patients. *Applied Neurophysiology*. 43: 259–262.

Burchiel, K.J. 1995. Thalamotomy for movement disorders. *Neurosurgical Clinics of North America*. 6: 55–71.

Cahn, D.A., Heit, G., Sullivan, E.V., Shear, P.K., Wasserstein, P., Lim, K.O. and Silverberg, G.D. 1997. Three-month followup of posterior ventral pallidotomy (abstract). *Journal of the International Neuropsychological Society*. 3: 60.

Cahn, D.A., Sullivan, E.V., Shear, P.K., Heit, G., Lim, K.O., Marsh, L., Lane, B., Wasserstein, P. and Silverberg, G.D. In press. Neuropsychological and motor functioning following unilateral anatomically-guided posterior ventral pallidotomy: Preoperative performance and three-month follow-up. *Neuropsychiatry, Neuropsychology, and Behavioral Neurology*.

Caparros-Lefebvre, D., Blond, S., Pécheux, N., Pasquier, F. and Petit, H. 1992. Évaluation neuropsychologique avant et après stimulation thalamique chez 9 parkinsoniens. *Revue Neurologique*. 148: 117–122.

Crosson, B. 1984. Role of the dominant thalamus in language: A review. *Psychological Bulletin*. 96: 491–517.

Cullum, C.M., Lacritz, L.H., Frol, A.B., Brewer, K.K., Giller, C. and Dewey, R. 1997. Effects of pallidotomy on cognitive function in Parkinson's disease (abstract). *Journal of the International Neuropsychological Society*. 3: 61.

Dogali, M., Fazzini, E., Kolodny, E., Eidelberg, D., Sterio, D., Devinsky, O. and Berić, A. 1995. Stereotactic ventral pallidotomy for Parkinson's disease. *Neurology*. 45: 753–761.

Favre, J., Taha, J.M., Nguyen, T.T., Gildenberg, P. and Burchiel, K.J. 1996. Pallidotomy: A survey of current practice in North America. *Neurosurgery*. 39: 883–892.

Fazzini, E., Dogali, M., Beric, A., Eidelberg, D., Sterio, D., Gianutsos, J., Newman, B., Kluger, A., Perrine, K., Loftus, S., Chin, L., Samelson, D. and Kolodny, E. 1995. The effects of unilateral ventral posterior medial pallidotomy in patients with Parkinson's disease and Parkinson's plus syndromes. In *Therapy of Parkinson's disease*, 2nd ed., ed. W.C. Koller and G. Paulson, pp. 353–379. New York: Marcel Dekker.

Fernandez, P.M. and Dujovny, M. 1996. Pallidotomy: Current developments. *Critical Reviews in Neurosurgery*. 6: 133–139.

Ffrench-Constant, C., Kiernan, B.W., Milner, R. and Scott-Drew, S. 1994. Developmental studies of oligodendrocyte precursor cell migration and their implications for transplantation as therapy for multiple sclerosis. *Eye*. 8: 221–223.

Fields, J.A., Wilkinson, S.B., Pahwa, R., Miyawaki, E., Koller, W.C. and Tröster, A. I. 1997. Globus pallidus stimulation in Parkinson's disease: Neurobehavioral functioning before and three months after electrode implantation (abstract). *Neurology*. 48: A431-A432.

Fox, M.W., Ahlskog, J.E. and Kelly, P.J. 1991. Stereotactic ventrolateralis thalamotomy for medically refractory tremor in post-levodopa era Parkinson's disease patients. *Journal of Neurosurgery*. 75: 723–730.

Gálvez-Jiménez, N., Lozano, A.M., Duff, J., Trépanier, L., Saint-Cyr, J.A. and Lang, A.E. 1996. Bilateral pallidotomy: Amelioration of incapacitating levodopa-induced dyskinesias but accompanying cognitive decline (Abstract). *Movement Disorders*. 11 (Suppl. 1): 242.

Goetz, C.G., Tanner, C.M., Penn, R.D., Stebbins, G.T., Gilley, D.W., Shannon, K.M., Klawans, H.L., Comella, C.L., Wilson, R.S. and Witt, T. 1990. Adrenal medullary transplant to the striatum of patients with advanced Parkinson's disease: 1-year motor and psychomotor data. *Neurology*. 40: 273–276.

Goldman, M.S., Ahlskog, J.E. and Kelly, P.J. 1992. The symptomatic and functional outcome of stereotactic thalamotomy for medically intractable essential tremor *Journal of Neurosurgery*. 76: 924–928.

Goldman, M.S. and Kelly, P.J. 1992. Symptomatic and functional outcome of stereotactic ventralis lateralis thalamotomy for intention tremor. *Journal of Neurosurgery*. 77: 223–229.

Green, J., Vitek, J.L., Bakay, R.A.E., Freeman, A., Evatt, M.L., McDonald, W.M. and DeLong, M.R. 1997. Pallidotomy for treatment of Parkinson's disease: Preliminary neuropsychological findings (abstract). *Journal of the International Neuropsychological Society*. 3: 67.

Harbaugh, R.E., Roberts, D.W., Coombs, D.W., Saunders, R.L. and Reeder, T.M. 1984. Preliminary report: Intracranial cholinergic drug infusion in patients with Alzheimer's disease. *Neurosurgery*. 15: 514–518.

Hays, P., Krikler, B., Walsh, L.S. and Wolfson, G. 1966. Psychological changes following surgical treatment of parkinsonism. *American Journal of Psychiatry*. 123: 657–663.

Iacono, R.P., Carlson, J.D., Kuniyoshi, S., Mohamed, A., Meltzer, C. and Yamada, S. 1997. Contemporaneous bilateral pallidotomy (electronic manuscript). *Neurosurgical Focus*. 2 (3): manuscript 5.

Iacono, R.P., Shima, F., Lonser, R.R., Kuniyoshi, S., Maeda, G. and Yamada, S. 1995. The results, indications and physiology of posteroventral pallidotomy for patients with Parkinson's disease. *Neurosurgery*. 36: 1118–1127.

Itakura, T., Komai, N., Ryujin, Y., Ooiwa, Y., Nakai, M. and Yasui, M. 1994. Autologous transplantation of the cervical sympathetic ganglion into the Parkinsonian brain: Case report. *Neurosurgery*. 35: 155–158.

Johansson, F., Malm, J., Nordh, E. and Hariz, M. 1997. Usefulness of pallidotomy in advanced Parkinson's disease. *Journal of Neurology, Neurosurgery and Psychiatry*. 62: 125–132.

Jurko, M.F. and Andy, O.J. 1964. Psychological aspects of diencephalotomy. *Journal of Neurology, Neurosurgery and Psychiatry*. 27: 516–521.

Jurko, M.F. and Andy, O.J. 1973. Psychological changes correlated with thalamotomy site. *Journal of Neurology, Neurosurgery and Psychiatry*. 36: 846–852.

Kocher, U., Siegfried, J. and Perret, E. 1982. Verbal and nonverbal learning ability of Parkinson patients before and after unilateral thalamotomy. *Applied Neurophysiology*. 45: 311–316.

Krayenbühl, H., Siegfried, J., Kohenof, M. and Yasargil, M.G. 1965. Is there a dominant thalamus? *Confinia Neurologica*. 26: 246–249.

Kumar, R., Lozano, A.M., Duff, J., Sime, E., Saint-Cyr, J. and Lang, A.E. 1997. Comparison of the effects of micro-electrode-guided posteroventral medial pallidotomy (PVMP) and globus pallidus internus (GPi) deep brain stimulation (DBS). (Abstract). *Neurology*. 48: A357.

Kuntzer, T., Ghika, J., Pollak, P., Benabid, A.-L., Limousin, P., Krack, P., Zurn, A.D., Tseng, J. and Aebischer, P. 1996. Treatment of Parkinson's disease. *European Neurology*. 36: 396–408.

Kurth, M.C., Kopyov, O.V., Jacques, D.B., Caviness, J.N., Duma, M., Eagle, S. and Lieberman, N. 1997. Safety of fetal tissue transplantation for Huntington's disease (abstract). *Neurology*. 48: A138.

Laitinen, L.V. 1995. Pallidotomy in Parkinson's disease. *Neurosurgical Clinics of North America*. 6: 105–112.

Laitinen, L.V., Bergenheim, A.T. and Hariz, M.I. 1992. Leksell's posteroventral pallidotomy in the treatment of Parkinson's disease. *Journal of Neurosurgery*. 76: 53–61.

Leroy, A., Michelet, D., Mahieux, F., Geny, C., Defer, G., Monfort, J.-C., Degos, J.-D., N'Guyen, J.-P., Peschanski, M. and Cesaro, P. 1996. Examen neuropsychologique de 5 patients parkinsoniens avant et après greffe neuronale. *Revue Neurologique*. 152: 158–164.

Levita E., Riklan, M. and Cooper, I.S. 1964. Verbal and perceptual functions after surgery of subcortical structures. *Perceptual and Motor Skills*. 18: 195–202.

Limousin, P., Pollak, P., Benazzouz, A., Hoffman, D., LeBas, J.-F., Broussolle, E., Perret, J.E. and Benabid, A.-L. 1995. Effect on parkinsonian signs and symptoms of bilateral subthalamic stimulation. *Lancet*. 345: 91–95.

Lindvall, O. 1995. Neural transplantation. *Cell Transplantation*. 4: 393–400.

López-Lozano, J.J., Bravo, G., Brera, B., Millán, I., Dargallo, J., Salmeán, J., Uría, J., Insausti, J. and the Clínica Puerta de Hierro Neural Transplantation Group. 1997. Long-term improvement in patients with severe Parkinson's disease after implantation of fetal ventral mesencephalic tissue in a cavity of the caudate nucleus: 5-year follow up in 10 patients. *Journal of Neurosurgery*. 86: 931–942.

Louw, D.F. and Burchiel, K.J. 1998. Ablative therapy for movement disorders: complications in the treatment of movement disorders. *Neurosurgery Clinics of North America*. 9: 367–373.

Lund-Johansen, M., Hugdahl, K. and Wester, K. 1996. Cognitive function in patients with Parkinson's disease undergoing stereotaxic thalamotomy. *Journal of Neurology, Neurosurgery and Psychiatry*. 60: 564–571.

Madrazo, I., Franco-Bourland, R.E., Castrejon, H., Cuevas, C. and Ostrosky-Solis, F. 1995. Fetal striatal homotransplantation for Huntington's disease: First two case reports. *Neurological Research*. 17: 312–315.

Marsden, C.D. and Obeso, J.A. 1994. The functions of the basal ganglia and the paradox of stereotaxic surgery in Parkinson's disease. *Brain*. 117: 877–897.

McFie, J. 1960. Psychological effects of stereotaxic operations for the relief of parkinsonian symptoms. *Journal of Mental Science*. 106: 1512–1517.

Obeso, J.A., Guridi, J. and DeLong, M. 1997. Surgery for Parkinson's disease. *Journal of Neurology, Neurosurgery and Psychiatry*. 62: 2–8.

Ojemann, G.A., Hoyenga, K.B. and Ward, A.A. 1971. Prediction of short-term verbal memory disturbance after ventrolateral thalamotomy. *Journal of Neurosurgery*. 35: 203–210.

Olanow, C.W., Freeman, T.B. and Kordower, J.H. 1997. Transplantation strategies for Parkinson's disease. In *Movement disorders: Neurologic principles and practice*, ed. R.L. Watts and W.C. Koller, pp. 221–236. New York: McGraw-Hill.

Ostrosky-Solis, F., Quintanar, L., Madrazo, I., Drucker-Colin, R., Franco-Bourland, R. and Leon-Meza, V. 1988. Neuropsychological effects of brain autograft of adrenal medullary tissue for the treatment of Parkinson's disease. *Neurology*. 38: 1442–1450.

Pahwa, R., Wilkinson, S., Smith, D., Lyons, K., Miyawaki, E. and Koller, W.C. 1997. High frequency stimulation of the globus pallidus for the treatment of Parkinson's disease. *Neurology*. 49: 249–253.

Perret, E. and Siegfried, J. 1969. Memory and learning performance of Parkinson patients before and after thalamotomy. In *Third Symposium on Parkinson's disease*, ed. F.J. Gillingham and I.M.L. Donaldson, pp. 164–168. Edinburgh: E. and S. Livingstone.

Philpott, L.M., Kopyov, O.V., Lee, A.J., Jacques, S., Duma, C.M., Caine, S., Yang, M. and Eagle, K.S. 1997. Neuropsychological functioning following fetal striatal transplantation in Huntington's chorea: Three case presentations. *Cell Transplantation*. 6: 203–212.

Riklan, M., Diller, L., Weiner, H. and Cooper, I.S. 1960. Psychological studies on effects of chemosurgery of the basal ganglia in parkinsonism. I. Intellectual functioning. *Archives of General Psychiatry*. 2: 22–31.

Riklan M. and Levita, E. 1970. Psychological studies of thalamic lesions in humans. *Journal of Nervous and Mental Disease*. 150: 251–265.

Riklan, M., Levita, E. and Cooper, I.S. 1966. Psychological effects of bilateral subcortical surgery for Parkinson's disease. *Journal of Nervous and Mental Disease*. 141: 403–409.

Riordan, H.J., Flashman, L.A. and Roberts, D.W. 1997. Neurocognitive and psychosocial correlates of ventroposterolateral pallidotomy surgery in Parkinson's disease (electronic manuscript). *Neurosurgical Focus*. 2 (3): manuscript 7.

Rossitch, E., Zeidman, S.M., Nashold, B.S., Horner, J., Walker, J., Osborne, D. and Bullard, D.E. 1988. Evaluation of memory and language function pre- and postthalamotomy with an attempt to define those patients at risk for postoperative dysfunction. *Surgical Neurology*. 29: 11–16.

Sass, K.J., Buchanan, C.P., Westerveld, M., Marek, K.L., Farhi, A., Robbins, R.J., Naftolin, F., Vollmer, T.L., Leranth, C., Roth, R.H., Price, L.H., Bunney, B.S., Elsworth, J.D., Hoffer, P.B., Redmond, D.E. and Spencer, D.D. 1995. General cognitive ability following unilateral and bilateral fetal ventral mesencephalic tissue transplantation for treatment of Parkinson's disease. *Archives of Neurology*. 52: 680–686.

Selby, G. 1967. Stereotactic surgery for the relief of Parkinson's disease. Part 2. An analysis of the results in a series of 303 patients (413 operations). *Journal of the Neurological Sciences*. 5: 343–375.

Shapiro, D.Y., Sadowsky, D.A., Henderson, W.G. and VanBuren, J.M. 1973. An assessment of cognitive function in postthalamotomy Parkinson patients. *Confinia Neurologica*. 35: 144–166.

Siegfried, J. and Lippitz, B. 1994. Bilateral chronic electrostimulation of ventroposterolateral pallidum: A new therapeutic approach for alleviating all parkinsonian symptoms. *Neurosurgery*. 35: 1126–1130.

Soukup, V.M., Ingram, F., Schiess, M.C., Bonnen, J.G., Nauta, H.J.W. and Calverley, J.R. 1997. Cognitive sequelae of unilateral posteroventral pallidotomy. *Archives of Neurology*. 54: 947–950.

Spiegel, E.A. and Wycis, T. 1954. Ansotomy in paralysis agitans. *Archives of Neurology and Psychiatry*. 71: 598–614.

Spiegel, E., Wycis, H., Orchinik, C. and Freed, H. 1955. Thalamic chronotaraxis. *Archives of Neurology and Psychiatry*. 73: 469–471.

Svennilson, E., Torvik, A., Lowe, R. and Leksell, L. 1960. Treatment of parkinsonism by stereotactic thermolesions in the pallidal region. *Acta Psychiatrica et Neurologica Scandinavica*. 35: 358–377.

Tasker, R.R. 1998. Deep brain stimulation is preferable to thalamotomy for tremor suppression. *Surgical Neurology*. 49: 145–154.

Thompson, L.L., Cullum, C.M., O'Neill, S. and Freed, C.R. 1996, November. *Effects of fetal cell transplantation on cognitive and psychological functioning in Parkinson's disease*. Paper presented at the Annual Meeting of the National Academy of Neuropsychology, New Orleans, 1 November, 1996.

Tronnier, V.M., Fogel, W., Kronenbuerger, M. and Steinvorth, S. 1997. Pallidal stimulation: An alternative to pallidotomy? (electronic manuscript). *Neurosurgical Focus*. 2 (3): manuscript 10.

Tröster, A.I., Fields, J.A., Koller, W.C. and Wilkinson, S.B. 1997a. Effects of chronic electrical stimulation of the left VIM thalamic nucleus on language and memory in a patient with Parkinson's disease (abstract). *Journal of Neuropsychiatry and Clinical Neurosciences*. 9: 148.

Tröster, A.I., Fields, J.A., Wilkinson, S.B., Busenbark, K., Miyawaki, E., Overman, J., Pahwa, R. and Koller, W.C. 1997b. Neuropsychological functioning before and after unilateral thalamic stimulating electrode implantation in Parkinson's disease (electronic manuscript). *Neurosurgical Focus*. 2 (3): manuscript 9.

Tröster, A.I., Fields, J.A., Wilkinson, S.B., Pahwa, R., Miyawaki, E. and Koller, W.C. 1997c. A comparison of neurobehavioral functioning before and three months following unilateral and bilateral globus pallidus stimulating electrode implantation for medically refractory Parkinson's disease (abstract). *Stereotactic and Functional Neurosurgery*. 67: 88.

Tröster, A.I., Fields, J.A., Wilkinson, S.B., Pahwa, R., Miyawaki, E., Lyons, K.E. and Koller, W.C. 1997d. Unilateral pallidal stimulation for Parkinson's disease: Neurobehavioral functioning before and three months after electrode implantation. *Neurology*. 49: 1078–1083.

Turnbull, I.M., McGeer, P.L., Beattie, L., Calne, D. and Pate, B. 1985. Stimulation of the basal nucleus of Meynert in senile dementia of the Alzheimer type. *Applied Neurophysiology*. 48: 216–221.

Uitti, R.J., Wharen, R.E., Turk, M.F., Lucas, J.A., Finton, M.J., Graff-Radford, N.R., Boylan, K.B., Goerss, S.J., Kall, B.A., Adler, C.H., Caviness, J.N. and Atkinson, E.J. 1997. Unilateral pallidotomy for Parkinson's disease: Comparison of outcome in younger versus elderly patients, *Neurology*. 49: 1072–1977.

Van Buren, J.M., Li, C.-L., Shapiro, D.Y., Henderson, W.G. and Sadowsky, D.A. 1973. A qualitative and quantitative evaluation of Parkinsonians three to six years following thalamotomy. *Confinia Neurologica*. 35: 202–235.

Van Manen, J., Speelman, J.D. and Tans, R.J.J. 1984. Indications for surgical treatment of Parkinson's disease after levodopa therapy. *Clinical Neurology and Neurosurgery*. 86: 207–212.

Vilkki, J. and Laitinen, L.V. 1974. Differential effects of left and right ventrolateral thalamotomy on receptive and expressive verbal performances and face-matching. *Neuropsychologia*. 12: 11–19.

Vilkki, J. and Laitinen, L.V. 1976. Effects of pulvinotomy and ventrolateral thalamotomy on some cognitive functions. *Neuropsychologia*. 14: 67–78.

Vitek, J.L. 1997. Stereotaxic surgery and deep brain stimulation for Parkinson's disease and movement disorders. In *Movement disorders: Neurologic principles and practice*, ed. R.L. Watts and W.C. Koller, pp. 237–255. New York: McGraw-Hill.

Von Falkenhayn, I., Ceballos-Baumann, A.O., Moringlane, J.R., Alesch, F., Pinter, M., Barcia, J.L., Tormos, J.M. and Pascual-Leone, A. 1997. Effects of subthalamic nucleus (STN) and globus pallidus internus (GPI) stimulation on procedural learning (abstract). *Neurology*. 48: A118.

Wester, K. and Hauglie-Hanssen, E. 1990. Stereotaxic thalamotomy – experiences from the levodopa era. *Journal of Neurology, Neurosurgery and Psychiatry*. 53: 427–430.

23

Memory dysfunction in neurodegenerative disease: ethical and legal issues

MARTIN D. ZEHR

INTRODUCTION

The progressive impairment of memory functions constitutes the primary clinical symptom of most of the neurodegenerative conditions which are the subject of this book. The study of memory dysfunction in this context, in which certain degrees and subtypes of impairment are considered to be abnormal and the direct product of specific neuropathological changes is certainly a welcome change from the time when clinical observations associated with these conditions were considered to be an inevitable byproduct of 'normal aging' (Ruscio and Cavarrochi 1984). This book itself is evidence of the fact that so-called 'senility' is not an inevitable consequence of aging, such that the term itself, along with such professional colloquialisms as 'organic brain syndrome', now have an antique quality which renders the speaker of such terms 'scientifically incorrect'. The accelerating biomedicalization of the dementias during the past two decades can be directly attributed to the dual impact of cutting-edge research, such as the recent work indicating an association of specific alleles for apolipoprotein E with probable Alzheimer's disease (AD) (Reiman et al. 1996; Chapters 17 and 18) and the impetus provided by changing population demographics characteristic of modern industrialized societies. Projections that the proportion of the population aged 85 years and older will be as high as 18% by the year 2040 (Taeuber 1990) have legitimized epidemiological questions regarding the inevitability of dementing conditions (Drachman 1994). Concomitant with these developments is an increasing awareness of the social, legal and ethical issues associated with all of the neurodegenerative disease processes resulting in dementia (Binstock et al. 1992) and a healthy skepticism regarding any tendency to biomedicalize the dementias to the exclusion of these concerns (Lyman 1989). The very nature of the cognitive changes associated with these neurodegenerative processes has implications which are qualitatively different from most common ailments associated with aging for the individual's functional status. In their advanced stages, all neurodegenerative conditions eventually result in motor or cognitive impairment which necessitates significant adjustments in living circumstances, but with the latter there is also the nascent possibility of changes so extreme that autonomous existence in any sense becomes problematic. The demented patient, in extremis, is at times described by family and friends as 'no longer here' or by institutional caregivers in the past tense, with references to the 'former self' (Turnbull 1990).

COGNITIVE IMPAIRMENT AND LEGAL CAPACITY

For the affected adult, changes in memory function associated with neurodegenerative disease processes have potential implications for changes in the individual's legal status. When the impairment of memory functions progresses to the point at which the ability to perform routine activities of daily living becomes questionable, it is necessary to consider the potential of compensatory mechanisms for the maintenance of the individuals's independence. In the early or intermediate stages of a neurodegenerative disease process, compensation is available through such mechanisms as routinized reliance on external reminders, such as a weekly-based organizing dispenser to assist with adequate adherence to a medication regimen, or delegation of responsibilities to significant others, e.g. shifting the management of finances to a spouse, child or close friend, whether through informal arrangements or by way of legal conveyance of authority. Increasingly, professional assistance, based on current knowledge of memory functioning, is being specifically tailored to the memory-related problems of these patients and their family members (Scogin and Prohaska 1993). Implicit in all of these measures is the assumption that the affected individual has an awareness of the nature, if not the extent, of his cognitive impairment, that there is a concomitant realization of the necessity of making compensatory adjustments and, finally, that there is adequate motivation to seek assistance and consider the recommendations of professionals and family members alike.

It is at this juncture of considerations of cognitive impairment and ability to function in the everyday environment that the research-based questions of neurodegenerative disease processes intersect with what are primarily legal and ethical considerations, i.e. capacity and autonomy. In the legal context, capacity or autonomy is typically described in reference to its absence, such as in the following statutory definition of an incapacitated person, in a civil, as opposed to a criminal, frame of reference as:

one who is unable by reason of physical or mental condition to receive and evaluate information or to communicate decisions to such an extent that he lacks capacity to meet essential requirements for food, clothing, shelter, safety, or other care such that serious physical injury, illness, or disease is likely to occur.

(SECTION 475. 010 REVISED STATUTES OF MISSOURI, 1985).

(see also, Uniform Probate Code, 1969, Section 5–101(1), upon which most statutory definitions of capacity in the United States are based). Such legal definitions incorporate the notion of capacity as a unitary, indivisible concept although, in practice, the legal system commonly recognizes separate competencies or degrees of competency, as, for example, in provisions for conservatorship, in which authority for making financial decisions is legally conferred to another, versus all-encompassing guardianships. Statutes in most states have been adopted during recent years which incorporate references to specific types of disabilities and degrees of cognitive incapacity and the legal system has now become more amenable to the use of data from the behavioral sciences which describe, for example, various types of memory deficits and their implications for actual functioning in everyday situations (Anderer 1990).

The neuropsychologist who becomes involved, directly or otherwise, in determinations of capacity or disability, should then be expected to be able to explain, for example, the difference between the subtle decline in episodic memory that accompanies aging and the severe impairment of episodic memory thought to be associated with structural damage in the region of the hippocampus, which is seen with AD (Tomlinson et al. 1970). In addition, differences in the types and severity of memory dysfunction which are distinguishing characteristics of specific neurological conditions have potential implications for recommendations regarding assistance needs. Thus, for example, while patients in advanced stages of AD or Korsakoff's syndrome show little or no ability to learn or retain new information, evidence shows that patients with Huntington's disease (HD), whose memory impairment is thought to reflect retrieval difficulties, can actually derive significant benefit from rehearsal and externally generated cues for recall (Delis et al. 1991). In contrast, the effects of practice, except in the earliest stages, have been shown to be relatively minimal for patients with AD (Heun et al. 1995). These types of research findings have clear implications for everyday living situations, e.g. differential expectations of benefits to be derived from posted notes and other such memory aids, and thus can have an impact on legal determinations of capacity designed to provide the individual with a maximum degree of autonomy. On the other hand, the professional who becomes involved in the making of such determinations should always be acutely aware of the fact that there exists no isomorphic relationship between controlled normative-based assessments of memory impairment and the ability of a particular individual to cope with the demands of everyday existence. Available research underscores the conclusion that the relationship between neuropsychological test data and the capacity to perform routine living skills remains problematic (Searight and Goldberg 1991), although batteries of neuropsychological tests including significant memory components have been shown to be substantially correlated with functional task performance in patients with AD (Baum et al. 1996). The latter study also supports the conclusion that, in AD, procedural memory, i.e. the ability to perform well-routinized motor activities, remains relatively intact (Chapters 12 and 20). More circumscribed research utilizing neuropsychological testing has substantiated predictive relationships between formal testing and everyday memory functions with more direct implications for assessments of functional competency (Little et al. 1986).

Despite the difficulties inherent in any attempt to apply research-based findings to legal issues involving questions of competency, or capacity, circumscribed efforts have yielded potentially useful information relevant to specific situations. Daniel Marson and colleagues have, for example, shown that deficits in semantic memory and word fluency measures are associated with competency status for different legal standards, with specific reference to the capacity to consent to treatment (Marson et al. 1995a, b, 1996). These researchers assessed the ability of normal older control subjects and patients with probable AD, when presented with two clinical vignettes requiring decisions regarding medical treatment, to respond in a manner indicating the following progressively complex legal standards:

(1)   The capacity to *evidence* a treatment choice, regardless of the appropriateness of the decision.

(2)   The capacity to make the *reasonable* treatment choice.

(3)   The capacity to *appreciate* the emotional and cognitive consequences of a treatment choice.

(4)   The capacity to provide *rational reasons* for a treatment choice.

(5)   The capacity to *understand* the treatment situation and choices.

(Marson et al. 1995a, p. 951. Italics in original). Although these studies clearly indicated the predictive value of neuropsychological test measures for the assessment of the various levels of capacity, the results of these studies showed that, for the most stringent legal standard, which required an 'understanding' of the treatment situation, measures of conceptualization from the Mattis Dementia Rating Scale and of visual confrontation naming (or semantic memory) from the Boston Naming Test, were better predictors of level five competence than was short-term memory per se. The authors concluded that this finding was likely attributable to the 'well-known floor effects demonstrated by AD patients' on memory tests (1996, p. 670), but another explanation is just as plausible under the circumstances. Without a significantly long time interval between stimulus presentation and recall testing, short-term memory impairment might be expected to have relatively less impact on the capacity to reason and to respond to the demand for a decision than might abstract reasoning ability

and word fluency. Thus, even with significant short-term memory impairment, such patients may provide relatively consistent choices indicating adequate comprehension of the treatment situation and choices. If the situation requires no additional response, an 'adequate' choice made under such circumstances may be construed as evidence of competency. If, however, the patient makes an otherwise appropriate choice which requires more than a passive acceptance of treatment alternatives, e.g. independent and consistent adherence to a medication regimen, then only a limited form of competence is demonstrated; the patient with significant short-term memory impairment could not, under these circumstances, be deemed capable of meeting essential care needs without assistance, especially if short-term memory deficits are accompanied by a conspicuous lack of awareness of the extent or nature of the impairment. Such lack of awareness would effectively preclude reliance on otherwise adequate compensatory measures and the individual exhibiting a pronounced lack of awareness of cognitive deficits will undoubtedly be unable to acknowledge the need for assistance with routine activities or the necessity to delegate responsibilities to others through informal arrangements or legal conveyances such as a durable power of attorney.

This example illustrates the possibility, perhaps even the likelihood, that a comprehensive empirically based measure of capacity, applicable across a wide variety of situations and for any given individual, cannot be devised. It also underscores the point that a diagnosis of neurodegenerative disease of any type, or short-term memory deficits in particular, is not, and should not be, the equivalent of a legal determination of capacity. The law usually does not presume that any medical or psychiatric diagnosis is synonymous with any legal incompetency (Grisso 1986). Even significant impairment of memory functions is not by itself a sufficient basis for a determination of capacity because awareness of such deficits, in combination with extra-cognitive factors, such as differences in willingness to delegate responsibilities and the existence of available support systems, will ultimately determine whether, in a strictly legal sense, an individual has the requisite 'capacity to meet essential requirements for food, clothing, shelter, safety or other care . . .' Thus, it would not only be inappropriate, as capacity determinations are ultimately legal questions, but also unethical, to make any statements regarding global capacities of an individual based solely on evidence of significant memory deficits. On the other hand, where warranted by clinical observations and testing evidence, conclusions regarding an individual's ability to accomplish specific tasks, e.g. manage finances, cook with a gas oven or adhere to a medication regimen without supervision or assistance, are quite appropriate and likely necessary, to ensure an optimal level of ability to fulfill basic living requirements.

ASSESSMENT OF DRIVING ABILITY

A major issue encountered on a regular basis by clinicians working with patients with suspected dementia concerns their ability to reliably operate a motor vehicle in a safe manner. While initial evidence bearing on this issue may consist of the anecdotal accounts of worried family members, more objective indicators in the form of test data with established and generally accepted normative ranges are certainly preferable, especially as any recommendations based on assessment may ultimately result in the termination of what is, from the patient's perspective, an important liberty interest. The neuropsychology literature contains few references to formal studies addressing this question, although it has in recent years increasingly drawn the attention of formal neuropsychological study (Hopewell and Van Zomeren 1990). For example, there is tentative evidence that traditional testing instruments, such as the Wisconsin Card Sorting Test, can be used to predict criterion performance consisting of a simulated driving situation (Chatel et al. 1993). In a recent study comparing simulated driving performance in AD and normal control groups, it was found that the patients were significantly more likely to have crashes and 'close calls' than controls. Several measures of visuospatial skill and attention (e.g. Rey-Osterrieth Complex Figure copy, Trailmaking Test, WAIS-R Block Design, Benton Facial Recognition Test) were found to be strong predictors of crashes (Rizzo et al. 1997). Similarly, actual driving performance in a small sample of patients with Parkinson's disease was strongly related to performance on tests of visual perception, vigilance, choice reaction time, and information processing speed (Heikkilä et al. 1998).

With reference to both AD and vascular dementia, there is evidence that short-term memory, in conjunction with impaired visual tracking ability, is correlated with actual driving ability to such an extent that recommendations regarding actual road testing should be considered

for some patients (Fitten et al. 1995). A corollary ethical issue of concern to the professional addressing this question is the matter of the duty to advise the patient and family members when there is evidence to suggest that an individual likely cannot drive in a safe manner. In practice, however, this may be less of a problem than expected. I have frequently found that family members and, at times, even the involved individual, are relieved to receive the recommendation from a third-party professional that driving activity should be limited to specific conditions or predicated on successful completion of an appropriate road test, or even cease altogether. The professional may in some instances have an understandable reluctance to make such recommendations, based on assumptions regarding potential personal liability, but recommendations based in part on objective evidence and made in 'good faith', the applicable legal term of art, are unlikely to result in any such liability. Indeed, most jurisdictions recognize the good faith duty of the professional to make such reports when safety issues are paramount.

PROFESSIONAL COMPETENCE AS AN ETHICAL ISSUE

Whether addressing a question of ability to perform a specific skill or more global capacities, psychologists and other professionals making predictive statements or recommendations on the basis of testing data should, of course, consider their own respective competencies. In a discussion of the application of the 1992 revision of the Ethics Code of the American Psychological Association to clinical neuropsychology, Binder and Thompson (1995) make reference to the boundaries of competence of the individual practitioner that should govern the scope of professional activities and note that these boundaries should also limit the types of conclusory statements which are potentially within the professional's area of expertise. When making statements regarding capacity based on cognitive assessment, admonitions to stay well within a circumscribed area of competence are particularly important, given the potential consequences of expressed opinions regarding such questions. In part this is because the label of incompetence or incapacity, once applied to an individual, invariably results not only in the deprivation of specific legal rights, but also has potentially devastating psychological effects on the person and changes the manner in which others react to that individual (Winick 1995). This cautionary note is underscored by evidence that psychologists who are increasingly working with an older adult population, i.e. those most likely to see clinical evidence of neurodegenerative disease processes, may be lacking basic factual information pertaining to AD (Bailey and Johnston 1994). For clinicians whose work requires them to address questions associated with dementing conditions, it is also important to be familiar with some of the generally accepted distinctions between the major neurodegenerative disease processes. An example of this type of information is the relative degree of motor impairment associated with conditions such as Parkinson's or Lewy body disease (Wagner and Bachman 1996) versus AD. The clinician should also be cognizant of the potential for reversibility or a slowing of the progression of impairment, through the timely initiation of appropriate measures, in dementias with etiologies associated with thyroid deficiencies or multi-infarct conditions. In particular, the potential reversibility of conditions such as multi-infarct dementia has important implications in areas such as competency determinations, as discussed earlier. Thus, the informed clinician, through the use of periodic serial testing in such cases, can provide valuable objective evidence of changes in memory functioning associated with concomitant amelioration of the underlying cause(s) which can have a direct bearing on the issue of legal status.

It is imperative that the professional who purports to have competency specific to working with populations in which the presence of a neurodegenerative process is a frequent diagnostic question be aware of age-specific issues relevant to testing (Chapter 16). In particular, the professional should be aware of the potential impact of variables such as age and formal education on interpretation of test data and avail himself of such data as that provided by Heaton and colleagues (1991, 1992), whose work is of inestimable value in making the use of the Halstead-Reitan Neuropsychological Test Battery and the Wechsler Adult Intelligence Scale-Revised more applicable to the assessment of older adults. Other investigators, like Ryan, Paolo and their colleagues (1990, 1992, 1995, 1996), have specifically focused their efforts on developing normative data for instruments such as the WAIS-R designed to make them more useful to those who work with elderly populations, i.e. individuals 75 years and older, and showing how test-retest changes in WAIS-R indices differ for the elderly. Similarly, Paolo et al. (1997) have extended the normative

and reliability data for memory measures such as the California Verbal Learning Test so that they might be more powerful to those working with the elderly. The clinician should also be aware that some testing instruments in common use have undergone revisions which now incorporate normative data for assessment of older individuals. Examples of the latter are the recent revision of the Rey Complex Figure Test (Meyers and Meyers 1995) which can be administered to adults aged 18–89 years, and the revision of the Wechsler Memory Scale (Wechsler, 1997). The availability of such age-related normative data, however, is not sufficient justification for the use of a particular instrument when addressing questions regarding dementia-related cognitive impairment. Even such widely used assessment instruments as the Mini-Mental State Exam, for which there exists normative data for ages 18–85 years (Crum et al. 1993), are inappropriate by themselves for assessment of the memory impairment associated with progressive dementias (Tombaugh and McIntyre 1992).

INFORMED CONSENT FOR TREATMENT AND RESEARCH PARTICIPATION

An issue of particular relevance to both the authors and readers of this volume concerns the consent to treatment and research participation by individuals with a form of neurodegenerative disease which may bring their capacity to provide informed consent into question. In a review of 99 separate studies in which research subjects consisted largely of individuals diagnosed with probable AD, High (1993) found a significant lack of any uniform standard for assessing the capacity of individuals to consent to research participation. This was even the case when such consent was conveyed by proxy, and there was no significant reliance on consent based upon formal conveyance, e.g. guardianship or durable powers of attorney. High concluded that, 'for any informed consent process, including proxy consent, to work well, effective communication is paramount. No researcher or ethicist should minimize the importance of effective communication among investigators, subjects and family surrogates' (High 1993, p. 175). At present there exist no consistent standards for ascertaining whether consent by the individual or proxy constitutes informed consent, but the work by Marson and his colleagues provides a reasonable starting point from which it could be determined whether a potential research subject understands, as a first step, that their participation is optional, i.e. that they can choose whether or not to be a research subject, and whether the individual understands the nature of the study and the known or predictable consequences of their participation.

High et al. (1994), in a comprehensive review of the primary ethical and legal issues confronting those researchers whose work involves the participation of individuals with AD, have provided a number of recommendations relevant to such research which are equally applicable when working with patients who are cognitively impaired as a result of the effects of any of the major neurodegenerative disease processes. Based on a 2-year project conducted at the University of Kentucky Alzheimer Disease Center, the review contains the following recommendations designed to ensure adherence to accepted standards of competent scientific research while simultaneously providing for the informed consent of the patient or his proxy:

(1)   Study populations, wherever possible, should include relevant demographic characteristics with proportionate representation. Such characteristics include ethnic and cultural background, as well as less obvious features such as institutionalized status.

(2)   Research instruments employed to assess cognitive status generally or circumscribed functions such as short-term memory should be devoid of cultural bias, to the extent possible.

(3)   Formal documents used for the purpose of obtaining informed consent should be readily comprehensible to the individual subject or proxy and the potential subject should have assistance available to answer any related questions.

(4)   Research protocols should have a predetermined and specified means for determining a subjects's capacity for providing informed consent on a task-specific basis.

(5)   For potential research participants who do not meet the criteria sufficient to warrant a determination of capacity, informed consent should be obtained through joint consultation with the subject and his authorized proxy, e.g. durable power of attorney or legal guardian.

(6)   Researchers should encourage potential research subjects to execute advance directives for research participation in future projects, as long as the potential subject is currently competent and willing to execute such instructions.

(7)   Potential conflicts of interest should be avoided in the care and recruitment of patients for research protocols. Sources of potential conflicts include financial or other benefits to be obtained by the researcher in conjunction with the adoption of a particular research or clinical care protocol.

(8)   Investigators should avoid making unwarranted claims regarding the benefits of research participation to potential subjects and should make every effort to minimize any risks associated with the research.

(High et al., 1994 p.73). With respect to the latter recommendation, High and his colleagues hold the opinion that in some instances involving research with potential risks and no discernible benefits to the cognitively impaired subject, adequate justification may nevertheless exist 'if the anticipated knowledge sought is deemed to be of vital importance for understanding and alleviating the disease in the future and the specific research protocol is reasonably likely to generate such knowledge' (High et al. 1994, p. 72).

Well-designed studies which incorporate the above recommendations are nevertheless susceptible to potential problems regarding disclosure of risk which are unrelated to the particular research or treatment protocol. For example, if we assume that the subject population for a research project is representative of the general population, in conformance with the first recommendation cited above, then there is an unspecified risk that a control group subject will, in the course of the study, manifest signs, through laboratory or clinical observation, of a neurodegenerative disease process, not necessarily the condition which is the focus of the study. When this occurs, the investigators must deal with an issue of disclosure which they may not have anticipated. Does the research participant in this situation have a right to receive relevant diagnostic information? The answer to this question in most cases will undoubtedly be affirmative, especially where a high degree of certainty exists regarding the presence of pathology, or where the condition is potentially amenable to treatment. In all cases, however, concerns of individual autonomy will dictate that the subject is entitled to disclosure of the information necessary to make a decision pertaining to further diagnostic work or treatment. This is especially true when we consider that presumptive capability to provide informed consent to participate in the research protocol ab initio implies, in most cases, presumptive capability to consent to treatment. Under such circumstances, failure to disclose opinions regarding the presence of a neurodegenerative process can be construed as a deprivation of the individual's decision-making capability without due process. This particular problem can be obviated, however, through the use of prior informed consent in a broader form which includes explicit reference to the risk, through research participation, of detection of conditions which would then be disclosed to the subject. Finally, it is important to emphasize that because many primary investigators in these situations may not be physicians, appropriate precautions should be taken when communicating observations and opinions to research subjects. These should, for example, be couched in probabilistic statements congruent with the investigator's own opinion regarding the likelihood that the observations on which the communication is based constitute evidence of pathology.

The question of informed consent is, of course, not confined to situations involving the participation of human subjects in research protocols. Where there exists a question of dementia, there may also be a question regarding the individual's capacity to provide informed consent to medical treatment. The legal notion of informed consent requires that the patient's permission in such instances be based on a reasonable and adequate explanation of the proposed treatment or procedure, including its likely consequences. This presupposes, of course, the capacity of the individual to understand, in at least general terms, the purpose and nature of the proposed treatment (Mills and Daniels 1987). While questions of capacity are ultimately legal, not medical, or psychological questions, courts will routinely rely on the advice of professionals to assist, when necessary, in making such determinations. In the medical context, such questions are frequently addressed on the basis of shifting, inconsistent and even contradictory standards, such that 'even well-trained (professionals) lack a firm, consistent basis for evaluating competency' (Macklin 1987). Most professionals who work with dementia patients lack any formal preparation in their training concerning the question of capacity and as a consequence, not surprisingly, have been found to disagree frequently in judgments of capacity (Marson et al. 1994). Even those who criticize the lack of a consistent basis for making such determinations, however, have at times begged the question, or rather, substituted another equally elusive

concept, as Macklin does for example when, in the context of a well-justified critique of the use of mental status tests to assess capacity, states, '. . . I am convinced that a person's ability to grant informed consent to treatment is a *commonsense* notion that does not require special psychiatric expertise to evaluate, . . .' (Macklin 1987, p. 85; italics added). Assumption of this position necessarily entails either (1) an abandonment of any attempt to develop a conception of capacity that can be applied in a uniform manner, or (2) the adoption of an equally daunting quest, the search for uniformly applicable referents to the nebulous and elusive concept of 'commonsense'. A better alternative, however, will result from the search for explicit, empirically valid criteria which provide replicable standards for addressing legal questions while simultaneously assuring that the individual is not subject to the curtailment of any civil rights as a result of the application of unspecifiable standards. The work of Marson and his colleagues referred to above represents a good example of the latter approach.

Scientists or practitioners who seldom or never become involved in such ethical-legal quandaries while working with individuals with neurodegenerative conditions should nevertheless be wary of the possibility that their work could, in an entirely unanticipated manner, have an impact on questions of capacity. To illustrate this possibility we need only note that every healthcare worker who records a patient-based observation in a medical record is creating evidence which may potentially be employed in a contemporaneous or *future* capacity determination. In such cases, when reports, progress notes, etc. are not prepared with the intention of addressing legal issues such as competency, it must nevertheless be assumed that such records may ultimately be used for this purpose and the professional may have no control over such use of written reports. However remote it might seem, because of this possibility, it is imperative that caution be used when employing terms or words that can be interpreted with reference to competency issues (Zehr 1994).

These standards for consent by individuals with varying types and degrees of cognitive impairment can hardly be considered to be onerous in application and are in fact analogous to those routinely applied in clinical situations specifically with AD patients. With AD, treatments of questionable efficacy and limited applicability are the rule rather than the exception, as no routinely effective treatment for AD yet exists (Chapter 21). The understandable desperation of patients with AD and their families, however, invariably leads to inquiries and requests regarding the implementation of experimental treatment protocols. Under such circumstances, where no immediate emergency presumably exists, patients, in the presence of invited family members and friends (invited by the patient) can be provided with an oral cost/benefit analysis of the protocol and simultaneously furnished with supporting written material upon which reflection and further questions can be based (e.g. Farlow et al. 1992; Growdon 1992). In this particular situation, another ethical issue exists regarding the predisposition of the particular clinician with respect to the use of a quasi-experimental medication, where the benefit to be derived is either doubtful, minimal or, at best, temporary. In this situation the most ethical approach likely consists of as complete disclosure of the benefits and risks as possible, noting any reservations but also underscoring the participation of the patient in such treatment protocol as ultimately a matter of personal choice. Of course, the scope of professional competence in regard to treatment issues includes a healthy skepticism regarding unverified causal explanations for such disease processes as, for example, the aluminum hypothesis that was popular a few years ago (Weiner 1987).

In cases involving patients with late-stage neurodegenerative disease, especially AD, the question to be addressed may not be one regarding capacity to make an informed decision. When it is evident that the patient lacks this capacity, the surrogate decision makers or caregivers must, by necessity, adopt a procedure, formally and explicitly, to be implemented as the need for treatment decisions arises in conjunction with the progression of the disease process. The potential legal problems inherent in such situations are obvious when there exists no advance directive or durable power of attorney designating a particular individual with proxy decision-making authority, but even in cases where this has been done, issues regarding the perspective and process of treatment decisions will remain. Thus, the surrogate decision maker may confront a situation in which a substituted judgment cannot easily be made because there is not even a modicum of certainty regarding the supposed preference of the patient. In such cases, where the patient's preferences prior to the time at which capacity ends cannot be fathomed, treatment decisions may be made on the basis of the perceived best interest of the patient. When such a change in perspective becomes necessary and even if it does not, it is neverthe-

less imperative that the decision maker obtain as much information regarding the treatment alternatives as practically possible, so that the consent, whether direct or by proxy, is truly *informed*. In situations involving late-stage Alzheimer's patients, where care is often administered in hospital, nursing home or hospice settings, it is incumbent on the treatment staff of the facility to take the initiative to work with family members or other surrogate decision makers to formulate a treatment plan which attempts to deal with common issues in advance. Ideally, the institutional staff should also attempt to make clear the channels for obtaining information or discussing concerns when unanticipated situations or emergencies arise in the course of treatment. A model for consensus decision making with institutionalized late-stage AD patients is provided by Hurley and her colleagues (Hurley et al. 1995). In this consensus model, the family caregiver or surrogate decision maker becomes the focus of staff efforts to increase satisfaction with decisions on behalf of the patient through active discussion of alternatives and likely outcomes in conjunction with continuing support for the proxy, who in many instances is experiencing significant anxiety associated with the prospect of making end-of-life decisions.

INFORMATION DISCLOSURE AND THE DEMENTIA PATIENT

Under the presumption that the patient with suspected neurodegenerative disease-based dementia is nevertheless competent until shown convincingly to be otherwise, he/she is entitled to disclosure of the conclusions regarding the existence of a disease entity, even when that conclusion is necessarily probabilistic, as is the case with any formal diagnosis of AD at the present time. There are occasionally instances in which family members may request that the term AD not be specifically employed when addressing the patient, but in evaluating such circumstances the clinician should nevertheless keep in mind the fact that it is the patient's information which would be withheld. It could be argued in this situation that providing the patient with an explanation of the neurological substrate of his/her cognitive deficits, in conjunction with a description of the nature and extent of the deficits, as well as the possible clinical course and prognosis, is in fact the equivalent of informing the patient that his/her symptoms are likely attributable to AD. Such argument, however, is defective because it fails to take into account the fact that the term AD is, like any diagnostic label, a shorthand term for a pathological process consisting of a cluster of specific symptoms with a presumed etiology and treatment, even if unknown. Failure to provide the patient with the specific diagnostic label in effect precludes the patient who is capable and motivated from seeking any information regarding the disease process and also from seeking available information regarding community resources. The patient presumably has the right to understand the disease process and its implications for changes in living circumstances and the planning thus required. In addition, the patient is also entitled to information pertaining to treatment alternatives and his/her right to execute advance directives, legal instruments which ensure that the patient's treatment preferences are respected in the event of future incapacity. Federal legislation, effective since 1991 and known as the Patient Self Determination Act (PSDA) (Public Law No. 101–508, Sections 4206, 4571), mandates that health care workers inform patients, in writing, of their legal right to execute advance directives in accordance with applicable state law. The intent of the PSDA is to explicitly reinforce the assumption of patient autonomy and opportunity to be involved in treatment decisions while the patient is presumed to be competent to make his/her preferences known. The PSDA was enacted following the decision of the United States Supreme Court in the so called 'right to die' case, *Cruzan v. Director, Missouri Department of Health*, 110 S. Ct. 2841 (1990), but is nevertheless of particular importance with respect to dementia patients, as a substantial number of such patients reside in nursing home settings. It is likely, however, that in many cases, the rights and preferences of dementia patients in such settings are ignored or unsolicited. Bradley and her colleagues (1997), in a study involving nursing home residents in three separate Connecticut facilities, found that in approximately 70% of admissions to such facilities where information regarding the PSDA was provided, the information was forwarded to someone other than the resident, even when the resident was judged to be alert and oriented. In some cases the failure to provide the information as required by the PSDA was based solely on subjective impressions of perceived cognitive impairment of the resident. Such findings underscore the prevalent notion that dementia, even when unverified by objective means, invariably implies incapacity, or at least justifies the usurpation of the patient's autonomy and

legal rights. These findings should, however, serve as an impetus for the development and standardized application of such instruments as those developed by Marson et al. and their use as a minimal prerequisite for any substantive reduction in patient autonomy and legal rights.

Disclosure of the existence and nature of a dementing process is invariably an emotionally difficult situation, but I would note that, in my experience, patients are usually somewhat aware of the nature, if not the extent, of their deficits, often also aware of the possibility of AD before any specific mention is made and likely as concerned regarding the reaction of family members as the family is with respect to the patient's reaction. One risk that the clinician should be cognizant of in the postassessment conference with the patient and family members is the possibility of severe depression. The potential for suicide with such patients exists, although it is relatively rare; Knight (1994) has offered the anecdotal observation that suicide may be a risk in patients with multi-infarct dementia and dementia pugilistica. For some neurodegenerative conditions, e.g. multiple sclerosis and HD, an increased risk for both clinical depression and suicide which warrants psychological intervention has been established (Stenager and Stenager 1992). In a review of studies whose subject matter was the relation between suicide frequency and a number of neurological conditions which included multiple sclerosis, HD and PD, Stenager and Stenager (1992) have cited a number of methodological problems or errors, most common of which was small sample size, which render interpretation of the stated conclusions as, at best, problematic. I have personally observed a significant number of patients, particularly those with early-stage dementia, with coexisting clinical depression, presumably related to the fact that such patients are more likely to have an awareness of the extent of present and future loss of capacity than patients in more advanced stages of the disease process. In contrast, I have only on rare occasions encountered a case in which a clinically significant depression appeared to be in part attributable to the formal disclosure of a dementing condition as a precipitating factor. In at least one neurodegenerative condition, HD, there is evidence derived from the Canadian Collaborative Study of Predictive Testing, conducted in 1988, that individuals who were informed of the increased risk of developing the disease, following genetic testing, did not generally show signs of significant depression at the time their risk was disclosed or at 12-month follow-up assessment (Wiggins et al. 1992).

Looking beyond the issue of disclosure of the neuro-degenerative process to the patient and information regarding its probable course, is there any requirement that the clinician discuss any of the extraclinical issues referred to in this chapter, e.g. subjects such as the conveyance of durable power of attorney? Strictly speaking, the answer to this question is no, i.e. the professional's duty may encompass only the communication of clinical findings and data-based opinions regarding the particular neurodegenerative condition and its treatment. The clinician is not, technically speaking, acting in the capacity of agent or representative of the legal system and therefore, presumably, has no legal obligation to discuss with the patient such matters as the possibility of conveying durable power of attorney to ensure that the patient's wishes are considered should he/she reach the point at which some form of proxy decision making becomes necessary. Certainly, however, for the professional who works on a regular basis with such patients, professional competence should entail an awareness of the potential impact of disease-based cognitive impairment on the patient's legal status. While medical treatment for such conditions as AD at this time is limited and can be described as palliative, the best professional advice may consist of prescriptions for changes in living circumstances that allow the patient an optimal level of autonomy with available assistance and supervision as needed. Alleviating the patient's suffering, in a broader context, then, includes provision for assistance in decision making when and if needed. It follows then, that the professional's ethical, if not legal, obligation to the patient under such circumstances includes the duty to advise the patient and family members of the option of conveying, through assistance of legal counsel, durable power of attorney in an attempt to simultaneously alleviate the burden of everyday functioning of the patient while ensuring that the patient's expressed or known preferences are considered. In addition, as a final important consideration, the professional's awareness of these issues and communication of their relevance to the patient and family members can obviate the necessity for later expensive and burdensome courtroom proceedings, such as those required for guardianship, when no prior durable power of attorney has been conveyed. As physicians, neuropsychologists and similarly situated professionals will generally be the first to have contact with patients with neurodegenerative conditions, they are in the best position to provide the patient and family members with information bearing on these ethical and legal issues when it will have its greatest potential beneficial impact (Overman and Stoudemire 1993).

Advances in detection and prediction of various forms of dementia will invariably be accompanied by additional disclosure-related issues. With forms of neurodegenerative disease for which there are known, or yet to be discovered, genetic predispositions, such as Huntington's chorea, there is the issue of genetic counseling for prospective parents and the personal dilemmas to be confronted by those who are in a position to know, if they should choose to know, whether they are likely future victims. With respect to such conditions as HD, sickle-cell anemia, and Tay–Sachs disease, the high predictability of detection through genetic testing has already become accepted to the extent that it is widely publicized in the popular press (Ubell 1997). In some respects, however, the availability of genetic testing for a neurodegenerative condition such as HD may be regarded as somewhat of a mixed blessing, as certainty regarding the likelihood of disease occurrence can be accompanied by serious psychological consequences for the affected individual and immediate family members. A diagnosis of HD affects every member of the family and at least one observer has argued that genetic testing for HD should be viewed as a family, not an individual, issue (Hayes 1992).

Presymptomatic testing for AD comparable in predictive accuracy to that available for HD is not yet available, although the recent work with apolipoprotein E suggests the possibility of discovery of a reliable genetic marker in the next few years. At present, evidence indicates that apolipoprotein E genotyping does not provide sufficient sensitivity and specificity to be used alone as a diagnostic test of AD, although it does improve the specificity of the diagnosis (Mayeux et al. 1998). Without commensurate developments in treatment, however, the potential ability to predict susceptibility to eventual cognitive impairment poses the same type of ethical dilemma confronted by those whose familial background indicates the possibility of HD, i.e. from a clinician's perspective, is there a duty to provide unsolicited disclosure of the probability of future impairment? The client, especially one who has a responsible family, social or professional role to maintain, confronts a mirror-image ethical quandary under such circumstances, i.e. is there a duty to find out what chances of neurodegenerative disease exist, even when such predictions are probabilistic at best? The number and complexity of similar ethical questions associated with neurodegenerative diseases will inevitably increase with the advent of additional clinical and research findings. It is also inevitable that the advances in medical care and improvements in diet that have resulted in the dramatic proportional increase in the elderly population during this century will require a continuing simultaneous awareness of these ethical issues on the part of both clinicians and research scientists.

REFERENCES

Anderer, S.J. 1990. A model for determining competency in guardianship proceedings. *Medical and Psychological Disability Law Reporter*. 14: 107–114.

Bailey, W.T. and Johnston, S.J. 1994, November. *Knowledge about Alzheimer's disease among licensed psychologists in Illinois*. Paper presented at the Annual Scientific Meeting of the Gerontological Society of America, Atlanta.

Baum, C., Edwards, D., Yonan, C. and Storandt, M. 1996. The relation of neuropsychological test performance to performance of functional tasks in dementia of the Alzheimer type. *Archives of Clinical Neuropsychology*. 11: 69–75.

Binder, L.M. and Thompson, L.L. 1995. The ethics code and neuropsychological assessment practices. *Archives of Clinical Neuropsychology*. 10: 27–46.

Binstock, R.H., Post, S.G. and Whitehouse, P.J. 1992. *Dementia and aging: Ethics, values and policy choices*. Baltimore: The Johns Hopkins University Press.

Bradley, E., Walker, L., Blechner, B. and Wetle, T. 1997. Assessing capacity to participate in discussions of advance directives in nursing homes: Findings from a study of the Patient Self Determination Act. *Journal of the American Geriatrics Society*. 45: 79–83.

Chatel, D.M., Bieliauskas, L.A., Green, P.A., McSweeney, A.J. and Warner, J.E. 1993, August. *Cognitive predictors of driving ability in the elderly*. Paper presented at the American Psychological Association Convention, Toronto, Canada.

Crum, R.M, Anthony, J.C., Bassett, S.S. and Folstein, M.F. 1993. Population-based norms for the Mini-Mental State Examination by age and educational level. *Journal of the American Medical Association*. 269: 2386–2391.

Delis, D.C., Massman, P.J., Butters, N., Salmon, D.P., Kramer, J.H. and Cermak, L. 1991. Profiles of demented and amnesic patients on the California Verbal Learning Test: Implications for the assessment of memory disorders. *Psychological Assessment: A Journal of Consulting and Clinical Psychology*. 3: 19–26.

Drachman, D.A. 1994. If we live long enough, will we all be demented? *Neurology*. 44: 1563–1565.

Farlow, M., Gracon, S.I., Hershey, L.A., Lewis, K.W., Sadowsky, C.H. and Dolan-Ureno, J. 1992. A controlled trial of tacrine in Alzheimer's disease. *Journal of the American Medical Association*. 268: 2523–2529.

Fitten, L.J., Perryman, K.M., Wilkinson, C.J., Little, R.J., Burns, M.M., Pachana, M., Mervis, J.R., Malmgren, R., Siembieda, D.W. and Ganzell, S. 1995. Alzheimer and vascular dementias and driving: A prospective road and laboratory study. *Journal of the American Medical Association*. 273: 1360–1365.

Grisso, T. 1986. *Evaluating competencies*. New York: Plenum Press.

Growdon, J. H. 1992. Treatment for Alzheimer's disease? *New England Journal of Medicine*. 327: 1306–1308.

Hayes, C.V. 1992. Genetic testing for Huntington's disease: A family issue. *The New England Journal of Medicine*. 327: 1449–1451.

Heaton, R.K. 1992. *Comprehensive norms for an expanded Halstead-Reitan Battery: A supplement for the Wechsler Adult Intelligence Scale-Revised*. Odessa FL: Psychological Assessment Resources.

Heaton, R., Grant, I. and Matthews, C. 1991. *Comprehensive norms for an expanded Halstead-Reitan Battery: Demographic corrections, research findings and clinical applications*. Odessa FL, Florida: Psychological Assessment Resources.

Heikkilä, V.-M., Turkka, J., Korpelainen, J., Kallanranta, T. and Summala, H. 1998. Decreased driving ability in people with Parkinson's disease. *Journal of Neurology, Neurosurgery and Psychiatry*. 64: 325–330.

Heun, R., Bierbauer, J. and Benkert, O. 1995. Visual memory in Alzheimer patients: Effects of practice, retention interval and severity of cognitive decline. *Dementia*. 6: 117–120.

High, W.M. 1993. Advancing research with Alzheimer disease subjects: Investigators' perceptions and ethical issues. *Alzheimer Disease and Associated Disorders*. 7: 165–178.

High, W.M., Whitehouse, P.J., Post, S.G. and Berg, L. 1994. Guidelines for addressing ethical and legal issues in Alzheimer disease research: A position paper. *Alzheimer Disease and Associated Disorders*. 8 (Suppl. 4): 66–74.

Hopewell, C.A. and Van Zomeren, A. H. 1990. Neuropsychological aspects of motor vehicle operation. In *The neuropsychology of everyday life: Assessment and basic competencies*, ed. D.E. Tupper and K.D. Cicerone, pp. 307–334. Boston: Kluwer Academic Publishers.

Hurley, A.C., Volicer, L., Rampusheski, V.F. and Fry, S.T. 1995. Reaching consensus: The process of recommending treatment decisions for Alzheimer's patient's. *Advances in Nursing Science*. 18: 33–43.

Knight, B.G. 1994. Providing clinical interpretations for older clients and their families. In *Neuropsychological assessment of dementia and depression in older adults: A clinician's guide*, ed. M. Storandt and G.R. VandenBos, pp. 141–154. Washington: American Psychological Association.

Little, M., Williams, J.M. and Long, C. 1986. Clinical memory tests and everyday memory. *Archives of Clinical Neuropsychology*. 1: 323–333.

Lyman, K.A. 1989. Bringing the social back in: A critique of the bio-medicalization of dementia. *The Gerontologist*. 29: 597–605.

Macklin, R. 1987. *Mortal choices: Ethical dilemmas in modern medicine*. Boston: Houghton Mifflin.

Marson, D., Chatterjee, A., Ingram, K. and Harrell, L. 1996. Toward a neurologic model of competency: Cognitive predictors of capacity to consent in Alzheimer's disease using three different legal standards. *Neurology*. 46: 666–672.

Marson, D., Cody, H., Ingram, K. and Harrell, L. 1995a. Neuropsychologic predictors of Alzheimer's disease using a rational reasons legal standard. *Archives of Neurology*. 52: 955–959.

Marson, D., Ingram, K., Cody, H. and Harrell, L. 1995b. Assessing the competency of patients with Alzheimer's disease under different legal standards. *Archives of Neurology*. 52: 949–954.

Marson, D., Schmitt, F., Ingram, K. and Harrell, L. 1994. Determining the competency of Alzheimer patients to consent to treatment and research. *Alzheimer Disease and Associated Disorders*. 8 (Suppl. 4): 5–18.

Mayeux, R., Saunders, A.M., Shea, S., Mirra, S., Evans, D., Roses, A.D., Hyman, B.T., Crain, B., Tang, M.-X. and Phelps, C.H. for the Alzheimer's Disease Centers Consortium on Apolipoprotein E and Alzheimer's disease. 1998. Utility of the apolipoprotein E genotype in the diagnosis of Alzheimer's disease. *New England Journal of Medicine*. 338: 506–511.

Meyers, J.E. and Meyers, K.R. 1995. *Rey Complex Figure Test and Recognition Trial*. Odessa FL: Psychological Assessment Resources, Inc.

Mills, M.J. and Daniels, M.L. 1987. Medical-legal issues. In *Principles of medical psychiatry*, ed. A. Stoudemire and B.S. Fogel, pp. 463–476. Orlando: Grune and Stratton.

Overman, W.H. and Stoudemire, A. 1993. Legal, financial and ethical issues in Alzheimer's disease and other dementias. In *Neuropsychology of Alzheimer disease and other dementias*, ed. R.W. Parks, R.F. Zec and R.S. Wilson, pp. 615–625. New York: Oxford University Press.

Paolo, A.M. and Ryan, J.J. 1995. Selecting WAIS-R norms for persons 75 years and older. *The Clinical Neuropsychologist*. 9: 1–6.

Paolo, A.M. and Ryan, J.J. 1996. Stability of WAIS-R scatter indices in the elderly. *Archives of Clinical Neuropsychology*. 11: 503–511.

Paolo, A.M., Tröster, A.I. and Ryan, J.J. 1997. California Verbal Learning Test: Normative data for the elderly. *Journal of Clinical and Experimental Neuropsychology*. 19: 220–234.

Reiman, E.M., Caselli, R.J., Yun, L.S., Chen, K., Bandy, D., Minoshima, S.,Thibodeau, S.N. and Osborne, D. 1996. Preclinical evidence of Alzheimer's disease in persons homozygous for the ε4 allele for apolipoprotein E. *New England Journal of Medicine*. 334: 752–758.

Rizzo, M., Reinach, S., McGehee, D. and Dawson, J. 1997. Simulated car crashes and crash predictors in drivers with Alzheimer's disease. *Archives of Neurology*. 54: 545–551.

Ruscio, D. and Cavarocchi, N. 1984. Getting on the political agenda: How an organization of Alzheimer families won increased federal attention and funding. *Generations*. 9: 12–15.

Ryan, J.J. and Paolo, A.M. 1992. Verbal-performance IQ discrepancies on the WAIS-R: An examination of the old-age standardization sample. *Neuropsychology*. 6: 293–298.

Ryan, J.J., Paolo, A.M. and Brungardt, T.M. 1990. Standardization of the Wechsler Adult Intelligence Scale-Revised for persons 75 years and older. *Psychological Assessment*. 2: 404–411.

Scogin, F. and Prohaska, M. 1993. *Aiding older adults with memory complaints*. Sarasota, Florida: Professional Resource Press.

Searight, H. and Goldberg, M., 1991. The Community Competence Scale as a measure of functional daily living skills. *Journal of Mental Health Administration*. 18: 128–134.

Stenager, E.N. and Stenager, E. 1992. Suicide and patients with neurologic diseases: Methodological problems. *Archives of Neurology*. 49: 1296–1303.

Taeuber, C. 1990. Diversity: The dramatic reality. In *Diversity in aging: Challenges facing planners and policymakers in the 1990s*, ed. S. Bass, E. Kutza and F. Torres-Gill, pp. 1–45. Glenview, Illinois: Scott, Foresman and Co.

Tombaugh, T.N. and McIntyre, N.J. 1992. The Mini-Mental State Examination: A comprehensive review. *Journal of the American Geriatrics Society*. 40: 922–935.

Tomlinson, B.E., Blessed, G. and Roth, M. 1970. Observations on the brains of demented old people. *Journal of Neurological Sciences*. 11: 205–242.

Turnbull, S. 1990. Ethical issues in the care of the patient with Alzheimer's disease. In *Alzheimer's disease: A handbook for caregivers*, ed. R.C. Hamdy, J.M. Turnbull, L.D. Norman and M.M. Lancaster, pp. 85–93. St. Louis, Missouri: The C.V. Mosby Company.

Ubell, E. 1997. Should you consider gene testing? *Parade Magazine*. New York: Parade Publications.

Wagner, M.T. and Bachman, D. L. 1996. Neuropsychological features of diffuse Lewy body disease. *Archives of Clinical Neuropsychology*. 11: 175–184.

Wechsler, D. 1997. *Wechsler Memory Scale – Third Edition*. San Antonio: The Psychological Corporation.

Weiner, M.A. 1987. *Reducing the risk of Alzheimer's*. New York: Stein and Day.

Wiggins, S., Whyte, P., Huggins, M., Adam, S., Theilmann, J., Bloch, M., Sheps, S., Schecter, M. and Hayden, M. 1992. The psychological consequences of predictive testing for Huntington's disease. *New England Journal of Medicine*. 327: 1401–1405.

Winick, B. 1995. The side effects of incompetency labeling and the implications for mental health law. *Psychology, Public Policy and Law*. 1: 6–42.

Zehr, M. 1994, July. *Legal considerations in the cognitive intellectual assessment of older adults*. Paper presented at the International Congress of Applied Psychology, Madrid, Spain.

24 Memory in neurodegenerative disease: clinical perspectives

THOMAS BENKE

INTRODUCTION

Impairment of memory is the hallmark and often among the first symptoms of the majority of neurodegenerative diseases. Thus, knowledge regarding memory and its deficits has become of major interest to individuals who are confronted with a person developing dementia, be it as medical staff, research personnel or, in a more social and immediate fashion, as a family member or caregiver. As evident in this book, there are several approaches to study the structure and impairments of memory. The *biological perspective* focuses on the brain as the host of memory; the *cognitive perspective* describes the varieties of memory and its pathology and the *clinical perspective* is concerned with the effects of neurodegenerative disorders on the brain, on memory functions and with their consequences for the patient. Among these three approaches, clinical memory research is the most pragmatic. Naturally, it is also the least homogeneous because it encompasses a number of domains such as research on normal aging, clinical investigations, neuropsychological assessment methods, pathology, treatment and epidemiology. Thus, despite the advantage it is afforded by being able to make use of theoretical frameworks emanating from experimental work, a high percentage of clinical questions remains unanswered. In the clinical perspectives section of this volume, some important issues regarding clinical memory research in dementia are updated, reviewed and discussed. The result is a state-of-the-art summary of the clinical research into dementia-related memory impairment; however, due to their critical modus operandi, the chapters in this section have also become a register of unanswered questions and research topics which need to be tackled in the future.

METHODOLOGICAL AND PRACTICAL ISSUES

Most clinicians would agree that the assessment of memory in elderly persons serves several important aims: the detection of memory impairment in relation to pre-morbid performance levels or performance in an age and education matched population; the evaluation of the extent and character of memory impairment; the differentiation of intrinsic, disease-related memory deficits from those caused by age, mood changes or other confounding factors; and finally an estimation of the impact of memory impairment on a patient's life. Not all aims of memory testing apply to a given patient. Table 24.1 summarizes some of the most important issues addressed by memory assessment in dementia as viewed from the clinical standpoint characterizing this overview.

Comorbidity of memory impairment with other cognitive deficits

The commonly agreed upon features of amnesia include a severe and permanent learning deficit (i.e. anterograde amnesia) and a variable loss of memory for information predating the onset of brain damage (i.e. retrograde amnesia) in the presence of normal intelligence and unimpaired attention (Parkin and Leng 1993). It is self-evident that the neuropsychological evaluation of a person's memory will yield a measure of amnesia. The measure of amnesia may not, however, be a pure measure of memory dysfunction. In a state like dementia, amnesia is not the only cognitive problem. All diagnostic criteria for dementia require that the memory loss be accompanied by deficits in other domains of cognition, some of which clearly interact in a reciprocal manner with memory. Although the coexistence of memory and other cognitive impairment is an almost invariable feature in more advanced disease stages, it is occasionally already observed early in the disease.

Memory involves many complex subsystems by means

Table 24.1. *Issues in the evaluation of memory in dementia*

Problem/study area	Challenge to memory assessment
Comorbidity of amnesia with other deficits	Develop memory measures capable of separating primary from secondary memory impairment
Universal risk factors for, and prevalence of, dementia	Develop cross-culturally valid screening and memory tests
Differential diagnosis of dementia	Develop/employ assessment procedures that are valid, reliable, responsive, sensitive, specific and have adequate normative data for the elderly with and without cerebral dysfunction
Preclinical detection	
Age-related memory alterations	
Impact of depression and mood state on memory	Rule out confounding factors
Impact of amnesia on everyday functions	Develop/use ecologically valid memory tests
Treatment of memory dysfunction	Develop/use tests sensitive to treatment effects and to deficits across the entire disease span
Changes in memory over the disease course	

of which an organism registers, stores, retains and retrieves some previous exposure to an event or experience (Lezak, 1995). These functions are highly specific but they do not work in isolation from other mental abilities and from mood states. Performing a memory test requires, for example, sensory-perceptual functions like hearing or seeing and it is well known that visual and auditory functions are often compromised in elderly persons (Chapter 16). Howieson and Lezak (1995) discuss the contribution of other cognitive functions to performance on memory tests. Performance on memory tests may vary as a function of intelligence. Virtually all memory tests place demands on directed and sustained attention which are necessary for proper registration of the information to be learned. It is well known that distinguishing between a primary memory disorder and an impairment of attention and concentration secondarily disrupting memory is often difficult. Furthermore, a memory test may require the examinee to draw upon verbal abilities like lexical-semantic knowledge or language comprehension and nonverbal abilities like visuospatial functions. Executive functions like planning, problem solving, the development of strategies, self-monitoring or decision making may play a crucial role in the performance on a memory test (Chapters 8 and 9). Finally, depression and mood state may influence performance on certain memory measures (Chapter 19). As demented patients often suffer from impairments of verbal, spatial and/or 'frontal' functions, a comorbidity of amnesia with other cognitive deficits is the rule rather than

the exception. Consequently, it must be clear to the investigator that a detailed separation of memory impairments from other cognitive problems is often impossible and that the resulting memory measures in dementia may only represent an approximation of the severity of memory impairment per se. For the reason of comprehensiveness and to gain insight into possible cognitive comorbidity, neuropsychological investigations in a patient with presumed or confirmed dementia should include a thorough investigation of language, visuospatial and frontal functions as well as an assessment of mood state (Chapter 18), as a minimum supplement to memory testing.

Risk factors

What do we know about populations developing memory disorders and dementia at a higher than average rate and about risk factors specific to a given cohort? Can we make any predictions about the risk for dementia from factors like age, education, occupation, gender or previous disease? The answer to these questions is particularly relevant to the future of social medicine and geriatric neurology. In their chapter on psychosocial and biological risk factors for dementia and memory loss, Jacobs and Schofield (Chapter 14) critically reviewed community-based epidemiological studies of dementia. The overall picture of risk factors for dementia is heterogeneous and depends on the given variables and the type of dementia under investigation. Age is consistently recognized as the single most important risk factor for dementia in Alzheimer's disease (AD),

Parkinson's disease (PD) and for cerebrovascular disorders. The investigation of relationships between dementia and risk factors other than age has yielded less consistent results. Several studies have claimed that extent of education is inversely associated with the development of dementia in AD and cerebrovascular disease, but this finding may be the result of a selection bias. A history of a head injury emerged as a risk factor for AD in several, but not all investigations. Similarly, other factors like ethnicity, gender and depression have only inconsistently been associated with dementia.

What has become increasingly recognized as a risk factor for various dementing disorders is the role of certain inheritance patterns and neurogenetic dispositions, such as the apolipoprotein E ε4 allele in a subgroup of patients with AD (Strittmatter and Roses 1995; Stern et al. 1997) and some other dementias (Schneider et al. 1995), or the length of the trinucleotide repeat expansion in HD, which is highly correlated with the rate of cognitive decline (Brandt et al. 1996). Although there is still a lack of screening tests which reliably predict the development of neurodegenerative disease, it seems likely that the rapid increase of neurogenetic knowledge will ultimately be translated into a promising clinical tool for the early detection and prediction of dementia.

Taken together, present knowledge leads one to hypothesize that several biological and psychosocial factors may modulate the neurodegenerative disease process. A caveat is that many epidemiological studies are subject to biases in case recruitment and ascertainment and, consequently, have not reliably identified demographic risk factors for memory loss and dementia. Clearly, this problem remains to be solved in future demographic studies.

Prevalence

Risk factors for dementia can also be identified by examining the prevalence rates of neurodegenerative diseases within certain geographical and ethnic boundaries. This approach tries to identify possible genetic and environmental factors underlying dementing disorders from their distribution in geographical and cultural areas. For example, the local and racial distribution of multiple sclerosis, another frequent and chronic neurological disorder, presents a riddle to epidemiologists. Geographical surveys of multiple sclerosis show high, medium and low risk areas (Kurtzke 1980; Ebers and Sadovnick 1994). High-prevalence areas with multiple sclerosis rates of more than

100 per 100 000 inhabitants comprise certain latitudes including northern and central Europe, the former Soviet Union, southern Canada, the northern United States and southeastern Asia. In contrast, other regions like Japan and the rest of Asia have prevalence rates of less than 25 per 100 000, indicating a racial distribution gradient. The white population of South Africa, in which multiple sclerosis-prevalence is moderate, is surrounded by a black population in which multiple sclerosis is virtually unknown. Interestingly, persons migrating after a critical age seem to retain the risk of the original geographical region; this raises speculations regarding exposure to an environmental agent at a critical age. In addition, putative epidemic factors have been related to the development of multiple sclerosis after analysis of the incidence rates from originally multiple sclerosis-free areas like the Faroe Islands and Iceland. These isolated areas had recorded no multiple sclerosis cases until they had sudden and dramatic appearances of multiple sclerosis coupled with military occupations during World War II. Thus, epidemiological studies of multiple sclerosis have identified several risk factors, among them racial distribution, environmental and age gradients and possibly transmissible agents. Even without the evidence of direct links between these factors and the outbreak of the disease, epidemiological approaches are certainly among the most crucial in the detection of a disease's cause.

The present knowledge about the epidemiology of dementia is far less advanced than that about multiple sclerosis. As pointed out in Chapter 15 by Monsch, Taylor and Bondi, the number of cross-cultural studies reaching valid comparisons of the dementia rates in two or more cultures or continents is low due to a lack of proper screening instruments which can be used for cross-cultural comparisons. Unlike multiple sclerosis, which has the advantage of being diagnosable by clinical features and relatively simple laboratory test results which are relatively invariant across cultures, dementia assessment is far more complex as it is largely based on culture-dependent psychometric screening procedures. Monsch and colleagues raise a number of methodological issues, among them the use of inconsistent clinical diagnostic criteria and practices and the lack of neuropsychological assessment procedures which are valid for detection of dementia in different cultures. Many cognitive tests are still hampered by biases regarding their construction, translation, items in use and administration procedures. Furthermore, cross-cultural comparisons have revealed different profiles of performance even on simple cognitive screening tests like the Mini-Mental State Examination (Folstein et al. 1975), thus highlighting the role of culture-specific education, training and experiences in test performance. It is clear that cross-ethnic and cross-cultural dementia prevalence studies are still inconclusive at present and unfortunately there is no satisfying answer to questions regarding the differentiation of neurodegenerative disorders in different ethnic and cultural groups.

Assessment

The accurate diagnosis of dementia is necessary to identify treatable causes, as well as to prognosticate and allow long-term planning. The clinical diagnosis of a syndrome like AD, HD or other neurodegenerative disorders includes diagnostic reasoning. Diagnostic reasoning in medicine is fed by disease-specific information, the most important sources of which are careful history taking and the proper use and evaluation of investigative procedures, including neuropsychological assessment. In addition, reaching a diagnosis of dementia is assisted by extrapolation from prevalence rates for a specific syndrome. Specifically, prevalence rates have been shown to be essential diagnostic aids by virtue of providing positive or negative predictive values. Positive predictive values indicate that a patient with a positive test result actually has the disease, whereas a negative predictive value is the probability that a patient with a negative test result does not have the disease. Positive predictive values and negative predictive values are calculated using the prevalence of the disease in a base population, in conjunction with a given diagnostic test's sensitivity and specificity (Fletcher et al. 1982). Thus, prevalence rates, predictive values and test procedures share an important functional relationship in the diagnosis of dementia.

As disease prevalence and test sensitivity and specificity significantly influence positive predictive values and negative predictive values, the selection of proper tests and knowledge about the confidence limits for the results of a given diagnostic procedure becomes crucial (Sox et al. 1988). Even when sensitivity and specificity are high (i.e. 90%), the positive predictive values can be less than 50% when the prevalence of a disease is low or, conversely, the negative predictive values can be less than 50% when the prevalence of a disease is high (Gifford et al. 1996).

It can be concluded from this theoretical background that one of the central problem areas for research into memory disorders in dementia regards the methodology which is employed to measure memory deficits and in particular the sensitivity, validity and reliability of test procedures. The demands upon psychometric test materials are well known: they have to be reliable, i.e. these instruments are supposed to measure a given variable in an accurate, consistent, reproducible way. Forms of reliability include internal consistency (the extent to which items comprising a scale measure the same construct), test-retest, inter-rater and parallel forms reliability. Furthermore, neuropsychological test materials have to be valid, i.e. they should be able to measure what they were intended to measure. Finally, as memory impairment progresses in neurodegenerative disorders, memory tests must have the ability to detect clinically important changes in a reliable way.

In his chapter on the psychometric issues involved in clinical memory assessment, Paolo (Chapter 16) compares the usefulness and the properties of memory tests in the diagnosis of dementia. A critical review of popular and frequently used memory assessment devices shows that few tests meet the most important psychometric demands. A considerable number of tests have limitations, such as small normative samples, poor or unknown test-retest reliability, inadequate internal consistency or low subtest reliabilities. Many tests only offer limited information on individual memory functions like learning, recall, recognition or the occurrence of specific errors observed in memory disorders (e.g. intrusions, perseverations, etc.). Some tests, like the California Verbal Learning Test (CVLT; Delis et al. 1987) do provide data concerning specific learning and memory parameters (Elwood 1995); however, normative data have only recently been extended beyond age 80 years (Paolo et al. 1997). As the majority of memory tests were designed for normal, nondemented elderly, they do not meet the explicit requirements of demented patients. Only a few memory tests are designed to serve both clinical and research purposes. Most authors of cross-cultural or multi-national studies of dementia have been confronted by the problem that memory tests designed in one language and normed in one culture may not be applicable to the group under investigation. In sum, there is no standard test for dementia fulfilling all the desired psychometric properties.

Preclinical detection

How early can dementia be detected and which measures best characterize and capture the latency phase of dementia? A group of studies has dealt with the emergence of memory decline in the earliest stages of dementia and the methods that best differentiate the effects of normal aging from pathological changes. Prior to the appearance of a full dementia syndrome, a preclinical period of cerebral structural and metabolic changes seems to precede overt, diagnosable manifestations of dementia, often by many years. This period has increasingly become a target of interest, as little is known about its duration, significance and predictive power in various dementia syndromes. Thus, researchers have tried to identify cognitive markers of incipient dementia, especially in subjects with certain genetic predispositions.

Bondi and Monsch (Chapter 17) summarize what is presently known about the preclinical detection of AD and discuss the theoretical background of neurocognitive development in elderly persons. Epidemiological studies with follow-up assessments have demonstrated that the subsequent development of AD can be predicted by cognitive markers, particularly by memory assessment procedures. The existence of a preclinical stage receives further support from the finding that the memory test performance of nondemented elderly individuals who have an increased risk for developing AD (due to a positive family history or due to a certain genotype like the apolipoprotein ε4), is poorer than that of elderly individuals without such risk factors. Similarly, a decline of cognitive performance has been found in carriers of the huntingtin gene who were still without signs or symptoms of HD (Foroud et al. 1995). The degree of cognitive deficit was found to be proportional to the number of trinucleotide repeats in the HD allele. Whereas a substantial percentage of AD patients seems to display discrete forms of memory impairment and other cognitive deficits in their preclinical stage (Jacobs et al. 1995a), the neuropsychological characteristics of preclinical dementia in PD is characterized by poor performance on letter and verbal fluency tasks, whereas tests of memory, orientation, reasoning, naming and constructional skills are less sensitive predictors of subsequent dementia (Jacobs et al. 1995b). Further complementary studies about the preclinical stages of dementia may help to develop more valid disease models.

Memory changes in normal aging and dementia

How can age-related changes in cognition be differentiated from disease-specific symptoms? This question highlights the need for memory assessment procedures with high dis-

criminative ability. Many elderly subjects experience age associated memory impairment (AAMI), or what has been called benign senescent forgetfulness. AAMI often includes a gradual worsening of name finding, of remembering to do multiple tasks or of recalling object locations.

Welsh-Bohmer and Ogrocki (Chapter 18) review memory changes encountered in normal and demented elderly. These authors point to the fact that AAMI, although being discernible from dementia-associated amnesia, is poorly understood. It is unclear whether AAMI is a benign entity, a risk factor for dementia, or if it is located at one end of a continuum and therefore a prodromal stage of dementia-associated amnesia with unclear pathogenesis. Most clinicians agree that the line between incipient dementia and cognitive changes associated with normal aging is a fuzzy one and one that can only be drawn by a comprehensive neuropsychological evaluation which, in addition to memory evaluation, includes a standardized assessment of functions like intelligence, language, visuospatial abilities and executive and sensorimotor functions.

It has been shown that memory assessment plays a special role in the differentiation of AAMI from dementia and that memory assessment can also serve the purpose of differentiating dementia syndromes by revealing different profiles and patterns of amnesia (e.g. in AD and subcortical types of dementia). Due to the diagnostic utility of memory testing, clinicians have been encouraged to evaluate assorted memory functions, like storage, encoding, retrieval, or rate of forgetting and to include assessment procedures for various types of memory like episodic, semantic and procedural memory.

Depression

The impact of depression on memory and other aspects of cognition has been demonstrated in many studies (Starkstein et al. 1989; Burt et al. 1995). Fields and colleagues' overview (Chapter 19) highlights that the association between memory impairment and depression is complex, requiring consideration of issues such as the heterogeneity of memory impairment in the depressed elderly, case ascertainment methods, the patterns of memory dysfunction observed in depression versus dementia, the biological correlates of depression, the effects of antidepressive therapy on memory performance, age-related factors and the role of depression in cortical versus subcortical dementias. A review of research related to these topics makes it evident that only some questions can be answered with confidence. It is generally accepted that depression plays a different role in various dementias: PD or HD have a seemingly higher prevalence of depression than AD and the initial degree of depression in PD may even predict subsequent declines in cognitive performance and abilities of daily living (Starkstein et al. 1992; Tröster et al. 1995). Indeed, evidence to date suggests that PD may be unique among dementias in that depression has been shown to clearly impact memory only in PD. The differential diagnosis between the memory impairment found in major depression versus dementia, particularly AD (e.g. Gainotti and Marra 1994) is another important clinical issue: the assessment of various memory functions such as recall, recognition, strategy use, remote memory or metamemory appear especially important in differential diagnosis.

Everyday memory functions

What are the practical consequences of memory loss for a patient with dementia? A major concern in the assessment of memory is the relationship between the assessment procedures used in the clinic and the impact of memory impairment on everyday life. An apparently poor correspondence between psychometrically or clinically derived estimates of memory impairment and functioning in everyday settings is a frequent criticism voiced by those in rehabilitation settings. This criticism is now recognized as a problem not only in dementia assessment but in clinical neuropsychology in general.

Basically, the decision whether to use more experimentally or ecologically relevant test materials is made according to the purpose of the assessment. Of course, the majority of persons who are routinely and primarily involved in the care and management of demented patients think that the assessment of cognitive functions should be routinely driven by ecological rather than cognitive theoretical issues. This argument is based primarily on the observation that memory tests of highly abstract, nonrealistic character do not reflect the patient's actual abilities, deficits or needs in his or her personal environment.

There remains a need for the development of ecologically based memory tests. The Rivermead Behavioural Memory Test (RBMT; Wilson et al. 1985) is one of the few tests which has been developed primarily with ecological validity in mind, i.e. it seeks to provide measures of the practical effects of impaired memory and can thus be used for monitoring memory changes with treatment (Lezak

1995). The RBMT includes mostly practical memory tasks such as name-face associations, remembering a hidden belonging, an appointment, a newspaper article, faces and routes, to deliver a message, as well as an orientation section. The test has four parallel forms and supplemental norms have been developed for the 70–94-year age range (Cockburn and Smith 1989).

Despite these apparent advantages, the RBMT is also noted to have several shortcomings. As the RBMT only has a two or three-point scoring range, it has been criticized for lacking sensitivity at both the high and low ends of memory functioning and being most relevant for patients with moderate memory disorders (Lezak 1995). Although widely applied to amnesias of various etiologies, few studies have evaluated the RBMT in dementia. Beardsall and Huppert (1991) compared the clinical utility of three subtests of the RBMT (story recall, route recall, name-face association) with that of a 16-word list memory task and that of the memory items of the Cambridge Cognitive Examination (CAMCOG; Roth et al. 1986) comprising recall of familiar objects, recall of a name and address, as well as recall of three words. These tests were evaluated in a community sample of elderly subjects divided into those with and without dementia based on the MMSE, the CAMDEX and a standardized, structured psychiatric interview and examination using DSM–III–R and ICD–10 criteria for dementia (Roth et al. 1986). The results showed that a combination of clinical, laboratory and psychometric memory tests best discriminated demented from nondemented individuals. A subset of five memory tests was found to produce the most economical differentiation between subjects with and without dementia: recall of objects, free recall of a word list and three behavioural memory tasks (immediate and delayed recall of a route and delayed recall of a name-face association). The authors concluded that everyday memory tests appear to be the most useful for assessment when the purpose is the basic diagnosis of dementia.

In another study in a similar setting the ability to remember to carry out actions (as measured by three RBMT tests) was evaluated as an early indicator of dementia (Huppert and Beardsall 1993). The target tasks were remembering an appointment, remembering a personal belonging and remembering to deliver a message. Minimally and mildly-to-moderately demented patients performed significantly more poorly than normals on all three of these measures of prospective memory. The results of both RBMT studies thus show that ecologically valid memory tests such as the RBMT may provide a good means of detecting mild-to-moderate dementia. Furthermore, these face-valid tests seem to be readily accepted by elderly and demented examinees.

Preserved skills

Are there special, isolated skills that remain undisturbed in demented patients? In addition to its theoretical implications, the question of preserved cognitive skills in dementia is closely related to the management of neurodegenerative disorders. A number of case reports have described the selective sparing of certain skills in dementia, such as musical skills, painting, calculating, imagery, playing complex games like chess or bridge, or solving jigsaw puzzles (Chapter 20; Obler and Fein 1988).

The diagnoses of patients with selectively spared skills covered a large range of neuropsychiatric conditions, among them dementia, autism or 'idiocy', making the identification of a potential cerebral substrate for preserved skills difficult. Several hypothetical interpretations have been offered for isolated, outstanding cognitive performances in demented subjects. Some researchers believe that the preservation of cognitive skills largely reflects a preservation of remote procedural memory, which is known to be intact in many forms of dementia and enables demented subjects to perform well-routinized activities. An alternative, not undisputed explanation, is that the retention of isolated skills might be due to a greater 'cognitive reserve'. A third account claims that preserved skills result from enhanced access to semantic memory which may remain relatively intact for a limited time in some forms of dementia. A more detailed understanding of preserved skills in dementia is hampered by the lack of systematic research in this field. It may therefore be rewarding to study the mechanisms of retained skills in greater detail for practical reasons, namely for the development of individually tailored interventional techniques which may help to improve the quality of life of patients and caregivers by capitalizing on the patients' preserved cognitive skills.

Treatment

Is there a therapy for the memory disorder in dementia? Successful interventions for amnesia and other cognitive deficits are of substantial importance for a patient's quality of life and for reducing caregiving burden and costs. A recent study of the potential savings in illness costs attainable from treatment of deficits in cognition and memory has estimated that large savings in the costs of caring for moderately and severely demented home-dwelling patients could be achieved from disease interventions that have even only minor effects on patients' cognitive status (Ernst et al. 1997).

Memory rehabilitation includes the use of various memory aids and pharmacological treatments (Wilson 1987). Internal, cognitive-based memory aids such as mnemonics require a variety of other cognitive skills like motivation, concentration, attention, language, mental imagery, as well as the ability to develop new strategies and are therefore not often suitable for patients with more advanced dementia. Despite these limitations, Camp et al. (1996) have found that a significant percentage of patients with mild-to-moderate cognitive impairment due to AD were able to improve their performance on two everyday, prospective memory tasks. Interestingly, the amount of memory improvement was not related to severity of dementia or demographic features, supporting the contention that the type of memory involved appears to be related to implicit rather than declarative memory.

A large variety of external memory aids has been developed to alleviate the effects of amnesia in everyday life, ranging from simple notepads and organizers, mechanical aids, electronic reminders and dictation machines to sophisticated computer software (for a review, see Kapur 1995). Remembering to apply or use these external memory aids in crucial situations, and managing their technical requirements, certainly poses a major problem to most patients with advanced dementia. This may explain why there are practically no systematic studies that have explored the benefit of these aids in dementia. Given the apparently limited applicability of memory aids to patients with dementia, the treatment of amnesia in neurodegenerative disorders has mainly relied on pharmacological agents.

Giron and Koller (Chapter 21) provide a critical update of available drug treatments and their limitations. Three important issues need to be considered in evaluating drug treatments: the population being treated, the properties of the drug and the rationale for the treatment. Heterogeneity of treatment populations is a frequent obstacle in treatment studies because it is difficult to select a sufficiently large, homogeneous cohort of patients with a clear-cut diagnosis, a similar disease stage and similar premorbid cognitive abilities, who also have few pre-existing diseases and are not taking other drugs potentially confounding the results of a therapeutic trial.

Another important issue concerns the pharmacological properties of the drug, such as its pharmacodynamic profile, in vitro and in vivo effects and its kinetics, tolerability and adverse effects. To cite a well-known example, the application of cholinergic drugs in dementia has often been hampered by these drugs' short half-life and their considerable side-effects. Another problem concerns the neurobiological and behavioural specificity of memory-enhancing drugs. Memory deficits in AD or PD are associated with multiple neurotransmitter changes. Thus, although AD and PD are primarily associated with cholinergic and dopaminergic dysfunction, respectively, it must be kept in mind that levels of other neurotransmitters like serotonin or glutamate are also affected; therefore, cholinergic treatment or dopamine substitution may improve only certain aspects of memory (Lombardi and Weingartner 1995). The fact remains that despite the large number of drug trials in the past decade, most cholinergic therapies have yielded only limited palliation in AD and other forms of dementia. A new generation of cholinergic agents and other novel drugs may yield better results.

A further issue in drug treatment of amnesia regards the dependent measure in the drug therapy – the memory impairment itself. Treatment effects can be evaluated in various ways and different forms of improvements may be accomplished, only some of which may be truly beneficial for the patient. Without wishing to make a case against systematic, theory-driven research, it is beyond doubt that a drug's benefit for cognitively impaired patients will have to be measured at the behavioural level, rather than by documenting drug effects on laboratory tests or solely in a clinical setting.

Other aspects

Wilkinson and Tröster (Chapter 22) provide a comprehensive overview of the effects of surgical interventions on memory and cognition in neurodegenerative disorders. This chapter deals with the indications, effects and techniques of stimulation, ablation and transplantation procedures which have been primarily developed to alleviate the motor symptoms of PD. Some interventions, especially in early series, have been followed by impairments of speech and memory, or by psychic disturbances. As neuro-transplantation and nonablative surgical procedures are

becoming increasingly important in the therapy of PD, and as transplantation or grafting of genetically engineered cells will likely become important in AD and multiple sclerosis, one aim of future research will have to be an expansion of knowledge about possible cognitive side-effects and risks related to these techniques. A second aim of research will be to develop a consensus regarding patient selection criteria. These criteria will serve to select patients most likely to benefit from the therapy and to exclude patients at risk for post-operative cognitive morbidity (for example, those with pre-existing cognitive deficits). Compared to the large body of knowledge regarding the technical and neurological aspects of surgical therapies, there is a lack of systematically derived neuropsychological and quality of life outcome data.

A number of rarely discussed but important ethical issues are summarized by Zehr (Chapter 23). This chapter deals with concepts like a demented individual's legal and functional status, degrees of mental competency and ethical issues involved in the treatment and management of demented patients. Although the legal standards discussed apply, by necessity, to only a restricted geographical area, the ethical issues are universally important and relevant. For relatives and caregivers, these issues are of undoubted significance in the many decisions and adjustments to be made in the life of patients with dementing disorders. For patients, a clear medico-legal concept is necessary to protect their fundamental rights.

CONCLUSION

The *Clinical Perspective* section of this book is concerned with what is presently known and hypothesized about the clinical, epidemiological and therapeutic aspects of memory impairment in dementia. The vast amount of data and observations on dementia have undisputedly multiplied exponentially during the past decade. Still it is difficult to escape the question whether we know anything fundamental about dementia. Is there a clearer vision about its etiology? Can we expect considerably more successful treatments, at least for some of the many variants of dementia in the future? Almost every worker dedicated to this field has experienced the uneasy feeling that the basic principles of dementia are incompletely understood, even in highly prevalent and well-studied dementia syndromes. Similarly, health care professionals and relatives and caregivers of patients, remain frustrated that the currently available management and treatment strategies are merely palliative and fail to stop disease progression. Consequently, we have to accept that work on dementia is far from complete.

Another related question is whether clinical research has made any relevant contributions to the basic understanding of dementias. Even without being blind to the many flaws and weaknesses of clinical research, my personal opinion is that some progress has been made. A meta-analysis of the clinical achievements in dementia research indicates that clinical research is now at a stage where it has identified its Achilles heel and can focus on the most important target areas. Clinical research has identified and classified subtypes of dementias; it has accumulated data on risk factors, prevalence rates and the socio-cultural appearance of dementia. Clinical findings have also set in motion the developments in neurogenetics, one of the most promising future research areas in the detection and probably also the treatment of dementia. Clinical observations have listed unexplained phenomena which can exclusively be observed in demented patients and which have led to further in-depth and fruitful studies concerning the biological and cognitive aspects of dementia. It is clear that so far clinical research has several achievements to its credit. There is no doubt that this knowledge only represents a beginning, or an intermediate state, and that it needs comprehensive elaboration to meaningfully serve patients with dementia.

REFERENCES

Beardsall, L. and Huppert, F.A. 1991. A comparison of clinical, psychometric and behavioural memory tests: Findings from a community study of the early detection of dementia. *International Journal of Geriatric Psychiatry*. 6: 295–306.

Brandt, J., Bylsma, F.W., Gross, R., Stine, O.C., Ranen, N. and Ross, C.A. 1996. Trinucleotide repeat length and clinical progression in Huntington's disease. *Neurology*. 46: 527–531.

Burt, D.B., Zembar, M.J. and Niederehe, G. 1995. Depression and memory impairment: A meta-analysis of the association, its pattern and specificity. *Psychological Bulletin*. 117: 285–305.

Camp, C.J., Foss, J.W., Stevens, A.B. and O'Hanlon, A.M. 1996. Improving prospective memory task performance in persons with Alzheimer's disease. In *Prospective memory: Theory and applications*, ed. M. Brandimonte, G.O. Einstein and M.A. McDaniel, pp. 351–367. Mahwah, NJ: Lawrence Erlbaum.

Cockburn, J. and Smith, P.T. 1989. *Rivermead Behavioural Memory Test (Suppl. 3): Elderly people*. Reading, UK: Thames Valley Test Company.

Delis, D. C., Kramer J.H., Kaplan, E. and Ober, B.A. 1987. *The California Verbal Learning Test: Research Edition, Adult Version*. San Antonio: The Psychological Corporation.

Ebers, G.C. and Sadovnick, A.D. 1994. The role of genetic factors in multiple sclerosis susceptibility. *Journal of Neuroimmunology*. 54: 1–17.

Elwood, R.W. 1995. The California Verbal Learning Test: Psychometric characteristics and clinical application. *Neuropsychology Review*. 5: 173–201.

Ernst, R.L., Hay, J.W., Fenn, C., Tinklenberg, J. and Yesavage, J.A. 1997. Cognitive function and the costs of Alzheimer's disease. *Archives of Neurology*. 54: 687–693.

Fletcher, R.H., Fletcher, S.W. and Wagner, E.H. 1982. Diagnostic tests. *Clinical epidemiology: The essentials*. Baltimore: Williams and Wilkins.

Folstein, M.F., Folstein, S.E. and McHugh, P.R. 1975. 'Mini mental state examination': A practical method for grading the cognitive state of patients for the clinician. *Journal of Psychiatric Research*. 12: 189–198.

Foroud, T., Siemers, E., Kleindorfer, D., Bill, D.J., Hodes, M.E., Norton, J.A., Conneally, P.M. and Christian, J.C. 1995. Cognitive scores in carriers of Huntington's disease gene compared to noncarriers. *Annals of Neurology*. 37: 657–664.

Gainotti, G. and Marra, C. 1994. Some aspects of memory disorders clearly distinguish dementia of the Alzheimer's type from depressive pseudo-dementia. *Journal of Clinical and Experimental Neuropsychology*. 16: 65–78.

Gifford, D.R., Mittman, B.S. and Vickrey, B.G. 1996. Diagnostic reasoning in neurology. *Neurologic Clinics*. 14: 223–238.

Howieson, D.B. and Lezak, M.D. 1995. Separating memory problems from other cognitive problems. In *Handbook of memory disorders*, ed. A.D. Baddeley, B.A. Wilson and F.N. Watts, pp. 411–426. New York: Wiley.

Huppert, F.A. and Beardsall, L. 1993. Prospective memory impairment as an early indicator of dementia. *Journal of Clinical and Experimental Neuropsychology*. 15: 805–821.

Jacobs, D.M., Marder, K., Côté, L.J., Sano, M., Stern, Y. and Mayeux, R. 1995b. Neuropsychological characteristics of preclinical dementia in Parkinson's disease. *Neurology*. 45: 1691–1696.

Jacobs, D.M., Sano, M., Dooneif, G., Marder, K, Bell, K.L. and Stern, Y. 1995a. Neuropsychological detection and characterization of preclinical Alzheimer's disease. *Neurology*. 45: 957–962.

Kapur, N. 1995. Memory aids in the rehabilitation of memory disordered patients. In *Handbook of memory disorders*, ed. A.D. Baddeley, B.A. Wilson and F.N. Watts, pp. 533–556. New York: Wiley.

Kurtzke, J.F. 1980. The geographical distribution of multiple sclerosis: An update with special reference to Europe and the Mediterranean region. *Acta Neurologica Scandinavica*. 62: 65–80.

Lezak, M.D. 1995. *Neuropsychological assessment*, 3rd ed. New York: Oxford University Press.

Lombardi, W.J. and Weingartner, H. 1995. Pharmacological treatment of impaired memory function. In *Handbook of memory disorders*, ed. A.D. Baddeley, B.A. Wilson and F.N. Watts, pp. 533–556. New York: Wiley.

Obler, L.K. and Fein, D. 1988. *The exceptional brain: Neuropsychology of talent and special abilities*. New York: Guilford Press.

Paolo, A.M., Tröster, A.I. and Ryan, J.J. 1997. California Verbal Learning Test: Normative data for the elderly. *Journal of Clinical and Experimental Neuropsychology*. 19: 220–234.

Parkin, A.J. and Leng, R.C. 1993. *Neuropsychology of the amnesic syndrome*. Hillsdale, NJ: Lawrence Erlbaum Associates.

Roth, M., Tym, E., Mountjoy, C.Q., Huppert, F.A., Hendrie, H., Verma, S. and Goddard, R. 1986. CAMDEX: A standardised instrument for the diagnosis of mental disorder in the elderly with special reference to the early detection of dementia. *British Journal of Psychiatry*. 149: 698–709.

Schneider, J.A., Gearing, M., Robbins, R.S., de l'Aune, W. and Mirra, S.S. 1995. Apolipoprotein E genotype in diverse neurodegenerative disorders. *Annals of Neurology*. 38: 131–135.

Sox, H.C., Blatt, M.A. and Higgins, M.C. 1988. *Medical decision making*. Stoneham, MA: Butterworth-Heinemann.

Starkstein, S.E., Mayberg, H.S., Leiguarda, R., Preziosi, T.J. and Robinson, R.G. 1992. A prospective longitudinal study of depression, cognitive decline and physical impairments in patients with Parkinson's disease. *Journal of Neurology, Neurosurgery and Psychiatry*. 55: 377–382.

Starkstein, S.E., Preziosi, T.J., Berthier, M.L., Bolduc, P.L., Mayberg, H.S. and Robinson, R.G. 1989. Depression and cognitive impairment in Parkinson's disease. *Brain*. 112: 1141–1153.

Stern, Y., Brandt, J., Albert, M., Jacobs, D., Liu, X., Bell, K., Marder, K., Sano, M., Albert, S., Del-Castillo Castaneda, C., Bylsma, F., Tycko, B. and Mayeux, R. 1997. The absence of Apolipoprotein ε4 allele is associated with a more aggressive form of Alzheimer's disease. *Neurology*. 41: 615–620.

Strittmatter, W.J. and Roses, A.D. 1995. Apolipoprotein E and Alzheimer's disease. *Proceedings of the National Academy of Sciences*. 92: 4725–4727.

Tröster, A.I., Stalp, L.D., Paolo, A.M., Fields, J.A. and Koller, W.C. 1995. Neuropsychological impairment in Parkinson's disease with and without depression. *Archives of Neurology*. 52: 1164–1169.

Wilson, B. 1987. *Rehabilitation of memory*. New York: Guilford.

Wilson, B., Cockburn, J. and Baddeley, A.D. 1985. *The Rivermead Behavioural Memory Test*. Reading, UK: Thames Valley Test Company.

Index

Note: page numbers in *italics* refer to figures and tables